Molecular Biology of Cardiovascular Diseases

FUNDAMENTAL AND CLINICAL CARDIOLOGY

Editor-in-Chief
Samuel Z. Goldhaber, M.D.

*Harvard Medical School
and Brigham and Women's Hospital
Boston, Massachusetts*

Associate Editor, Europe
Henri Bounameaux, M.D.

*University Hospital of Geneva
Geneva, Switzerland*

1. *Drug Treatment of Hyperlipidemia*, edited by Basil M. Rifkind
2. *Cardiotonic Drugs: A Clinical Review, Second Edition, Revised and Expanded*, edited by Carl V. Leier
3. *Complications of Coronary Angioplasty*, edited by Alexander J. R. Black, H. Vernon Anderson, and Stephen G. Ellis
4. *Unstable Angina*, edited by John D. Rutherford
5. *Beta-Blockers and Cardiac Arrhythmias*, edited by Prakash C. Deedwania
6. *Exercise and the Heart in Health and Disease*, edited by Roy J. Shephard and Henry S. Miller, Jr.
7. *Cardiopulmonary Physiology in Critical Care*, edited by Steven M. Scharf
8. *Atherosclerotic Cardiovascular Disease, Hemostasis, and Endothelial Function*, edited by Robert Boyer Francis, Jr.
9. *Coronary Heart Disease Prevention*, edited by Frank G. Yanowitz
10. *Thrombolysis and Adjunctive Therapy for Acute Myocardial Infarction*, edited by Eric R. Bates
11. *Stunned Myocardium: Properties, Mechanisms, and Clinical Manifestations*, edited by Robert A. Kloner and Karin Przyklenk
12. *Prevention of Venous Thromboembolism*, edited by Samuel Z. Goldhaber
13. *Silent Myocardial Ischemia and Infarction: Third Edition*, Peter F. Cohn
14. *Congestive Cardiac Failure: Pathophysiology and Treatment*, edited by David B. Barnett, Hubert Pouleur, and Gary S. Francis

15. *Heart Failure: Basic Science and Clinical Aspects*, edited by Judith K. Gwathmey, G. Maurice Briggs, and Paul D. Allen
16. *Coronary Thrombolysis in Perspective: Principles Underlying Conjunctive and Adjunctive Therapy*, edited by Burton E. Sobel and Désiré Collen
17. *Cardiovascular Disease in the Elderly Patient*, edited by Donald D. Tresch and Wilbert S. Aronow
18. *Systemic Cardiac Embolism*, edited by Michael D. Ezekowitz
19. *Low-Molecular-Weight Heparins in Prophylaxis and Therapy of Thromboembolic Diseases*, edited by Henri Bounameaux
20. *Valvular Heart Disease*, edited by Muayed Al Zaibag and Carlos M. G. Duran
21. *Implantable Cardioverter-Defibrillators: A Comprehensive Textbook*, edited by N. A. Mark Estes III, Antonis S. Manolis, and Paul J. Wang
22. *Individualized Therapy of Hypertension*, edited by Norman M. Kaplan and C. Venkata S. Ram
23. *Atlas of Coronary Balloon Angioplasty*, Bernhard Meier and Vivek K. Mehan
24. *Lowering Cholesterol in High-Risk Individuals and Populations*, edited by Basil M. Rifkind
25. *Interventional Cardiology: New Techniques and Strategies for Diagnosis and Treatment*, edited by Christopher J. White and Stephen R. Ramee
26. *Molecular Genetics and Gene Therapy of Cardiovascular Diseases*, edited by Stephen C. Mockrin
27. *The Pericardium: A Comprehensive Textbook*, David H. Spodick
28. *Coronary Restenosis: From Genetics to Therapeutics*, edited by Giora Z. Feuerstein
29. *The Endothelium in Clinical Practice: Source and Target of Novel Therapies*, edited by Gabor M. Rubanyi and Victor J. Dzau
30. *Molecular Biology of Cardiovascular Disease*, edited by Andrew R. Marks and Mark B. Taubman

ADDITIONAL VOLUMES IN PREPARATION

Ultrasound Imaging in Coronary Artery Disease: Clinical Applications and Decision Making, edited by Robert J. Siegel

Dedicated to Marnie, Joshua, Daniel, and Sarah
—A.R. Marks

Molecular Biology of Cardiovascular Diseases

edited by

Andrew R. Marks
Mark B. Taubman

Mount Sinai School of Medicine
New York, New York

MARCEL DEKKER, INC.   NEW YORK · BASEL · HONG KONG

Library of Congress Cataloging-in-Publication Data

Molecular biology of cardiovascular disease / edited by Andrew R.
Marks, Mark B. Taubman.
    p. cm. — (Fundamental and clinical cardiology ; v.30)
    Includes bibliographical references and index.
    ISBN 0-8247-9405-2 (hardcover : alk. paper)
    1. Cardiovascular system—Diseases—Molecular aspects. I. Marks,
Andrew R. II. Taubman, Mark B. III. Series.
    [DNLM: 1. Cardiovascular Diseases—physiopathology.
  2. Cardiovascular Diseases—genetics. 3. Cardiovascular Diseases-
-immunology. 4. Cardiovascular system—physiology. W1 FU538TD
v.30 1997/WG 120 M7175 1997]
RC669.9.M656 1997
616.1'071—dc21
DNLM/DLC
for Library of Congress

96-40406
CIP

The publisher offers discounts on this book when ordered in bulk quantities. For more information, write to Special Sales/Professional Marketing at the address below.

This book is printed on acid-free paper.

MARCEL DEKKER, INC.
270 Madison Avenue, New York, New York 10016

Current printing (last digit):
10 9 8 7 6 5 4 3 2 1

PRINTED IN THE UNITED STATES OF AMERICA

Foreword

Cardiovascular science has moved rapidly in the past fifteen years. Perhaps, at this time, the most exciting changes are concerning the field of molecular biology. Thus, molecular and cell biology is competing with the excitements of the impact of risk factor modification and interventional cardiology over this period of time. Today, more and more of the trainees in cardiology are aiming towards careers in basic cardiovascular investigations.

Molecular Biology of Cardiovascular Disease provides an outstanding introduction to the power and breadth of molecular and cellular biology as it applies to the cardiovascular system. All the major areas of interest are covered, including a concise and practical guide to techniques, as well as thoughtful and insightful chapters by leading cardiovascular scientists in each of the major areas of cardiovascular disease, including vascular biology, ion channels, cell growth, and signaling.

For the novice, this is an eminently readable text that will serve as a guide into the excitement of the new science in cardiology. The book is also a resource for the more experienced cardiovascular scientist as it presents detailed accounts of some of the major advances in recent years. Thus, for the expert in vascular biology, there are valuable reviews of important discoveries, but also chapters covering basic areas that may be less familiar such as ion channel structure and function, genetics, and signal transduction.

Dr. Andrew R. Marks and Dr. Mark B. Taubman, both physician cardiologists at the Mount Sinai Cardiovascular Institute, are nationally and internationally recognized as molecular and cell biologists. Together with other recognized experts, they have put together a book that serves an important function as we stand on what is going to be a marvelous journey into the next decade of scientific discoveries in cardiovascular biology. Despite multiple authors, the book appears as having been written by an integrated group of investigators. Indeed, over the years, most of the expert contributors in the book have interacted with Drs. Marks and Taubman on a research basis. This integration of effort results in a continuity from chapter to chapter that is rewarding to the reader.

I feel proud, as a member of the cardiovascular research team of Drs. Marks and Taubman, to have had the opportunity to write this foreword for an excellent contribution.

Valentin Fuster, M.D., Ph.D.
Director, Cardiovascular Institute
Arthur M. & Hilda A. Master Professor of Medicine
Dean for Academic Affairs
Mount Sinai Medical Center

Preface

Literature searches in any of the fields addressed in this book yield thousands of references per year. The pace of research in cardiovascular molecular and cellular biology has indeed quickened. Our aim has been to provide thoughtful, forward-looking summaries of exciting discoveries in important areas of investigation.

The book has three major parts. Part I is a primer in molecular biology that should be useful to both novices and more experienced investigators. Basic concepts are explained in simple terms so that a cardiologist or a trainee without prior knowledge can follow them. In most cases these introductory chapters have been written by cardiologists trained in molecular and cellular biology. Thus, the approach differs from standard primers in molecular biology designed for graduate students and postdoctoral fellows. Part I does not replace the excellent manuals found in every basic science laboratory, but provides explanations for the terms and techniques used in the later parts of this book so the reader does not constantly have to refer to other sources to understand the experimental approaches. Moreover, specialized approaches that are particularly important to investigators in the cardiovascular fields—and may not be addressed in standard laboratory manuals—are presented in detail. These include Chapter 4, by Drs. Hasegawa and Kitsis entitled "Gene Transfer into Adult Cardiac Myocytes in Vivo by Direct Injection of DNA"; Chapter 5, by Dr. Kohtz, "Studies of Cardiac Myocytes in Culture"; and Chapter 6, by Dr.

Gelb, "Congenital Heart Disease: Gene Defects and Molecular Biological Studies."

Part II focuses on transmembrane signaling in cardiocytes, with chapters on small signaling molecules, including Chapter 7, "Molecular Biology of Nitric Oxide Synthases," by Drs. Michel, Lamas, and Sase; and Chapter 8, "Signaling Through Heterotrimeric G Proteins," by Drs. Chen, Harry, and Iyengar. This part also includes work on the major voltage-gated ion channels that are responsible for cardiac excitability: Chapter 9, "Molecular Physiology of Cardiac Sodium Channels," by Drs. England and Tamkun; Chapter 10, "Molecular Properties of Cardiac Potassium Channels in Health and Disease" by Drs. Langan and Logothetis; and Chapter 11, "Plasma Membrane Calcium Channels," by Dr. Marks. In Chapter 12, Dr. Marks focuses on the structure and function of calcium release channels that regulate cardiac contractility; and in Chapter 13, Drs. Schulze and Lederer cover "Advances in the Molecular Characterization of the Na^+/Ca^{2+} Exchanger."

Part III addresses topics of interest in the field of vascular biology and the regulation of cellular growth. Chapter 14, "Tyrosine Kinases in the Regulation of Vascular Smooth Muscle Function," by Drs. Corson and Berk, addresses the role of receptor tyrosine kinases that are, in general, growth factor receptors in modulating signaling relevant to cell growth. Chapter 15, "Myocardial Growth Factors," by Drs. MacLellan, Hawker, and Schneider, focuses on the signaling molecules that stimulate the growth factor receptors and play important roles in heart failure and cardiac development. Chapter 16, "Gene Therapy and the Vessel Wall" by Dr. Marmur, addresses the unique aspects of the cardiovascular system that make it particularly well suited to introducing exogenous genes that can be expressed in cardiac tissues. The growth in our understanding of the importance of the extracellular matrix in cardiovascular pathophysiology is addressed in Chapter 17, by Drs. Weintraub and Taubman. Drs. Pereira, Zhang, and Ramirez describe the discovery of the cause of Marfan's disease and the molecular biology of fibrillin in Chapter 18. Chapter 19, by Dr. Taubman, focuses on the emerging understanding of the role of thrombosis— and, in particular, tissue factor—in atherosclerotic diseases. Dr. Fisher's work on lipoproteins, Chapter 20, addresses an area in which molecular biology has had enormous impact in the past decade on both diagnosis and treatment of cardioavascular disease. The final chapter, "Platelets and Cardiovascular Disease," by Drs. Grimaldi and French, considers the role of molecular approaches in developing potent new therapies for treating and preventing platelet-mediated cardiovascular disease.

In all cases we have attempted to cover the basics, to address clinically relevant questions wherever possible, and to provide a perspective as to where the challenges and opportunities for important advances will be in the next five to ten years. The book is accessible to cardiology students, fellows, and cardiologists and should serve as a useful overview for experienced scientists.

We thank our colleagues who contributed the chapters that made this book possible. We also thank the members of our laboratories, many of whom contributed chapters, provided time-tested methods for Part I, and performed the experiments discussed in our own chapters.

Andrew R. Marks
Mark B. Taubman

Contents

Foreword   Valentin Fuster   *iii*
Preface   *v*
Contributors   *xiii*

Part I.   Overview of Methodology and Introduction to Techniques

1. **DNA and RNA**   **1**
   Loewe O. Go

2. **Cloning and Expression**   **33**
   Andrew R. Marks

3. **Expression Cloning and Screening for Unknown Genes**   **51**
   Mark E. Lieb

4. **Gene Transfer into Adult Cardiac Myocytes in Vivo by Direct
   Injection of DNA**   **67**
   Koji Hasegawa and Richard N. Kitsis

5. **Studies of Cardiac Myocytes in Culture: A Developmental
   Perspective**   **81**
   D. Stave Kohtz

6. Congenital Heart Disease: Gene Defects and Molecular
   Biological Studies   111
   Bruce D. Gelb

Part II. Transmembrane Signaling

7. Molecular Biology of Nitric Oxide Synthases   141
   Thomas Michel, Santiago Lamas, and Kazuhiro Sase

8. Signaling Through Heterotrimeric G Proteins   161
   Yibang Chen, Anya Harry, and Ravi Iyengar

9. Molecular Physiology of Cardiac Sodium Channels   173
   Sarah K. England and Michael M. Tamkun

10. Molecular Properties of Cardiac Potassium Channels in
    Health and Disease   197
    Marie-Noelle S. Langan and Diomedes E. Logothetis

11. Plasma Membrane Calcium Channels   237
    Andrew R. Marks

12. Structure and Function of Calcium Release Channels   251
    Andrew R. Marks

13. Advances in the Molecular Characterization of the Na^+/Ca^{2+}
    Exchanger   275
    Dan H. Schulze and W. J. Lederer

Part III. Signaling in Disease States

14. Tyrosine Kinases in the Regulation of Vascular Smooth
    Muscle Function   291
    Marshall A. Corson and Bradford C. Berk

15. Myocardial Growth Factors   327
    W. Robb MacLellan, James Hawker, and Michael D. Schneider

16. Gene Therapy and the Vessel Wall   379
    Jonathan D. Marmur

17. The Extracellular Matrix and Smooth Muscle Cell Migration   401
    Andrea S. Weintraub and Mark B. Taubman

18. Microfibril Pathology and Cardiovascular Manifestations in
    Marfan Syndrome   431
    Lygia V. Pereira, Hui Zhang, and Francesco Ramirez

19. **The Role of Tissue Factor in Arterial Thrombosis and Atherosclerosis**   447
    Mark B. Taubman

20. **Regulation of the Production of Lipoproteins Containing Apolipoprotein B**   471
    Edward A. Fisher

21. **Platelets and Cardiovascular Disease**   489
    Christine M. Grimaldi and Deborah L. French

Appendix: *Genetic Cardiovascular Disease*   *517*

Index   *523*

Contributors

Bradford C. Berk, M.D., Ph.D. Professor, Division of Cardiology, Department of Medicine, University of Washington, Seattle, Washington

Yibang Chen, Ph.D. Research Associate, Department of Pharmacology, Mount Sinai School of Medicine, New York, New York

Marshall A. Corson, M.D. Assistant Professor, Division of Cardiology, Department of Medicine, University of Washington, Seattle, Washington

Sarah K. England, Ph.D. Research Instructor, Department of Molecular Physiology and Biophysics, Vanderbilt University School of Medicine, Nashville, Tennessee

Edward A. Fisher, M.D., Ph.D. Director of Lipoprotein Research and Associate Professor of Medicine, Cardiovascular Institute, Mount Sinai School of Medicine, New York, New York

Deborah L. French, Ph.D. Assistant Professor of Medicine, Division of Hematology, Mount Sinai School of Medicine, New York, New York

Bruce D. Gelb, M.D. Assistant Professor, Departments of Pediatrics and Human Genetics, Mount Sinai School of Medicine, New York, New York

Loewe O. Go, M.D.   Instructor of Medicine, The Cardiovascular Institute, Mount Sinai School of Medicine, New York, New York

Christine M. Grimaldi, Ph.D.   Research Associate, Department of Medicine, Mount Sinai School of Medicine, New York, New York

Anya Harry, Ph.D.   Department of Pharmacology, Mount Sinai School of Medicine, New York, New York

Koji Hasegawa, M.D., Ph.D.   Postdoctoral Research Fellow, Departments of Medicine (Cardiology) and Cell Biology, Albert Einstein College of Medicine, Bronx, New York

James Hawker, Ph.D.   Postdoctoral Fellow, Department of Medicine, (Cardiology), Baylor College of Medicine, Houston, Texas

Ravi Iyengar, Ph.D.   Professor, Department of Pharmacology, Mount Sinai School of Medicine, New York, New York

Richard N. Kitsis, M.D.   Assistant Professor, Departments of Medicine (Cardiology) and Cell Biology, Albert Einstein College of Medicine, Bronx, New York

D. Stave Kohtz, Ph.D.   Assistant Professor, Department of Pathology, Mount Sinai School of Medicine, New York, New York

Santiago Lamas, M.D., Ph.D.   Department of Protein Structure and Function, Center for Biological Investigations, Madrid, Spain

Marie-Noelle S. Langan, M.D., F.R.C.P.(C)   Assistant Professor of Medicine, Division of Cardiology, Mount Sinai School of Medicine, New York, New York

W. J. Lederer, M.D., Ph.D.   Professor, Departments of Physiology and Molecular Biology and Biophysics, University of Maryland School of Medicine, Baltimore, Maryland

Mark E. Lieb, M.D.   Instructor of Medicine, The Cardiovascular Institute, Mount Sinai School of Medicine, New York, New York

Diomedes E. Logothetis, Ph.D.   Assistant Professor of Physiology and Biophysics, Mount Sinai School of Medicine, New York, New York

W. Robb MacLellan, M.D.   Assistant Professor, Department of Medicine (Cardiology), Baylor College of Medicine, Houston, Texas

Andrew R. Marks, M.D.   Irene and Dr. Arthur Fishberg Professor of Medicine (Cardiology), Departments of Medicine, Physiology and Biophysics, and Brookdale Center for Molecular Biology, Mount Sinai School of Medicine, New York, New York

Jonathan D. Marmur, M.D.   Assistant Professor, Department of Medicine, Mount Sinai School of Medicine, New York, New York

Thomas Michel, M.D., Ph.D., F.A.C.C.   Associate Professor of Medicine, Cardiovascular Division, Brigham and Women's Hospital and Harvard Medical School, Boston, Massachusetts

Lygia V. Pereira, Ph.D.   Associate Professor, Departamento de Biologia, Instituto de Biociências, Universidade de São Paulo, São Paulo, Brazil

Francesco Ramirez, Ph.D.   Professor, Department of Molecular Biology, Mount Sinai School of Medicine, New York, New York

Kazuhiro Sase, M.D., Ph.D.   Research Fellow in Medicine, Cardiovascular Division, Brigham and Women's Hospital and Harvard Medical School, Boston, Massachusetts

Michael D. Schneider, M.D.   Professor, Departments of Medicine, Cell Biology, and Molecular Physiology & Biophysics, Baylor College of Medicine, Houston, Texas

Dan H. Schulze, Ph.D.   Associate Professor, Department of Microbiology and Immunology, University of Maryland School of Medicine, Baltimore, Maryland

Michael M. Tamkun, Ph.D.   Associate Professor, Department of Molecular Physiology and Biophysics, Vanderbilt University School of Medicine, Nashville, Tennessee

Mark B. Taubman, M.D.   Irene and Dr. Arthur Fishberg Professor of Medicine (Cardiology), Department of Medicine, Brookdale Center for Molecular Biology, Mount Sinai School of Medicine, New York, New York

Andrea S. Weintraub, M.D.   Assistant Professor, Department of Pediatrics, Mount Sinai School of Medicine, New York, New York

Hui Zhang, M.D., Ph.D.   Pediatric Resident, Department of Pediatrics, Long Island College Hospital, Brooklyn, New York

Molecular Biology of Cardiovascular Diseases

DNA and RNA

Loewe O. Go
Mount Sinai School of Medicine
New York, New York

STRUCTURE OF NUCLEIC ACIDS

The central dogma in molecular biology is that the genetic information stored in deoxyribonucleic acids (DNAs) is first transcribed to ribonucleic acids (RNAs) and then translated to proteins (Fig. 1). By definition, a gene is a portion of DNA that codes for a specific polypeptide or protein, and hence the gene is the functional unit of genetic information. Our current understanding of how the genetic code works has been made possible by breakthroughs and insights into the structure and function of nucleic acids and proteins. This chapter provides a concise introduction to nucleic acid structure and the basic techniques used in molecular biology to manipulate nucleic acids. It is meant to facilitate the reading of the rest of this book by a novice in the field of molecular biology. For more detailed information, the reader is referred to standard textbooks (1–3) and technique protocol manuals (4, 5).

Structure of DNA and Genes

DNAs are linear polymers of nucleotides. Each nucleotide is composed of a phosphate group, a deoxyribose sugar, and one of four nitrogenous bases: two

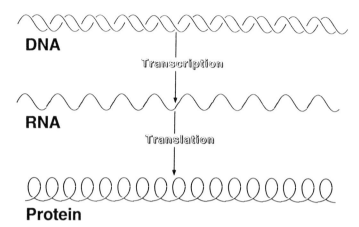

DNA

Transcription

RNA

Translation

Protein

Figure 1 Central dogma of molecular biology. The flow of genetic information goes from double-stranded DNA to single-stranded RNA to protein. The process of copying the information from DNA to RNA is called transcription, while converting that information from RNA to protein is called translation.

purines, adenine (A) and guanine (G), and two pyrimidines, thymine (T) and cytosine (C) (Fig. 2). The nucleotides are linked by the phosphate groups at the 5′ and 3′ carbon positions of the deoxyribose sugar, forming phosphodiester bonds in the sugar–phosphate backbone and giving rise to polarity (i.e., 5′ or 3′ end) (Fig. 3). In eukaryotes, DNA resides in the nucleus and exists as a double helix composed of two polynucleotide strands coiled around each other in antiparallel fashion (one is 5′ to 3′, while the other is 3′ to 5′) and are held together by hydrogen bonding between bases (Fig. 4). The hydrogen bonding between complementary base pairs (bp) is highly specific and follows Chargaff's rules: adenine forms two hydrogen bonds only with thymine (A=T), while guanine forms three hydrogen bonds only with cytosine (G≡C).

Complementary bp hydrogen bonding maintains the double helix, allowing DNA to remain stable under various physiological conditions. Exposure to near-boiling temperatures or extremes of pH causes the two strands to separate or denature, while annealing or renaturation of the two strands occurs when conditions return to normal. Since G-C bps form more hydrogen bonds than A-T bps, DNA helices composed predominantly of G-C bps are more stable than those containing mostly A-T bps, and thus G-C-rich DNA requires higher temperatures to denature. The genetic information is stored in the actual sequence of the nucleotides, while the specific base pairing between complementary strands permits duplication of the information. These properties are exploited in molecular biology techniques described later.

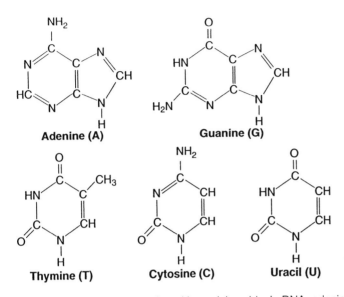

Figure 2 Common bases found in nucleic acids. In DNA, adenine (A) and guanine (G) are the purine bases while thymine (T) and cytosine (C) are the pyrimidine bases. In RNA, the pyrimidine uracil (U) replaces the thymine (T) found in DNA.

DNA is packaged inside eukaryotic cells into chromosomes, which are basically very long, tightly coiled negatively charged DNA helices associated with positively charged histone proteins in repeating units called nucleosomes (Fig. 5). On the average, a human chromosome is 120 million bp long and contains multiple genes, with each gene located on a particular site (or locus) of the chromosome. All eukaryotic chromosomes are paired (except for the sex chromosomes), and since the two chromosomes almost always have identical organization of the gene loci, they are called homologous. The genes in homologous chromosomes that occupy the same locus and code for the same protein are called alleles. Homologous alleles that differ in their actual base sequences give rise to polymorphism.

Reproduction requires duplication of the entire DNA molecule, or DNA replication. This entails separation of the double helix strands and utilization of both strands as templates for the sequential ligation of complementary deoxyribonucleotides (dNTPs), an energy-requiring process mediated by the enzyme DNA polymerase. DNA synthesis by this enzyme is preceded by the binding of a primer (a short nucleotide segment complementary to a section of the parent template) and always proceeds in the 5′ to 3′ direction of the daughter strand. Since the parent strands have opposite polarity, DNA synthesis beginning at a

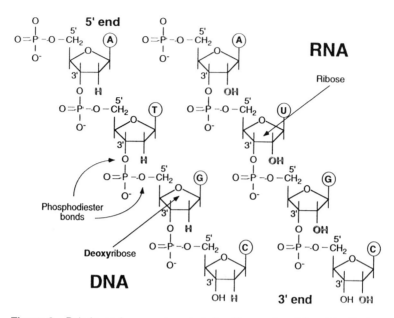

Figure 3 Polarity and sugar–phosphate backbone of nucleic acids. Each nucleotide in a DNA or RNA is composed of a phosphate group, a deoxyribose sugar for DNA (where oxygen is taken out in the 2′ carbon position) or ribose sugar for RNA, and one of the nitrogenous bases. The nucleotides are linked by the phosphate groups at the 5′ and 3′ carbon positions of the sugar, forming phosphodiester bonds in the sugar–phosphate backbone and giving rise to polarity (i.e., 5′ or 3′ end). Note that phosphate groups confer a net negative charge on nucleic acids.

replication fork is continuous only on the parent strand with a 3′ to 5′ orientation (leading strand), and discontinuous on the parent strand with a 5′ to 3′ orientation, occurring in a retrograde piecemeal fashion (lagging strand). These short segments of new DNA, called Okazaki fragments, start with RNA primers that are eventually replaced and the fragments joined together by the enzyme DNA ligase (Fig. 6). Generation of new double-stranded DNA molecules is thus semiconservative: one strand is conserved from the parent molecule while the other is newly synthesized. The proofreading and self-correcting capabilities of DNA polymerase limit the error of replication to one nucleotide for every 10^9 assembled. Uncorrected errors result in gene mutations, which may either be silent (e.g., mutation in a noncoding region of DNA) or produce abnormal protein expression and function.

   In contrast to reproduction, maintenance of cell integrity requires duplication of only certain portions of the DNA that contain the information to direct the synthesis of specific proteins: in other words, transcription of DNA into a

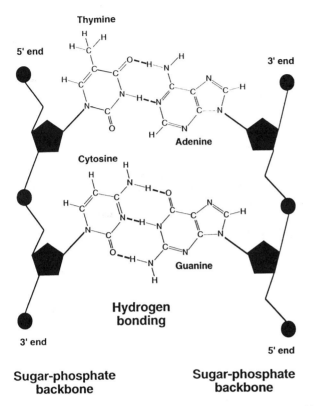

Figure 4 Double-strand nature of DNA. In eukaryotes, DNA polynucleotide strands are held together by hydrogen bonding between bases in antiparallel fashion (one is 5′–3′, while the other is 3′–5′). The hydrogen bonding between complementary base pairs (bp) is highly specific and follows Chargaff's rules: adenine forms two hydrogen bonds only with thymine in DNA and with uracil in RNA, while guanine forms three hydrogen bonds only with cytosine. This specific base pairing between complementary strands permits duplication of genetic information.

messenger RNA (mRNA) template. These functional units of genetic information are referred to as genes. Each gene is composed of a coding region for the polypeptide, and noncoding sequences on both 5′ and 3′ ends (or upstream and downstream respectively) that initiate, regulate, and terminate transcription (Fig. 7). The coding region often contains intervening noncoding sequences, or introns, which separate the actual sequences which code for the polypeptide, or exons. Sequences on the 5′ end include promoters, enhancers, and silencers, which regulate the activity of RNA polymerase and determine the rate of transcription. In most eukaryotes, the promoter sequence located 25–30 bp up-

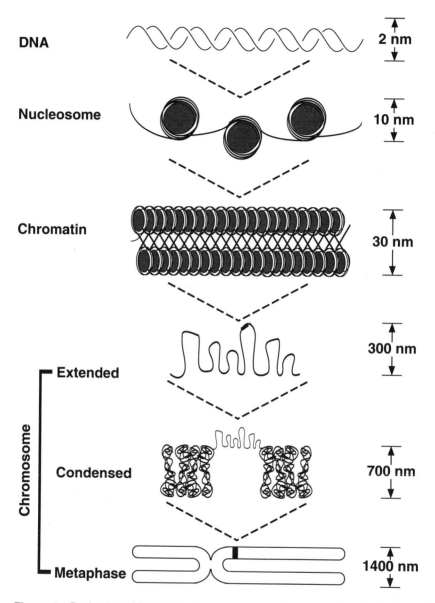

DNA

Nucleosome

Chromatin

Chromosome
   Extended

   Condensed

   Metaphase

2 nm

10 nm

30 nm

300 nm

700 nm

1400 nm

Figure 5 Packaging of DNA into chromosomes in eukaryotes. Negatively charged DNA helices are tightly coiled around positively charged histone proteins in repeating units called nucleosomes. Nucleosomes are then packaged into strands of chromatin, and the chromatin strands undergo further compaction into chromosomes (which are easily visible only during metaphase). How the tightly packaged DNA becomes selectively decompacted and exposed for transcription remains relatively unexplored. Relative sizes of molecules are shown on the right column.

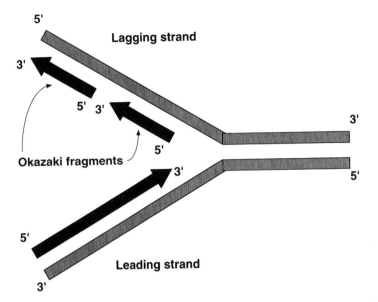

Figure 6 DNA replication fork. Since the double helix parent strands have opposite polarity and synthesis of daughter strands always proceeds in the 5'–3' direction, DNA replication is continuous only on the parent strand with a 3'–5' orientation (leading strand), and discontinuous in a retrograde piecemeal fashion on the parent strand with a 5'–3' orientation (lagging strand). These short DNA segments, called Okazaki fragments, start with RNA primers that are eventually replaced and the fragments joined together by the DNA ligase. Generation of new double-stranded DNA is thus semiconservative.

stream of the transcription initiation site is rich in A and T (TATA or Hogness box) or CCAAT box, and is the binding site for RNA polymerase. Enhancers and silencers, as their names imply, are *cis*-acting sequences located further upstream of promoters, which, upon binding to certain proteins called transcription factors (*trans-* acting factors), lead to the enhancement or inhibition of transcription, respectively. The 3' end includes terminator nucleotide sequences as well as the AATAAA sequence, which identifies the site on the primary transcript RNA that is cleaved and where a variable length of adenine nucleotides is attached, called the poly(A) tail.

The complete collection of DNA sequences in an organism, genes and otherwise, is referred to as the genome. Of the total DNA in the human genome, which contains about 3 billion bp, it has been estimated that fewer than 5% encodes for proteins, and fewer than 50% are single copied. Repetitive sequences of varying complexity and length make up about 55% of the human

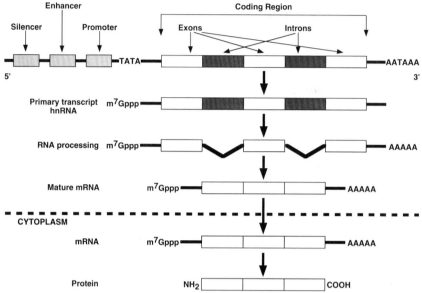

Figure 7 Gene structure, stages of transcription, and translation. A gene is a functional unit of genetic information that consists of a coding region flanked by noncoding sequences on both 5′ and 3′ ends that initiate, regulate, and terminate transcription. The 5′ regulatory sequences include silencers, enhancers, and promoters, as well as the TATA box where RNA polymerase binds. The coding region is composed of exons (expressed sequences that code for protein) and introns (intervening noncoding sequences), while the 3′ end includes terminator nucleotide sequences and the AATAAA site, which is eventually cleaved off the RNA and to which the poly(A) tail is attached. The primary transcript or heterogenous nuclear RNA (hnRNA) is synthesized in the nucleus by RNA polymerase II and then undergoes extensive processing. RNA processing include capping with a 7-methylguanosine at the 5′ end of the mRNA (m^7Gppp), polyadenylation at the 3′ end (AAA), and splicing together of the coding exons to form a mature messenger RNA (mRNA). Mature mRNA exists to the cytoplasm and is translated into a polypeptide. The mRNA is read from 5′ to 3′ end, corresponding to the amino terminus (NH_2) and carboxy terminus (COOH) of the protein.

genome. Examples of highly repetitive sequences are the ~300 nucleotide Alu family sequences (so-called because they contain a site recognized by the restriction endonuclease *Alu* I) that appear approximately every 5,000 bp and make up about 5% of the genome, and the L1 transposable element that make up about 4% of the genome. The actual functions of these high copy noncoding sequences remain a mystery. Examples of repetitive sequences that do perform functions are the preribosomal RNA genes, which exist as multiple copies in tandem with spacer DNA in between the copies and are selectively amplified when ribosomes are in demand (such as during oogenesis).

Structure of RNA

Similar to DNAs from which they are transcribed, RNAs are also linear polymers of nucleotides but with three differences: (a) RNAs are generally single-stranded (Fig. 1), (b) the pyrimidine uracil (U) replaces thymine (T) (Fig. 2), and (c) the sugar in the RNA backbone is ribose instead of deoxyribose (Fig. 3). In eukaryotes, the synthesis of three types of RNAs is carried out by specialized enzymes. RNA polymerases I and III transcribe ribosomal (rRNA) and transfer (tRNA) RNAs, respectively (RNA products necessary for protein synthesis) while RNA polymerase II transcribes the protein-encoding mRNAs. Transcription of RNA also requires transient separation of the double helix DNA strands and proceeds from 5′ to 3′ direction, but unlike replication only the 3′ to 5′-oriented DNA strand (antisense) is used as the template. The RNA is hence a copy of the sense strand. Elongation of RNA proceeds with addition of ribonucleotides (rNTPs) until the termination site of DNA template is reached, followed by separation of RNA from the DNA template.

As implied in the previous review of gene structure, the primary transcript RNA (also called heterogeneous nuclear RNA or hnRNA) contains noncoding sequences and requires extensive processing in the nucleus before it can emerge in the cytoplasm in its mature form. Such posttranscriptional processing includes (a) capping with a 7-methylguanosine at the 5′ end of the mRNA (m⁷Gppp), (b) attaching a poly(A) tail at the 3′ end (polyadenylation), and (c) removal of the introns and splicing together of the coding exons to form a coherent functional mRNA (Fig. 7). The 5′ capping is universal in eukaryotic mRNAs and appears to facilitate ribosome binding and translation, while 3′ polyadenylation seems to facilitate the exit of mRNA into the cytoplasm and to enhance its stability. RNA splicing is also thought to be essential for mature mRNA exit; in addition, it also provides opportunities to generate a variety of different protein isoforms from a single gene via alternative splicing.

Unlike DNAs, which remain quite stable due to their double helix structure, single-stranded mRNAs are more susceptible to degradation by cytoplasmic ribonucleases (RNAses) and thus lasts only for a few minutes to hours. A single mRNA on the average encodes about 1400 copies of the polypeptide. In contrast, rRNAs (and to a lesser extent tRNAs) are much more stable due to their secondary and tertiary structures formed by the significant amount of intrastrand hydrogen bonding between segments (Fig. 8) as well as associated ribosomal proteins in the case of rRNAs. The composition of the total RNA in the cell reflects the relative stability of these types of RNA, with 80% be-

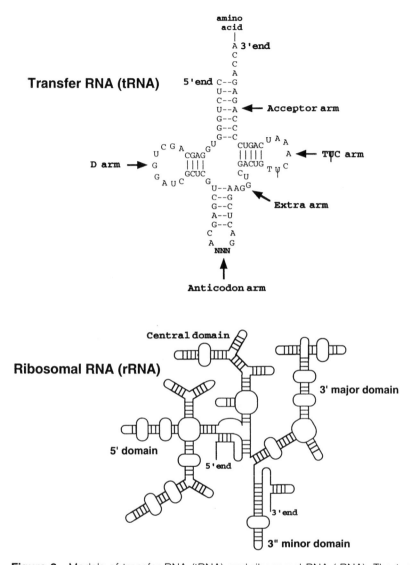

Figure 8 Models of transfer RNA (tRNA) and ribosomal RNA (rRNA). The typical tRNA has a cloverleaf structure comprised of the amino acid receptor site at the 3′ end with the CCA sequence (receptor arm), the anticodon sequence located at another exposed site (anticodon arm), and several other stems/loops (D arm, TUC arm, and sometimes an extra arm). The anticodon arm contains the triplet nucleotide sequence that "reads" the genetic message of mRNA by anticodon–codon base-pairing, and each amino acid is represented by at least one tRNA. In contrast, rRNA has a much more complex secondary and tertiary structure, with multiple domains due to significant amount of intrastrand hydrogen bonding. This more complex structure of tRNA and rRNA relative to mRNA, as well as association of ribosomal proteins with rRNA, accounts for their increased stability.

ing rRNA, 15% tRNA, and less than 5% mRNA. (The preponderance of 28S and 18S rRNAs in mammalian cells makes them useful in assessing the quality and relative quantity of total RNA isolated, but the presence of poly[A] tails in mRNAs permits their selective isolation from the other more abundant RNAs, as discussed later in the section on molecular biology techniques.)

The Genetic Code

The conversion of genetic information in the mRNA into a sequence of amino acids during protein synthesis, referred to as translation, is based on the genetic code (Table 1). The triplet nature of the genetic code was initially proven by Brenner and Crick in 1961 and completely deciphered by 1966. Each sequence of three nucleotides or codon is recognized by the protein manufacturing complex as representing one of the 20 naturally occurring amino acids. Given that 4 different nucleotides produce 64 possible combinations of triplet codons, there

Table 1 The Genetic Code

1st Letter (5′end)	2nd Letter				3rd Letter (3′end)
	U	C	A	G	
U	Phe	Ser	Tyr	Cys	U
U	Phe	Ser	Tyr	Cys	C
U	Leu	Ser	Stop	Stop	A
U	Leu	Ser	Stop	Trp	G
C	Leu	Pro	His	Arg	U
C	Leu	Pro	His	Arg	C
C	Leu	Pro	Gln	Arg	A
C	Leu	Pro	Gln	Arg	G
A	Ile	Thr	Asn	Ser	U
A	Ile	Thr	Asn	Ser	C
A	Ile	Thr	Lys	Arg	A
A	Met & Start	Thr	Lys	Arg	G
G	Val	Ala	Asp	Gly	U
G	Val	Ala	Asp	Gly	C
G	Val	Ala	Glu	Gly	A
G	Val	Ala	Glu	Gly	G

RNA codon bases are abbreviated as follows: U = uracil; C = cytosine; A = adenine; G = guanine.
Amino acids are abbreviated as follows: Ala = alanine; Arg = arginine; Asn = asparagine; Asp = aspartic acid; Cys = cysteine; Gln = glutamine; Glu = glutamic acid; Gly = glycine; His = histidine; Ile = isoleucine; Leu = leucine; Lys = lysine; Met = methionine; Phe = phenylalanine; Pro = proline; Ser = serine; Thr = threonine; Trp = tryptophan; Tyr = tyrosine; Val = valine.

is considerable redundancy or degeneracy of the genetic code, with several amino acids represented by more than one codon (Table 1). Many variations in the third position of the codon do not change the amino acid translated. In addition, the codon AUG serves as the start codon that initiates translation as well as the codon for methionine, while the codons UAA, UAG, and UGA serve as stop codons that signal the end of translation.

The order of the codons in the mRNA from the 5′ to 3′ direction determines the sequence of amino acids in the protein from the amino (NH_2) terminus to the carboxyl (COOH) terminus (Fig. 7). The process of mRNA translation utilizes multiple proteins and RNA species including tRNAs and ribosomes (multienzyme-rRNA complexes). The tRNAs are a family of about 40 different species, each about 80 nucleotides long and structurally folded such that the anticodon (a sequence of three nucleotides complementary to the codon) is exposed at one end of the molecule and the specific amino acid acceptor site is located at the 3′ end with CCA nucleotide sequence (Fig. 8). Each tRNA serves as a mediator, first by being covalently bonded to the appropriate amino acid (or "charged") via highly specific aminoacyl-tRNA synthetase, and second by bringing its amino acid to the appropriate location in the translation complex through a codon–anticodon interaction between the mRNA and itself. Mature mRNA exiting into the cytoplasm is bound serially by ribosomes beginning at the 5′ end and supplies the sites for aminoacyl-tRNA recognition and binding, peptide bond formation, and translocation. In effect, these polyribosomes act as the "factories" for protein synthesis (Fig. 9).

Under physiological conditions, translation of mRNA begins with an initiator methionine (usually at an AUG preceded by a purine rich sequence) and proceeds until one of the termination codons is encountered; this translatable portion is called the open reading frame. Frameshift mutations arising from an insertion or deletion of a nucleotide result in incorporation of incorrect amino acids (missense) and often premature termination due to a new in-phase termination codon (nonsense) (Fig. 10). On the other hand, point mutation or substitution of a nucleotide may be silent if (a) the same amino acid is incorporated due to the degeneracy of the genetic code, or (b) the amino acid replacement occurs in a noncritical section of the protein (Fig. 10). In rare cases mutations result in proteins with altered functions that prove advantageous for the organism, thus providing a mechanism for evolutionary adaptations to occur.

GENERAL TECHNIQUES OF MOLECULAR BIOLOGY

This section describes some common techniques utilized in studying nucleic acids and explains the rationale behind the methods. These methods include how

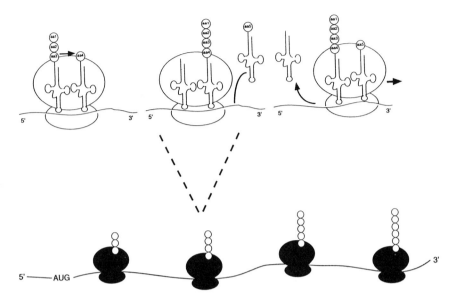

Figure 9 Polyribosomes. Ribosomes (made up of rRNAs and proteins) serially bind mRNA in cytoplasm beginning at the 5′ end and supply the sites for aminoacyl-tRNA recognition and binding, peptide bond formation, and translocation as they proceed downstream. Such complexes, which act as the "factories" for protein synthesis, are known as polyribosomes. aa1, aa2, aa3, and aa4 refer to amino acids linked in sequence, and AUG is the start site in mRNA for protein synthesis.

to purify DNA or RNA, use of restriction enzymes and reverse transcriptase, gel electrophoresis, sequencing and labeling of DNA, Southern and Northern blotting and hybridization, and how to quantify mRNA levels. One important property of nucleic acids, which is exploited in most of these techniques and hence is useful to remember, is the specific base pairing of the complementary strands of DNA to each other or of DNA to RNA.

Preparation of DNA

In general, it is easier to purify DNA than RNA due to the much better stability conferred by the double helix structure of the former and to the susceptibility of the latter to ubiquitous RNAses. Genomic DNA can in principle be obtained from any batch of cells by following sequential steps of cell lysis, decontamination of other macromolecules, and recovery of DNA whether from prokaryotes (e.g., bacteria *Escherichia coli*) or eukaryotes (e.g., human leukocytes). Cells are initially incubated in buffers containing ionic detergents (e.g.,

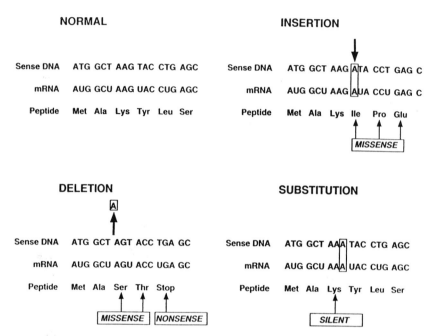

Figure 10 Effect of mutations. Insertion or deletion of a nucleotide produces frame-shift mutations that lead to changes in amino acid translation (missense) and often premature termination due to a new in-phase termination codon (nonsense). Some-times substitution of a nucleotide may be silent if (a) the same amino acid is incor-porated due to the degeneracy of the genetic code, or (b) the amino acid replace-ment occurs in a noncritical section of the protein.

sodium dodecyl sulfate [SDS] or N-laurosylsarcosine [Sarkosyl]) and proteases (e.g., proteinase K) to promote cell lysis and protein degradation (6). Ethyl-enediaminetetraacetic acid (EDTA) is included in the buffers to inhibit DNAses. The protein contaminants are further denatured and extracted with an equal volume of organic solvent mixture, most commonly phenol/choloroform, which maximizes aqueous phase yield (7). The DNA solubilized in the aqueous phase is selectively precipitated by adding 2–3 volumes of chilled 100% ethanol in the presence of relatively high (0.3–0.5 M) salt concentration (e.g., sodium or ammonium acetate) and is pelleted by centrifugation. The DNA pellet is rinsed with 70% ethanol to remove the salts and residual organic molecules, dried, and resuspended in water (or Tris-EDTA buffer with ethanol for long-term storage). The usual yield is 100 µg DNA from 10 ml blood or from 1 g tis-sue.

Residual RNA may be removed by incubation with RNAse, followed by another round of organic extraction and ethanol precipitation to recover the DNA. In certain situations, further purification of DNA after deproteination may be required (such as in the presence of large amounts of polysaccharides from plants and bacteria), and is accomplished by additional incubation with the detergent cetyltrimethylammonium bromide (CTAB), which complexes with both polysaccharides and residual proteins and allows their subsequent organic extraction (8). Large amounts of pure DNA (0.5–2 mg) can be isolated by scaling up the lysis and extraction procedures followed by prolonged high-speed centrifugation (300,000–500,000 × g) on cesium chloride gradient (1 g/ml), which separates the high-molecular-weight DNA from the RNA and other macromolecules. The DNA band stained with ethidium bromide is visualized under ultraviolet (UV) light and removed manually, the ethidium bromide extracted by butanol, and the DNA recovered by ethanol precipitation. Purifying DNA from contaminants in aqueous phase can be accomplished more rapidly using commercially available glass beads (9). Addition of 2–3 volumes of high-salt (6 M sodium iodide) causes DNA to bind efficiently to the small glass beads, which can then be pelleted. The DNA/glass bead pellet is washed several times with 50% ethanol in Tris-EDTA to remove salt and other impurities, and the DNA is eluted into water by gentle heating. The glass bead method works best for purifying small amounts (5–15 µg) of DNA at least 500 bp in length.

The amount of DNA in solution is traditionally determined using absorption spectroscopy. Nucleic acids have peak absorbance readings ($Å$) at 260 nm wavelength and thus both DNA and RNA are quantified the same way and cannot be differentiated. Because of different specific absorption coefficients, an A260 of 1 corresponds to approximately 50 µg/ml for double-stranded DNA, 40 µg/ml for single-stranded DNA and RNA, and ~20 µg/ml for short synthetic DNA or oligonucleotides. Since proteins have peak absorption at 280 nm, the ratio between readings at 260 and 280 nm provides a rough indication of nucleic acid purity. Highly purified DNA and RNA have A260/A280 ratios of 1.8 and 2.0, respectively; contaminants such as protein and phenol lower this ratio. If the DNA is heavily contaminated or the amount isolated is not enough for accurate spectrophotometry (<0.25 µg/ml), an alternative way to estimate the quantity of DNA is to compare the intensity of red–orange fluorescence (560 nm) emitted by ethidium bromide dye staining the sample with the fluorescent intensities of a similarly stained series of standards. Ethidium bromide intercalates between the stacked bases of nucleic acids and fluoresces under UV radiation (260–360 nm) in proportion to the total mass of nucleic acid, thus allowing detection of very small quantities of DNA (1–5 ng) in solution or via gel electrophoresis (see below).

Preparation of RNA

Purifying RNA essentially follows similar protocols except for one important caveat: all reagents and laboratory ware to be used must be kept free of RNAse activity. RNAses are quite stable and ubiquitous, and most require no cofactors to remain active. Hence all reagents that come into contact with RNA (e.g., water, salt buffers, cesium chloride solution) must first be treated with diethylpyrocarbonate (DEPC), which inactivates RNAses by covalent modification, then the excess DEPC is hydrolyzed off by autoclaving. Laboratory ware is made RNAse-free by baking at 300°F for a few hours or rinsing with chloroform, and gloves are worn routinely since hands are a major source of contaminating RNAse.

In addition to detergents, cell lysis is performed in the presence of much stronger denaturing agents such as 4 M guanidinium isothiocyanate (10) and 1% (v/v) β-mercaptoethanol in order to inactivate released RNAses immediately. This is followed by a brief centrifugation to pellet cellular debris, then shearing of chromosomal DNA in the lysis mixture to reduce viscosity. For purifying large amounts of full-length RNA, the lysis mixture is subjected to prolonged high-speed centrifugation (150,000 × g) over a cesium chloride cushion (5.7 M) that pellets the higher-density RNA while the high salt concentration precipitates the DNA along with denatured macromolecules at the interface (11). The RNA pellet is rinsed free of salt and residual organic molecules with 70% ethanol (RNAse free) and the RNA recovered by ethanol precipitation. For isolating small quantities of RNA from eukaryotic cells, nonionic detergents (e.g., Nonidet P-40) may be used for the initial lysis since they release only cytoplasmic contents while preserving nuclei integrity, thus permitting pelleting of nuclei (which contain most of the DNA) and denatured proteins via centrifugation (12). The RNA content is then determined by spectroscopy as for DNA. Yield is approximately 200 µg RNA from 1 g tissue.

Total RNA isolated by these methods consists largely of rRNA and tRNA, with less than 5% being mRNA. However, mRNAs can be selectively isolated since most have a poly(A) tail. Total RNA is first denatured (e.g., 65°C for few minutes) to disrupt any secondary structure and expose the poly(A) tails, then is passed several times through a cellulose column composed of deoxythymidine oligonucleotides that binds poly(A)-containing mRNA (13). The mRNA is eluted from the oligo(dT) column by reducing the salt concentration, which destabilizes the dT:rA hybrids, and is finally recovered by ethanol precipitation. Enriching the mRNA fraction is useful for constructing complementary DNA libraries (see below and Chap. 2) as well as studying low-level messages.

Enzymatic Manipulation and Analysis of Nucleic Acids

Restriction Endonucleases

Major breakthroughs in genetic engineering over the past 20 years were made possible by the discovery and utilization of various enzymes that catalyze specific reactions on nucleic acids. Chief among these are the restriction endonucleases, which are enzymes that recognize short sequences within double-stranded DNA and cleave the DNA at or near these recognition sites either in a nonspecific fashion (type I) or in an exact manner than produces discrete fragments of well-defined length and sequence (type II). Over 600 type II restriction enzymes have been isolated, generally from prokaryotic organisms in which they serve a protective role by degrading foreign DNA (e.g., bacteriophage). These organisms protect their own genomes by methylating adenine or cytosine nucleotides within the endonuclease recognition sequences, which renders them resistant to cleavage.

Typical restriction enzyme recognition sequences are 4–8 bp in length and exhibit dyad symmetry or palindrome (Table 2). Some type II restriction enzymes cut with staggered cleavages that create overhanging single-stranded 5′ ends (e.g., *Msp I* and *Eco* RI) or 3′ ends (e.g., *Hha* I and *Kpn* I) referred to as cohesive or "sticky" ends (Table 2). Such ends can then anneal to other ends produced by the same enzyme via complementary base pairing and be covalently ligated by DNA ligase (Fig. 11). Other enzymes (e.g., *Hae* III and *Sma* I) cut at the axis of symmetry and produce flush or "blunt" ends that do not link together normally (Table 2). Restriction endonucleases are quantified in terms of units (U), and in principle 1 U enzyme completely digests 1 μg DNA in 1 h using appropriate reaction parameters. Such parameters include the required divalent cations (usually Mg^{2+}) and optimal buffered pH, ionic concentration, and temperature (which are usually supplied or instructed by commercially available restriction enzyme kits). Contaminated DNA may require more enzyme (up to 10–20 U/μg) or increased reaction volume to dilute the impurities. It is also important to remember that the reaction volume should be at least 10 times the enzyme volume since the glycerol in the enzyme storage buffer may interfere with the enzymatic activity. Nonoptimal conditions such as low ionic strength may result in less specific recognition of sequences and multiple cuts by the enzyme, or "star" activity (14).

The ability to cleave DNA at discrete nucleotide sequences has been utilized in diverse applications such as (a) making physical maps of DNA based on the locations of cleavage sites (restriction mapping, Fig. 12); (b) analyzing DNA by digesting it into a series of fragments (restriction fragments) that can then be subjected to electrophoretic separation, sequenced, and/or labeled as

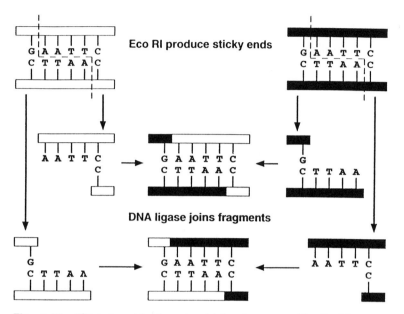

Figure 11 "Sticky" end ligation of restriction fragments. The EcoRI enzyme makes staggered cuts in two different DNA (one could be mammalian and the other a vector), leaving identical cohesive or "sticky" ends. The ends of such restriction fragments can then anneal to each other and be covalently joined by DNA ligase, resulting in a recombinant DNA molecule.

probes for Southern or Northern blotting (see below); and (c) creating recombinant DNA by generating segments of mammalian and vector DNA that anneal to each other (see Chap. 2).

Reverse Transcriptase

Another important discovery is the enzyme reverse transcriptase isolated from retroviruses such as avian myeloblastosis virus (AMV) or Moloney murine leukemia virus (MMLV). Reverse transcriptase synthesizes complementary DNA (cDNA) from an mRNA template using an appropriate primer and dNTPs (15). This unique ability to reverse the genetic flow of information enabled scientists to bypass the tedious and often fruitless structure–function analysis of genomic DNA (given that less than 5% of the genome codes for proteins), and go directly to making copies of the active coding sequences based on purified mRNA. The initial cDNA copies are single-stranded and contain the antisense sequence. DNA polymerase is then used to synthesize the sense strands and produce much more stable duplex cDNAs that can then be manipulated further

Table 2 Some Restriction Endonucleases and Their Cleavage Sequences

Microorganism	Enzyme	Recognition Sequence and Cleavage Site	Notes
Haemophilus aegyptius	*Hae* III	5'—G G|C C—3' 3'—C C|G G—5'	1
Moraxella species	*Msp* I	5'—C|C G G—3' 3'—G G C|C—5'	2
Haemophilus haemolyticus	*Hha* I	5'—G C G|C—3' 3'—C|G C G—5'	3
Desulfovibrio desulfuricans	*Dde* I	5'—C|T N A G—3' 3'—G A N T|C—5'	4
Serratia marcescens	*Sma* I	5'—C C C|G G G—3' 3'—G G G|C C C—5'	1
Escherichia coli RY 13	*Eco* RI	5'—G|A A T T C—3' 3'—C T T A A|G—5'	2
Klebsiella pneumonia OK8	*Kpn* I	5'—G G T A C|C—3' 3'—C|C A T G G—5'	3
Bacillus stearothermophilus ET	*Bst*E II	5'—G|G T N A C C—3' 3'—C C A N T G|G—5'	4
Bacillus species M	*Bsp* M I	5'—A C C T G C (N)$_4$|—3' 3'—T GGACG (N)$_8$—5'	5
Nocardia otitidis-caviarum	*Not* I	5'—G C|G G C C G C—3' 3'--C G C C G G|C G—5'	6

1. Blunt ends produced by cleavage.
2. Single-stranded 5' ends produced by cleavage.
3. Single-stranded 3' ends produced by cleavage.
4. Base pair N represents any purine-pyrimidine pair.
5. Cleavage does not occur within recognition sequence, but at whatever sequence lying 3' to the recognition site.
6. Eight-base pair recognition sequence occurs very infrequently, and thus cutting mammalian DNA with this enzyme produces few fragments.

as with any other DNA (i.e., restriction mapping, sequencing, labeling, or even cloning; see Chap. 2). By definition, the cDNAs made from mRNAs contain only the exons, but no introns nor other noncoding sequences, and thus are quite different from their genomic counterparts.

Gel Electrophoresis

Separation of DNA restriction fragments (or total RNA that naturally include a variety of mRNAs with different lengths) is traditionally accomplished by being loaded into a well of a gel and subjected to electrophoresis (16). Nucleic acids are negatively charged molecules with a fairly constant charge to mass

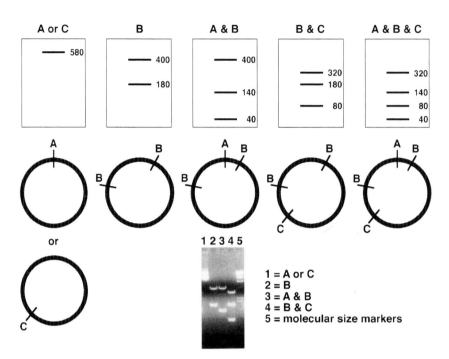

Figure 12 Restriction mapping and gel electrophoresis. Circles represent plasmid DNA; A, B, C represent restriction enzymes with different cleavage sites on the plasmid; rectangles represent gels in which the digested DNA are loaded and subjected to electrophoresis. Enzymes A or C cuts at one site and produces a single linear band with size of 580, while enzyme B cuts at two sites and hence results in two smaller-sized bands that add up to 580. Double digestions reveal that A cuts the smaller B fragment further, while C cuts the larger B fragment. By studying these patterns of digestion, one can construct a restriction map of the DNA. Inset shows part of the actual gel electrophoresis of this restriction digest. Negatively charged nucleic acid fragments migrate toward the positive pole (anode) of an electric field at a rate inversely proportional to their lengths: the longer the fragment, the slower its migration. DNA fragments in the gel stained with ethidium bromide fluoresce under UV light. The size of the fragments is determined by comparing their positions to simultaneously run standard molecular weight or size markers.

ratio, and hence migrate toward the positive pole (anode) of a constant electric field at a rate inversely proportional to their lengths (i.e., the longer the fragment, the slower its migration). Depending on the concentration of agarose, which determines its matrix pore size, agarose gels are used to separate the DNA fragments ranging from 100 to 300,000 bp or 30 kb (Table 3). Pulsed field electrophoresis can separate even longer fragments (up to 2,000,000 bp

Table 3 Gel Concentrations for Separating Nucleic Acid Fragments

Agarose Gel (%)	Size Fragments Separated (kb)
0.3	5–60
0.5	1–30
0.7	8–12
1.0	0.5–10
1.2	0.4–7
1.5	0.2–3
2.0	0.1–2

Acrylamide Gel (%)	Size Fragments Separated (bp)
3.5	100–1000
5.0	100–500
8.0	60–400
12.0	50–200
20.0	5–100

or 2 Mb). Polyacrylamide urea gels that denature DNA have very small pore sizes are able to separate DNA fragments from 5 to 1,000 bp at high voltage, and are thus ideal sequencing gels (see below).

The DNA fragments in the gel are visualized with UV light by staining with ethidium bromide (mixed in the gel and/or in the electrophoretic running buffer) and their sizes determined by comparing their positions to simultaneously run standard sequences with known specific lengths, often referred to as molecular weight or size markers (Fig. 12). Genomic DNA restriction digests separated by gel electrophoresis often appear as a smear since the ethidium bromide stains all fragments (Fig. 13). It should be noted that circular DNA (e.g., plasmid), may assume several structural conformations that migrate differently during electrophoresis: compact supercoiling (form I) migrates faster than linearized (form III) or relaxed supercoiling (form II), and thus give rise to the illusion of two or more different fragments from the same DNA (Fig. 12) (17).

For RNA electrophoresis, 1% formaldehyde/agarose gels in special buffer containing 3-(N-morpholino)-porpanesulfonic acid (MOPS) are used to denature RNA (18) and maintain its stability during size-fractionation. Due to the abundance of rRNAs in mammalian total RNA, the UV-induced fluorescence of the ethidium bromide intercalated into the RNA is concentrated in the regions of 28S and 18S rRNA (Fig. 14). The 28S and 18S rRNA bands are often used as size markers (corresponding to 4.7 kb and 1.9 kb, respectively), and the sharpness and intensities of their fluorescence give a rough indication of degree of RNA degradation and relative quantity of RNA loaded. Gel electro-

Genomic DNA
Gel Electrophoresis

Southern Blot Analysis
of DNA Restriction Fragments

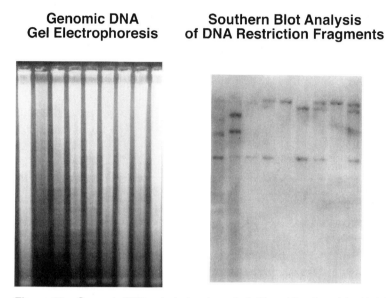

Figure 13   Genomic DNA gel electrophoresis (left) and Southern blot (right). Human genomic DNA digested with EcoRI is separated by electrophoresis in agarose gel, with each vertical lane corresponding to a separate individual in a family. Note the smear characteristic of ethidium bromide stained digested genomic DNA. The corresponding Southern blot hybridized to a specific collagen cDNA probe shows different patterns that reflect the restriction fragment length polymorphisms (RFLP) present in this family.

phoresis of enriched poly(A) RNA fraction usually reveals ethidium bromide fluorescent smear starting at ~20 kb and becoming maximal between 10 and 5 kb, with no rRNA bands visualized.

Sequencing of DNA

There are two traditional methods of sequencing DNA that rely on two different panels of reagents specific for the four bases. The Maxam and Gilbert chemical method (19) involves the isolation of single-stranded DNA labeled at the 5′ end with ^{32}P radioisotope by a kinase (see below) and aliquoting the DNA into four separate reactions, each containing a chemical that cleaves the DNA at one or two specific bases (Fig. 15). Each reaction is controlled so that each chemical cuts most DNA strands only once at the recognized base, thus generating a series of fragments with sizes varying according to the locations of this particular base. Concurrent electrophoresis of the treated DNA on four lanes of a polyacrylamide gel produces a distribution of labeled fragments (detected by autoradiography) as a function of their terminal bases. The base se-

RNA Gel Electrophoresis

**Northern Blot
Analysis**

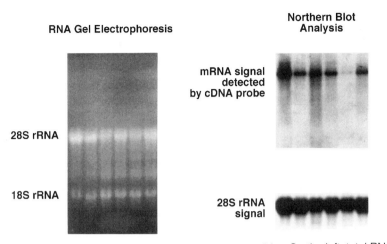

mRNA signal
detected
by cDNA probe

28S rRNA

18S rRNA

28S rRNA
signal

Figure 14 RNA gel electrophoresis and Northern blot. On the left, total RNA is size-fractionated in formaldehyde/agarose gel, followed by ethidium bromide staining. Each vertical lane corresponds to a different RNA sample. Note that in contrast to the previous genomic DNA gel, this gel has two very distinct bands that are characteristic of ethidium bromide staining of the normally abundant 28s and 18s mammalian ribosomal RNAs (which make up about 85% of total RNA). On the right, the corresponding Northern blot hybridized to a specific calcium release channel cDNA probe reveals different levels of mRNA expression in the individual samples, even though total RNA loading was fairly uniform as gauged from the 28s rRNA signals.

quence of the DNA from 5′ to 3′ end is obtained by reading the lane location of successive bands from the bottom to the top of the sequencing gel autoradiograph.

A second DNA sequencing procedure called the Sanger and Coulsen method (20) involves synthesizing copies of the primed DNA in four reactions, each containing one of the four ^{32}P-labeled 2′,3′-dideoxynucleotides (ddNTPs) in the presence of DNA polymerase and excess unlabeled dNTPs (Fig. 16). Incorporation of a ddNTP at any point where its corresponding dNTP should have been placed terminates chain elongation, thus randomly producing DNA copies of various lengths but all ending with the particular nucleotide. Separating the four reaction mixtures by gel electrophoresis followed by autoradiography reveals the base sequence in a manner similar to the first method.

Generation of Labeled Nucleic Acids

Isolating a specific DNA or RNA is most quickly achieved by utilizing a labeled single-stranded nucleic acid fragment of known sequence (a probe) that can form complementary hydrogen bonding with the molecule of interest, a

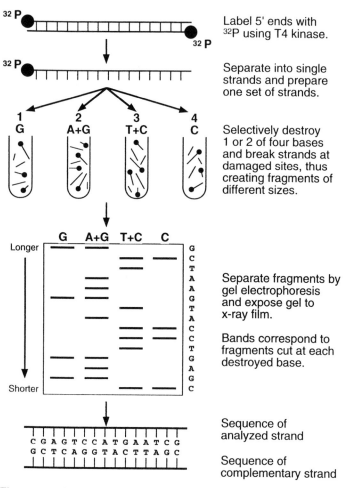

Label 5' ends with
^{32}P using T4 kinase.

Separate into single
strands and prepare
one set of strands.

Selectively destroy
1 or 2 of four bases
and break strands at
damaged sites, thus
creating fragments of
different sizes.

Separate fragments by
gel electrophoresis
and expose gel to
x-ray film.

Bands correspond to
fragments cut at each
destroyed base.

Sequence of
analyzed strand

Sequence of
complementary strand

Figure 15 Maxam and Gilbert DNA sequencing method. This method requires 5'
end labeling of the DNA of interest with P^{32}, denaturing and isolating one set of
strands, and aliquoting these into four base-specific chemical cleavage reactions as
illustrated to generate various fragments. These fragments are subjected to polyacrylamide gel electrophoresis and their radioactive signals detected by exposing the gel
to x-ray film. Base sequence of the DNA from 5' to 3' end is obtained by reading the
lane location of successive bands from the bottom to the top of the sequencing gel
autoradiograph.

process referred to as molecular hybridization. Various labels or "tags" in
current usage include ^{32}P isotope that is detected by its radioactivity, fluorescent or biotinylated compounds, and covalently linked enzymes (e.g., horseradish peroxidase). In practice, most probes are labeled DNA since RNA is

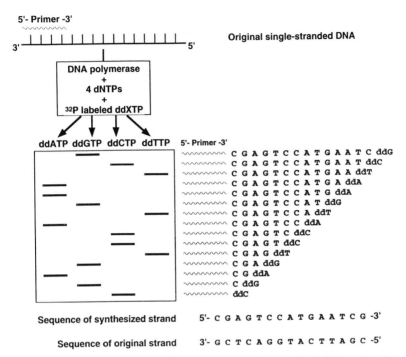

Figure 16 Sanger and Coulsen DNA sequencing method. This method requires copying the primed DNA in four reactions, each containing one of four ^{32}P-labeled 2′,3′-dideoxynucleotides (ddNTPs) in the presence of DNA polymerase and excess unlabeled dNTPs. Since ddNTP lacks the 3′ carbon hydroxyl group, incorporation of a ddNTP terminates elongation at any point where its corresponding dNTP should have been placed. Variable-sized DNA copies ending with the particular nucleotide are randomly produced. Gel electrophoresis to separate these fragments followed by autoradiography reveals the base sequence of the synthesized strand.

easily degraded, and have a radioisotope as the label due to its high sensitivity.

One technique of labeling DNA called nick translation (21) utilizes DNA polymerase I to nick the DNA sugar–phosphate backbone at many sites, exposing 3′ hydroxyl groups to which the polymerase adds ^{32}P-labeled dNTPs serially while concurrently removing downstream nucleotides via its 5′–3′ exonuclease activity. The label is thus randomly incorporated into the duplex DNA, producing probes with only moderate radioactivity to mass ratio (specific activity). Another related method called random hexamer labeling (22) generates probes of very high specific activity ($>10^8$ cpm/µg) by first denaturing the DNA, adding random hexadeoxynucleotide primers and all four dNTPs of which one is labeled (e.g., α-P^{32} dCTP), then using the Klenow fragment of DNA polymerase I successively to incorporate nucleotides and produce a complementary radiolabeled DNA. Klenow fragment is the large portion cleaved off by subtilisin from DNA polymerase I and only exhibits 5'–3' polymerase (but not exonuclease) activity. A third technique called kinase or end labeling (23) utilizes the enzyme T4 polynucleotide kinase to exchange the free 5' end phosphate groups of the nucleic acid chain with labeled phosphates obtained from γ-P^{32} ATP. Although this method produces probes with only moderate specific activity, its reaction conditions are quite favorable to maintaining the stability of single-stranded molecules and hence it is commonly used for labeling oligonucleotides or RNA. For all three methods, the excess ^{32}P-labeled nucleotides are separated from the probes by passing the reaction mixture through a Sephadex G-50 spin column in which the beads preferentially bind nucleotides while allowing nucleic acid chains to go through.

On certain occasions, an RNA rather than a DNA probe is required. In this case, template DNA containing the sequence of interest must first be inserted into a vector (bacteriophage) carrying the appropriate promoter, then digested with a restriction enzyme that generates 5' overhanging ends flanking the promoter and probe sequence (3' overhanging ends are undesirable as they provide potential initiation sites for transcription of sense RNA). The template DNA is then transcribed by bacteriophage RNA polymerase in the presence of RNAse inhibitors and all four rNTPs, of which one is labeled (e.g., α-P^{32} UTP), thus producing a discrete antisense RNA probe complementary to the mRNA (sense) strand (24). High yield and specific activity (10^9 cpm/μg) of RNA probes is obtained due to the extreme efficiency of bacteriophage RNA polymerases (200–300 NTPs/min). The RNA probe is purified from contaminating DNA template, proteins, and excess ^{32}P NTPs by DNAse I treatment, phenol/choroform extraction, and spin column passage.

Southern Blotting

This procedure is named after E. M. Southern, who discovered in 1975 that following separation and denaturation of DNA restriction fragments by gel electrophoresis, the single-stranded DNA can be transferred from the gel to a nitrocellulose (NC) filter by a flow of buffer through capillary action, and the separated DNA fixed on the filter can then be hybridized with specific probes (25). This technique was a major innovation: it provided important size and structural information about the DNA of interest. The Southern transfer apparatus (Fig. 17) consists of a tray filled with buffer, usually 10X standard saline citrate; the wick consisting of several sheets of thick filter paper, usually Whatman 3mm, on top of a support; DNA-containing gel on top of the supported sheets; NC or nylon filter cut to size and overlaid on gel; several sheets

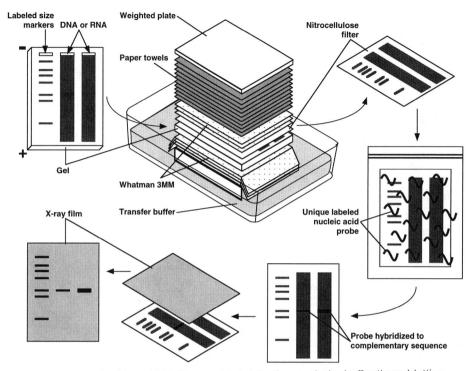

Figure 17 Nucleic acid blotting and hybridization analysis. In Southern blotting, DNA restriction fragments are loaded onto the gel, while in Northern blotting, RNA is loaded. The nucleic acid fragments separated by electrophoresis are then transferred from the gel onto a nitrocellulose filter by a flow of buffer through capillary action using a Southern transfer apparatus as illustrated (see text for details of apparatus). The flow of buffer is maintained perpendicular to the face of the gel and hence the pattern of DNA or RNA separation is imprinted or "blotted" on the filter. The filter or blot is incubated overnight with a specific radiolabeled nucleic acid probe that hybridizes with its complementary sequence of interest. After excess radioactivity is washed off, the blot is exposed to x-ray film to detect the probe-nucleic acid hybrid signals.

of Whatman 3mm cut to size and overlaid on filter; stack of paper towels fitted on top, which provides the capillary force to draw up the buffer through the gel to the filter; and a weighted plate (500 g) pressing down on paper towels. Parafilm is sometimes placed around all sides of the gel so that the buffer is forced to pass through the gel and not around it, thus avoiding "short circuit." The flow of buffer carrying DNA to the filter is maintained perpendicular to the face of the gel and hence the pattern of DNA separation is imprinted on the filter. Nylon membranes are much less brittle and last longer, but are prone to give high background signals after hybridization. Although the binding of DNA to either NC or nylon filter occurs by an unknown mechanism, the DNA is permanently fixed on the filter by vacuum baking at 80°C for 2 h or by brief UV crosslinking.

Before the DNA bound to the filter is hybridized to a probe, it is often useful to incubate the filter for 6–24 h with a prehybridization solution containing random denatured genomic DNA fragments (e.g., sonicated calf thymus DNA) essentially to block nonspecific binding sites that may contribute to background signals. Hybridization is then performed by incubating the filter with the denatured radiolabeled DNA probe in a hybridization buffer for 12–24 h, which in practice takes place in heat-sealed polyethylene bags submerged in water baths. Hybridization buffers almost always include formamide, since it permits lower incubation temperatures and thus less degradation of nucleic acids. Optimal incubation temperature for hybridization depends on several factors, including formamide content (standard 50%), salt concentration, total G + C content of the hybridizing sequences, and the anticipated degree of nucleotide sequence matching or homology between the probe and DNA (26). The higher the expected homology, the higher the hybridization temperature can be set to reduce nonspecific binding. As a general rule, in the presence of 50% formamide, 42°C is optimal for hybridizing sequences with 95–100% homology; this drops to 37°C for sequences with 90–95% homology, and to 32°C for sequences with 85–90% homology. The filter is then washed to remove excess radioactivity from nonspecific binding and subjected to autoradiography to detect probe-DNA hybrid signals (Fig. 17). Autoradiography is performed by exposing the filter on x-ray film at –80°C with intensifying screen or on special radioactivity detection systems such as Storage Phosphor Screen. The filter can be stripped of the probe by heating in a detergent solution (0.1% SDS) that breaks hydrogen bonding, thus permitting the blotted DNA to be rehybridized to new probes. A sample Southern blot is shown in Fig. 13.

Northern Blotting

This technique is virtually identical to Southern blotting except that denatured RNA rather than DNA is size fractionated on formaldehyde/agarose gels and transferred to filters for hybridization. RNA blotting, developed by Alwine in 1977, was initially jokingly called "Northern" and the name has stuck (27). This procedure is useful for determining whether a specific mRNA is expressed in RNA samples obtained from particular cells or tissues, for identifying the sizes of isoforms of the mRNA transcript, for estimating the abundance of the particular mRNA, and for examining the regulation of the mRNA expression by various hormonal metabolic stimuli or in normal vs. disease states (Fig. 14).

In other words, this is a powerful tool to study gene expression at the level of transcription.

After hybridization of an RNA blot to a specific probe and identification of the radioactive signal by autoradiography, the steady-state level of the specific mRNA of interest is quantified by measuring the strength of the signal. This is accomplished either by laser densitometry of the signal from the x-ray film autoradiograph or actual radioactivity counting using special equipment such as the Phosphorimager, which measures the amount of β-particles emitted by the probe-mRNA hybrid. Important caveats to remember when comparing mRNA levels in different samples by Northern blot analysis are that (a) the degree of RNA degradation is inversely related to the intensity of the signals; (b) the values measured by either scanning technique are relative, not absolute, amounts of mRNA; and (c) each signal value obtained must be normalized to the RNA level in each sample of housekeeping proteins (e.g., glyceraldehyde-3-phosphate dehydrogenase) or constitutive molecules (e.g., 28S rRNA) to control for variability in the amount of total RNA blotted for each sample (Fig. 14) (28, 29).

Methods to Quantify mRNA

In addition to Northern blot analysis, there are several other methods of assessing mRNA levels. If the DNA probe is highly specific for the mRNA (as determined by the presence of a single band on Northern blot analysis), size fractionation of RNA can be bypassed and serial dilutions of total RNA can be immobilized on a filter for subsequent hybridization and autoradiography. Although this technique of slot or dot blot analysis (30) does not allow size identification of the mRNA, it does provide more precision (given that the mRNA signal is measured based on several dilutions) and sensitivity (especially for partially degraded mRNA).

Another technique called ribonuclease protection assay uses a labeled sequence-specific antisense RNA molecule as the probe to hybridize with the RNA sample in solution before analysis on a sequencing gel. The RNA probe is incubated overnight with the denatured RNA sample in hybridization buffer, and subsequent treatment with RNAse digests the excess unattached probes, while those annealed to homologous sequences of RNA remain protected. The labeled RNA–RNA fragments are electrophoresed on a sequencing gel and the band radioactivity counted to assess mRNA abundance. The disadvantage of this technique is the RNA probes are easily degraded, but the advantages are the higher sensitivity afforded by tighter binding of RNA to each other (as compared with DNA to RNA) and by the substantial amount and specific activity of RNA probes generated by bacteriophage RNA polymerases (24).

A third method called primer extension analysis involves designing an oligonucleotide primer specifically for the mRNA of interest, labeling the 5′ end of the primer with ^{32}P using T4 polynucleotide kinase, annealing an excess of 5′ end-labeled primer to the RNA, and extending the primer to the 5′ end of the mRNA by using reverse transcriptase and dNTPs. Denaturation and electrophoresis of the DNA-RNA hybrid on a sequencing gel permit quantification of mRNA by radioactivity counting of the DNA band representing extension product. Primer extension analysis takes advantage of cDNA stability and is especially useful in studying the relative abundance of isoform mRNAs, which often have near identical sizes.

To determine whether changes in mRNA levels reflect a change in its synthesis as opposed to its degradation or transport from nucleus to cytoplasm, the technique called nuclear runoff transcription assay is performed (12). In essence, RNAs undergoing initiation of synthesis in isolated nuclei just prior to cell lysis are labeled to high specific activity by continuing transcription in the presence of ^{32}P rNTPs. A minimum number of clean intact nuclei ($\geq 5 \times 10^6$) is required in order to achieve adequate incorporation of the ^{32}P into total RNA (1×10^6 cpm). The labeled RNAs are then purified and hybridized to the specific cDNAs of interest that have been previously linearized, denatured, and immobilized on a dot blot. The RNA-cDNA hybrids that give high radioactivity counts indicate the genes being highly transcribed in the cells during the particular condition before lysis. On the other hand, the hybrids that give weak signals but represent genes with high steady-state mRNA levels suggest slowed degradation by inference. The greatest advantage of this technique is allowing the state of transcription for many different genes to be determined simultaneously.

COMMENTS

The key to understanding nucleic acid biology, although complex at first glance, is to recall the basic concepts presented in the first part of this chapter: the simple units called nucleotides make up the sequences that carry the genetic information, that specific base pairings occur between them that provide the capacity for recognition as well as fidelity for duplicating the information, and that the useful information is always relayed in specific orientations. These principles are exploited by the various molecular biology techniques to investigate and manipulate nucleic acids as described in the second part of the chapter. We hope that subsequent chapters will bring to light the potentially broad applications of these techniques in elucidating selected areas of cardiovascular biology.

REFERENCES

1. Alberts B, Bray D, Lewis J, Raff M, Roberts K, Watson J, eds. Molecular Biology of the Cell, 3rd ed. New York: Garland Publishing, 1994.
2. Darnell J, Lodish H, Baltimore D, eds. Molecular Cell Biology, 2nd ed. New York: Scientific American Books, 1990.
3. Lewin B: Genes. New York: Oxford University Press, 1994.
4. Ausubel F, Brent R, Kingston R, Moore D, Seidman J, Smith J, Struhl K, eds. Current Protocols in Molecular Biology. New York: John Wiley & Sons, 1994.
5. Sambrook J, Fritsch E, Maniatis T, eds. Molecular Cloning: A Laboratory Manual, 2nd ed. Cold Spring Harbor, NY: Cold Spring Harbor Laboratory Press, 1989.
6. Gross-Bellard M, Oudet P, Chambon P. Isolation of high-molecular-weight DNA from mammalian cells. Eur J Biochem 1973; 36:32–38.
7. Marmur J. A procedure for the isolation of deoxyribonucleic acid from microorganisms. J Mol Biol 1961; 3:208–218.
8. Murray M, Thompson W. Rapid isolation of high-molecular-weight plant DNA. Nucl Acids Res 1980; 8:4321–4325.
9. Vogelstein B, Gillespie D. Preparative and analytical purification of DNA from agarose. Proc Natl Acad Sci USA 1979; 76:615–619.
10. MacDonald R, Swift G, Przbyla A, Chirgwin J. Isolation of RNA using guanidinium salts. Methods Enzymol 1987; 152:219–227.
11. Glisin V, Crkvenjakov R, Byus C. Ribonucleic acid isolated by cesium chloride centrifugation. Biochemistry 1974; 13:2633–2637.
12. Marzluff W. Transcription of RNA in isolated nuclei. Methods Cell Biol 1978; 19:317–331.
13. Aviv H, Leder P. Purification of biologically active globin messenger RNA by chromatography on oligothymidylic acid-cellulose. Proc Natl Acad Sci USA 1972; 69:1408–1412.
14. Fuchs R, Blakesley R. Guide to the use of type II restriction endonucleases. Methods Enzymol 1983; 100:3–38.
15. Baltimore D. Viral RNA-dependent DNA polymerase. Nature 1970; 226:1209–1211.
16. Southern E. Gel electrophoresis of restriction fragments. Methods Enzymol 1979; 68:152–176.
17. Johnson P, Grossman L. Electrophoresis of DNA in agarose gels: optimizing separations of conformational isomers of double- and single-stranded DNAs. Biochemistry 1977; 16:4217–4224.
18. Lehrach H, Diamond D, Wozney J, Boedtker H. RNA molecular weight determinations by gel electrophoresis under denaturing conditions: a critical reexamination. Biochemistry 1977; 16:4743–4751.
19. Maxam A, Gilbert W. A new method of sequencing DNA. Proc Natl Acad Sci USA 1977; 74:560–564.
20. Sanger F, Coulson A. A rapid method for determining sequences in DNA by primed synthesis and DNA polymerase. J Mol Biol 1975; 94:444–448.

21. Rigby P, Dieckmann M, Rhodes C, Berg P. Labeling deoxyribonucleic acid to high specificity in vitro by nick translation with DNA polymerase I. J Mol Biol 1977; 113(1):237–251.

22. Feinberg A, Vogelstein B. A technique for radiolabeling DNA restriction endonuclease fragments to high specific activity. Anal Biochem 1983; 132:6–13.

23. Chaconas G, and van de Sande J. 5'-^{32}P labeling of RNA and DNA restriction fragments. Methods Enzymol 1980; 65:75–88.

24. Melton D, Krieg P, Rebagliati M, Maniatis T, Zinn K, Green M. Efficient in vitro synthesis of biologically active RNA and RNA hybridization probes from plasmids containing a bacteriophage SP6 promoter. Nucl Acids Res 1984; 12:7035–7056.

25. Southern E. Detection of specific sequences among DNA fragments separated by gel electrophoresis. J Mol Biol 1975; 98:503–517.

26. Meinkoth J, Wahl G. Hybridization of nucleic acids immobilized on solid supports. Anal Biochem 1984; 138:267–284.

27. Alwine J, Kemp D, Stark G. Method for detection of specific RNAs in agarose gels by transfer to diazobenzyloxymethyl-paper and hybridization with DNA probes. Proc Natl Acad Sci USA 1977; 74:5350–5354.

28. Brilliantes A, Allen P, Takahashi T, Izumo S, Marks A. Differences in cardiac calcium release channel (ryanodine receptor) expression in myocardium from patients with end-stage heart failure caused by ischemic versus dilated cardiomyopathy. Circ Res 1992; 71:18–26.

29. Go L, Moschella M, Watras J, Handa K, Fyfe B, Marks A. Differential regulation of two types of intracellular calcium release channels during end-stage heart failure. J Clin Invest 1995; 95:888–894.

30. Kafatos F, Jones C, Efstratiadis A. Determination of nucleic acid sequence homology and relative concentrations by a dot hybridization procedure. Nucl Acids Res 1979; 7:1541–1552.

2

Cloning and Expression

Andrew R. Marks
Mount Sinai School of Medicine
New York, New York

INTRODUCTION TO CLONING

Cloning DNA is fundamentally a series of purification steps that result in isolation of a unique sequence of DNA. The key to most isolations of cDNA or genomic DNA clones is to synthesize a radioactive "probe," usually representing a small portion of the DNA sequence that you wish to isolate. This radioactive probe is then used in a series of "screenings" or purifications that result in the isolation of a single species of DNA sequence or a clone. Other strategies for cloning include using antibodies as probes and isolating clones based on their functional (rather than structural) properties.

Probes are often cDNA sequences deduced from partial amino acid sequences obtained by sequencing small regions of a purified protein. Other commonly used sources of sequence information for making probes for cloning are the data banks of the known sequences of all the genes and cDNAs that have been isolated to date. Another strategy that is often used is to design a probe based on the sequence of a highly conserved region of a protein and use it to "fish" out closely related, but not identical, sequences.

Essentially two types of cloning are most frequently used: genomic cloning is used to obtain structural information about genes; and cDNA cloning provides structural information about mRNAs that encode proteins. cDNA cloning is somewhat more complex technically in that it requires copying of mRNA sequences into complementary DNA (cDNA) using the enzyme reverse transcriptase. However, genomic cloning provides much larger pieces of DNA, often necessitating huge DNA sequencing efforts. cDNA clones contain essentially only the necessary information required to encode the protein product of a gene (i.e., the "coding sequence" contained in "exons"). Genomic clones contain this information, but also the genetic information required to regulate turning genes on and off ("transcription") as well as large amounts of structural information that is never expressed as functional protein. The sequences containing information not encoding protein sequence are referred to as untranslated sequences and they include the introns that separate individual exons in the gene and unprocessed mRNA. During processing the introns are removed and the mature mRNA contains only exons and small amounts of 5' and 3' untranslated sequences that are required to initiate and terminate translation of the mRNA by polyribosomes.

METHODS USED IN CLONING

The methods described here are designed to provide brief overviews of representative strategies that can be used to clone cDNAs and genes. Each cloning project presents its own potential stumbling blocks, and the best strategy when starting out is to confer with an experienced cloner *before* taking the plunge. The level of detail presented here would be sufficient to point the way, but the essential details (e.g., ingredients for commonly used solutions) can be found in several outstanding laboratory manuals, at least one of which should be a standard source in any laboratory working with RNA and DNA (8). When manufacturers are mentioned they are presented merely as recommendations; for commonly used reagents there are almost always multiple excellent sources. When detailed information is provided it is done so because we have found that among the many protocols available for a given experiment, one stands out as being more reliable.

CONSTRUCTING A cDNA LIBRARY

Total RNA is isolated from the tissue of interest using the guanidinium–thiocyanate lysis buffer followed by centrifugation over a cesium chloride cushion. Poly A$^+$ RNA is subsequently isolated using two passes over an oligo-dT column. Double-stranded cDNA is synthesized from this poly A$^+$ RNA using either oligo-dT or random oligonucleotide primers (use of random synthetic oligonucleotide hexamers increases the representation of 5' ends of mRNAs that

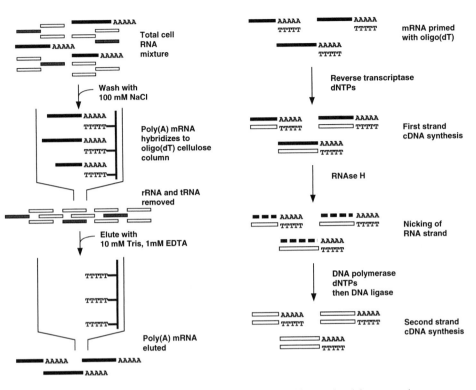

Figure 1   Schematic illustration of the steps involved in synthesizing complementary DNA (cDNA) starting with total cellular RNA.

might have significant secondary structures, reverse transcriptase (Life Sciences, FL.) and DNA polymerase (New England Biolabs, MA) (Fig. 1). This double-stranded cDNA can be size selected (>1 Kilobase [kb]) using a Sephacryl-200 (Pharmacia) spin column, EcoRI adapters are ligated and the cDNA is subcloned into a suitable vector (e.g., λZAPII vector, Stratagene) and packaged using Gigapack Gold (Stratagane). The resulting cDNA libraries (one random primed and one oligo-dT primed) should contain ~90% inserts with an average size of ≥2.5 kb (Fig. 2).

LABELING PROBES

cDNA Probes

Fifty nanograms of plasmid DNA are placed in 10 μl nuclease-free H_2O and boiled in a 1.5 ml eppendorf tube for 5 min to denature the DNA followed by

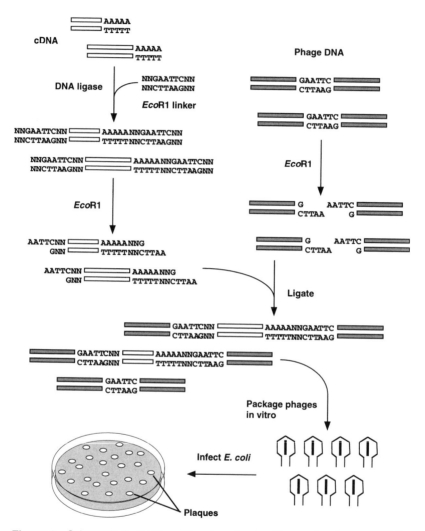

Figure 2 Schematic illustration of the steps involved in constructing a cDNA library. Construction of a genomic library involves the same steps except that a piece of genomic DNA is inserted into the phage vector instead of a piece of cDNA.

submersion of the tube in ice water for 2 min. Following the denaturation, a random priming labeling reaction is performed in 25 µl reaction volume by adding 10 µl labeling buffer (6 µg/ml hexadeoxy-ribonucleotides, 440 mM HEPES pH 6.6, 110 mM Tris pH 8.0, 11 mM MgCl$_2$, 22 mM β-mercaptoethanol, 44 mM each of dATP, dGTP, and dTTP), 5 µl α ^{32}P dCTP, and 5 units DNA polymerase I-Klenow fragment.) After a 1 h incubation at 37° C the probe is purified as follows. The reaction mixture is loaded on a Sephadex G-50 column in a 1 ml syringe and washed with 150 µl TE buffer pH 8.0 by centrifugation at $500 \times$ g for 30 s. A 1 µl aliquot of the probe is taken and mixed with 5 ml liquid scintillation solution and measured in the scintillation counter. The probe is denatured in a boiling H_2O bath for 5 min and then transferred directly to ice cold hybridization buffer with a minimum final concentration of 1 million cpm/ml solution.

Oligonucleotide Probes

Five hundred nanograms of a synthetic oligonucleotide (18–25 bases in length) are mixed with 50 mM Tris-HCl pH 7.8; 10mM $MgCl_2$, 5mM DTT, 0.1 mM spermidine, 100 µCi γ-^{32}P ATP (3000 Ci/mM) (New England Nuclear [NEN]), and 20 U T4 polynucleotide kinase in 50 µl reaction volume. The reaction is incubated at 37° C for 1 h and probe purification carried out as described above for the cDNA probe. For primer extension assays, the labeled oligonucleotide probes are electrophoretically separated using an 8% denaturing polyacrylamide gel. The radioactive bands on the gel are excised, transferred to an Eppendorf tube, and eluted in 300 µl elution buffer containing 0.5 M NH_4OAc, 1 mM EDTA, and 0.2% sodium dodecyl sulfate (SDS). A one microliter aliquot of the probe is taken for measurement of radioactivity using a scintillation counter.

cRNA Probes

Five to ten micrograms of the plasmid of interest are linearized with an appropriate restriction enzyme so that the bacteriophage T7, T3, or SP6 promoter on the vector can be used to direct the synthesis of a radiolabeled antisense cRNA probe with a defined length. The linearized DNA is purified with phenol, phenol/chloroform, followed by chloroform and precipitated with 75% ETOH. The DNA pellet is then dissolved in deithyl pyrocarbonate (DEPC) treated with H_2O (DEPC inactivates RNAses). One microgram of this template DNA is mixed with 20mM DTT, 1 mM ATP, 1 m GTP, 1mM CTP, 40 mM Tris-HCl (pH 7.5), 10mM $MgCl_2$, 50 ng/ml BSA, 25 U ribonuclease inhibitor, 5 µl α-^{32}P CTP (800 Ci/mmol), and 10 U of the appropriate RNA polymerase (T7, T3, or SP6), and then incubated for 40 min in a 25° C water bath. Two units of DNAase I are added to the reaction to remove template DNA. Probes are electrophoretically separated on a 6% denaturing polyacrylamide gel at 200 volts for 1.5 h. Radioactive bands of expected length localized by autoradiography are excised and transferred into an Eppendorf tube containing 300 µl elution buffer (0.5M NH_4OAc, 1mM ethylene diaminotetraacetic acid (EDTA), and 0.2% SDS). The cRNA probe is eluted for 30 min at room temperature with gentle shaking (vortex, speed 4). A 1 µl aliquot of the probe is taken to measure radioactivity using a scintillation counter and the remainder of the probe can be stored at $-20°$ C until use within 1 week.

ISOLATION OF cDNA CLONES

When a specific cDNA probe, labeled to a specific activity of 1×10^9 cpm/ µg, is used to screen an oligo dT or random primed cDNA library it is common to screen approximately 1 million plaques (assuming that 90% of the plaques contain cDNa inserts). Lawns of bacteria are grown on agarose plates and infected with phage that lyse the bacteria and form plaques. These phage-infected bacteria are then transferred to the nitrocellulose filters by laying the nitrocellulose sheet on top of the bacteria and lifting them slowly off, followed by immersion of the filters in denaturing (alkaline) solution and neutralization (buffered) solution sequentially for 5 min each step. Filters are then air dried and baked at 80°C in a vacuum oven for 2 h and then soaked in prehybridization and hybridization solutions as mentioned in the section on Southern analysis. A final washing of the filters is done at 60° C for 20 min in buffer containing 0.2X SSC and 0.1% SDS. Positive clones are identified by exposing the dried filter paper to autoradiographic film for 1–3 days. Films are then aligned with the agarose plates and the radioactive plaques are identified and removed from the plates. The process is repeated until a single pure colony is isolated. Phage DNA is then prepared for subcloning into a plasmid vector and the DNA is sequenced.

Polymerase Chain Reaction

The polymerase chain reaction (PCR) potentially speeds up the cloning process by allowing one to bypass many steps (Fig. 3). The potential negatives are introducing errors in the sequence (this is less of a problem when polymerases that also have editing functions) and amplifying sequence that you do not want. If you know the sequence of the cDNA that you want to clone, or can make an educated guess based on data from closely related species or homologous mRNAs (for example, members of a conserved gene family), a set of primers can be synthesized that will allow you to amplify the sequence you want from a pool of cDNA. Single-stranded cDNA is synthesized as described above and used as the template for a reaction that includes two primers (forward or sense, and reverse or antisense), a mixture of all four dNTPs, and a temperature-stable DNA polymerase with its buffer. Three reaction temperatures are set (a) annealing (usually between 37°C and 65°C) that allows the primers to anneal to the template; (b) extension (usually ~72°C) that allows the polymerase to direct

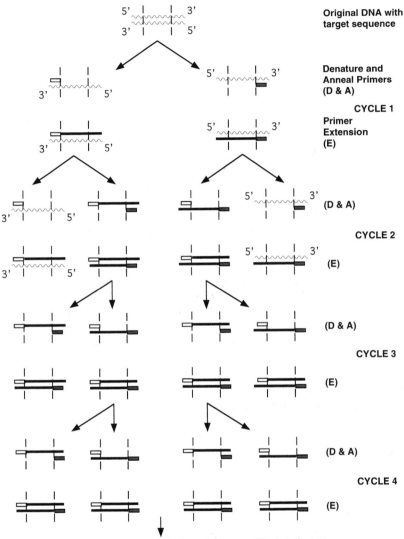

After 32 cycles, target sequence (short product) is amplified >10⁶ - fold

Figure 3 Schematic illustration of the amplification of a target sequence using heat-stable DNA polymerases and temperature cycling.

the synthesis of a new second strand of cDNA; (c) denaturation (usually ~95°C) that denatures the newly synthesized double-stranded cDNA resulting in 2X single-stranded templates. This cycle is then repeated approximately 30 times to achieve about a 1 million-fold amplification of the sequence of interest. If the synthetic primers also contain built in restriction sites, the amplified cDNA can easily be subcloned into a plasmid vector and sequenced.

Rapid Amplification of cDNA

Rapid amplification of cDNA ends (RACE) (3) allows one to clone either the 5' or the 3' part of a cDNA if one has isolated and sequenced the middle portion. This frequently happens when cDNAs are very long or when secondary structures in the template mRNA inhibit synthesis of the first-strand cDNA. In general because the reverse transcriptase reactions are performed at relatively low temperatures (usually 37–42°C), complex secondary structures in mRNA can be resistant to denaturation and the transcriptase may "fall off" the template, resulting in partial cDNAs. A typical strategy for RACE to clone a missing 5' end involves synthesis of nested primers, for example, three specific antisense 20 oligonucleotide primers located as close to possible as the most 5' available cDNA sequence. One microgram of mRNA from the tissue of interest is reverse transcribed using the most 3' primer of this set. An oligo dG tail can be added to this specific first strand cDNA, which is then used as the template for PCR amplification. For the PCR amplification, the second-most 3' of the set of antisense primers is used and a sense primer that includes an oligo dC plus a specific sequence including a restriction site. The most 5' of the three antisense synthetic oligonucleotides is radioactively labeled with ^{32}P γ ATP and hybridized to Southern blots of the PCR product to confirm its identity. PCR products hybridizing to these probes are subcloned into a plasmid vector and sequenced. The situation is reversed to isolate a missing 3' piece of cDNA: the nested primers are based on the sequence of the most 3' available cDNA and used as sense primers in the PCR reaction, oligo dT-primed first-strand cDNA is used as the template, and the antisense primer for the PCR reaction is a synthetic oligonucleotide that contains an oligo dT sequence plus a restriction site.

Genomic Cloning

Genomic DNA from the species of interest is digested with Sau3A and cloned into a suitable phage vector (e.g., the BamH I site of EMBL3). Recombinants are grown in Le392 bacterial host and screened using suitable probes labeled as described above. Positive clones are purified to homogeneity as described above. Genomic clones are then restriction mapped and sequenced using standard procedures (8). In general, a reasonable strategy for isolating a gene is to screen two genome equivalents of the species of interest. For most mammals, screening of several hundred thousand recombinants is more than sufficient.

METHODS USED TO CHARACTERIZE cDNA

RNAse Protection

RNAse protection is used to map the 5′ end of an mRNA. RNAse protection is performed using cRNA probes labeled with ^{32}P CTP and the appropriate RNA polymerase. RNA transcription to prepare cRNA probes is carried out in 20 μl the buffer containing 1 μg template DNA, 10 mM DTT, 0.5 mM of each of the ATP, GTP, and TTP, 1X transcription buffer (Ambion), 25 units RNAase inhibitor, 50 μCi[α-^{32}P]CT and 10 units of the proper RNA polymerase. The reaction is incubated at 25° C for 1 h and the DNA template removed with 2 units of Dane I at 37° C for 15 min. The reaction is then mixed with equal volume of loading buffer and run on a 5% of denaturing polyacrylamide gel for 1 h at 200 V. After electrophoresis, the gel is covered with plastic wrap and exposed to x-ray film for 1–5 min at room temperature in the dark. One corner of the film and the gel are aligned so as to localize the probe precisely. The area of the gel indicating the probe is excised and eluted in 350 μl buffer containing 0.5 M NH$_4$OAc, 1mM EDTA, and 0.1% SDS at room temperature with gentle shaking on the vortex at dial 3 for 25 min. Hybridizations of total RNA (usually 10–20 μg) with the radiolabeled cRNA (2×10^4 cpm) are performed in solution (80% deionized formamide, 40 mM PIPES pH 6.4, 400 mM NaOAc pH 6.4, mM EDTA) overnight at 45°C in a 20 μl reaction volume. Following incubation, reactions are digested with RNase A (0.33 units/μl)/RNAse T1 (100 units/μl) at 37°C for 30 min with 300 μl of a solution containing 10 mM Tris (pH 7.5), 300 mM NaCl, and 0.005 mM EDTA. Reactions are stopped with 10 μl 10% SDS and 50 μl proteinase K (1 mg/ml) followed by incubation for 15 min at 37°C. Protected fragments are ethanol-precipitated, resuspended in loading buffer, and size fractionated on 6–8% polyacrylamide gels under denaturing conditions at 200 V for 4 h in Tris–borate EDTA buffer. Gels are dried and exposed to x-ray film at –80°C with one intensifying screen.

Primer Extension

Primer extension assays are used to map the start site of transcription when cloning a novel mRNA. Primer extension assays are performed using 10 fmol gel-purified 14 or 16 nucleotide synthetic primer 5′ end-labeled with T4 polynucleotide kinase. Conditions for hybridization of the primer to the target RNA species can vary but an example is as follows: (20 μl volume), 0.4 M NaCl, 40 mM PIPES (pH 6.5), 1 mM EDTA, and 80% formamide at 30° C for 12 h. After precipitation with 1/2 volume of 7.5 M NH$_4$OAc, reverse transcriptase is added at 37° C for 1 h in the presence of 0.1 mM each of dTTP, dCTP, dGTP, and dATP to synthesize extended product. After RNAse treatment, phenol/chloroform extraction, and ethanol precipitation, the pellet is resuspended in 8 µl loading buffer, denatured at 100° C for 3 min, and size fractionated on a 6–8% polyacrylamide gel electrophoresis (PAGE). Gels are dried and exposed to x-ray film at –80°C with one intensifying screen for 48 h.

In Vitro Synthesis of mRNA

In vitro synthesis of 5′ cap mRNA suitable for injection into *Xenopus* oocytes for expression or for expression using rabbit reticulocyte lysate is performed following the maufacturer's protocol (e.g., mCAP Stratagene)]. This method is used because the 5′ cap structure of in vitro mRNA transcripts increases the yield and stability of the synthesized RNA and also enhances the translation efficiency both by rabbit reticulocyte lysate and of microinjected *Xenopus* oocytes. Plasmid DNA to be used as the template is banded twice on a CsCl gradient to provide extremely pure DNA. The DNA is linearized using an appropriate restriction enzyme, treated with proteinase K, ethanol-precipitated, and centrifuged under the RNAase-free conditions. One µg of this DNA template is transcribed in a solution containing 200 mM Tris pH 7.5, 250 mM NaCl, 40 mM $MgCl_2$, and 10 mM spermidine in the presence of rNTPs and cap analog. T3, T7, or SP6 RNA polymerase is then added to the reaction and incubated at 37° C for 30 min. DNAase I is used to remove the DNA template. The reaction is then extracted with phenol/chloroform and ethanol precipitated in the presence of the 0.3 M sodium acetate pH 5.0. The resulting pellet is then washed with 80% ethanol and dried. The concentration of the RNA sample is determined with a spectrophotometer at 260 nM ultraviolet (UV).

Isolation of RNA and Northern Hybridizations

Total RNA is prepared from cells or from tissue using the guanidinium isothiocyanate/cesium chloride centrifugation method. Cells are harvested, resuspended in 8 ml lysis buffer (2M guanidinium isothiocyanate, 0.1% lauryl sarcosyl, and 0.01% of 2-mercaptoethanol), and sheared by several passages through a 22 gauge needle. The suspension is then layered over 5.7 M cesium chloride and centrifuged overnight at 40,000 X g at 40°C. The resulting RNA pellet is ethanol precipitated and resuspended in DEPC-treated water. All operations are done on ice. RNA is quantitated by spectrophotometry at 260 nm.

Northern hybridizations are performed on RNA (usually ∼20 µg) or mRNA (usually ∼1–5 µg) that is size-fractionated on formaldehyde–agarose gels. RNA is transferred onto nitrocellulose filters overnight using 10X SSC transfer buffer. Filters are baked, prehybridized overnight in buffer containing

1X Denhardt's solution (0.02% polyvinylpyrrolidone/0.02% Ficoll/0.02% bovine serum albumin), 5X SSC (1X = 0.15M NaCl/0.015M sodium citrate, pH 7.0), 0.025M sodium phosphate (pH 7.4), sonicated calf thymus DNA (50 mg/ml), 0.1% SDS, and 50% (vol/vol) formamide, and hybridized with cDNA probes in the same buffer mixture overnight at 42°C. Blots are then washed to a final stringency of 0.2X SSC/0.1% SDS at 65°C for 15 min. Filters are exposed at –80°C on x-ray films (X-OMAT, AR, Eastman KODAK, Rochester, NY) with a single intensifying screen or at room temperature on a storage phosphorscreen (Molecular Dynamics).

Solution Hybridization Assays

Northern Analysis

Twenty to fifty micrograms of total cellular RNA are vacuum-dried, resuspended in 5 ml H_2O, and mixed with 15 ml RNA loading buffer containing 8% of formaldehyde; 67% formamide; 1X Mops; 2mM EDTA; 5.7% glycerol; 0.1% SDS; and 0.01% of the dyes bromophenol blue and xylene cyanol. The RNA is electrophoretically size-separated on a 1% agarose gel containing 20 mM Mops pH 7.4, 1 mM EDTA, and 3% formaldehyde. The electrophoresis is performed for 15 h at 30 mA in 1X Mops buffer with circulation to provide resolution of high-molecular-weight mRNAs. The gel is denatured in solution of 0.05N NaOH and 0.15M NaCl for 30 min and neutralized in 0.1 M Tris pH 7.5 and 0.15M NaCl for 30 min. RNA is transferred onto nitrocellulose filters overnight in 10X SSC buffer (1X = 0.15 M NaCl/0.015 M sodium citrate, pH 7.0). Following the transfer, the filter is photographed, UV crosslinked with 120 mJ, and baked at 80° C in the vacuum for 2 h. The filter is then prehybridized in a solution containing 5X SSC; 0.266 mg/ml; calf-thymus DNA; 25 mM sodium phosphate pH 6.4; 50% formamide; and 0.1% each of the following: SDS, BSA, Ficoll, and PVP in a 42° C water bath overnight. The prehybridization solution is removed and the filter then hybridized in a solution containing 5X SSC; 0.1 mg/ml calf-thymus DNA; 50 mM sodium phosphate pH 6.4; 0.1% SDS; 50% formamide; and 0.02% of the following: BSA, Ficoll, and PVP at 42° C overnight. The filter is washed twice with 2X SSC and 0.1% SDS at room temperature for 10 min, twice with 1X SSC and 0.1% SDS at 42° C for 20 min, and once in 0.2X SSC and 0.1% SDS for 15–20 min at 50–65° C. The filter is air dried, wrapped with plastic wrap, and exposed to film (X-OMAT, AR, Eastman KODAK, Rochester, NY) with a single intensifying screen at –80° C for the desired time period and developed in M35AX-Omat Kodak machine.

Southern Analysis

Ten micrograms of genomic DNA are digested with 100 units restriction enzyme in a 100 μl reaction volume at 37° C overnight. The reactions are phenol/chloroform extracted and ethanol precipitated. The pellet is dissolved in H_2O and mixed with loading buffer containing 0.25% of bromophenol blue; 0.25% of xylene cyanol and 40% (W/V) sucrose. The sample is run on a 0.7% agarose gel at 100 V for 5 h. Capillary DNA transfer onto nitrocellulose filters is conducted overnight in 10X SSC buffer. Prehybridization and hybridization are performed as described for Northern analysis. Final washing is in 0.2X SSC and 0.1% SDS solution at 60° C for 15 min. Films are autoradiographed using a single intensifying screen at –80° C for the desired time period.

Western Analysis and Antibody Production

Synthetic peptides, based on the amino acid sequence of the protein of interest, are coupled to keyhole lympet hemocyanin with glutaraldehyde and used to immunize two rabbits (5). After three immunizations at 2 week intervals, serum is collected. The IgG fraction is purified, and the antibodies affinity-purified using cyanogen bromide-activated sepharose beads to which the antigenic peptide has been coupled. The resulting sequence-specific polyclonal antibodies are suitable for immunoblotting.

A 30–35 μg of protein sample is separated on 6–8% SDS-PAGE according to Laemmli (6). Prestained molecular weight standards (Bethesda Research Laboratories) are used to monitor gel migration. The proteins are transferred to a PVDF (polyvinylidene difluoride) membrane (Du Pont) overnight at 4° C and 0.3 A in a buffer containing 25 mM Tris, 200 mM glycine, and 15% methanol. The membrane is then air-dried, wet with methanol, and rinsed with water. PBST solution pH 7.5 (80 mM of disodium hydrogen orthophosphate anhydrous, 20 mM sodium dihydrogen orthophosphate, 100 mM sodium chloride, and 0.1% Tween-20) supplemented with 5% dry milk is used to block the membrane at room temperature for 1 h. Primary antiserum is generally diluted 100–2000-fold with PBST buffer and incubated with the membrane for 1 h at room temperature with gentle shaking. After extensive washing with PBST buffer, the membrane is incubated in horseradish peroxidase-labeled antirabbit IgG solution at room temperature for 1 h. The membrane is washed thoroughly with PBST 6 times, and then incubated in the detection solution (supplied by the ECL kit, Amersham) for 1 min and exposed to a Hyperfilm-MP for the desired period of time.

EXPRESSION IN INSECT CELLS

Construction of Recombinant Vectors

Materials and methods for manipulating Baculovirus DNA (AcNPV) and Sf9 cells are described in the literature from the manufacturers of the Baculogold expression system (Pharmingen). We have found it useful to modify the baculo-virus transfer vector, pVL941 by incorporating a polycloning site. The pVL941 vector is digested with BamH1 and ligated to preannealed oligonucleotide linkers (sense and antisense linkers are combined in equimolar amounts, incubated at 95°C for 5 min, and allowed to cool slowly to room temperature) with the following sequences: sense: 5'-GATCCGCGAATTCTCACTAGTCGACGC-GTGATCTAGACGGAATTCGCG-3', and anti-sense: 5'-GATCCGCGAATTC-CGTCTAGATCACGCGTCGACTAGTGAGAATTCGCG-3', to yield pVL941-Link. Although the manufacturers do not recommend trying to use this or similar vectors for cDNA larger than ~8 kb, we have had success expressing cDNAs as large as 16 kb with this system. (1). Once you have cloned your cDNA into a suitable baculovirus transfer vector, it is cotransfected with bacu-lovirus gold DNA into Sf9 cells. Three days after transfection Sf9 clones con-taining recombinant Baculovirus and the cDNA of interest are isolated either by plaque assays or by dilutional cloning. Sf9 clones containing Baculovirus expressing recombinant protein can be identified by immunoblots. Individual viral isolates are subsequently amplified and used to reinfect Sf9 cultures. Sf9 cells are maintained in monolayer culture at 27°C in TNM-FH medium supple-mented with 10% fetal calf serum, 2.5 µg/ml "Fungizone," and 50 µg/ml gentamycin. Details of Baculovirus expression protocols are contained in an excellent manual (7).

Isolation of Sf9 Membranes

Sf9 cells are harvested, centrifuged for 2 min at 1000 rpm on a desktop cen-trifuge, and resuspended at a concentration of 1X 10^7 cells/ml in 50 mM Tris-Cl (pH 7.25), 250 mM sucrose. Cells are homogenized with 30 strokes in a Dounce homogenizer and the suspension then centrifuged at 4500X g for 15 min. The supernatant is centrifuged at 142,000X g for 45 min. The resulting membrane pellet is resuspended at a final concentration of 5–10 mg/ml in 20 mM Tris-Cl (pH 7.25) and 300 mM sucrose. All operations are carried out on ice and all solutions contained the following protease inhibitors: 0.1 mM phenyl-methylsulfonyl flouride (PMSF), 1 mM aprotinin, 10 µg/ml pepstatin, 10 µgml leupeptin, 10 µg/ml aprotinin.

EXPRESSION IN *XENOPUS LAEVIS* OOCYTES

Oocyte Expression

Oocytes are isolated from *Xenopus laevis* using standard techniques (2). Oocytes are defolliculated during a 2 h incubation in 2 mg/ml collagenase at room tem-perature in Ca^{2+}-free ND96 solution (96 mM NaCl, 2mM KCl, 1 mM $MgCl_2$, and 5 mM HEPES, pH 7.5). Oocytes are examined under a dissecting microscope and healthy-looking stage V and stage VI cells (2) are selected and maintained at 21 °C in enriched ND96 solution for 1 day prior to injection with in vitro transcribed RNA. Oocytes are microinjected according to the methods described by Gurdon (4). Approximately 5–20 ng of in vitro synthesized 5' capped mRNA in 50 nl volume is injected into each oocyte followed by incubation for 5 days at 18°C in Barth's medium. Functional expression of many proteins can be confirmed using appropriate assays such as measuring changes in intracellular calcium concentrations in response to receptor binding and direct measurement of ionic currents of expressed ion channels.

DNA Preparation

Following isolation of phage or plasmid clones, a variety of techniques can be used to purify quantities of DNA sufficient for sequencing and other manipulations. We have found several of the following protocols to be most useful. In particular we have had excellent results using modifications of standard procedures that reduce the amount of starting material (thus decreasing the time and cost of DNA purification) but still result in high-quality DNA suitable for sequencing.

Plasmid Isolation

MicroPlasmid Prep ("Zippy Prep")

This method can be used when it is only necessary to know the gross relative size of a plasmid, for example, when selecting plasmids for sequence analysis following an Exo III digestion. An individual bacteria colony is removed from the transformation plate (e.g., Exo III digestion-generated plasmid transformants) using the tip of a toothpick and resuspended in 20 µl lysis buffer containing 1 mg/ml lysozyme, 1 mg/ml RNAase A, 50 mM Tris-HCl pH 8.0, and 50 mM EDTA in a 1.5 ml Eppendorf tube and incubated for 5 min at room temperature. An equal volume of TE-equilibrated phenol is added, the tube is vortexed for 30 s and then centrifuged for 5 min at 14,000 rpm. A 10 µl aliquot of the supernatant is carefully removed from the top layer and run on a 1% agarose gel.

One-Step Miniprep

One-half milliliter of overnight bacteria culture is transferred into a 1.5 ml Eppendorf tube and an equal volume of phenol/chloroform/isoamylalcohol (25:24:1) added. The tube is vortexed for 1 min at maximum speed and then centrifuged at 14,000 rpm for 5 min. Approximately 0.45 ml of the upper aqueous phase is transferred to a new Eppendorf tube and mixed with 0.5 ml isopropanol, vortexed, and centrifuged immediately thereafter at 14,000 rpm for 5 min. The supernatant is discarded and the pellet washed twice with 70% ethanol. The pellet is dried and resuspended in 100 µl TER buffer containing 10 mM Tris, pH 7.5, 1 mM EDTA, and 20 mg/ml RNAase A. Five to ten microliters of that DNA are digested with the appropriate restriction enzyme for analysis.

Midiprep

A bacterial colony, or 5 µl of frozen bacteria stock, is inoculated into 50 ml of the proper medium supplemented with the proper antibiotic in a 250 ml flask and incubated overnight at 37° C with vigorous shaking (250 rpm). The cells are pelleted in a 50 ml tube and resuspended in 3.6 ml solution I containing 5 mg/ml lysozyme, 50 mM glucose, 25 mM Tris-Cl pH 8.0, and 10 mM EDTA. The cell suspension is incubated at room temperature for 5 min and 7.2 ml of solution II containing 0.2 N NaOH and 1% SDS is added. The tube is inverted 20 times and then chilled on ice for 5 min. Solution III (5.4 ml) containing 3M KOAc and 11.5% of glacial acetic acid is added, the tube is inverted 20 times, and then chilled on ice for another 5 min. Following a spin at 4K for 15 min at 4° C, the supernatant is transferred to a 30 ml Corex tube, mixed with 0.6 volumes of isopropanol, and incubated at room temperature for 15 min. The DNA is pelleted at 10K for 15 min at 4°C. The supernatant is discarded and the pellet is dissolved in 4.4 ml TE (pH 7.4). CsCl (4.6 g) and 100 µl ethidium bromide (10 mg/ml) are added and mixed well. The sample is loaded into a 13 × 51 mm polyallomer quick-seal centrifuge tube and centrifuged in a VTi 65.1 rotor at 65K for 4 h or 54K for 15 h at 20°C. The lower band is removed (~0.6 ml) with an 18 gauge needle under long-wavelength UV and transferred to an Eppendorf tube. The sample is extracted four times with an equal volume of TE (pH 8.0)-saturated butanol to remove all ethidium bromide. The aqueous phase is transferred into a 15 ml Corex tube and 3 volumes of TE (pH 8.0) and 2.5 volumes of 100% ethanol are added. After 20 min incubation on ice, the plasmid is pelleted at 10K for 15 min at 4° C. The supernatant is discarded and the pellet is redissolved in 400 µl TE (pH 8.0) and transferred to an Eppendorf tube. The DNA is extracted once with phenol/chloroform, chloroform, and then precipitated with 2.5 vol ethanol in the presence of 0.3 M sodium acetate. The DNA pellet is then washed with 75% ethanol, dried in Speedvac and dissolved in 200 µl H₂O.

Superminiprep

This modified miniprecipitation method is used to prepare plasmid DNA for sequence analysis. Three milliliters of overnight bacterial culture are pelleted in an Eppendorf tube. The pellet is resuspended in 100 µl solution I containing 50 mM glucose, 25 mM Tris pH 8.0, 10mM EDTA, and 10 mg/ml lyso-zyme and vortexed briefly. Following a 10 min incubation at room tempera-ture, solution II (200 μl) containing 1% SDS and 0.2 N NaOH is added to the bacterial suspension and mixed by multiple inversions. This mixture is incubated for 5 min on ice. Two hundred microliters of solution III containing 3M KOAc and 11.5% of glacial acetic acid are then added, mixed briefly by vortexing, and incubated for 5 min on ice. The samples are centrifuged at full speed for 5 min , the supernatant transferred to a new tube, and recentrifuged for 5 min to obtain particle-free lysate. The supernatant is precipitated with two volumes of 100% ethanol, and centrifuged for 2 min (12,000g at room temperature). The pellet is dissolved in 200 μl H_2O, RNAase A added to a final concentration of 50 μg/ml, and the reaction incubated for 30 min at 37° C. Then the reaction is digested with proteinase K at a final concentration of 0.5 μg/ml, and incu-bated for 30 additional min at 42° C. The reaction mixture was then extracted twice with 200 μl phenol/chloroform (70:30), and once with 200 μl pure chlo-roform. DNA is precipitated with 2.5 volume of 100% ethanol without add-ing any extra salt, mixed by inversion, and centrifuged for 3 min (12,000/g at room temperature). The pellet is washed with 75% ethanol, dried in Speedvac, and redissolved in 20–50 μl H_2O. DNA concentration is determined spectro-photometrically at 280/260 nM. Typically 50–100 μg of plasmid DNA is iso-lated by this method and 10 μg is used for each sequencing reaction.

Phage DNA Isolation

Ten microliters of an overnight culture of host bacterial cells are grown in a 50 ml conical tube with antibiotics (e.g., ampicillin) in the appropriate media. This culture is added to 500 ml fresh media without antibiotics in a 2 L flask and incubated at 37° C, shaking at 250 rpm. After 2 h, when the bacteria is in its logarithmic growth phase, 1×10^{10} pfu of phage is added. The culture is incubated at 37° C with shaking for an additional 6–8 h. When lysis occurs, 10 ml chloroform is added to the culture and incubated for an additional 15 min. The culture is subsequently transferred to a centrifuge bottle and spun at 5000X g at 20° C for 20 min. DNAase I and RNAase (each to a final concentration of 1 μg/ml) are added to the supernatant. The nuclease reaction is incubated for 30 min at room temperature. Solid polyethylene glycol (PEG 8000) is added to a final concentration of 10% and crystal sodium chloride added to a final concentration of 1M with slow stirring on a magnetic stirrer at room tempera-ture. The solution is placed on ice for 1 h and then centrifuged at 10,000X g for 15 min at 4° C. The pellet is resuspended in 3 ml buffer L3 from the Qiagen phage precipitation kit (Qiagen Inc.). The manufacturer's instructions (after step 4) for the Qiagen kit are then followed. The resulting phage is dis-solved in 200 μl H_2O.

Genomic DNA Isolation

A total of 10^8 to 10^9 cells are collected by centrifugation at 1000X g for 5 min. The pellet is washed once in 10 ml PBS and resuspended in 10 volumes of lysis buffer containing 10 mM Tris pH 7.4, 10 mM EDTA, 150 mM NaCl, 0.4% SDS, and 1 mg/ml proteinase K. The reaction was incubated for 3 h at 50° C with periodic swirling. An equal volume of TE-saturated phenol (pH 8.0) is added and the tube gently inverted 50 times to extract the DNA followed by a quick spin at 200 X g for 2 min. The organic phase, including the interface, was discarded. The phenol extraction was repeated two more times. The aqueous phase DNA was dialyzed overnight at 4° C against 4 L of a solution (50 mM Tris-HCl pH 8.0, 10 mM EDTA, and 10 mM NaCl) with four changes. The sample was then incubated with 100 µg/ml DNAase-free RNAase at 37° C for 2 h. The DNA is gently extracted twice with phenol/chloroform and then dialyzed extensively against TE pH 8.0 with frequent change of the solution at 4°C for 2 days.

REFERENCES

1. Brillantes A-M B, Ondrias K, Scott A, Kobrinsky E, Ondriasova E, Moschella MC, Jayaraman T, Landers M, Ehrlich B E, Marks A R. Stabilization of calcium release channel (ryanodine receptor) function by FK-506 binding protein. Cell 1994; 77:513–523.
2. Dumont JN. Oogenesis in *Xenopus laevis* (Daudin), I. Stages of oocyte development in laboratory maintained animals. J Morphol 1972; 136:153–180.
3. Frohman MA, Dush MK, Martin GR. Rapid production of full-length cDNAs from rare transcripts: amplification using a single gene-specific oligonucleotide primer. Proc Natl Acad Sci 1988; 85:8998–9002.
4. Gurdon JB, Lane DC, Woodland HR, Marbaix G. Nature 1971; 233.
5. Harlow E, Lane D. Antibodies, A Laboratory Manual. Cold Spring Harbor, NY: Cold Spring Harbor Laboratory, 1988.
6. Laemmli UK. Nature 1970; 227:680–685.
7. O'Reilly D, Miller L, Luckow V. Baculovirus Expression Vectors: A Laboratory Manual. New York: WH Freeman, 1992.
8. Sambrook J, Fritsch EF, Maniatis T. Molecular Cloning: A Laboratory Manual. Cold Spring Harbor, NY: Cold Spring Harbor Laboratory Press, 1989.

3

Expression Cloning and Screening for Unknown Genes

Mark E. Lieb
Mount Sinai School of Medicine
New York, New York

The previous chapter introduced the techniques used to isolate genomic and cDNA clones using radiolabled probes. These techniques involve the use of a radiolabled probe derived from a known sequence to identify a clone whose sequence is not known. The use of these techniques is therefore restricted to situations in which some specific information about the sequence of the gene to be cloned can be inferred. The present chapter will outline how basic cloning strategies have been extended to use in situations in which no assumptions can be made about the sequence of the gene to be cloned. Subsequently, these will be refered to as "unknown" genes, that is, genes for which there is no prior information about their potential sequence. A distinction should be made between these techniques and the large-scale projects underway to sequence entire genomes. The techniques outlined in this chapter are designed to identify expressed genes with specific attributes of interest, while the genome projects are geared to obtain large stretches of sequence from entire chromosomes.

OVERVIEW

Most projects involving the cloning of an "unknown" gene are primarily concerned with identifying the gene's protein product. The isolation of a novel protein traditionally involved the progressive purification of a series of crude protein fractions from a tissue until a relatively pure preparation of the protein could be isolated. Once this frequently Herculean task was accomplished, the amino acid sequence of the protein could then be determined. As described in the previous chapter, once partial amino acid sequence is obtained for a protein, this sequence can be used to design the radiolabeled probes needed to clone the gene that encodes the protein. In general, with the appropriate probe, the actual cloning of a gene or cDNA requires a small fraction of the time and effort needed to isolate a novel protein. The strategies outlined below, are used to allow the identification of "unknown" genes by cloning their cDNAs directly, without the need to isolate the protein they encode.

Most mammalian cells are assumed to make approximately 10,000 different proteins. Each protein is encoded by a unique mRNA and, for most purposes, the amount of a given protein made should be proportional to the number of copies of the unique mRNA in the cell at a given time. Thus, the cell might contain hundreds of mRNA molecules encoding a relatively abundant protein, but only several copies of an mRNA molecule encoding a rare protein. As might be inferred, identifying clones corresponding to low-abundance mRNAs presents a greater challenge and has led to a variety of modifications of the basic techniques to increase the chances of identifying a rare clone.

Two general strategies exist for cloning unknown genes: (a) expression-based cloning strategies to purify a specific cDNA using an assay related to the protein's function; and (b) differential cloning strategies, which allow isolation of cDNAs more highly expressed under one condition when compared to a second condition. The choice between these two general strategies depends on the nature of the protein being cloned and its hypothesized function. Expression cloning entails identifying a clone based upon a specific property of its corresponding protein. It has the distinct advantage of leading to the isolation of a clone that produces a protein with the property of interest, and it is the technique of choice when at least one property of the protein is well defined and can be easily measured (e.g., as is often the case with a transcription factor, growth factor or cytokine, ion channel, or cell surface receptor). In practice, however, the properties of an unidentified protein may not be well defined or not easily measurable using expression systems. In these situations, differential cloning strategies are frequently employed. Various refinements of the methods for differential cloning in recent years have made these techniques increasingly easier to perform, allowing the relatively rapid identification of clones representing differences in mRNA expression between two experimental conditions.

EXPRESSION CLONING STRATEGIES

Expression cloning involves four general steps: (a) the generation of a cDNA library, (b) expressing that library in cells that will produce the protein of interest, (c) screening pools of cells with a biological assay to detect a specific property of the protein being sought, and (d) recovery of the cDNA clone that encodes the protein.

As described in the previous chapter, cloning involves sequential rounds of purification until the single clone of interest is isolated from a background of thousands to millions of clones. Part of what makes cDNA cloning with radiolabeled DNA probes so powerful is that it is sensitive enough to allow the screening of millions of clones at once to detect a specific clone of matching sequence. In general, because expression cloning methods do not have as high a level of sensitivity, a series of relatively small pools of clones are screened to detect a pool of clones that can produce the protein of interest. The "positive" pool is then split into a series of smaller pools, which are screened again. The process is repeated until a single pure clone is obtained.

The simplest form of expression cloning involves the screening of a cDNA library expressed in bacteria, using an antibody directed against the protein of interest as a probe. A number of the lambda phage vectors used in the previous chapter for cloning by in situ plaque hybridization are designed to allow expression of the peptide corresponding to the cloned insert in bacteria. Under the appropriate conditions, an inducible promoter in the cloning vector causes production by the bacteria of mRNA transcripts complementary to the sequence of the cloned insert. The bacteria, grown in a lawn on agar plates, will then produce the corresponding protein. Nitrocellulose lifts made from the plates can be screened with a labeled antibody against the desired protein in a similar manner to the way a labeled DNA probe was used in the previous chapter. Of course, with modern cloning techniques, if one has purified a peptide to the point at which antibodies can be generated, it would generally be more straightforward to obtain partial amino acid sequence and clone the cDNA using synthetic oligonucleotide probes. Even where an antibody against the protein exists, the bacteria may not make the appropriate posttranslational modifications required to produce an antigenically recognizable protein. Eukaryotic expression systems, such as frog oocytes or COS cells, can allow expression of proteins with the correct posttranslational processing, which can then be detected with either an antibody or a biological assay based upon function.

The frog oocyte system was the first eukaryotic system widely applied to expression cloning of cDNAs encoding mammalian proteins. A cDNA library is constructed in a plasmid vector that contains the appropriate recognition site for a bacterial RNA polymerase. The plasmid library is used to transform bacteria and divided into smaller pools of clones. The plasmid DNA is recovered from an aliquot of the bacteria, and the purified plasmids are used to generate RNA transcripts for each cDNA in the pool of clones by in vitro transcription. The synthesized mRNA is then injected into frog oocytes, and the injected oocytes are assayed for the presence of the functional protein. When a pool of clones is identified that can confer the desired function on the oocytes, the plasmid-containing bacteria in that pool are further subdivided. Each subdivided pool of clones can be amplified by allowing the bacteria to replicate, the plasmid DNA is again recovered from a portion of the bacteria, and the process of in vitro transcription and injection of the mRNA into oocytes is repeated. Through repeated rounds of subdividing and rescreening, eventually a pure clone can be isolated. A strategy of this nature allowed the cloning of the human thrombin receptor (1) when efforts failed to isolate the putative receptor by methods of protein purification had failed.

Expression systems that use cultured mammalian cells (Fig. 1) are less labor intensive, because they allow the same general cloning strategy to be used without the need to synthesize separately the mRNA and manually inject it into cells. Instead, plates of cultured mammalian cells can be transfected directly with aliquots of the cDNA library constructed in an appropriate plasmid vector. Transfected cells will produce the protein encoded by the plasmid without requiring any further intervention. For example, plasmid libraries constructed in mammalian expression plasmids containing the SV40 origin of replication allow high levels of expression of proteins corresponding to the cDNA inserts when they are transfected into COS cells. COS cells are a line of cultured mammalian cells that constitutively express high levels of the SV40 large T antigen. The large T antigen causes high levels of replication of transfected plasmids containing the SV40 origin of replication. COS cells transfected with clones from the plasmid library will produce the corresponding mRNAs, and cDNA clones corresponding to full-length mRNAs can generally be expected to cause production of high levels of mature proteins (with the appropriate mammalian posttranslational processing). Cultured plates of cells transfected with pools from the cDNA library can then be screened to identify pools of clones that make the protein of interest. The method for screening the transfected COS cells depends upon the nature of the protein's function. For a secreted protein such as a growth factor, screening involves assaying the cell culture medium for the activity being sought. For a cell surface protein such as a growth factor receptor, screening can be performed by assaying for binding of the radiolabeled ligand. The second strategy has been used to clone vascu-

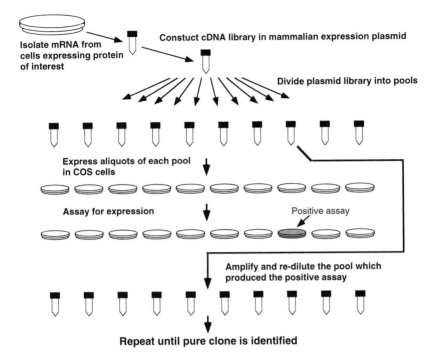

Isolate mRNA from cells expressing protein of interest

Constuct cDNA library in mammalian expression plasmid

Divide plasmid library into pools

Express aliquots of each pool in COS cells

Assay for expression

Positive assay

Amplify and re-dilute the pool which produced the positive assay

Repeat until pure clone is identified

Figure 1 Expression cloning in mammalian cells. Messenger RNA is isolated from cultured cells thought to express the protein of interest, and used to construct a cDNA library in a mammalian expression plasmid containing the SV40 origin of replication. The library is divided into smaller pools of clones, and an aliquot from each pool is transfected into COS cells. COS cells are used in this case because they consitutively express high levels of the SV40 large T antigen, which causes high levels of replication of transfected plasmids containing the SV40 origin of replication. The plates are assayed for the expression of the protein of interest. The library pool corresponding to the plate with the positive assay is then rediluted, amplified if necessary, and the new pools are used to transfect COS cells again. The cycle is repeated until a pure clone is obtained.

lar angiotensin II receptors (2). The sensitivity of the technique can be enhanced by using photographic emulsion for in situ visualization of the cells binding the radiolabeled ligand. This method was used to clone TGF-beta type III and type II receptors from a rat vascular smooth muscle cell library (3,4). It is interesting to note that the protein expression levels of COS cells tranfected with the plasmid containing the SV40 origin of replication were high enough to allow positive clones to be identified, even though COS cells constitutively express the TGF-beta III receptor at high levels (5). In spite of this strategy, constitutive expression by COS cells of the protein being cloned can create difficulties with expression cloning. Other problems may arise when additional proteins are required in order to detect the functional protein, as may be the case with G-protein coupled receptors or multimeric ion channels. A recent review article is a useful starting point for further reading about expression cloning of mammalian proteins (6).

YEAST TWO-HYBRID SYSTEM

Expression cloning to identify proteins that can interact with a protein of interest can be accomplished using the yeast two-hybrid system (7), an extremely powerful tool for studying protein–protein interactions. The system was developed by taking advantage of certain properties of the yeast protein GAL4 (8). GAL4 is a transcriptional activator that binds to a specific segment of yeast DNA, causing expression of particular yeast genes. The region of the GAL4 protein responsible for binding to DNA (the binding domain), and the region responsible for actually activating transcription (the activation domain), are structurally distinct. These two domains of the GAL4 protein, when they are artificially introduced into the yeast using expression plasmids, will not activate transcription unless they can be caused to associate with each other. It is possible to cause the binding domain and the activation domain of the GAL4 protein to interact by linking them to proteins that *are* able to interact. For example, assume two hypothetical proteins A and B are able to interact with each other, and the cDNAs encoding these proteins are available. Two yeast expression plasmids could be created. The first plasmid would contain the cDNA for protein A inserted after the cDNA encoding the GAL4-binding domain. Transfected into the yeast host, this plasmid would cause the yeast to synthesize a fusion protein containing the GAL4-binding domain at one end, and protein A at the other end. The second plasmid would be designed to produce a fusion protein with protein B at one end and the GAL4-activation domain at the other end. When both of these plasmids are expressed in the yeast, the association between proteins A and B would cause the binding and activation domains of the GAL4 to be brought together, enabling them to bind to DNA and activate transcription.

To clone cDNAs that produce proteins that interact with a protein of interest, a cDNA library is constructed in a plasmid vector designed to express the cDNA inserts as fusion proteins with the GAL4 activation domain. The cDNA encoding the known protein to be studied is cloned into a second plasmid that will express the protein as a GAL4-binding domain fusion protein. The two plasmids are cotransfected into a strain of yeast that has been altered to contain a reporter gene under the control of the GAL4 recognition site. Colonies of yeast are screened for expression of the reporter gene. The plasmid DNA can be recovered from these colonies and studied further. The development of the yeast two-hybrid cloning strategy has allowed the identification proteins that interact with numerous target proteins (9) and has engendered a significant amount of active investigation in a variety of fields.

DIFFERENTIAL CLONING STRATEGIES

Differential Screening

The basic protocol for screening cDNA libraries for differentially expressed genes (Fig. 2) is an extension of the standard methods used for cloning by in situ plaque hybridization. First, mRNA is isolated from cells or tissues hypothesized to express the mRNA(s) of interest and is used to construct a cDNA library in a bacteriophage vector as described in the previous chapter. Second, the phage library is plated in a bacterial lawn on agar plates so that clonal plaques containing isolated pools of concentrated phage are produced on the surface of the agar. Third, duplicate nitrocellulose "lifts" are made by sequentially laying nitrocellulose filters on the surface of of the agar plates, and the

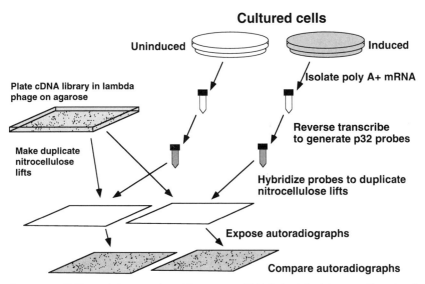

Cultured cells

Uninduced   Induced

Plate cDNA library in lambda phage on agarose

Isolate poly A+ mRNA

Make duplicate nitrocellulose lifts

Reverse transcribe to generate p32 probes

Hybridize probes to duplicate nitrocellulose lifts

Expose autoradiographs

Compare autoradiographs

Figure 2 Differential screening. Messenger RNA is isolated from cultured cells grown under the two conditions to be compared and used as a template for reverse transcriptase to generate single-stranded, ^{32}P-labeled cDNA probes. These two probes are individually hybridized to duplicate nitrocellulose lifts from a lambda phage cDNA library on agarose plates. Autoradiographs from the two filters are visually compared to identify clones that produce a significantly stronger signal with probes from one of the two conditions.

plates are stored at 4°C to allow later recovery of the plaques of interest. Finally, the filters are hybridized to probes generated to represent all of the mRNAs expressed under the two conditions being compared.

Probes for Use in Differential Screening

Probes for use in differential screening are designed to hybridize to *all* of the clones corresponding to mRNAs expressed in the cells or tissues under the conditions studied. To create these "fully representative" probes, RNA is extracted from cells or tissues under the two conditions to be compared and mRNA is isolated. Single-stranded, radioactive, cDNA probes are then synthesized by reverse transcribing the mRNA from each condition. Since reverse transcriptase will make a single cDNA copy of each mRNA molecule, the amount of specific radioactivity incorporated for each species of cDNA in the radiolabeled probe should be directly proportional to the level of each mRNA expressed in the cells at the time the RNA was isolated. These probes are hybridized separately to the duplicate nirtocellulose filters. When autoradiographs of the duplicate filters are examined, the signal for plaques corresponding to differentially expressed mRNAs should be more intense on one autoradiograph than the other. The autoradiographs are aligned to the original agar plates to allow identification and recovery of the plaques of interest. The recovered plaques are plated on new plates, and the process repeated with this substantially smaller pool of clones until pure clones that consistently demonstrate a differential signal are isolated.

We have used a protocol for differential cloning based on the method of Lau and Nathans (10) to identify PDGF- (platelet-derived growth factor) inducible genes in vascular smooth muscle cells (11). While the methods for in situ plaque hybridization are well described in the previous chapter and in standard laboratory manuals (12), certain specific details as they relate to differential cloning are worthy of mention. In standard cDNA cloning, only a small proportion of plaques will hybridize to the radioactive probe. In differential cloning, because the probes are generated from total mRNA, virtually every plaque from the agar plates will produce a signal. Only a small proportion of the plaques will correspond to differentially expressed mRNAs. Thus, relatively minor irregularities in the surfaces of the agar plates can lead to variations that may lead to significant difficulties interpreting the autoradiograms of the hybridized filters. Measures should taken to ensure that the plates are poured on a level surface and that the filters are handled in a consistently careful manner. In our laboratory, for each round of screening, ~ 10,000 plaques were plated at a density of ~ 300 plaques per plate on square 10 cm gridded petri dishes (Falcon #1012). Denaturation and neutralization steps were carried out by placing the filters, DNA side up, on 3 mm chromatography paper (Whatman), saturated with the appropriate denaturing and neutralization solutions. The two sets of 24 nitrocellulose filters were hybridized separately with their respective probes. Although attempts can be made to adjust for differences in overall signal intensity between the two sets of lifts by varying their individual exposure times, in our experience a subjective adjustment by the observer while examining the autoradiograms is just as effective. Clones that were judged to have a significant difference in signal intensity by visual inspection were cored from the agar and eluted in SM buffer. A bacterial lawn in top agarose was grown on the surface of a new set of agar plates, and eluates from each clone were then spotted directly onto a lawn of bacteria using a sterile pipette tip in a grid array. Pairs of duplicate nitrocellulose lifts were made from these secondary plates and hybridized to the two different probes. Clones that repeatedly showed differences in signal strength with the two probes through several rounds of replating were recovered from the plates and studied further. In our initial screening of ~118,000 clones, approximately 800 plaques were identified that gave differential signals. Of these, 45 continued to give differential signal in subsequent rounds of hybridization and were recovered for further study. Ultimately, five of these corresponded to mRNAs regulated by PDGF.

Subtractive Cloning Strategies

Although there are variations in the method described for differential screening outlined above, an inherent difficulty with all of them is the substantial "background" of nondifferentially expressed plaques present in the initial rounds of screening. To reduce the magnitude of this problem, a number of methods of subtractive hybridization have been developed to enrich both cDNA libraries and probes for clones of interest. An example of one method for generating a subtracted probe is shown in Figure 3. Single-stranded cDNA is synthesized from mRNA isolated under conditions in which the gene(s) of interest are thought to be induced. The single-stranded cDNA is then hybridized, in solution, to an excess of mRNA isolated from the uninduced condition and double-stranded DNA-RNA hybrids are removed by passage through hydroxyapatite. The process can be repeated to enrich further the cDNA for induced sequences. The remaining cDNA is used to construct a "subtracted" cDNA library. In a similar fashion, the radiolabeled cDNA probes used to screen the library can be hybridized to an excess of cold mRNA or double-stranded cDNA to remove noninduced transcripts. An example of the application of this technique was the cloning of the myogenic factor MyoD1 (13) by using fibroblast mRNA to "subtract" cDNA from proliferating myoblasts. A variety of novel variations on the basic technique of subtractive hybridization have been described that involve

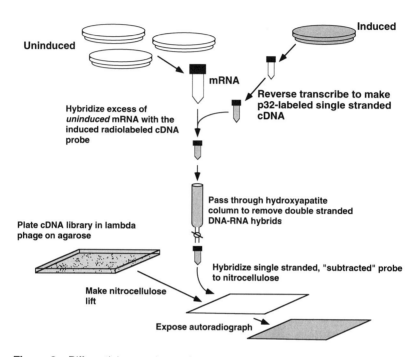

Figure 3 Differential screening: subtracted probes. Messenger RNA is isolated from cultured cells grown under the two conditions to be compared. The mRNA from the condition in which the unknown gene is thought to be induced is used as a template to generate a single stranded P32 labeled cDNA. The cDNA is then hybridized in solution to an excess of mRNA from the condition in which the unknown gene is not induced. The double-stranded cDNA-mRNA hybrids are removed by passage through a hydroxyapatite column. The single-stranded, "subtracted" cDNA probe that is recovered is enriched for sequences present at higher levels under the induced condition. The subtracted probe is then used to screen a cDNA library in lambda phage using standard techniques.

incorporating chemically modified nucleotides into the noninduced cDNA to allow the hybrids to be removed with easier-to-use techniques than hydroxyapatite columns. Subtractive libraries created in appropriate expression vectors can be used as a starting point for the expression cloning strategies earlier in this chapter. It should be noted that subtractive strategies are useful only in situations where it is known in which of the two conditions the gene expression is elevated. A number of these novel methods are commercially available as kits, with improvements and variations on the theme being introduced each year. Although we have no firsthand experience with these commercial products, at the present time a kit from a reliable vendor is probably the best starting point for a subtractive screening project, particularly for laboratories that do not routinely work with RNA.

Differential Display of mRNA

A PCR-based method for identifying differentially expressed mRNAs was recently described (14) that has a number of advantages over the differential screening techniques described above and has become an increasingly popular method for differential cloning. The basic strategy for differential display (Fig. 4) is to use PCR of reverse-transcribed mRNA to produce short cDNA fragments corresponding to every mRNA present. If the banding pattern produced by gel electrophoresis of these PCR products is reproducible, then the pattern produced by using mRNA from different tissues (or cells) can be compared to identify differentially expressed mRNAs. The bands that differ can be recovered from the gel, further amplified by PCR, and then ligated into plasmid vectors for DNA sequencing. In theory, to compare completely the mRNA expression patterns of two different tissues, ~10,000 DNA bands would need to be compared. To make this logistically possible, the primers for reverse transcription and PCR are designed to produce a limited pool of amplified products, in the size range that can be conveniently resolved on standard acrylamide gels. A series of primers, each designed to amplify a conveniently small portion of the total number of mRNA species present, are used in separate reactions in the presence of radiolabeled nucleotides and the products of each reaction are analyzed in separate lanes of the electrophoresis gel. In this way, the bands produced by thousands of different mRNA species can be examined on the autoradiograph of a single gel, and the banding pattern produced by mRNA from different tissues can be compared in adjacent lanes of the same gel.

The mRNA differential display technique has a number of potential advantages over conventional differential cloning strategies. First, because of the sensitivity of PCR, the reverse transcription step can be carried out using the oligo dT primer directly on total RNA, without the need for isolating mRNA. Second, the reproducibility of the banding pattern allows each successive experiment to serve as a control for subsequent experiments. This differs from the techniques for differential screening using plaque hybridization, in which the actual pattern of plaques is entirely nonreproducible. Third, primers can be selected to allow display of a banding pattern representing virtually the entire population of mRNAs present, allowing the total number of genes differentially expressed genes to be estimated. In addition, the method is not necessarily restricted to pairwise comparisons, since the same primers can potentially be used to amplify cDNA from a variety of experimental conditions, with the

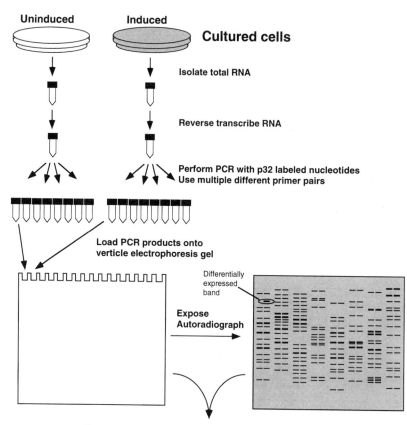

Figure 4 Differential display of mRNA. Total RNA is isolated from culture cells or tissues obtained under the two conditions to be compared. The total RNA is used as a template for reverse transcriptase, using oligo dT primers that have been modified so that only a fraction of the total population of mRNA present is primed. The single-stranded cDNA from each condition is used as a template for PCR in the presence of radiolabeled nucleotides, using a series of arbitrary primers designed to amplify a still smaller fraction of the population of expressed mRNAs. The PCR products from each primer pair are separated by polyacrylamide gel electrophoresis. The lanes of the gel are loaded so that adjacent lanes contain the PCR products from the two different cultured cells (or tissues), amplified with identical primers. The autoradiograph of the gel is examined to identify bands that are differentially expressed between the two conditions. In the figure, a single band present in the second lane, but not the first lane, has been circled. This band would be expected to correspond to an mRNA expressed only in the induced cells. The autoradioraph is used to find the exact location of the band on the gel so that it can be recovered and subjected to further analysis.

banding patterns compared in serial lanes of a single electrophoresis gel. The necessary primers, reagents, and instructions for performing mRNA differential display are available in a single kit (GenHunter Corporation, Brookline, MA). A review and discussion of mRNA differential display, along with a detailed laboratory protocol (including suggested sequences for the PCR primers), has recently been published (15).

Considerations

It is critical to recognize that all of the differential cloning techniques will only do what they are designed to do: to identify mRNAs that are expressed at different levels when two different conditions are compared. As the techniques become more refined, this goal becomes easier and easier to accomplish. It remains critical, however, to choose experimental conditions that are likely to show differences meaningful to the hypothesis being tested. Comparisons between cells or tissues that are too similar might fail to demonstrate detectable differences, while some conditions may have so many differences that meaningful interpretation becomes impossible. The choice of which differential cloning technique to use is dependent upon the nature of the experiment and the facilities and expertise available. Standard differential screening and differential display of mRNA would seem to be applicable to similar situations: in which there are likely to be a number of differentially expressed genes, and the identification of any of these genes would be interesting. The differential display technique is technically more straightforward, and offers the potential advantages outlined above. It should be kept in mind, however, that the sensitivity for either of these techniques for identifying a given differentially expressed gene is unknown, and one method might be able to identify a given gene where the other might fail. When it is anticipated that a only a small number of mRNAs will be differentially expressed between the conditions, subtractive cloning strategies have the advantage of allowing successive rounds of enrichment to be carried out by repeating the subtraction process. This is particularly applicable when the mRNA of interest is expressed only at low levels.

Sequence Analysis

Access to facilities for computer analysis of DNA sequences and comparison to current databases are essential parts of any differential cloning project. Fortunately, a number of publicly available resources exist over the Internet to allow the user to ascertain rapidly if a cloned sequence shares homology with any known sequences. A useful introduction to computer analysis of DNA sequence exists in a standard lab manual (16). Access to the Internet to allow homology searches of the comprehensive sequence databases maintained at the National Center for Biotechnology Information (NCBI), National Library of Medicine in Bethesda, MD. Servers running implementations of the BLAST algorithm for sequence similarity searches (17) can be accessed by e-mail (detailed instructions may be obtained by sending an e-mail message to blast@ncbi.nlm.nih.gov, with the word "help" in the body of the message) and through the NCBI Web site (www.ncbi.nlm.nih.gov).

While a detailed discussion of sequence homology searches is beyond the scope of this chapter, several points are worthy of mention as they relate to searches involving sequence from unknown clones. First, the sensitivity of homology searches can be greatly increased by comparing peptide, rather than nucleotide, sequences since peptide sequences are obviously more highly conserved. To facilitate these comparisons when the correct reading frame of a partial clone might not be known, the BLAST server provides an option in which the nucleotide query sequence submitted is translated into all six possible reading frames, and compared to a comprehensive database that has also been translated into all open reading frames. This will frequently be the only method that might allow detection of the similarity between homologous sequences from distantly related organisms. If a search performed in this manner fails to yield the identity of the query sequence, the search should be repeated as a nucleotide search, since if the query sequence is of poor quality (multiple insertion and deletion errors), the protein translations may occasionally become too garbled to allow the program to detect the homology. Second, it should be recognized that the initial sequences cloned from oligo dT primed libraries may be from the 3′ untranslated region of the mRNA. This is likely to be particularly true of the initial clones obtained from mRNA differential display, in which the technique is specifically designed to amplify only the few hundred bases adjacent to the poly-A tail of the mRNA. Because the conservation of sequence homology outside of the coding region may be very low between different species, searches using the sequence from the fragments initially recovered from the differential display gels may fail to identify the similarity of the gene to its homolog in another species. Novel clones of this sort can be used as probes to identify longer clones using the standard cloning methods described in the previous chapter. The databases can then be reinterrogated with the longer sequences to see if homologous genes have been described.

REFERENCES

1. Vu T, Hung D, Wheaton V, Coughlin S. Molecular cloning of a functional thrombin receptor reveals a novel proteolytic mechanism of receptor activation. Cell 1991; 64:1057–1068.
2. Murphy TJ, Alexander RW, Griendling KK, Runge MS, Bernstein KE. Isolation

of a cDNA encoding the vascular type-1 angiotensin II receptor. Nature 1991; 351(6323):233–236.

3. Lin HY, Wang XF, Ng-Eaton E, Weinberg RA, Lodish HF. Expression cloning of the TGF-beta type II receptor, a functional transmembrane serine/threonine kinase. Cell 1992; 68(4):775–785.

4. Wang XF, Lin HY, Ng-Eaton E, Downward J, Lodish HF, Weinberg RA. Expression cloning and characterization of the TGF-beta type III receptor. Cell 1991; 67(4):797–805.

5. Lin HY, Wang XF. Expression cloning of TGF-beta receptors. Mol Reprod Dev 1992; 32(2):105–110.

6. Simonsen H, Lodish HF. Cloning by function: expression cloning in mammalian cells. Trends Pharmacol Sci 1994; 15(12):437–441.

7. Chien CT, Bartel PL, Sternglanz R, Fields S. The two-hybrid system: a method to identify and clone genes for proteins that interact with a protein of interest. Proc Natl Acad Sci USA 1991; 88(21):9578–9582.

8. Fields S, Song O. A novel genetic system to detect protein–protein interactions. Nature 1989; 340(6230):245–246.

9. Fields S, Sternglanz R. The two-hybrid system: an assay for protein-protein interactions. Trends Genet 1994; 10(8):286–292.

10. Lau L, Nathans D. Identification of a set of genes expressed during the G0/G1 transition of cultured mouse cells. EMBO J 1985; 4:3145–3151.

11. Green R, Lieb M, Weintraub A, Gacheru S, Rosenfield C, Shah S, Kagan H, Taubman M. Identification of lysyl oxidase and other platelet-derived growth factor-inducible genes in vascular smooth muscle cells by differential screening. Lab Invest 1995; 73(4):476–482.

12. Sambrook J, Fritsch E, Maniatis T. Molecular Cloning: A Laboratory Manual, 2nd ed. Cold Spring Harbor, NY: Cold Spring Harbor Laboratory Press, 1989.

13. Davis RH, Weintraub H, Lassar A. Expression of a single transfected cDNA converts fibroblasts to myoblasts. Cell 1987; 51:987–1000.

14. Liang P, Pardee A. Differential display of eukaryotic messenger RNA by means of the polymerase chain reaction. Science 1992; 257:967–971.

15. Warthoe P, Bauer D, Rohde M, Strauss M. Detection and identification of expressed genes by differential display. In: Diffenbach C, Dveksler G, eds. PCR Primer: A Laboratory Manual. Cold Spring Harbor, NY: Cold Spring Harbor Laboratory Press, 1995:421–438.

16. Cherry J. Computer manipulation of DNA and protein sequences. In: Current protocols in molecular biology, Ausubel F, Brent R, Kingston R, Moore D, Seidman J, Smith J, and Struhl K, ed. New York: John Wiley & Sons, 1995:7.7.1–7.7.16.

17. Altschul S, Gish W, Miller W, Myers E, Lipan D. Basic local alignment search tool. J Mol Biol 1990; 215:403–410.

4

Gene Transfer into Adult Cardiac Myocytes in Vivo by Direct Injection of DNA

Koji Hasegawa and Richard N. Kitsis
Albert Einstein College of Medicine
Bronx, New York

INTRODUCTION

Cardiac myocytes are highly differentiated cells with chronotropic, contractile, and metabolic properties specialized for the maintenance of the circulation. Far from being static, however, these characteristics undergo rapid and dramatic modifications in response to a wide variety of humoral, neural, and mechanical stimuli (reviewed in 1). These changes are mediated, in large part, by alterations in the expression of specific genes. Therefore, a detailed knowledge of cardiac gene regulation is essential for understanding the molecular basis of the cardiac myocyte phenotype and the signal transduction pathways through which it is modulated by extracellular signals.

The majority of cardiac gene regulation studies have employed transient transfections into cultured cardiac myocytes derived from late fetal or neonatal rats. It is necessary to make primary cultures for these kinds of studies because of the absence of a phenotypically suitable established cardiac cell line. Although this approach has provided valuable insights into cardiac gene regulation and physiology, it has several potential limitations. First, a general concern with using any cell culture-based system for gene regulation experiments is that differences in phenotype and gene regulation have been documented in the same cells when studied in culture vs. in the intact organism (reviewed in 2). More specific to this particular system is the unresolved question of whether fetal and neonatal cardiac myocytes are appropriate models for disease processes primarily affecting adult cells. (Although adult cardiac myocytes can be cultured, these cells are particularly resistant to nonviral-mediated gene transfer techniques.) Second, it is very difficult to model in culture many complex physiological and pathological stimuli of particular relevance to heart disease (e.g., hemodynamic overload). For these reasons, alternative approaches have been developed that allow cardiac myocyte gene regulation to be studied in the hearts of live adult rodents. These include direct gene transfer into the myocardium (the subject of this chapter) and generation of transgenic mice.

CHARACTERISTICS OF CARDIAC GENE TRANSFER BY DIRECT INJECTION

Genes can be transferred into and expressed in striated (cardiac and skeletal) myocytes by the macroscopic injection of naked, closed, circular plasmid DNA into muscle tissue of intact animals. The essential features of this approach include those reviewed below.

Striated Myocyte Specificity

Although it remains unclear how DNA presumably placed into the extracellular space can gain entry into a cell, histochemical studies using the *lac Z* reporter gene have demonstrated that this process occurs efficiently only in striated muscle cells (3–7). In addition, for a given amount of input DNA, expression levels are 10–100 times higher in cardiac than in skeletal myocytes (5).

Absence of Chromosomal Integration of the Injected DNA

Southern blot analysis of injected DNA demonstrates that most, if not all, of the injected DNA remains in an episomal state (3). Because of the nonuniform nature of gene transfer (see below), it is difficult to estimate the copy number of injected DNA on a per cell basis. Indirect evidence, including high levels of expression in relatively few cells and the observation of competition phenomena among coinjected promoters (see below), suggests that the transfected cells contain multiple copies of DNA.

Localization of Injected DNA

A single injection of DNA results in the transfection of 10^3–10^4 myocytes ($\sim 0.03\%$ of the total in the heart), most of which are localized to a 3 mm region surrounding the needle track (6,7).

Time Course of Expression

Expression in cardiac muscle is detectable at low levels at 1 day postinjection. Between 5 and 14 days, it is maximal. Following this, expression decreases in a significant proportion of animals (6). Expression has been noted to persist for months after injection in some animals, however (3,4).

Regulated Expression of Injected Gene

The expression of an injected construct driven by promoter sequences from a cardiac gene is regulated in parallel with that of the endogenous cardiac gene from which the promoter was derived (5). This fact permits the direct injection of reporter constructs to be used to study gene regulation in vivo.

DIRECT INJECTION OF GENES TO STUDY CARDIAC GENE REGULATION

We have recently reviewed the experimental methodology involved in performing cardiac gene injections (7) and this information will not be repeated here. We will summarize, however, several conceptual issues important in designing these kind of experiments.

Use of Reporters

For the purposes of promoter analysis, the basic approach of gene transfer into adult cardiac myocytes in vivo involves a single injection of closed, circular DNA into the lateral–apical wall of the left ventricle. Two constructs are simultaneously coinjected. The first consists of the cellular promoter under study driving a reporter gene. The second contains a constitutive promoter fused to a different reporter gene. The activities of the two reporters are assayed in a homogenate of the heart 4–14 days following injection. The activity of the reporter driven by the cellular promoter is then normalized to that of the reporter directed by the constitutive promoter to control for differences in the efficiency of gene transfer and possible global effects of the stimulus under study on general RNA and protein turnover. We have found the firefly luciferase (*luc*) (8) and bacterial chloramphenicol acetyl transferase (CAT) (9) reporters most useful in these studies because they are easy to assay, quite sensitive, quantitative with linearity over a reasonable range, and not present in wild-type mammalian cells. Since luciferase is more sensitive than CAT, we have generally linked it to the cellular promoter of interest, while CAT has been used in the internal control plasmid. However, the opposite combination could be used as well. Although the bacterial β-galactosidase gene is useful for histochemical studies, it is not optimal in colorimetric assays of cardiac tissue homogenates because of background color resulting from trapped blood.

Quantities of DNA

The direct injection of DNA presents a relatively large quantity of DNA to a limited number of myocytes. As a result, there exists the theoretical possibility of competition among DNA molecules for gaining entry into the cell and/ or among the same and different promoters for commonly needed transcriptional machinery. Indirect evidence in support of this hypothesis is provided by the amount of reporter gene expression resulting from various input doses of a construct consisting of 613 base pairs (bp) of rat α-cardiac myosin heavy chain (MHC) 5′ flanking sequence driving *luc*. In the dose range between 0 and 5 µg ($\sim$1.5 pmol), the amount of *luc* activity in cardiac homogenates increases linearly. When the dose of DNA exceeds 5 µg for this construct, the increment in reporter expression per amount of input DNA becomes smaller. Competition for transcription factors may influence measurements not only of basal levels of promoter activity but also of its responsiveness to a stimulus. For example, the expression of a directly injected *luc* construct containing a promoter derived from the rat β-cardiac MHC gene increases in response to hemodynamic overload in parallel with that of the endogenous β-MHC gene. However, this increment in reporter gene transcription can be blunted by the coinjection of large amounts of a construct containing an unrelated promoter (e.g., pRSVCAT consisting of Rous sarcoma virus long terminal repeat sequences driving CAT) (Hasegawa and Kitsis, unpublished). Therefore, it is advisable to perform preliminary dose–response studies with 1.0–5.0 µg of the construct containing the promoter under study coinjected with 0.2–1.0 µg of the constitutively expressed construct. The goal is to define a dose range at which competition effects can be minimized while still maintaining reporter gene expression in an easily detectable range.

Timing of Sacrifice

Expression of directly injected genes in cardiac muscle is maximal and stable between 4 and 14 days postinjection. Therefore, the hearts should usually be harvested between these time points. In addition, in promoter mapping studies, it is also important to consider the time course of stimulus-induced changes in the expression of the endogenous gene under study. Temporal changes in the steady-stage level of the mRNA encoded by the endogenous gene can easily be obtained and this information is often helpful. However, even with this information, there often remains some uncertainty as to when the most dramatic stimulus-induced changes in promoter activity occur due to the fact that steady-state mRNA levels also reflect posttranscriptional changes. Therefore, it is wise to evaluate changes in promoter activity at several time points before selecting a specific one at which to perform promoter mapping studies. Two obvious time points that should be assessed in these pilot experiments are when the rate of change in the expression of the endogenous gene is maximal and when the levels of the endogenous mRNA become most abundant.

Quantity of Supernatant to be Assayed

The quantity of supernatant to be assayed depends on several factors. The most important is that the resulting reporter activity be detectable and within the linear range of the assay. With supernatant prepared from homogenates of tissue as opposed to cultured cells, another factor also influences this decision. A lack of linearity is sometimes observed between the amounts of supernatant assayed and reporter gene activity detected. We hypothesize that this nonlinearity results from nonspecific inhibition of the reporter assay by impurities in the crude supernatant. In our hands, this effect appears to be more marked with luciferase than with CAT assays, perhaps because we routinely preheat aliquots to be assayed for CAT activity at 65°C for 10 min. (Note: The CAT protein is heat-stable. In contrast, even gentle heating of luciferase will rapidly result in complete loss of function.) Therefore, in reporter gene assays of tissue, it is prudent to use as small amount of supernatant as necessary to produce a reasonable signal. In addition, a uniform volume of each sample should be assayed to minimize variation resulting from this nonlinearity. Since we routinely homogenize tissues in a volume of buffer proportional to the sample mass, this is equivalent to assaying a fixed amount of protein. However, it is not necessary to use the same volume of supernatant for both luciferase and CAT assays.

Variability and Normalization

Due to variability among injections, there is often a 5–10-fold variability in the activities of each of the reporter genes when injecting a group of animals in the same physiological state with the same constructs. However, following normalization of the activity of the reporter gene driven by the cellular promoter under study to that of the reporter gene driven by the constitutive promoter, this variability decreases to less than twofold. When four to six animals are studied for each cellular promoter construct in each physiological state, we find that differences in promoter activity greater than two- to threefold can be discriminated with statistical certainty.

STUDIES OF CARDIAC GENE REGULATION USING THE DIRECT INJECTION APPROACH

Several laboratories including our own have used cardiac DNA injections to identify *cis*-acting regulatory elements involved in mediating changes in the transcription of specific cardiac genes in response to pathophysiological stimuli in vivo. Examples include thyroid hormone-induced changes in myosin heavy chain gene expression (10) and induction of *c-fos* (11) and β-myosin heavy chain gene expression (Hasegawa and Kitsis, manuscript submitted) by hemodynamic overload. Although some of the findings of these studies agree with those of cell culture studies, others diverge significantly. This underscores the importance of an in vivo approach to study pathophysiological regulation of cardiac genes.

Thyroid Hormone-Induced Changes in α-Myosin Heavy-Chain Gene Transcription

Thyroid hormone regulates the expression of cardiac myosin heavy-chain (MHC) genes in vivo and in cultured heart cells, stimulating the transcription of the α-MHC gene and repressing that of the β-MHC gene (12). These changes in transcription are mediated by the direct interaction of T_3-receptors with DNA sequences termed thyroid-responsive elements (TRE) (13). A TRE consisting of tandem hexameric direct repeats separated by a spacer of four nucleotides, is located between nt -149 to -134 (relative to the start of transcription) of the rat α-MHC (14). In addition, sequences flanking these 16 bp and, possibly, a second TRE located somewhat more proximally appear to play roles in modulating the effect of thyroid hormone on the transcription of this gene (15). Transfections into fetal rat cardiac myocytes have demonstrated that a promoter consisting of the 161 bp immediately upstream of the transcription initiation site of the rat α-MHC gene is inactive in the absence of thyroid hormone and activated 14-fold in its presence (16). We have tested the role of these sequences in mediating T_3-induced changes in α-MHC gene expression in vivo (10). In contrast to the cell culture results, the transcriptional activity of these sequences is easily detectable in the hearts of euthyroid animals and is not altered by either severe hypothyroidism or hyperthyroidism. On the other hand, the activity of a promoter containing 388 bp of rat α-MHC 5' flanking sequence is stimulated fourfold in vivo by the administration of thyroid hormone, a response abolished by point mutations in the TRE. Thus, although the TRE is required for positive thyroid hormone responsiveness, the sequences proximal to nt –161 by themselves are insufficient to mediate this response in vivo. Some sequences located between –161 and –388 also appear to be necessary. The discrepancies between these in vivo results and those of cell culture studies may reflect differences in the developmental states of the myocytes and/or between the cell culture and in vivo milieu.

The in vivo approach has also provided insight into another aspect of the regulation of α-MHC transcription by thyroid hormone: decreases in transcription that occur with thyroid hormone deficiency. Since all α-MHC promoters studied thus far are inactive in fetal cardiac myocytes grown in thyroid hormone-free media (16), cell culture experiments do not provide a means to determine which *cis*-acting elements are needed to mediate negative thyroid hormone responsiveness. The direct injection approach does, however. As discussed above, the activity of a promoter containing 388 bp of α-MHC upstream sequence increases in response to thyroid hormone in vivo. Despite appropriate positive responsiveness, this promoter lacks negative responsiveness as it remains as active in hypothyroid as in euthyroid myocardium. In contrast, the expression of the endogenous α-MHC gene decreases to extremely low levels in hypothyroid as compared with euthyroid heart muscle. Thus, these 388 bp lack sufficient information to be transcriptionally inactive during hypothyroidism. The transcriptional activity of a construct containing 2936 bp of α-MHC 5′ flanking sequence, on the other hand, is three to fourfold less in the hearts of hypothyroid than compared with euthyroid animals. This result suggests that sequences located considerably upstream of the TRE(s) in the proximal promoter play a role in the negative responsiveness of the α-MHC gene to thyroid hormone deficiency. This finding has subsequently been borne out in studies of transgenic mice carrying α-MHC driven reporter genes (17).

Hemodynamic Overload-Induced Changes in *c-fos* Transcription

Hemodynamic overload, resulting from excess pressure and/or volume, is of great clinical importance as it plays a role in the pathogenesis of virtually all disorders affecting cardiac muscle. The signal transduction pathways, through which this presumably heterogeneous collection of extracellular stimuli elicit changes in cardiac myocyte structure and function, have been and continue to be an area of intense study. Although their precise roles in mediating the effects of hemodynamic overload remain unclear, specific changes in the cardiac expression of two classes of genes have been noted to occur in temporal association with this stimulus. These include transient increase in the expression of a variety of immediate early genes within minutes to hours following the onset of experimental hemodynamic overload and the somewhat later reinduction of cardiac genes that are normally expressed predominantly during fetal life (1). The direct injection technique has provided a means by which to investigate the molecular basis of changes in the expression of these genes in response to hemodynamic overload.

Aoyagi and Izumo used this approach to define a *cis*-acting element in the c-*fos* promoter that is necessary and sufficient to induce the expression of this immediate early gene in response to pressure overload (11). Rat hearts were coinjected with a CAT construct driven by 356 bp of sequence upstream of the mouse c-*fos* gene and a luciferase gene spliced to the constitutively active cytomegalovirus promoter/enhancer as an internal control. Two days following injection, hearts were excised and studied as isolated, perfused (Langendorff) preparations. In the experimental group, acute pressure overload was induced by inflating an intraventricular balloon for 2 h. Controls underwent balloon placement without inflation. Pressure overload increased the relative CAT activity (CAT/luciferase ratio) by 3.5-fold (Fig. 1). The c-*fos* upstream sequences in the CAT construct contain two major inducible *cis*-acting elements: a Ca^{2+}/cAMP response element at nt $\sim$ –60 and a serum response element (SRE) at nt $\sim$ –300. Deletion of the 356 bp promoter to nt –71 resulted in complete loss of pressure overload-induced CAT expression, as did two sets of point mutations in the SRE in the context of the 356 bp promoter. These data demonstrate the necessity of the SRE and the insufficiency of the Ca^{2+}/cAMP element in mediating pressure overload-stimulated increases in c-*fos* transcription. One of the SRE point mutations, pm12, abolishes the ability of the serum response factor (SRF) to bind the SRE. The other SRE mutation, pm 18, preserves the ability of SRF to bind SRE but abrogates the binding of p62[TCF] to form a terniary complex and, thereby, results in the selective loss of protein kinase C-stimulated c-*fos* transcription. The lack of pressure overload-responsiveness in the expression of pm 18 suggests that the p62[TCF]-pathway is necessary for this response. In addition, a single copy of the SRE spliced a 56 bp minimal c-*fos* promoter was sufficient to confer pressure overload-responsive expression onto the CAT gene. Thus, the SRE is both necessary and sufficient to mediate pressure overload-induced increases in c-*fos* transcription.

Hemodynamic Overload-Induced Changes in β-Myosin Heavy Chain Transcription

As noted above, hemodynamic overload reinduces the expression of cardiac genes, which, under normal circumstances, are expressed predominantly during fetal life. These are exemplified by the β-myosin heavy chain (β-MHC) gene. While expressed at low levels in normal adult rodent ventricle (5), the abundances of β-MHC mRNA and protein begin to increase within days fol-

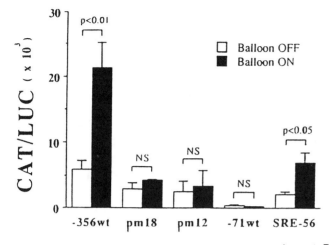

Figure 1 Mapping of the c-*fos* pressure response element. Relative expression of CAT in control (open bars) and pressure-overloaded (closed bars) states following the intracardiac injection of CAT constructs driven by the following mouse c-*fos* upstream sequences: 356 bp (–356 wt); 356 bp with a point mutation in the outer pallindromic arm of the SRE (pm 18); 356 bp with a point mutation in the SRE core (pm 12); 71 bp (–71 wt); and a single copy of the SRE spliced to the first 56 bp of upstream sequence (SRE-56). pCMVluc was coinjected as an internal control. The transcriptional activities of only –356 wt and SRE-56 increased in response to pressure overload indicating the necessity and sufficiency of the SRE for pressure overload-induced c-*fos* transcription. (From Ref. 11.)

lowing the onset of experimental hemodynamic overload and continue to increase in proportion to the degree of cardiac hypertrophy (18,19). Previous work to define the regulation of genes during cardiac hypertrophy has employed a model developed by Simpson and co-workers (20), in which cultured neonatal cardiac myocytes are stimulated to hypertrophy in response to α_1-adrenergic agonists. This model recapitulates the increases in myocyte volume and protein content and many of the changes in gene expression that characterize cardiac hypertrophy in vivo (1). This system has been used to map *cis*-acting elements that mediate increases in the transcription of β-MHC in response to α_1-adrenergic stimuli (21–23). These studies have clearly demonstrated that the M-CAT motif located between –215 and –196 of the rat β-MHC gene, which binds members of the TEF-1 family of transcription factors, is necessary and sufficient to mediate α_1-adrenergic-induced activation of the β-MHC promoter.

Since the physiological relevance of these studies to hemodynamic overload-induced hypertrophy in adult cardiac myocytes in vivo remains unclear, we have employed the direct injection approach to identify DNA sequences which modulate hemodynamic overload-induced changes in β-MHC transcription in the adult heart (Hasegawa and Kitsis, manuscript submitted). A construct containing 3542bp rat β-myosin heavy chain upstream sequence fused to the luciferase gene was coinjected along with pRSVCAT as an internal control. The following day, animals underwent either suprarenal abdominal aortic constriction or sham operation. Twelve days later, animals were sacrificed and cardiac homogenates assayed for reporter gene activities and the abundance of the endogenous β-MHC transcript. Aortic constriction resulted in 80% increase in the ratio of left ventricular mass to body mass as well as four-fold induction in the expression of the endogenous β-MHC gene. As shown in Figure 2, relative luciferase expression driven by the 3542bp β-MHC promoter was 3.1-fold higher in the aortic constricted as compared with the sham-operated group (p < 0.005). That this effect truly represents an increase in the promoter activity of these β-MHC sequences rather than merely alterations in the relative mRNA and protein stabilities of luciferase and CAT is demonstrated by the similar levels of reporter gene expression in sham and aortic constricted hearts coinjected with pRSVluc and pRSVCAT. In addition, the absence of an aortic constriction-induced change in the transcriptional activity of a promoter consisting of 2936 bp of rat α-MHC upstream sequence demonstrates that the hemodynamic overload responsiveness of the 3542 bp β-MHC promoter is specific for these sequences. These findings show that accumulation of β-myosin heavy-chain mRNA during hemodynamic overload is regulated primarily at the transcriptional level and that sequences in the 3542bp rat β-myosin heavy-chain gene promoter are sufficient to mediate this response. Additional data (not shown) have demonstrated that β-MHC sequences between –303 and –202 are both necessary and sufficient to mediate this response. These ~ 100 bp contain two M-CAT motifs, the more proximal of which is the element shown to be necessary and sufficient for α_1-adrenergic-induced increases in β-MHC transcription in cultured neonatal cardiac myocytes. In contrast, the simultaneous introduction of point mutations adequate to abolish TEF-1 binding into both M-CAT motifs does not abolish the hemodynamic overload responsiveness of a 333 bp β-MHC promoter in vivo. Thus, while the M-CAT box may play some role, it does not seem to be necessary for the transactivation of the β-MHC promoter by hemodynamic overload in adult cardiac myocytes in vivo. It is unclear at present whether differences with the in vitro findings reflect the extracellular environment of cells (culture vs. in vivo), the developmental stage of the cells (neonatal vs. adult), or the nature of the hypertrophic stimulus (α_1-adrenergic stimulation vs. hemodynamic overload). Nevertheless, these results underscore the importance of an in vivo system for studies concerned with the signal transduction of hemodynamic overload.

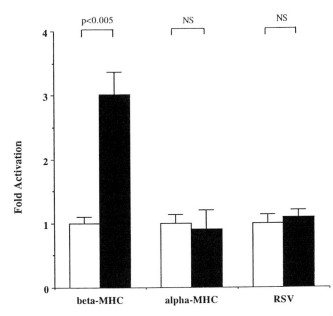

Figure 2 The transcriptional activity of a ~3.5 kb β-MHC gene promoter increases in response to hemodynamic overload. Left ventricles were injected with luciferase constructs driven by 3542 bp of rat β-MHC upstream sequence (beta-MHC), 2936 bp of rat α-MHC upstream sequence (alpha-MHC), or RSV long terminal repeat sequences (RSV). Each injection also included a small amount of pRSVCAT as an internal control. On the following day, animals were subjected either to sham operation (open bars) or suprarenal abdominal aortic constriction (closed bars). Twelve days later, cardiac homogenates were assayed for luciferase and CAT activities. For each set of injected constructs, the luc/CAT ratio (mean ± SE) of the aortic constricted animals is plotted relative to that of sham operated animals arbitrarily set to 1.0.

COMPARISON WITH TRANSGENIC APPROACH

Introduction of exogenous DNA into the germ line and the creation of transgenic animals has greatly advanced the study of gene regulation during development and in various induced states. Advantages of this approach over direct injections include (a) constant and permanent levels of reporter gene expression; (b) the absence of cell to cell variability in copy number of the transferred gene; and (c) geographic homogeneity of transgene expression within a tissue (although, in practice, patchiness of expression is sometimes found). In addition, although rigorous studies addressing this issue have not been performed, it appears that promoter competition issues may be less of a problem in transgenic animals that in gene injections. Despite these advantages, it remains laborious and costly to map promoters in transgenic mice. In part, this is due to the necessity of studying each construct in several independent lines to control for differences resulting from the chromosomal site of transgene integration. One reasonable approach for studying cardiac gene regulation in vivo is to combine the direct injection and transgenic approaches. The former can be used relatively quickly to screen putative regulatory regions for DNA sequences that may be of importance. These can then be tested selectively in transgenic mice.

SUMMARY

Genes can be transferred into cardiac myocytes in vivo by the simple macroscopic injection of plasmid DNA. Although this gene transfer technique is not adequate to modify the phenotype of the entire myocardium, it has proven useful in the study of gene regulation. An important factor to be considered in the interpretation of promoter mapping data obtained with this technique is the potential for competition among promoter sequences for transcription factors. Despite this and other limitations, the simplicity, speed, and relative economy of this approach compared with the generation of multiple transgenic lines make direct injections useful in the initial identification of functionally important regulatory sequences. This methodology complements the selective generation of transgenic animals for studies of cardiac gene regulation, and it may aid the investigator in using transgenic technology in the most efficient manner.

ACKNOWLEDGMENTS

This work was supported by a fellowship to KH from the Martin Foundation and by grants to RNK from the NIH (HL02699) and the American Heart Association, New York City Affiliate. RNK is the Charles and Tamara Krasne Faculty Scholar in Cardiovascular Research of the Albert Einstein College of Medicine.

REFERENCES

1. Chien KR, Knowlton KU, Zhu H, Chien S. Regulation of cardiac gene expression during myocardial growth and hypertrophy: molecular studies of an adaptive physiologic response. FASEB J 1991; 5:3037-3046.
2. Kitsis RN, Leinwand LA. Discordance between gene regulation in vitro and in vivo. Gene Exp 1992; 2: 313-317.
3. Wolff, JA, Malone RW, Williams P, Chong W, Acsadi G, Jani A, Felgner PI. Direct gene transfer into mouse muscle in vivo. Science 1990; 247: 1465-1468.
4. Acsadi G, Jiao SS, Jani A, Duke D, Williams P, Chong W, Wolff JA. Direct gene

transfer and expression into rat heart in vivo. New Biol 1991; 3: 71-81.

5. Kitsis RN, Buttrick PM, McNally EM, Kaplan ML, Leinwand LA. Hormonal modulation of a gene injected into rat heart in vivo. Proc Natl Acad Sci USA 1991; 88:4138-4142.

6. Buttrick PM, Kass A, Kitsis RN, Kaplan KL, Leinwand LA. Behavior of genes directly injected into rat heart in vivo. Circ Res 1992; 70: 193-198.

7. Kitsis RN, Buttrick PM, Kass AA, Kaplan ML, Leinwand LA. Gene transfer into adult rat heart in vivo. Methods Mol Gen 1993; 1:374-392.

8. Brasier AR, Tate JE, Habener JF. Optimized use of the firefly luciferase assay as a reporter gene in mammalian cell lines. Biotechniques 1989; 7: 1116-1122.

9. Gorman CM, Moffat LF, Howard BH. Recombinant genomes which express chrolamphenicol acetyl-transferase in mammalian cells. Mol Cell Biol 1982; 2:1044-1051.

10. Buttrick PM, Kaplan ML, Kitsis RN, Leinwand LA. Distinct behavior of cardiac myosin heavy chain gene constructs in vivo: discordance with in vitro results. Circ Res 1993; 72: 1211-1217.

11. Aoyagi T, Izumo S. Mapping of the pressure response element of the c-fos gene by direct DNA injection into beating hearts. J Biol Chem 1993; 268: 27176-27179.

12. Lompre A-M, Nadal-Ginard B, Mahdavi V. Expression of the cardiac ventricular α- and β-myosin heavy chain genes is developmentally and hormonally regulated. J Biol Chem 1984; 259: 6437-6446.

13. Glass CK, Franco R, Weinberger C, Albert VR, Evans RM, RosenfeldMG: A c-erb A binding site in rat growth hormone gene mediates trans-activation by thyroid hormone. Nature 1987; 329:738-741.

14. Umesono K, Murakami KK, Thompson CC, Evans RM. Direct repeats as selective response elements for the thyroid hormone, retinoic acid, and vitamin D_3 receptors. Cell 1991; 65: 1255-1266.

15. Flink IL, Morkin E. Interaction of thyroid hormone receptors with strong and weak cis-acting elements in the human α-myosin heavy chain gene promoter. J Biol Chem 1990; 265: 11233-11237.

16. Tsika RW, Bahl JJ, Leinwand LA, Morkin E. Thyroid hormone regulates expression of a transfected human α-myosin heavy chain fusion gene in fetal rat heart cells. Proc Natl Acad Sci USA 1990; 87: 379-383.

17. Subramanian A, Gulick J, Neumann J, Knotts S, Robbins J. Transgenic analysis of the thyroid-responsive elements in the α-cardiac myosin heavy chain gene promoter. J Biol Chem 1993; 268: 4331-4336.

18. Izumo S, Lompre A-M, Matsuoka R, Koren G, Schwartz K, Nadal-Ginard B, Mahdavi V. Myosin heavy chain messenger RNA and protein isoform transitions during cardiac hypertrophy: interaction between hemodynamic and thyroid hormone-induced signals. J Clin Invest 1987; 79: 970-977.

19. Chassagne C, Wisnewsky C, Schwartz K. Antithetical accumulation of myosin heavy chain but not α-actin mRNA isoforms during early stages of pressure-overload-induced rat cardiac hypertrophy. Circ Res 1993; 72: 857-864.

20. Simpson PC, McGrath A, Savion S. Myocyte hypertrophy in neonatal rat heart cultures and its regulation by serum and by catecholamines. Circ Res 1982; 51:

787-801.

21. Kariya K, Karns LR, Simpson PC. Expression of a constitutively activated mutant of the β-isozyme of protein kinase C in cardiac myocytes stimulates the promoter of the β-myosin heavy chain isogene. J Biol Chem 1990; 266: 10023-10026.

22. Kariya K, Karns LR, Simpson PC. An enhancer core element mediates stimulation of the rat β-myosin heavy chain promoter by an α_1-adrenergic agonist and activated β-protein kinase C in hypertrophy of cardiac myocytes. J Biol Chem 1994; 269: 3775-3782.

23. Kariya K, Farrance IKG, Simpson PC. Transcriptional enhancer factor-1 in cardiac myocytes interacts with an α_1-adrenergic- and β-protein kinase C-inducible element in the rat β-myosin heavy chain promoter. J Biol Chem 1993; 268:26658-26662.

5

Studies of Cardiac Myocytes in Culture: A Developmental Perspective

D. Stave Kohtz
Mount Sinai School of Medicine
New York, New York

INTRODUCTION

Some of the earliest studies of viable cardiac cells in culture were reported by Carrel in 1912 (1). An explant of fetal chicken heart (18d) was maintained on a silk veil in plasma for several weeks. The explant was observed contracting rhythmically, and the radial growth and migration of a cell population occurred over a period of several days. As the explant grew and released cells, Carrel washed it with buffer and replaced the plasma; hence, one important contribution of this early report was to demonstrate the importance of feeding to the long-term maintenance of cells in culture. However, growth of the explant was accompanied by a loss of contractile activity, until "pulsations" were no longer observed in the culture. To remedy this problem, Carrel dissected the explant again, removed a small central fragment, and placed it in fresh plasma. The fragment recovered contractile activity rapidly, and was maintained for several more days. Contractile activity was used in Carrel's studies as a parameter to demonstrate that cells in culture can retain their normal function. The cells that grew from the explant, however, did not contribute contractile activity.

The sequence of events observed by Carrel is consistent with those observed when a 0.5–2 mm explant of fetal myocardium from most vertebrates is cultured on tissue culture plasticware in a contemporary medium. It is now known that growth of the explant is associated with mitogenic stimulation of cells lacking the myocardial phenotype, such as fibroblasts. After attachment of the tissue fragment, cells bearing a mesenchymal phenotype are stimulated to proliferate and migrate radially. In contrast to the silk veil used by Carrel, tissue culture plastic provides a substrate for cell adhesion; hence, mesenchymal cells migrate out of the explant, proliferate, and form a surrounding monolayer. Although cardiac myocytes within an explant remain viable and contractile for extended periods in culture, they do not proliferate or migrate.

The profound display of function by myocardial cells in culture is both beautiful and limiting. Fetal, neonatal, and adult cardiac myocytes can be dissociated from fragments of cardiac tissue by proteases and chelating agents (reviewed below). Individual cardiac myocytes will attach and adhere to culture plasticware or plasticware coated with extracellular matrix components, and will display spontaneous contractile activity. The utility of these cells in electrophysiological, biochemical, or molecular biological experiments has been documented. Isolated cardiac myocytes, however, are near or at terminal differentiation, and do not proliferate appreciably in culture. This poses limitations on studies of myocardial cell biology. For example, only limited quantities of cultured cardiac cells can be generated for biochemical studies or molecular analyses of gene expression, and these cultures are neither clonal nor homogeneous. Significant is that the observation that myocardial cells in situ will take up and express exogenous DNAs has provided an alternative means for analyzing regulation of myocardial gene transcription (2).

CELL TYPES IN THE HEART

Although this chapter is concerned mainly with cells of the myocardial lineage, it is important to remember that the heart contains many cell types, several of which have been cultured successfully. The earliest cell lineages in the embryonic heart, the myocardial and endocardial lineages, are related. Cultures of avian embryonic endocardium and myocardium have been used successfully to study septum and valve development. A culture system developed by Markwald and colleagues has employed embryonic endocardium, myocardium, and collagen gels to identify factors controlling endocardial to mesenchymal transitions in developing valve and septal tissues (3, 4). The collagen gel serves as a surrogate cardiac jelly, and migration of mesenchymal cells derived from the embryonic endocardium is observed when embryonic myocardium is cultured on the opposite side of the gel. A factor that activates mesenchymal trans-

formation of embryonic endocardial cells (ES/130; 5) has been identified using this culture system. The ES/130 cDNA has been cloned and sequenced, and
expression of this gene is one of the earliest markers of commitment to the myocardial lineage (5). Embryonic cardiac myocytes in the heart tube secrete ES/
130, which apparently diffuses across the cardiac jelly and induces certain populations of endocardial cells to transform to a mesenchymal phenotype. Mesenchymal cells derived from the endocardium secrete and modify the extracellular matrix molecules of the forming valve and septal tissues, and remain resident
in these tissues in the adult heart (3). As they maintain the ability to proliferate, it is possible to culture these cells as fibroblasts.

   Cardiac myocytes, a subpopulation of the endocardial cells, and mesenchymal cells derived from these endocardial cells represent the three cell types of
the adult heart that arise directly or indirectly from precardiac mesoderm. In
the adult heart, a large fraction of endocardial cells are derived from vascular
endothelium. Mesenchymal cells are derived also from the epicardium, and
neural crest cells contribute significantly to the development of the outflow tracts
(6). Coronary vasculature also contributes endothelial, smooth muscle, and
mesenchymal cells. Fetal/neonatal heart tissue contains neuronal cells that will
frequently be retained in myocyte cultures. Although formally not part of the
heart tissue, the contribution of cells from the hemopoietic system is also apparent in cardiac cell cultures. However, a compendium of the culture experiments performed with each of the different cell types derived from heart would
be well beyond the scope of this chapter. Instead, the contributions of cell
culture models to understanding the ontogeny and development of cardiac myocytes will be emphasized. The phenotypes displayed by myocardial cells in
different culture systems will be compared to the phenotypes expressed by
cardiac myocytes and myocardial progenitors during development (Fig. 1).
Some of the cultured cell types presented below maintain a relatively stable
phenotype, whereas others are sensitive to extrinsic signals and can be induced
to differentiate. An important challenge for contemporary researchers of heart
development is to determine how these culture systems should be used to understand the molecular processes that control development of myocardial cell
lineages in situ.

DEVELOPMENTAL BIOLOGY OF CARDIAC MYOCYTES

The progression of committed precardiac mesodermal cells to contractile cardiac myocytes is completed early during embryonic development. In most vertebrate embryos, the population of noncontractile cardiac premyocytes (presumptive cardiac myoblasts) has differentiated entirely into contractile
embryonic cardiac myocytes by the appearance of the 25th pair of somites (7–

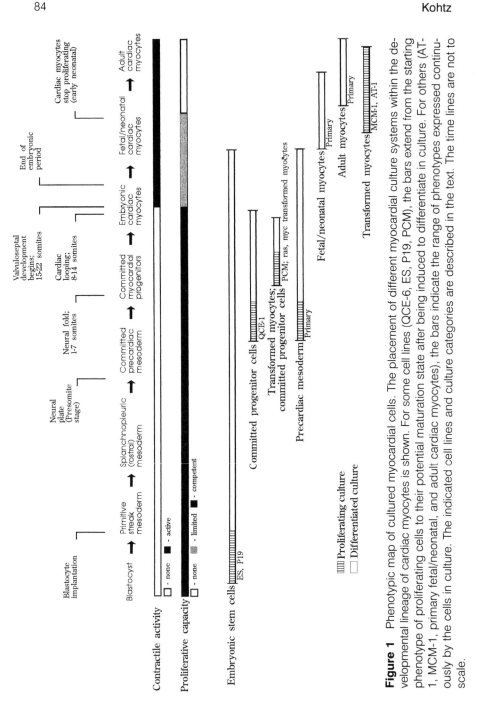

Figure 1 Phenotypic map of cultured myocardial cells. The placement of different myocardial culture systems within the developmental lineage of cardiac myocytes is shown. For some cell lines (QCE-6, ES, P19, PCM), the bars extend from the starting phenotype of proliferating cells to their potential maturation state after being induced to differentiate in culture. For others (AT-1, MCM-1, primary fetal/neonatal, and adult cardiac myocytes), the bars indicate the range of phenotypes expressed continuously by the cells in culture. The indicated cell lines and culture categories are described in the text. The time lines are not to scale.

9). Embryonic cardiac myocytes, although functional, undergo a mitogenic period before developing into terminal cardiac myocytes (10–12). When dissociated and maintained in culture, embryonic cardiac myocytes that continue to display a functional phenotype either will not undergo mitosis or will be restricted to very few divisions (13, 14, 85, 89). Hence, termination of mitogenesis of embryonic cardiac myocytes does not appear to require signals from the embryonic milieu; acquisition of the contractile phenotype initiates a program of terminal differentiation that is set to follow a limited period of mitogenic growth. Growth of the heart through the embryonic period, and through the fetal and early neonatal periods, results from both hyperplasia and hypertrophy of differentiated cardiac myocytes. The clonal progeny of chicken cardiac myocytes form vertically arrayed cones, and during the first week of avian myocardial development display an average cycling time of 16–18 h (15, 16). A single embryonic cardiac myocyte (derived from precardiac mesoderm) will give rise to a few hundred daughter cells, consuming approximately eight divisions before the termination of its mitogenic activity. After the early neonatal period in most vertebrates, growth of myocardial cells is entirely hypertrophic.

One consequence of this pattern of development is that the heart lacks a cell population equivalent to the satellite cells present in skeletal muscle. In the myocardial lineage, a proliferative committed cell type similar to the skeletal myoblast appears only briefly during embryonic development, and in contrast to skeletal muscle, a population of these cells is not retained. Consequently, cardiac muscle lacks both the ability to regenerate and a cell population equivalent to skeletal myoblasts that can be grown in culture and induced to differentiate into fully contractile cells. The myocardium also has an extremely low incidence of primary neoplasia (17), which may be at least partly associated with the early disappearance of committed myocardial progenitors. In most other tissues and in the hemopoietic system, native tumor cells have provided useful cell culture models for specific developmental processes and cell phenotypes. Of course, such models are lacking for the myocardium.

Skeletal muscle genes are expressed coordinately after depletion of extracellular growth factors, and most evidence indicates that expression of these genes in skeletal muscle is controlled by common rather than disparate transcriptional regulators (18–20). In addition, terminal withdrawal of skeletal myoblasts from the cell cycle and differentiation occur concurrently (21, 22). Differentiation of cardiac myocytes, in contrast, occurs before the final stages of terminal differentiation, and expression of contractile genes and assembly of the cardiac myofibrillar structures proceeds in phases that differ from those observed in skeletal muscle. Thus, skeletal muscle development is probably not a satisfactory model for cardiac muscle development. Although differentiation of cardiac myocytes occurs only during a brief period in embryonic development, discrete stages in the progression of immature progenitors to contractile myocytes have been identified based on morphology, changes in gene expression, and commitment in transplantation studies.

Bader and colleagues have identified experimentally an embryonic period during which mesoderm commits to the cardiac lineage (13, 14). Chicken embryos before and after gastrulation were dissociated into individual cells and plated, and the differentiation of cardiac myocytes from dissociated progenitors was evaluated by expression of cardiac isoforms of sarcomeric myosin heavy chain (sMHC). In cultures plated at clonal density, cardiac myocytes will develop from a fraction of postgastrulation mesoderm, but not from earlier embryonic cells. This and other studies (23) suggest that commitment to the cardiogenic lineage occurs in postgastrulated mesoderm, in a period immediately preceeding the presomitic phase and extending to the four-somite phase. Several experiments suggest that embryonic cells first committed to the cardiac lineage generate either cardiac myocytes or endocardial cells. A second event then restricts cells to either myocardial or endocardial phenotypes (24–27). Gene expression markers of entry into the cardiogenic lineage are limited. Immunohistological studies have shown that expression of the cell adhesion protein N-cadherin (28) is enhanced in nascent mesoderm destined for the cardiac lineage, and that expression of cytokeratins differentiates cardiogenic mesoderm from other mesoderm (29–31). Markers of subsequent entry into the myocardial lineage are also limited. The absence of markers for the endocardial or endothelial lineages, such as QH-1 (32) among cardiac progenitor cells, has been used as an indicator of commitment to the myocardial lineage (26).

Perhaps of greater utility for understanding early commitment to the myocardial lineage will be studies of the expression and function of the transcription factors controlling development of that lineage. Several transcriptional regulators have been shown to control muscle gene transcription in cultured cardiac myocytes. Some of these are expressed in several different cell lineages (e.g., SRF, USF, and Egr-1; 33–35), suggesting that they do not directly function in determination of the cardiac myocyte lineage. Others are expressed in cardiac myocytes and other types of muscle cells (e.g., MEF-2; 37–39). These genes appear to regulate tissue-specific gene expression in differentiated cardiac myocytes, but their role in determination of the cardiac myocyte lineage is unclear. The skeletal myogenic basic helix-loop-helix (bHLH) regulators (the MyoD family) are not expressed in cardiac muscle and do not function in the regulation of cardiac gene transcription (36, 40). In fact, ectopic expression of MyoD family members in cardiac muscle appears to result in transdetermination to the skeletal muscle phenotype (41). Transcriptional regulators have been identified that display at least partial restriction to cardiac myocytes and precardiac mesoderm. In *Drosophila*, expression of the tinman (*tin* or *msh-2*) gene is restricted to developing mesoderm, and genetic analysis has revealed that it is required for development of the heart, visceral musculature, and certain body wall muscles (42,43). In vertebrates, the *Nkx2-5* or *Csx-1* gene may be the homolog of *msh-2*, with expression restricted to precardiac mesoderm, tongue and stomach muscles, spleen, and pharyngeal floor (44–46). Targeted disruption of the *Nkx2-5* gene in mice interfered with morphogenic transformation of the heart tube, although a linear tube did develop that contained cells bearing a myocardial phenotype (46). Only selective loss of myofibrillar gene expression was observed, suggesting that *Nkx2-5* is not required for determination and differentiation of cardiac myocytes. Recent studies have intriguingly suggested that GATA-4 functions as a tissue-specific transcription factor in cardiac myocytes (47). Expression of anti-sense GATA-4 transcripts in differentiating P19 embryonal carcinoma cells blocks the development of cardiac myocytes, suggesting an important role for this gene in determination of the myocardial lineage (48). Finally, two basic helix-loop-helix proteins (dHAND and eHAND; 49) have been identified that function in avian cardiac morphogenesis. These proteins are expressed in the cardiac primordia and neural crest cells during early embryogenesis, and are essential for proper cardiac looping and assembly of septa and outflow tracts. However, a direct role for these transcriptional activators in development of the myocardial phenotype has not been demonstrated.

Differentiation of committed myocardial progenitor cells into functional embryonic cardiac myocytes proceeds through premyofibrillar and myofibrillar phases. These phases are defined by both gene transcription and by the assembly state of the sarcomeric protein components. Precardiac mesoderm in the embryo generates cells of either endocardial or myocardial lineages. Ablation studies have suggested that contact with endoderm is important for commitment of mesoderm to the myocardial phenotype in the embryo (50–53). Committed premyocardial cells have been identified by morphological and positional criteria in one- to seven-somite embryos (7–9).

Progression of these cells through the premyofibrillar phase of myocardial development is marked by induction of a subset of sarcomeric protein genes that includes α-actins, α-actinin, titin, and sarcomeric myosin heavy chain, but may exclude desmin (54). The premyofibrillar phase of cardiac myocyte differentiation is characterized by sarcomeric gene expression without sarcomere assembly. Titin and α actinin accumulate during this phase of myocardial differentiation in punctate densities throughout the cytoplasm, whereas accumulation of sMHC at this phase occurs more diffusely (55). Progression to the myofibrillar phase of cardiac myocyte differentiation is marked by the replacement of autonomous accumulations of sarcomeric proteins with organized structures (56).

The myofibrillar phase of cardiac myocyte differentiation may be classified into precontractile and contractile periods. Prior to the appearance of functional sarcomeres, rudimentary structures referred to as myofilaments appear in differentiating cardiac myocytes (57). The primary protein components of these structures include titin, myosin, and actin, although the molar quantities of these components probably differ from those in mature myofibrils (58, 59). Accumulations of myofilaments in the myocardium of nine-somite embryos appear as periodically aligned spots when visualized by immunofluorescence microscopy with titin antibodies (56). The corresponding structures visualized by electron microscopy appear as single or small groups of primitive Z structures (or dense bodies) laced by filaments (60). In addition, electron microscopic studies have revealed that plaques containing α-actinin assemble near the sarcolemma of differentiating cardiac myocytes (58). These structures may serve to organize the assembly of myofilaments in differentiating cardiac myocytes, and to align developing myofibrils in functional embryonic and fetal cardiac myocytes. Nascent myofibrils are assembled during the precontractile period, apparently organized by dense Z material placques (60). Although the development and organization of myofibrils in the contractile myocardium have been studied in some detail, the process of nascent myofibrillogenesis in precontractile cardiac myocytes in not well understood. It is presumed that the contractile phase begins when the assembling sarcomeres are sufficiently mature to function.

Changes in α-actin isoform expression during differentiation of cardiac myocytes provide a useful reference for assigning premyofibrillar, myofibrillar, embryonic/fetal, and adult phases. Expression of smooth muscle and cardiac α-actin genes is observed at the inception of the premyofibrillar phase, followed by skeletal α-actin expression (61). During myofibrillar differentiation cardiac myocytes in mice, smooth muscle, cardiac, and skeletal α-actin genes are expressed at the transition from precontractile to contractile stages (93). The initial contractile activity of cardiac myocytes in the heart tube resembles peristalsis, but the cells mature rapidly and pulsatile contractions are observed (with the onset of cardiac looping). Concurrently, smooth muscle α-actin expression is lost and only cardiac and skeletal isoforms persist (61, 62). In rodents, expression of skeletal muscle α-actin is a marker of the embryonic/fetal cardiac myocyte phenotype, whereas adult cardiac myocytes express predominantly the cardiac α-actin isoform (63–65). In addition, the murine ventricle expressed βMHC during the embryonic/fetal phase, switching to the αMHC isoform shortly after birth (66). Thus, βMHC expression marks the embryonic/fetal phenotype in rodent ventricular cardiac myocytes, whereas in humans and other larger mammals βMHC expression predominates in ventricular myocytes of both embryonic/fetal and adult hearts.

Expression of atrial and ventricle myocyte type-specific markers can be detected early after the cardiogenic mesoderm fuses to form the heart tube and prior to morphogenesis of the heart chambers (67, 68). Some studies have shown directly that atrial-specific gene transcription precedes septation of the developing heart (69). Transplantation studies have been performed to determine at which stage during their development cardiac myocytes commit to either atrial or ventricular lineages. When transplanted, undifferentiated progenitors (from the heart-forming fields, for example) assume the phenotype of the surrounding myocytes; in contrast, transplantation of differentiated (contractile) myocytes does not alter their atrial or ventricular phenotypes (70). Subdiversification of cardiac myocytes into, for example, atrial secretory or contractile populations, apparently occurs at latter stages of cardiac development, although this process has not been studied in detail.

FETAL/NEONATAL CARDIAC MYOCYTES IN CULTURE

The earliest cultures of cardiac myocytes were in the form of explants. Ventricles were minced into 1–3 mm pieces of tissue containing a heterogeneous assembly of cells that could include cardiac myocytes, mesenchymal cells, vascular endothelium, and smooth muscle cells. Explants were cultured from 8 day or later chicken embryoes (e.g., 1) The heart of an 8 day chicken embryo is well developed, equivalent in maturity to a vertebrate fetal heart. The chambers of the fetal heart are formed, ontogeny of the valve and septal tissues is nearly complete, and vascular tissues is infiltrating the myocardium. Cardiac myocytes at this stage of development are fully contractile, although they maintain a finite potential for mitogenic growth and display a fetal phenotype. Although cardiac myocytes at this stage of development have been referred to as embryonic, we will use the term *fetal/neonatal cardiac myocytes* instead, and will restrict the term *embryonic cardiac myocytes* to describe cardiac myocytes derived from embryonic myocardium or earlier progenitors. Fetal/neonatal cardiac myocytes in explants display a contractile phenotype, and as long as they remain in the explant this phenotype appears relatively stable after passage. Mesenchymal cells migrate out of the explant and proliferate; however, migration of cardiac myocytes is limited. The utility of explant cultures in biochemical, pharmacological, and eventually membrane and molecular studies is limited by their heterogeneity, and by difficulties in assessing the behavior of individual myocytes within the explant.

Explants of fetal/neonatal myocardium were later dissociated into individual cardiac myocytes by enzyme digestion or mechanical disruption. Enzymatic digestion alone or in combination with mechanical disruption has gained widespread use for generating primary cultures of fetal/neonatal cardiac myocytes. One of the earliest reports of enzymatic dissociation of cardiac myocytes employed trypsin to digest the minced myocardium of 8-day chicken "embryos" (73). The individual cardiac myocytes released displayed a contractile phenotype, but the cultures also contained many mesenchymal cells. Fetal/neonatal rat cardiac myocytes were subsequently isolated from minced newborn (1–3 days after birth) rat ventricle by digestion with trypsin (74, 75). These cells displayed a contractile phenotype, although spontaneous contractile activity was lost after passage. Multiple rounds of trypsin digestion were used to isolate fetal/neonatal cardiac myocytes from other vertebrate sources, most commonly neonatal hamster (76) and guinea pig ventricle (77). Isolation of cardiac myocytes from larger mammals, including humans, also has been reported (94). Several refinements have been introduced into the digestion protocols, including the successive or concurrent use of collagenase, DNAase, and hyaluronidase in addition to trypsin (78-90). Some of these steps are required for isolation of cardiac myocytes from adult hearts (reviewed below).

Culturing cells dissociated from fetal/neonatal myocardium in an appropriate culture medium supplemented with serum or growth factors permits cardiac myocytes to remain viable for several weeks in culture. However, this also results in proliferation of mesenchymal cells, or fibroblasts. For cultures of dissociated cardiac myocytes to be useful for biochemical or molecular studies, enrichment of the myocyte population to at least 20–50% of the total is required. The problem of contaminating mesenchymal cells has been addressed by several procedures. The most common, referred to as preplating (81), exploits the more rapid adhesion properties of dissociated mesenchymal cells to tissue culture plastic. The latter technique uses the more rapid adhesion of mesenchymal cells to plastic culture dishes to enrich the myocyte population. After digestion with proteases, dissociated cardiac myocytes and other cells are separated from larger tissue fragments by filtration and/or differential sedimentation. The cells are plated in culture medium supplemented with serum on plastic tissue culture dishes for 30–60 min. The nonadherent population is recovered from the culture medium by centrifugation, while the adherent population, which contains mainly mesenchymal cells, is either discarded or cultured as fibroblasts. The preplating procedure can be repeated, recovering the nonadherent fraction (enriched in cardiac myocytes) by centrifugation. Enrichment of the myocyte population also has been accomplished by discontinuous density gradient centrifugation of dissociated myocardial cells through media such as Ficoll or Percoll (91, 121, 124).

After enrichment, adhesion of fetal/neonatal cardiac myocytes to culture dishes is more efficient in medium containing serum. In addition, coating the culture plasticware with gelatin promotes attachment of the cells (84), although they will adhere to plasticware. After the myocytes adhere, usually 24–48 h later, the medium is replaced with low-serum medium. Proliferation of fibroblasts is attenuated by culturing the cells in low-mitogen medium, which may also be supplement with BrdU (79, 91). Maturation of fetal/neonatal cardiac myocytes is also promoted by low serum or serum free medium (86, 90, 91). In cultures of neonatal rat cardiac myocytes, mitogens inhibit expression of muscle creatine kinase, reduce the stability of sMHC and α-cardiac actin expression in the long-term, and prevent down regulation of skeletal α-actin expression (87). Some studies have suggested that high serum promotes dedifferentiation of fetal/neonatal cardiac myocytes (88, 90), while others have suggested that serum promotes acquisition of a phenotype corresponding to that assumed by mature cardiac myocytes in situ undergoing hypertrophic adaptation (80). Changes in gene expression induced by hypertrophic adaptation of adult cardiac myocytes to work overload suggest reversion from an adult to a fetal/neonatal phenotype. The changes include enhanced expression of ANF, β-myosin heavy chain, β-tropomyosin, and β_2 Na/K ATPase (63). In addition, expression of immediate early and early response genes (*c-fos, c-jun, c-myc,* and *Egr-1*) is induced by work overload (83, 98).

Culturing fetal/neonatal cardiac myocytes in high-serum medium appears to maintain the immature phenotype typical of hypertrophic myocytes; cultures maintained in low-serum medium appear to approach the more mature adult phenotype. In addition to serum, purified basic fibroblast growth factor (bFGF) and transforming growth factor β (TGFβ) also induce contractile gene expression in culture cardiac myocytes typical of the immature, hypertrophic phenotype (82, 95–97). Other studies have suggested that cultured fetal and neonatal cardiac myocytes incorporate thymidine and increase in number in response to treatment with bFGF, aFGF, and insulin growth factors I or II either alone or in combinations (100). Acidic fibroblast growth factor is deposited in the cardiac extracellular matrix and possibly secreted by cardiac myocytes, and some studies have suggested that it may regulate cardiac myocyte proliferation during development (99). In contrast, angiotensin II is secreted by cardiac myocytes under work overload, and by either a paracrine or autocrine mechanism appears to mediate hypertrophic growth of the cells by binding the AT1 receptor (111). The role of angiotensin II or possible homologs that may be expressed during embryonic development of the heart has not been explored. Finally, factors contributed by endoderm and ectoderm appear to influence the determination of cardiac progenitors in culture and in situ (50–52, 110). On the other hand, their role in the differentiation of cardiac myocytes is less clear (53). In general, the functions of diffusible factors in induction and maintenance of the myocardial phenotype as well as their role in the proliferation and growth of cardiac myocytes are poorly understood.

Commitment to the atrial or ventricular lineage occurs early during development of cardiac myocytes, and regional populations of myocytes are present in the early heart tube that will maintain either atrial or ventricular phenotypes upon transplantation to the opposite region (67, 68). The specific phenotypes of neonatal/fetal cardiac myocytes derived from atrium or ventricle, as indicated by the predominant expression of either αMHC (atrial) or βMHC (ventricle) isoforms, are stable in culture. The secretory characteristics of atrial and ventricular myocytes also differ significantly, and these differences are also maintained in culture. In particular, secretion of atrial natriuretic factor (ANF) from ventricular myocytes occurs constitutively, whereas secretion from atrial myocytes is regulated by exogenous factors (102). Studies of the regulation of ANF secretion by exogenous factors and drugs have been pursued using cultured atrial myocytes, which have been dissociated from fetal/neonatal rat atrium and enriched by methods similar to those used for ventricular myocytes. Fetal/neonatal atrial myocytes appear to increase in number after being plated (85); indeed, adult atrial myocytes have been reported to display mitogenic growth in vivo after certain types of injury (103). The growth potential of atrial may exceed that of ventricular myocytes; however, when isolated form fetal/neonatal hearts, neither type of cardiac myocyte has been shown to possess sufficient proliferative potential to justify a single passage. Finally, some studies have indicated that differentiation of ES cell in embroid bodies (reviewed below) leads to preferential development of venticular myocytes (112). This observation suggests that factors may be provided by the embryonic milieu that are essential for the development of atrial myocytes.

Shortly after birth in rodents, a switch from βMHC expression to αMHC expression is observed. The molecular basis of αMHC expression in rodent ventricle differs significantly from that of αMHC expression in atrial myocytes. Cultured rodent fetal/neonatal ventricle myocytes will continue to express βMHC when cultured in high- or low-serum medium lacking thyroid hormone, in contrast to atrial myocytes, which will express αMHC under these conditions (104, 105). In low-serum medium supplemented with thyroid hormone, however, rodent fetal/neonatal ventricular myocytes will mature and express αMHC (104). The role of thyroid hormone in the expression of αMHC in adult rodent ventricle and other muscle tissues has been well established at the molecular level (106). The role of mechanical stress on the phenotype of cardiac myocytes in culture has also been investigated. Fetal/neonatal rat cardiac myocytes have been cultured on flexible silicon rubber dishes (107, 108). By stretching the silicon dishes, mechanical stress is transmitted to the cultured cells. This culture system mimics work overload on cardiac myocytes, and induces secretion of angiotensin II (109). Angiotension II, by either an autocrine or paracrine mechanism, cooperates with mechanical stress to induce hypertrophic changes in cardiac myocytes (111, 113). Hypertrophic changes in gene expression (enhanced ANF expression) and cells size also are induced in cultured rat neonatal cardiac myocytes after treatment with α1-adrenergic agonists (117). It is interesting that isoproterenol-induced cardiac hypertrophy in rats does not induce detectable DNA synthesis in the myocyte population (71). Similar experiments, however, have not been performed yet with cultured rat cardiac myocytes.

ADULT CARDIAC MYOCYTES IN CULTURE

Isolation and maintenance in culture of cardiac myocytes from adult hearts are technically more demanding than equivalent procedures with hearts from fetal or neonatal animals. Early investigations with rodents showed that the viability and yield of cardiac myocytes dropped drastically when the postnatal age of the donor exceeded 5 days (74). Similar to fetal/neonatal cultures, enzymatically dissociated adult cardiac myocytes do not proliferate, and must be isolated from contaminating mesenchymal cells. In addition, culture conditions should be used that retard the growth of mesenchymal cells (see above). One of the first reports of viable adult cardiac myocytes in culture was achieved by mechanical disaggregation of a mouse heart in a blender (114). The released cells were maintained in phosphate-buffered saline supplemented with ATP and glucose, displayed a characteristic staircase morphology, and contracted spontaneously for 20 min after they were isolated. At about the same time, enzymatic digestion of adult rat myocardium was found to release myocytes, albeit less efficiently than similar digestions of fetal/neonatal myocardium (78, 115, 116). To improve the yield of cardiac myocytes and reduce the number of contaminating mesenchymal cells, adult rat hearts were first perfused with crude collagenase, then hyaluronidase (79). After perfusion digestion the hearts were minced, and digested further. Later investigators enriched the myocyte component of these preparations by Ficoll or Percoll density centrifugation, or elutriation (121–124). Adult cardiac myocytes have been isolated from many vertebrate species, and several reviews have described how these cells are used in investigations of the pharmacology and membrane dynamics of the adult myocardium (118–120).

Isolated adult cardiac myocytes do not attach or adhere well to plastic, and adhesion may be an important parameter in determining their viability in culture. Adhesion of adult cardiac myocytes is strongly dependent on the matrix material used, since these cells adhere poorly to tissue culture plastic. Systematic studies have shown that rat adult cardiac myocytes bind well to laminin and type IV collagen, but only weakly to fibronectin, type I, II, III, and V collagen, and gelatin (84). Isolation and maintenance of adult cardiac myocytes in culture have presented investigators with another problem. To dissociate myocytes from intercalated disks and the cardiac interstitium, the adult heart is perfused with a Ca^{2+}-free balanced salt buffer containing digestive enzymes, then minced and further digested in Ca^{2+}-free buffer. Returning the dissociated myocytes to medium containing physiological levels of Ca^{2+} results in a rapid and profound loss of viability, an effect generally referred to as the Ca^{2+} paradox. This term was applied originally to a similar form of cell death previously associated with the return of Ca^{2+} into perfused hearts (125), although direct evidence was lacking that the mechanisms of cell death were the same. Although the mechanism of Ca^{2+}-induced cell death of cultured adult cardiac myocytes is not completely understood, it is thought that reducing the extracellular concentration of Ca^{2+} disrupts normal membrane controls on transport of the ion (126-128, 132). Returning cells to physiological concentrations of Ca^{2+} results in a rapid influx of Ca^{2+} into the cells, possibly activating autolytic enzymes that mediate cell death. Protection of adult cardiac myocytes against Ca^{2+}-induced cell death has been accomplished by several procedures. Inclusion of 25 and 50 μM Ca^{2+} into the perfusion and digestion media has been shown to increase the viability (126, 129), followed by a graded return to physiological concentrations of Ca^{2+}. As an alternative, inclusion of other divalent cations (Cd^{2+}, Mn^{2+}, Co^{2+}, Mg^{2+}) has been shown to have a protective effect (128, 131). Reducing the concentration of Na^+ in the low-Ca^{2+} perfusion and/or digestion buffers and lowering the buffer temperature also improves the viability of released adult cardiac myocytes (128, 130–133). Finally, the addition of antioxidants (such as taurine) to these buffers has been shown to improve the viability and function of adult cardiac myocytes in culture (134).

CARDIAC MYOCYTES TRANSFORMED TO GROWTH

The severely limited growth potential of differentiated cardiac myocytes in culture has prompted investigators to explore possible techniques for transformation to growth and immortalization of the cells. As indicated above, primary neoplasias rarely arise from the myocardium, and the growth in culture of rhabdomyosarcoma cells bearing the myocardial (rather than the skeletal muscle) phenotype has not been documented. Transformation to growth of cardiac myocytes by SV40 T-antigen has been investigated. A prevailing feature of cardiac myocytes induced to proliferate by SV40 T-antigen is the maintenance of a differentiated phenotype; indeed, populations of cardiac myocytes expressing T-antigen have been shown to continue to exhibit contractile activity. In one study, rat neonatal cardiac myocytes in culture were infected with replication-defective human adenoviruses modified to express T-antigen (135). The infected myocytes were induced to replicate, while continuing to express sarcomeric proteins and display spontaneous contractile activity. The cells maintained both the capacity to replicate and their contractile activity in foci after a single passage; however, a permanent cell line was not established. In other studies, expression of SV40 T-antigen was targeted to atrial myocytes in transgenic mice. Constructs containing T-antigen driven by either the mouse protamine 1 (136) or the atrial natriuretic factor promoters (137) were integrated into the genome of transgenic animals. These animals developed atrial tumors; the tumor cells, although malignant, displayed the phenotype of contractile cardiac myocytes. The tumor cells from both types of transgenic mice proliferated in culture; those derived from mice with the protamine/T-antigen transgene generated a heterogeneous population of cells displaying the phenotypes of either cardiac myocytes or mesenchymal cells (136). Tumor cells derived from mice with the atrial natriuretic factor promoter/T-antigen transgene maintained consistently the contractile phenotype of cardiac myocytes in culture (137). The different behaviors of the tumor cells from these two transgenic mouse strains in culture may be attributed to the atrial natriuretic factor promoter, which displays a greater specificity for expression in myocytes.

Permanent cell lines have been established from the myocardial tumor cells of mice carrying the atrial natriuretic factor/T-antigen (AT-1 cells; 138, 139) or the protamine promoter/T-antigen transgenes (MCM-1 cells; 140). Studies of MCM-1 cells have revealed that approximately 25% of the cells express sarcomeric myosin heavy chain (136, 140); further studies will be required to establish the ontogeny of these cells in relation to those lacking sarcomeric myosin heavy chain. In addition, it has been shown that cultures of MCM-1 cells express functional M2 (cardiac) muscarinic acetylcholine receptors (140). AT-1 cells were initially established as a transplantable tumor line in syngeneic animals, since cells derived from the primary tumors did not proliferate in culture (139, 141). The transplanted tumors consisted of proliferating cells bearing the phenotype of differentiated cardiac myocytes and vascular cells, the latter of which were probably contributed by the host (137). Cells from the transplanted tumors proliferated in culture, and maintained a stable differentiated phenotype. The cultured tumor cells could be frozen and recovered, and from such cells the AT-1 cell line was derived. By biochemical, molecular, and histochemical criteria, AT-1 cells maintain phenotypic characteristics of differentiated cardiac myocytes in culture, including assembly of functional myofibrils, spontaneous contraction, and significant electrophysiological activity. These characteristics are remarkable, considering that they are maintained in a proliferating cell line. In addition to their uses for studies of cardiac myocyte physiology, these and any other similarly generated cell lines should provide insights into the mechanisms that restrict the proliferative growth of normal mature cardiac myocytes (101).

Expression of other viral proteins and oncogenes in cultured cardiac myocytes has been shown to activate their proliferation. Infection of fetal rat cardiac myocytes with replication-defective retroviral constructs expressing either v-myc or v-H-ras has been shown to transform the cells to growth (100). Stable clones of the transformed cells have been shown to express a limited subset of myocardial genes. Assembly of complete sarcomeres or spontaneous contractions was not observed. A noncontractile avian cardiac myocyte cell line has likewise been derived from myocytes infected with a defective retrovirus expressing v-myc (142). The utility of these cultured cell lines in studies of the regulation of myocardial gene expression and development has yet to be explored.

EMBRYONIC CARDIAC MYOCYTES: DIFFERENTIATION OF ES AND TERATOCARCINOMA CELLS

Single-cell analyses have been performed with cardiogenic mesoderm of developing embryos (13, 14). Avian mesodermal cells removed after gastrulation from the heart-forming fields will grow from clonal density into colonies containing cardiac myocytes. These cells can be removed from the postgastrulated embryo prior to the expression of cardiac myocyte markers, indicating that their development is completed in vitro. The committed mesodermal cells develop into mature cardiac myocytes (embryonic phenotype), suggesting that inductive signals are not required for the later phases of cardiac myocyte differentiation and maturation (13, 14). This conclusion contrasts results obtained with other culture systems (53), including studies using an immortalized cell line derived from the same precardiac mesoderm (26). Although it is possible that signals from the embryonic milieu are not required for the later stages of cardiac myocytes development, it is also possible that these signals are received some time prior to the actual onset of differentiation. The usefulness of this culture system for molecular or biochemical analysis of myocardial development is restructed by the small number of primary cells that can be recovered consistently and by the brevity of their growth phase (prior to differentiation). An immortalized cell line derived from these cells (26) should provide a limitless supply of material and may serve as an alternative to primary cardiogenic mesoderm for molecular studies.

Mesoderm derived from embryos prior to gastrulation also can develop in vitro; however, only cells plated in high-density cultures will develop into cardiac myocytes (13, 14). These results strongly suggest that heterotypic cell–cell interactions are required for myocardial development from pregastrula mesoderm. These cultures are functionally similar to embryonal stem (ES) cell cultures, which also generate cardiac tissue in vitro (143–145). ES cells are derived from the inner-cell mass of the blastocoel, and can be maintained indefinitely if grown on the appropriate feeder layer or in the presence of specific growth factors (146, 147). ES cells differentiate when removed from the feeder cells or cultured in low-mitogen medium. Differentiation of ES cells results in the assembly of laminated structures resembling embryonic endoderm, ectoderm, and mesoderm develop, while in long-term cultures functional groups of cells resembling embryonic cardiac myocytes become apparent within the embroid bodies. The foci of cardiac myocytes that develop within embroid bodies contract spontaneously and by morphological criteria have well-defined myofibrillar structures and intercalated disks (145, 146). Molecular evidence of the myocardial phenotype of these cells includes the expression of α- and β-myosin heavy chain genes, characteristic of atrial and ventricular cardiac myocytes, respectively (148). This culture system has considerable potential for study of the early phases of cardiac development, since generation manipulation of embroid bodies is relatively simple and can be performed on a large enough scale for biochemical and molecular analyses. A caveat of this system is heterogeneity; cardiac myocytes make up a small percentage of the total cells in the embroid body. It may be possible to isolate cardiac myocytes from embryoid bodies, and if appropriate markers were available, to isolate cardiac progenitors as well. Genetic studies are possible using this culture system, and studies of differentiation of ES cells in culture may allow closer examination of the development of mutants than would be possible in vivo. ES cell cultures could also be used to study the role of specific factors on different phases of myocardial development. Expression of specific genes could likewise be reduced or ablated by addition of antisense oligonucleotides, or the activity of cell surface receptors or their ligands altered by neutralizing antibodies. The critical feature of the ES cell culture system is that it allows access to coordinated developmental events that may be difficult to observe or manipulate in situ.

Teratocarcinoma cells represent the neoplastic variant of ES cells. The P19 embryonal carcinoma cell line differentiates into embryonic cardiac myocytes when cultured as aggregates in the presence of DMSO (149, 150). Cardiac myocytes that develop from P19 embryonal carcinoma cells assemble active sarcomeres and are contractile. As with ES cell cultures, however, cardiac myocytes make up only a small percentage of the total cells in a differentiated P19 culture.

DIFFERENTIATION OF PROGENITORS COMMITTED TO THE MYOCARDIAL LINEAGE

For some cell types, it is possible to grow progenitor cells committed to a specific phenotype under conditions that promote proliferation and suppress differentiation. The progenitor cells, which may be derived from normal stem cells, blasts, or tumor cells, can be grown indefinitely, and then induced to differentiate by altering the culture medium. Skeletal myoblasts, neuroblastoma cells, and leukemia cells have been grown in this manner, prompting some investigators to explore the potential growth and differentiation in culture of committed progenitors for cardiac myocytes. This approach has been hindered by the restricted access to committed, undifferentiated progenitors for cardiac myocytes, which appear only during a brief period in embryonic development (see above). In addition, primary tumors of the myocardium are extremely rare. Some anomalous cell lines have been described in the literature that resemble proliferating myocardial progenitors; eventually, most of these were found to exhibit more features of skeletal than of cardiac muscle.

Differentiation and maturation of rat neonatal cardiac myocytes are thought to proceed after their dissociation and maintenance in culture. Freshly cultured neonatal rat cardiac myocytes were maintained for different times in low-mitogen medium, then treated with high-serum medium (86). Cultures were maintained in low-serum medium for 2, 7, or 14 days after isolation, then treated with high-serum medium. Cultures maintained in low-mitogen medium for 2 days responded to high-serum medium with both DNA synthesis and mitogenic activity; cultures maintained in low-mitogen medium for 7 days responded to high-serum medium with DNA synthesis; cultures maintained in low-mitogen medium for 14 days responded to high-serum medium with greatly attenuated DNA synthesis. These results show that the differentiation of cardiac myocytes proceeds in culture through stages similar to those observed in vivo. In addition, it is apparent that cardiac myocytes isolated from fetal and neonatal animals can display some mitogenic activity in high-serum medium prior to entering a terminal state. Cells responding to high-serum medium displayed reduced expression of certain sarcomeric proteins. Although the extent of cardiac myocyte proliferation observed in these experiments was limited, the results suggested that the appropriate culture conditions could permit propagation of these cells prior to their terminal differentiation. The conditions that promoted proliferation also appeared to suppress the contractile phenotype of the cells.

In other studies, dissociated cells from human fetal myocardium were cultured in a high-mitogen medium containing serum and embryo extracts. Proliferating cells from these cultures were passaged, and no longer expressed markers of the cardiac myocyte phenotype. Culturing the cells in low-mitogen medium induced expression of the atrial natriuretic factor and cardiac α-actin genes (151). Significant accumulation of titin also was observed (Kohtz, unpublished). However, neither contractile activity nor significant accumulation of sarcomeric myosin heavy chain was observed in these cultures. Expression of this subset of myocardial genes resembled the progression from committed mesoderm to premyofibrillar cardiac myocytes. Additional environmental cues, not yet identified, appear necessary to induce maturation to a contractile phenotype. Cardiac cells cultured in this manner were referred to as presumptive cardiac myoblasts (PCMs), consistent with the interpretation that they maintained commitment to the cardiac myogenic lineage in the absence of appropriate signals to induce differentiation and maturation. Further investigations of PCM cells prepared from several 14–15 week gestational age hearts showed that cultures arose rarely that expressed significant sarcomeric myosin heavy chain upon mitogen withdrawal (152). The reasons for this variation among different preparations of human PCMs are not clear, although it is not surprising considering the inherent heterogeneity of autopsy material. Other recent experiments have shown that inhibition of GATA-4 expression blocks differentiation of cardiac myocytes in vitro (48). Expression of GATA-4 in vivo anticipates myofibrillar differentiation of cardiac myocytes, suggesting that commitment of progenitor cells to this lineage may indeed precede their differentiation. A conserved binding site for GATA-4 is contained within the ANF promoter, and GATA-4 localizes to secretory myocytes in the adult heart (48). These results support the notion that induction of ANF transcription by differentiating presumptive cardiac myocytes in culture (151) may mark an early event of cardiac myocyte differentiation (153). Studies of GATA-4 expression in these cells may provide further insights.

Since fetal or neonatal myocardium lacks an obvious population of satellite or stem cells, the origin of the presumptive cardiac myoblasts described above is enigmatic. It is possible that after dissociation and culturing in high-mitogen medium, a population of fetal cardiac myocytes reverts to a more primitive phenotype. As an alternative, mesenchymal cells isolated with the fetal cardiac myocytes may be induced to express markers of the myocardial phenotype by components of the mitogen rich medium. Supporting the latter possibility, cultures of adult cardiac fibroblasts have been shown to express some markers of the myocardial phenotype (e.g., cardiac α-actin) when exposed to transforming growth factor β (154). It is important (and difficult) in these cases to differentiate between myocardial cell lines and cell lines that merely share some properties with cardiac myocytes. Finally, one study has suggested that a population of proliferating cells can arise from dissociated human fetal myocardium in high-mitogen medium that returns to a contractile phenotype when cultured in low-mitogen medium (155). These studies are intriguing since the cultures proliferated well enough to be passed (although no permanent lines were established), and the differentiated cells in the low-mitogen cultures were clearly cardiac myocytes.

A successful culture system for committed cardiac progenitor cells has been described by Eisenberg and Bader (26). Cardiogenic mesoderm from Japanese quail embryo was treated in culture with the mutagen 20-methylcholanthrene. Serial cloning was performed to select cells expressing sarcomeric myosin heavy chain. Subsequently, a rapidly growing population of cells (QCE-6) was selected that expressed isoforms of α-actin but not other markers of differentiated cardiac myocytes. When these cells were treated with retinoic acid and transforming growth factors $\beta1$ and $\beta2$, differentiation into either the myocardial or endocardial lineages was observed. Expression of several sarcomeric proteins, including sarcomeric myosin heavy chain, titin, and cardiac troponin I, was observed in the cardiomyogenic component of the differentiated cultures, although these cells did not achieve a contractile state (perhaps due the lack of expression of certain myocardial proteins, such as C-protein; 26, 156). These results demonstrate that the lineages of cells in the endocardium and myocardium are closely related, and support the notion that additional signals are required for maturation of cardiac myocytes to the contractile phenotype. The QCE-6 cell line is clonal and immortal, and should prove to be an invaluable tool for studying the molecular events controlling early myocardial development.

FUTURE DIRECTIONS

The possibility that grafts of fetal cardiac myocytes could be introduced into murine adult myocardium has been suggested by recent studies of Field and colleagues (157). The grafted fetal cardiac myocytes integrated into the myocardium remained viable and appeared to be functional. Whether the use of this technique could result in physiological improvement of a human heart damaged by infarct or disease remains as a more difficult question, but several intriguing possibilities are suggested by this observation (72). Although fetal tissue represents a possible source of cardiac myocytes for transplantation, the ultimate source of spare cardiac myocytes could be the mesenchymal cells of the recipient. Skeletal myoblasts have been generated from fibroblasts by ectopic expression of the myogenic bHLH regulators (40). Similar master regulatory genes have not been isolated from cardiac muscle; in fact, somatic cell fusion of cardiac myocytes and fibroblasts has indicated that the fibroblast phenotype is dominant (158). Nonetheless, it is possible that future studies will reveal that artificial expression and possibly suppression of certain genes will transdetermine mesenchymal cells to the myocardial phenotype. To overcome both the difficulty of growing cardiac myocytes and the potential for rejection of allografts, mesenchymal cells (fibroblasts) then could be derived from the patient, grown to the quantity required for grafting, and transdetermined to the myocardial phenotype. Although at present this procedure may appear to include as much fantasy as fact, the quest to find genes controlling the myocardial phenotype and exploit their potential uses has only begun.

REFERENCES

1. Carrel A. On the permanent life of tissues outside of the organism. J Exp Med 1912; 15:516-528.
2. Kitsis RN, Buttrick PM, McNally EM, Kaplan ML, Leinwand LA. Hormonal modulation of a gene injected into rat heart in vivo. Proc Natl Acad Sci 1991; 88:4138-42.
3. Bernanke DH, Markwald RR. Migratory behavior of cardiac cushion tissue cells in a collagen–lattice culture system. Dev Biol 1982; 91: 235-245.
4. Mjaatvedt CH, Markwald RR. Induction of an epithelial-mesenchymal transition by an in vivo adheron-like complex. Dev Biol 1989; 136: 118-128.
5. Razaee M, Isokawa K, Halligan N, Markwald RR, Krug EL. Identification of an extracellular 130 kDa protein involved in early cardiac morphogenesis. J Biol Chem 1993; 268:144401-144411.
6. Kirby ML, Waldo KL. Neural crest and cardiovascular patterning. Circ Res 1995; 77:211-215.
7. Manasek FJ. Embryonic development of the heart. I. A light and electron microscopic study of myocardial development in the early chick embryo. J Morphol 1968; 125: 329-336.

8. Manacek FJ. Histogenesis of the embryonic myocardium. Am J Cardiol 1970; 25:149-168.

9. Stalsberg H. Regional mitotic activity in the pre-cardiac mesoderm and differentiated heart tube in the chick embryo. Dev Biol 1969; 20:28-45.

10. Rychterova V. Principle of growth in the thickness of the ventricular wall in the chick embryo. Folia Morphol 1971; 19:113-124.

11. Jeter JR, Cameron IL. Cell proliferation patterns during cytodifferentiation in embryonic chick tissues: liver, heart, and erythrocytes. J Embryol Exp Morphol 1971; 23: 403-422.

12. Rychter Z, Ostadal B. Mechanism of the development of coronary arteries in the chick embryo. Folia Morphol 1971; 19: 113-124.

13. Gonzalez-Sanchez AG, Bader D. In vitro analysis of cardiac progenitor cel differentiation. Dev Biol 1990; 139:197-209.

14. Montgomery MO, Litvin J, Gonzalez-Sanchez A, Bader D. Staging of commitment and differentiation of avian cardiac myocytes. Dev Biol 1994; 164:63-71.

15. Mikawa T, Borisov A, Brown AMC, Fischman DA. Clonal analysis of cardiac morphogenesis in the chicken embryo using replication-defective retrovirus: I. Formation of the ventricular myocardium. Dev Dyn 1992; 193:11-23.

16. Mikawa T, Cohen-Gould L, Fischman DA. Clonal analysis of cardiac morphogenesis in the chicken embryo using a replication-defective retrovirus. III. Polyclonal origin of adjacent ventricular myocytes. Dev Dyn 1992; 195:133-141.

17. Jennings RB, Steenbergen C, Hackel DB. The heart. In: Rubin E, Farber J, eds. Pathology. Philadelphia: JB Lippincott, 1994:551-552.

18. Emerson CP. Myogenesis and developmental control genes. Curr Opin Cell Biol 1990; 2:1065-1075.

19. Olson EN, Klein WH. bHLH factor in muscle development: dead lines and commitments, what to leave in and what to leave out. Genes Dev 1994; 8:1-8.

20. Grepin C, Dagnino L, Robitaille L, Haberstrohl L, Antakly T, Nemer M. A hormone-encoding gene identified a pathway for cardiac but not skeletal muscle gene transcription. Mol Cell Biol 1994; 14:3115-3129.

21. Clegg C, Linkhart T, Olwin B, Hauschka S. Growth factor control of skeletal muscle differentiation: commitment to terminal differentiation occurs in G_1 phase and is repressed by fibroblast growth factor. J Cell Biol 1987; 105:949-956.

22. Olson EN. Interplay between proliferation and differentiation within the myogenic lineage. Dev Biol 1992; 154:261-272.

23. Han Y, Dennis JE, Cohen-Gould L, Bader DM, Fischman DA. Expression of sarcomeric myosin in the presumptive myocardium of chicken embryos occur within sic hours of myocyte commitment. Dev Dyn 1992; 193:257-265.

24. Garcia-Martinez V, Schoenwolf GC. Primitive-streak origin of the cardiovascular system in avian embryos. Dev Biol 1993; 159:706-719.

25. Linask KK, Lash JW. Early heart development: dynamics of endocardial cell sorting suggests a common origin with cardiomyocytes. Dev Dyn 193; 195:62-69.

26. Eisenberg CA, Bader D. QCE-6: a clonal cell line with cardiac myogenic and endothelial cell potentials. Dev Biol 1995; 167:469-481.

27. Deruiter MC, Poelmann RE, Mentink MM, Vaniperen L, Gittenberger-Degroot AC. Early formation of the vascular system in quail embryos. Anat Rec 1993; 235:261-274.

28. Linask KK. N-cadherin localization in early heart development and polar expression of Na$^+$, K$^+$-ATPase, and integrin during pericardial coelom formation and epithelialization of the differentiating myocardium. Dev Biol 1992; 151:213-224.

29. Duband J-L, Volberg T, Sabanay I, Thiery JP, Geiger B. Spacial and temporal distribution of the adherens-junction-associated-associated molecule A-CAM during avian embryogenesis. Development 1988; 103:325-344.

30. Holtzer H, Schultheiss T, Dilullo C, Choi J, Costa M, Lu M, Holtzer S. Autonomous expression of the differentiation programs of cells in the cardiac and skeletal myogenic lineages. Ann N Y Acad Sci 1990; 599:158-169.

31. Kuruc N, Franke WW. Transient coexpression of desmin and cytokeratins 8 and 18 in developing myocardial cells of some vertebrate species. Differentiation 1988; 38:177-193.

32. Coffin JD, Poole TJ. Embryonic vascular development: immunohistochemical identification of the origin and subsequent morphogenesis of the major vessel primordia in quail embryos. Development 1988; 102:735-748.

33. Miwa T, Kedes L. Duplicate CarG box domains have positive and mutually dependent regulatory roles expression of the human cardiac α-actin gene. Mol Cell Biol 1987; 7:2802-2813.

34. Gupta MP, Gupta M, Zak R, Sukhatme VP. Egr-1, a serum-inducible zinc finger protein, regulates transcription of the rat α-myosin heavy chain gene. J Biol Chem 1991; 266:12813-12816.

35. Farrance IKG, Mar JH, Ordahl CP. M-CAT binding factor is related to the SV40 enhancer binding factor, TEF-1. J Biol Chem 1992; 267:17234-17240.

36. Olson E. Regulation of muscle transcription by the MyoD family: the heart of the matter. Circ Res 1993; 72: 1-6.

37. Zhu H, Nguyen VTB, Brown AB, Pourhosseini A, Garcia AV, van Bilsen M, Chien K. A novel tissue-restricted zinc finger protein (HF-1b) binds to the cardiac regulatory element (HF1B/MEF2) in the rat myosin light chain 2 gene. Mol Cell Biol 1993; 13:4432-4444.

38. Edmondson DG, Lyons GE, Martin JF, Olson EN. Mef2 gene expression marks the cardiac and skeletal lineages during mouse embryogenesis. Development 1994; 120: 1251-1263.

39. Navankasattusas S, Sawadogo M, van Bilsen M, Dang CV, Chien KR. A ubiquitous factor HF-1a) and a distinct muscle factor (Hf1b/MEF2) form an E-box-independent pathway for cardiac muscle gene expression. Mol Cell Biol 1992; 12:1469-1479.

40. Weintraub HR, Davis S, Tapscott S, Thayer M, Krause R, Benezra R, Blackwell TK, Turner D, Rupp R, Hollenberg S, Zhuang Y, Lassar A. The myoD gene family: nodal point during specification of the muscle cell lineage. Science 1991; 251:761-766.

41. Miner JH, Miller JB, Wold BJ. Skeletal muscle phenotypes initiated by ectopic MyoD in transgenic mouse heart. Development 1992; 114:853-860.

42. Azpiazu N, Frasch M. *tinman* and *bagpipe*: two homeo box genes that determine cell fates in the dorsal mesoderm of *Drosophila*. Genes Deve 1993; 7:1325-1340.

43. Bodmer R. The gene *tinman* is required for specification of the heart and visceral msucles in *Drosophila*. Development 1993; 188:719-729.

44. Komuro I, Izumo S. Csx: A murine homeobox-containing gene specfically expressed in the developing heart. Proc Natl Acad Sci 1993; 90: 8145-8149.

45. Tonissen KF, Drysdale TJ, Lints TJ, Harvey RP, Krieg PA. Xnkx2.5, a *Xenopus* gene related to Nkx-2.5 and *tinman*: evidence for a conserved role in cardiac development. Dev Biol 1994; 162:325-328.

46. Lyons I, Parsons LM, Hartley L, Li R, Andrews JE, Robb L, Harvey RP. Myogenic and morphogenetic defects in the heart tubes of murine embryos lacking the homeo box gene Nkx2-5. Genes Dev 1995; 9:1654-1666.

47. Lints TJ, Parsons LM, Hartley L, Lyons I, Harvey RP. Nkx-2.5: a novel murine homeobox gene expressed in early heart progenitor cells and their myogenic descendants. Development 1993; 119:419-431.

48. Grepin C, Robitaille L, Antakly T, Nemer M. Inhibition of transcription factor GATA-4 expression blocks in vitro cardiac muscle differentiation. Mol Cell Biol 1995; 15:4095-4102.

49. Srivastava D, Cserjesi P, Olson EN. A subclass of bHLH proteins required for cardiac morphogenesis. Science 1995; 270:1995-1999.

50. Kokan Moore NP, Bolender DL, et al. Secretion of inhibit beta A by endoderm cultured from early embryonic chicken. Dev Biol 1991; 146:242-245.

51. Orts-Llorca F. Influence of the endoderm on heart differentiation during the early stages of development of the chicken embryo. Arch Entwicklungsmech 1963; 154:533-551.

52. Sugi Y, Lough J. Anterior endoderm is a specific effector of terminal cardiac myocyte differentiation of cells from the embryonic heart forming region. Dev Dyn 1994; 200:155-162.

53. Yamakazi Y, Hirakow R. Factors required for differentiation of chick precardiac mesoderm cultured in vitro. Proc Jpn Acad 1991; 76:165-170.

54. Schaart G, Vieban C, Langmann W, Ramaekers F. Desmin and titin expression in early post-implantation mouse embryos. Development 1989; 107:585-596.

55. Tokuyasu KT, Maher PA. Immunocytochemical studies of cardiac myofibrillogenesis in early chick embryos. I. Presence of immunofluorescent titin spots in premyofibril stages. J Cell Biol 1987; 105:2781-2793.

56. Tokuyasu KT, Maher PA. Immunocytochemical studies of cardiac myofibrillogenesis in early chick embryos. II. Generation of α-actinin dots within titinspots a the time of the first myofibril formation. J Cell Biol 1987; 105:2795-2801.

57. Dlugosz AA, Antin FB, Nachmis VT, Holtzer H. The relationship between stress fiber-like structures and nascent myofibrils in cultured cardiac myocytes. J Cell Biol 1984; 99:2268-2278.

58. Wang SM, Greaser ML, Schultz E, Bulinski JC, Lin JC, Lessard JL. Studies on cardiac myofibrillogenesis with antibodies to titin, actin, tropomyosin and myosin. J Cell Biol 1988; 107:1075-1083.

59. Lim SS, Woodroofe N, Lemanski LF. An analysis of contractile proteins in developing chick heart by SDS polyacrylamide gel electrophoresis and electron microscopy. J Embryol Exp Morphol 1983; 77:1-14.

60. Markwald RR. Distribution and relationship of precursor Z material to organizing myofibrillar bundles in embryonic rat and hamster ventricular myocytes. J Mol Cell Cardiol 1973; 5:341-350.

61. Ruzicka DL, Schwartz RJ. Sequential activation of α-actin genes during avian cardiogenesis: vascular smooth muscle α-actin gene transcripts mark the onset of cardiomyocytes differentiation. J Cell Biol 1988; 107:2527-2586.

62. Vanderkerckhove J, Bugaisky G, Buckingham M. Simultaneous expression of skeletal muscle and heart proteins in various striated muscle tissues and cells. A quantitative determination of the two actin isoforms. J Biol Chem 1986; 261:1838-1943.

63. Nadal-Ginard B, Mahdavi V. Basic mechanisms of cardiac gene expression. Eur Heart J 1993; 14(supplement):2-11.

64. Gunning P, Ponte P, Blau H, Kedes L. α-Skeletal and α-cardiac actin genes are coexpressed in adult human skeletal muscle and heart. Mol Cell Biol 1983; 3:1985-1995.

65. Minty A, Blau H, Kedes L. Two-level regulation of cardiac actin gene transcription: muscle-specific modulating factors can accumulate before gene activation. Mol Cell Biol 1986; 6:2137-2148.

66. Lompre AM, Mahdavi V, Nadal-Ginard B. Expression of the cardiac ventricular α and β myosin heavy chain genes is developmentally and hormonally regulated. J Biol Chem 1984; 259:6437-6446.

67. Yutzey KE, Bader D. Diversification of cardiomyogenic cell lineages during early heart development. Circ Res 1995; 77:216-219.

68. Yutzey KE, Rhee JT, Bader D. Expression of the atrial-specific myosin heavy chain AMHC1 and the establishment of anteroposterior polarity in the developing chicken heart. Development 1994; 120:871-883.

69. Kubalak SW, Miller-Hance WC, O'Brien TX, Dyson E, Chien KR. Chamber specification of atrial myosin light chain-2 expression precedes septation during murine cardiogenesis. J Biol Chem 1994; 269:16961-16970.

70. Satin J, Fujii S, DeHaan R. Development of cardiac beat rate in early chick embryos is regulated by regional cues. Dev Biol 1988; 129:103-113.

71. Soonpaa MH, Field LJ. Assessment of cardiomyocyte DNA synthesis during hypertrophy in adult mice. Am J Physiol 1994; 266:H1439-H1445.

72. Soonpaa MH, Daud AI, Koh GY, Kulg MG, Kim KK, Wang H, Field LJ. Potential approaches for myocardial regeneration. Ann NY Acad Sci 1995; 752:446-454.

73. Cavanough MW. Pulsation, migration, and division in dissociated chick embryo heart cells in vitro. J Exp Zool 1955; 128:573-589.

74. Harary I, Farley B. Invitro studies of single isolated beating heart cells. Science 1960; 131:1674-1675.

75. Mark GE, Strassen FF. Pacemaker activation and mitosis in cultures of newborn rat heart ventricle cells. Exp Cell Res 1966; 44:217-233.

76. Andrus W, Strasser FF. Beating hamster heart cells in tissue culture. Exp Cell Res 1967; 47:613-616.

77. Stemmer P, Akera T, Brody TM, Rardon DP, Watanabe AM. Isolation and enrichment of Ca^{2+}-tolerant myocytes for biochemical experiments from guinea-pig heart. Life Sci 1989; 44:1231-1237.

78. Vahouny C, Wei R, Starkweather R, Davis C. Preparations of beating heart cells from adult rats. Science 1970; 167:1616-1618.

79. Orlowski J, Lingrel JB. Thyroid and glucocorticoid hormones regulate the expression of multiple Na^+/K^+ATPase genes in cultures neonatal rat cardiac myocytes. J Biol Chem 1991; 265:3462-3470.

80. Parker TG, Chow KL, Schwartz RJ, Schneider MS. Differential regulation of skeletal α-actin transcription in cardiac muscle by two fibroblast growth factors. Proc Natl Acad Sci 1990; 87:7066-7080.

81. Blondel B, Roijen I, Chenevel JP. Heart cells in culture: a simple method for increasing the proportion of myoblasts. Experientia 1971; 27: 356-358.

82. Parker TG, Packer SE, Schneider MD. Peptide growth factors can provoke "fetal" contractile protein gene expression in rat cardiac myocytes. J Clin Invest 1990; 85:507-514.

83. Chein K, Knowlton K, Zhu H, Chien S. Regulation of cardiac gene expression during myocardial growth and hypertrophy: molecular studies of an adaptive physiological response. FASEB J 1991; 5:3037-3046.

84. Borg TK, Rubin K, Lundgren E, Borg K, Obrink B. Recognition of extracellular matrix components by neonatal abd adult cardiac myocytes. Dev Biol 1984; 104:86-96.

85. Kardami E. Stimulation and inhibition of cardiac myocyte proliferation in vitro. Mol Cell Biochem 1990; 92:129-135.

86. Ueno H, Perryman B, Roberts R, Schneider MD. Differentiation of cardiac myocytes after mitogen withdrawal exhibits three sequential states of the ventricular growth response. J Cell Biol 1988; 107:1911-1918.

87. Claycomb WC. Culture of cardiac muscle cells in serum free media. Exp Cell Res 1980; 131:231-236.

88. Nag AC, Cheng M. Biochemical evidence for cellular dedifferentiation in adult rat cardiac muscle cells in culture: expression of isoenzymes. Biochem Biophys Res Commun 1986; 137:855-862.

89. Oberpriller JO, Oberpriller JC. Cell division in cardiac myocytes. In: Ferrans VJ, Rosenquist G, Weinstein C, eds. Cardiac Morphogenesis. New York: Elsevier Science, 1985: 12-22.

90. Simpson PA, McGrath A, Savion S. Myocytes hypertrophy in neonatal rat heart cultures and it regulation by serum and by catechoamines. Circ Res 1982; 51:787-801.

91. Brand T, MacLellan WR, Schneider MD. A dominant-negative receptor for type β transforming growth factors created by deletion of the kinase domain. J Biol Chem 268; 1993:11500-11503.

92. Matiuck NV, Swain JL. Proto-oncogenes and cardiac development. TCM 1992; 2:61-65.

93. Sugi Y, Lough J. Onset of expression and regional deposition of α-smooth and sarcomeric actin during avian development. Dev Dyn 1992; 193:116-124.

94. Claycomb WC, Delcarpio JB, Guice SE, Moses RL. Culture and characterization of fetal human atrial and ventricular cardiac muscle cells. In Vitro Cell Dev Biol 1989; 25:1114-1120.

95. Engelmann GL, Boehm KD, Birchenall-Roberts MC, Ruscetti FW. Transforming growth factor β1 in heart development.Mech Dev 1992; 38:85–97.

96. MacLellan WR, Brand T, Schneider MD. Transforming growth factor β in cardiac ontogeny and adaptation. Circ Res 1993; 73:783-791.

97. Schneider MD, McLellan WR, Black FM, Parker TG. Growth factors, growth factor response elements, and the cardiac phenotype. Basic Res Cardiol 1992; 87(Supplement 2):33-48.

98. Pollack PS, Houser SR, Budjak R, Goldman B. c-myc gene expression is localized to the myocyte following hemodynamic overload in vivo. J Cell Biochem 1994; 54:78-84.

99. Engelmann GL, Dionne CA, Jaye MC. Acidic fibroblast growth factor and heart development. Role in myocytes proliferation and capillary angiogenesis. Circ Res 1993; 72:7-19.

100. Engelmann GL, Birchenall-Roberts MC, Rucetti FW, Samarel AM. Formation of fetal cardiac cell clones by retroviral transformation: retention of select myocyte charateristics. J Mol Cell Cardiol 1993; 25:197-213.

101. Kim KK, Soonpaa MH, Daud AI, Koh GY, Kim JS, Field LJ. Tumor suppressor gene expression during normal and pathological myocardial growth. J Biol Chem 1994; 269:22607-22613.

102. Bloch K, Seidman J, Naffilan J, Fallon J, Seidman C. Neonatal atria and venctrciles secrete atrial natriuretic factor via tissue-specific pathways. Cell 1986; 47:695-702.

103. Rumyantsev PP. Interrelations of the proliferation and differentiation processes during cardiac morphogenesis and regeneration. Int Rev Cytol 1977; 51:187-273.

104. Nag AC, Cheng M. Expression of myosin isozymes in cardiac muscle cells in culture. Biochem J 1984; 221:21-26.

105. Gupta MP, Gupta M, Zak R, Sukhatre VP. Egr-1, a serum inducible zinc finger protein, regulates transcription of the rat cardiac α-MHC gene. J Biol Chem 1991; 266:12813-12816.

106. Izumo S, Mahdavi V, Nadal-Ginard B. All members of the MHC multigene family respond to thyroid hormone in a highly tissue-specific manner. Science 1986; 231:597-600.

107. Sadoshima J, Tkhashi T, Jahn L, Izumo S. Roles of mechano-sensitive ion channels, cytoskeleton, and contractile activity in stretch-induced immediate early gene expression and hypertrophy of cardiac myocytes. Proc Natl Acad Sci 1992; 89:9905-9909.

108. Sadoshima J, Jahn L, Takahashi T, Kulik TJ, Izumo S. Molecular charaterization of the stretch-induced adaptation of cultured cardiac cell. An invitro model of load-induced cardiac hypertrophy. J Biol Chem 1992; 267:10551-10560.

109. Sadoshima J, Xu Y, Slayter HS, Izumo S. Autocrine release of angiotensin II

mediates stretch-induced hypertrophy of cardiac myocytes in vitro. Cell 1993; 75:977-984.

110. Sater AK, Jacobson AG. The role of the dorsal lip in the induction of heart mesoderm. Development 1990; 108:461-470.

111. Sadishima J, Izumo S. Molecular charaacterization of angiotensin II-induced hypertrophy of cardiac myocytes and hyperplasia of cardiac fibroblast. Critical role of the AT1 receptor subtype. Circ Res 1993; 73:413-423.

112. Miller-Hance WC, LaCorbiere M, Fuller SJ, Evans SM, Lyons G, Schmidt C, Robbins J, Chien KR. In vitro chamber specification during embryonic stem cell cardiogenesis. Expression of the venticular myosin light chain-2 gene is independent of heart tube formation. J Biol Chem 1993; 268:25244-25252.

113. Sadoshima J, Izumo S. Mechanical stress rapidly activates multiple signal transduction pathways in cardiac myocytes: protential involvement of an autocrine/ paracrine mechanism. EMBO J 1993; 12:1681-1692.

114. Bloom S. Spontaneous rhythmic contraction of separated heart cells. Science 1970; 167:1727-1729.

115. Berry MN, Friend DS, Scheuer JS. Morphology and metabolism of intact muscle cells isolated from adult rat heart. Circ Res 1970; 26:679-687.

116. Powell T, Twist VW. A rapid technique for the isolation and purification of adult cardiac muscle cells that have respiratory control and a tolerance to calcium. Biochem Biophy Res Commun 1976; 72:327-333.

117. Knowlton KU, Michel MC, Itani M, Shubeita HE, Ishihara K, Brown JH, Chien KR. the α1-adrenergic receptor subtype mediates biochemical, molecular, and morphological features of cultured myocardial cell hypertrophy. J Biol Chem 1993; 268:15374-15380.

118. Stemmer P, Wisler PL, Watanabe AM. Isolated myocytes in experimental cardiology. In Fozzard HA et al. eds. The Heart and the Cardiovascular System. New York: Raven Press, 1992: 387-404.

119. Dow JW, Harding NGL, Powell T. Isolated cardiac myocytes. II. Functional aspects of mature cells. Cardiovasc Res 1981; 15:549-579.

120. Farmer BB, Mancina M, William ES, Watanabe AM. Isolation of calcium tolerant myocytes from adult rat hearts: Review of the literature and description of a method. Life Sci 1983; 33:1-18.

121. Nag A, Zak R. Dissociation of adult mammalian heart into single cell suspension: an ultrastructural study. J Anat 1979; 129:541-559.

122. Stemmer P, Akera T, Brody TM, Raidon DP, Watanabe AM. Isolation and enrichment of Ca^{2+}-tolerant myocytes for biochemical experiments from guinea pig heart. Life Sci 1989; 44:1231-1237.

123. Gupta R, Neumann J, Durant P, Watanabe A. α1-Adrenergic receptor-mediated inhibition of isoproterenol-stimulated protein phosphorylation in ventricular myocytes. Circ Res 1993; 72:65-74.

124. Zhu H, Garcia AV, Ross RS, Evans RS, Chien KR. A conserved 28-base-pair element (HF-1) in the rat cardiac myosin light chain 2 gene confers cardiac-specific and α adrenergic-inducible expression in neonatal rat myocardial cells. Mol Cell Biol 1991; 11: 2273-2281.

125. Zimmerman ANE, Huslmann WC. Paradoxical influence of calcium ions on the permeability of the cell membranes of the isolated rat heart. 1966; 211:646-647.

126. Crevey BJ, Langer GA, Frank JS. Role of Ca^{2+} in maintenance of rabbit myocardial cell membrane structural and functional integrity. J Mol Cell Cardiol 1984; 10:1081-110.

127. Frank JS, Langer GA, Nudd LM, Seraydarian K. The myocardial cell surface, its histochemistry, and the effect of sialic acid and calcium removal on its structure and cellular ionic exchange. Circ Res 1977; 41:702-714.

128. Frank JS, Rich TL, Beydler S, Kreman M. Calcium depletion in rabbit myocardium. Circ Res 1982; 51:117-130.

129. Alto LE, Dhalla NS. Role of changes in microsomal calcium uptake in the effects of reperfusion of Ca^{2+}-depressed rat hearts. Circ Res 1981; 48:17-24.

130. Alto LE, Dhalla NS. Myocardial cation contents during induction of calcium paradox. Am J Physiol 1979; 237:H713-H719.

131. Rich TL, Langer, GA. Calcium depletion in rabbit myocardium. Calcium paradox protection by hypothermia and cation substitution. Circ Res 1982; 51: 131-141.

132. Muir AR. The effects of divalent cations on the ultrastructure of the perfused rat heart. J Anat 1967; 101:239-261.

133. Bulkey BH, Nunnally RL, Hollis DP. "Calcium paradox" and the effect of varied temperature on its development. 1978; 39:133-140.

134. Kramer JH, Chovan JP, Schaffer SW. Effect of taurine on calcium paradox and ischemic heart failure. Am J Physiol 1981; 240:H238-H246.

135. Sen A, Dummon P, Henderson SA, Gerard RD, Chien KR. Terminally differentiated rat myocardial cells proliferate and maintain specific differentiated functions following expression of SV40 large T antigen. J Biol Chem 1988; 263:19132-19136.

136. Behringer RR, Peschon JJ, Messing A, Gartside CL, Hauschka SD, Palmiter RD, Brinster RL. Heart and bone tumors in transgenic mice. Proc Natl Acad Sci 1988; 85:2648-2652.

137. Field LJ. Atrial natriuretic factor SV40 T antigen transgenes produce tumors and cardiac arrhythmias in mice. Science 1988; 239:1029-1033.

138. Steinhelper ME, Lanson NA, Dresdner KP, Delcarpio JB, Wit Al, Claycomb WC, Field LJ. Proliferation in vivo and in culture of differentiated adult atrial cardiomyocytes from transgenic mice. Am J Physiol 1990; 259:H1826-H1834.

139. Delcarpio JB, Lanson NA, Field LJ, Claycomb WC. Morphological charaterization of cardiomyocytes isolated from a transplantatble cardiac tumor derived from transgenic mouse atria (AT-1 cells). Circ Res 1991; 69:1591-1600.

140. Morton ME, Brumwell C, Gartside CL, Hauschka SD, Nathanson NM. Characterization of muscarinic acetylcholine receptors expressed by an atrial cell line derived from a transgenic mouse tumor. Circ Res 1994; 74:752-756.

141. Kline RP, Sorota S, Dresdner KP, Steinhelper ME, Lanson NA, Wit AL, Claycomb WC, Field LJ. Spontaneous activity in transgenic mouse heart: comparison of primary atrial tumor with cultured AT-1 atrial myocytes. J Cardiovasc Electrophysiol 1993; 4:642-660.

142. Saule S, Merigaud JP, Al-Moustafa AEM, Ferre F, Rong PM, Amouyel P, Quatannens B, Stehelin D, Dieterlen-Lievre F. Heart tunors specifically induced in young avian embryos by the v-myc oncogene. Proc Natl Acad Sci 1987; 84:7982-7986.

143. Evans MJ, Kaufman MH. Establishment in culture of pluripotent cell from mouse embryos. Nature 1981; 292:154-156.

144. Martin GR. Isolation of a pluipotent cell line from early mouse embryos cultured in medium conditioned by teratocarcinoma stem cells. Proc Natl Acad Sci 1981; 78: 7634-7638.

145. Martin GR, Lock LF. Pluripotent cell lines derived from early mouse embryos cultured in medium conditioned by teratocarcinoma stem cells. In Silver LM, Martin GR, Strickland S, eds. Teratocarcinoma Stem Cells: Cold Spring Harbor Conference on Cell Proliferation. Cold Spring Harbor, NY: Cold Spring Harbor Laboratory, 1983: 635-663.

146. Doetschman TC, Eistetter H, Katz M, Schmidt W, Kemler R. The invitro development of blastocyst-derived embryonic stem cell lines: formation of visceral yolk sac, blood islands and myocardium. J Embryol Exp Morphol 1985; 87:27-45.

147. Wobus AM, Holzhausen H, Jakel P, Schoneich J. Charaterization of a pluripotent stem cell line derived from a mouse embryo. Exp Cell Res 1984; 152:212-219.

148. Robbins J, Doetschman T, Jones WK, Sanchez A. Embryonic stem cells as a model for cardiogenesis. TCM 1992; 2:44-50.

149. Rudnicki MA, Ruben M, McBurney MW. Regulated expression of a transfected cardiac actin gene during differentiation of multipotential murine embryonal carcinoma cells. Mol Cell Biol 1988; 8:406-417.

150. Rudnicki MA, Jackowski G, Saggin L, McBurney MW. Actin and myosin expression during development of cardiac muscle from cultured embryonal carcinoma cells. Dev Biol 1990; 138:348-358.

151. Kohtz DS, Dische NR, Inagami T, Goldman B. Growth and partial differentiation of presumptive human cardiac myoblasts in culture. J Cell Biol 1989; 109:1067-1078.

152. Goldman BI, Wurzel J. Effects of subcultivation and culture medium on differentiation of human fetal cardiac myocytes. In Vitro Cell Dev. Biol. 1992; 28A:109–119.

153. Zeller R, Bloch KD, Williams BS, Arceci RJ, Seidman CE. Localization of the atrial natriuretic factor gene during cardiac embryogenesis. Genes Dev 1987; 1:693-698.

154. Eghbali M, Tomek R, Woods C, Bhambi B. Cardiac fibroblasts are predisposed to convert into myocyte phenotype: specific effect of transforming growth factor β. Proc Natl Acad Sci 1991; 88:795-799.

155. Wang YC, Neckelmann N, Mayne A., Herskowitz A, Srinivasan A, Sell KW, Ahmed-Ansari A. Establishment of a human fetal cardiac myocyte cell line. In Vitro Cell Dev Biol 1991; 27A:63-74.

156. Kawashima M, Kitani S, Tanaka T, Obinata T. The earliest form of C-protein

expressed during striated muscle development is immunologically the same as cardiac-type C-protein. J Biochem 1986; 99:1037-1047.

157. Soonpa MH, Koh GY, Klug MG, Field LJ. Formation of intercalated disks between fetal cardiomyocytes and host myocardium. Science 1994; 264:98-101.

158. Evans SM, Tai LJ, Tan VP, Newton CB, Chien KR. Heterokaryons of cardiac myocytes and fibroblasts reveal the lack of dominance of the myocardial phenotype. Mol Cell Biol 1994; 14:4269-4279.

6

Congenital Heart Disease: Gene Defects and Molecular Biological Studies

Bruce D. Gelb
Mount Sinai School of Medicine
New York, New York

INTRODUCTION

Congenital heart defects (CHD) are present in nearly 1% of all newborns and continue to be a significant cause of death in infancy. Despite the substantial progress made in recent decades in the diagnosis and treatment for CHD, little advance was made in our understanding of the fundamental causes of CHD for a long period of time. Recently, molecular biological techniques have been applied to CHD, leading to the identification of two probable CHD genes (connexin43 and elastin) and the promise that more will soon follow. In this chapter, the results of a variety of molecular studies related to CHD will be reviewed. These include studies of chromosomal abnormalities resulting in CHD (haploinsufficiency of chromosome 22q11 and trisomy 21), studies of single gene defects associated with CHD, and the identification of CHD-causing genes in mice. As will be noted, single gene defects may underlie CHD occurring with gross chromosomal abnormalities and identification of single gene defects may uncover syndromes with previously unrecognized chromosomal defects.

CATCH SYNDROME

Congenital heart disease, especially conotruncal defects (truncus arteriosus, interrupted aortic arch type B, tetralogy of Fallot, conal septal ventricular septal defects), have been associated with both the DiGeorge and velocardiofacial (Shprintzen) syndromes. Recent molecular investigations have revealed that a high percentage of patients with both syndromes have microscopic or submicroscopic deletions at chromosome 22q11. The acronym CATCH-22 (Cardiac defects, Abnormal facies, Thymic aplasia/hypoplasia, Cleft palate, Hypocalcemia) was proposed by Wilson and co-workers to include the range of abnormalities associated with these deletions and to unify separate diagnostic entities that were overlapping even within individual families (1). As will be reviewed, deletions of chromosome 22q11 are responsible for isolated conotruncal heart defects in addition to causing the more complex syndromes. The various phenotypes will be reviewed separately, reflecting their history and the independent molecular studies that have been undertaken.

DiGeorge first described the association between thymic aplasia and absence of the parathyroid glands in certain immunologically impaired infants in 1965 (2). He attributed this combination of abnormalities to a common embryological origin of the defective structures from the third and fourth pharyngeal pouches. The associations with certain dysmorphic features and congenital heart disease in DiGeorge syndrome were noted subsequently. Van Mierop and Kutsche delineated the congenital heart defects in a study of 151 autopsy cases of DiGeorge syndrome (3). They found an interrupted aortic arch (type B) in 32% of all cases, truncus arteriosus in 25%, tetralogy of Fallot in 23%, isolated VSD in 7%, and no heart defect in 3%. Subsequent studies have found a similar incidence and distribution of cardiac lesions.

Gross chromosomal abnormalities have been identified in a minority of patients with DiGeorge syndrome but were crucial in identifying potential genetic loci containing genes responsible for this disorder. In 1981, de la Chapelle and co-workers reported a patient with an unbalanced translocation between chromosomes 20 and 22 resulting in monosomy for 22q11 (4). Subsequent reports of other unbalanced translocations confirmed the importance of monosomy 22q11 in DiGeorge syndrome (5). In a prospective series preceding the advent of molecular cytogenetics, Greenberg and co-workers found that 18% of patients with DiGeorge syndrome had chromosomal defects, primarily monosomy 22q11 but also monosomy 10p13 (5). The association with monosomy 10p13 has been confirmed in other patients (6).

Two research groups, one at the University of Pennsylvania under Beverly Emanuel and the other at the Institute of Child Health in London under Peter Scambler, initiated molecular studies of the chromosome 22q11 deletions in DiGeorge syndrome in an attempt to isolate the gene(s) responsible for various aspects of the phenotype including the congenital heart disease. After isolating DNA probes from the DiGeorge critical region, these groups have shown either by dosage analysis or fluorescent in situ hybridization (FISH) that more than 85% of patients with DiGeorge syndrome have deletions of 22q11 (7–10) (Fig. 1). The parent of origin for the deletion has been demonstrated to be irrelevant for DiGeorge syndrome (7, 11). A balanced translocation between chromosomes 2 and 22 was reported in a patient with "partial" DiGeorge syndrome (12). This translocation has recently been studied by two groups, resulting in the identification of several genes in the region (13, 14). The most promising candidate genes at present are DGCR3, which spans the breakpoint, and DGCR4, which may span the breakpoint.

Velocardiofacial syndrome (VCFS) was first described by Shprintzen in 1978 (15) and includes overt or submucosal cleft palate in almost all cases; facial anomalies including a squared nasal root with a narrow alar base, retrognathia, and malar flatness; and congenital heart disease in more than 80% of cases (16). Central nervous system abnormalities associated with VCFS include

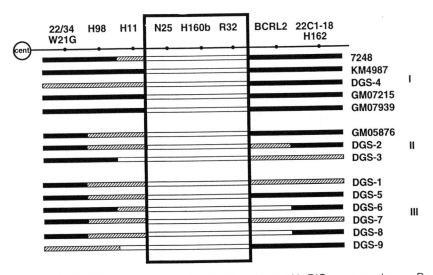

Figure 1 RFLP and dosage studies in 14 patients with DiGeorge syndrome. Patients are grouped by cytogenetic findings. Group I, (del)22(q11.21q11.23); II, possible deletion of 22q11; III, normal karotype. Probes are ordered from centromere (cent) on the left to telomere on the right. Fully blackened bars represent the presence of two copies of the locus; hatched bars represent uninformative or nonpolymorphic loci for which dosage has not been performed to determine copy number; unblackened bars represent deletions. The minimal region of overlap is indicated by the box and includes probes N25, pH160b, and pR32. (From Ref 7.)

learning disabilities in nearly all patients and a variety of psychiatric disorders presenting in adolescence or adulthood (16). The congenital heart defects commonly encountered with VCFS are ventricular septal defects, especially conal septal defects (56% of patients), tetralogy of Fallot (19%), and isolated right aortic arch (11%) (17).

Prompted by the clinical overlap with DGS, evidence for 22q11 microdeletions has been sought in VCFS patients (8, 18-20). By high-resolution cytogenetic analysis, approximately 20% of VCFS patients have 22q11 deletions that can be demonstrated (18). Molecular analyses including dosage studies, restriction fragment length polymorphism (RFLP) analysis, and FISH have demonstrated 22q11 deletions in approximately 75% of cases (8). Considerable phenotypic variability has been shown within families transmitting these submicroscopic deletions, which are presumed to be stable (21).

Several investigations studied a variety of patients with isolated conotruncal defects to determine whether 22q11 deletions also play an important causative role in these heart defects. Wilson and co-workers assembled nine pedigrees with at least two first-degree relatives with CHD (22). They demonstrated 22q11 deletions in the affected members from five of the families: two families had at least one member with neonatal hypocalcemia but the other three families had no other manifestations of CATCH syndrome. Of particular note, one transmitting mother with the deletion had only a patent ductus arteriosus and one transmitting father with the deletion had no cardiac malformations. Goldmuntz and co-workers evaluated 17 patients with conotruncal cardiac defects for 22q11 deletions (23). Fourteen patients had no major extracardiac malformations but most had minor dysmorphism. Five of these 14 patients had 22q11 deletions including one patient with a mother with repaired tetralogy of Fallot. None of the three patients with other major anomalies (one-Pierre Robin sequence with cleft palate, one tracheal stenosis, one cleft palate and imperforate anus) had a deletion. Johnson and co-workers screened 61 patients with conotruncal defects with FISH (24). They found 25 patients with 22q11 deletions, of whom 18 showed no evidence of DGS or VCF. Subsequent parental testing revealed three deletions among eight pairs. Finally, a prospective study of all newborns and infants presenting with conotruncal defects in a 2 year period within a defined region of the United Kingdom found 39 patients: 17 with dysmorphism including 9 with a facial appearance consistent with CATCH syndrome (25). Deletions were found in of nine CATCH patients, but none of the 19 nondysmorphic patients.

The genetic region at chromosome 22q11, which is deleted in VCF, was recently cloned in a yeast artificial chromosome (YAC) contig (overlapping clones spanning the region) by Bernice Morrow and co-workers (26). After isolating new DNA markers in the region, these investigators defined the deletions from 61 VCF patients (Fig. 2). They determined that 82% of patients were deleted for two markers that defined a 2 Mb region. Correlation with the phe-

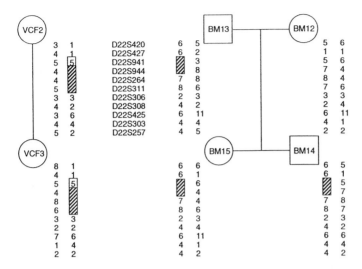

Figure 2   Genotype analysis of two familial cases of velocardiofacial syndrome. Haplotypes of 11 polymorphic loci were deduced for two families with affected parents and children. The hatched box represents the hemizygous region; the unhatched box denotes an uninformative marker. In the family shown on the left, an affected mother (VCF2) with a VSD passed on the 22q11 deletion to her daughter (VCF3) who also had a VSD. In the family shown on the right, an affected father (BM13) without CHD passed on the 22q11 deletion to a daughter (BM15) who also had no CHD and a son (BM14) who had an interrupted aortic arch with VSD and ASD. (From Ref. 26.)

notype was found for neither the size of the deletion nor, in familial cases, the parent of origin. The latter observation rules out a possible role for imprinting in the expression of VCF. In one family, one affected child had an interrupted arch while his affected father and sister had no cardiac defects; molecular analysis of the deletion was identical in all three individuals. Similar conclusions have been obtained in the molecular analyses of DiGeorge syndrome patients and families (11).

   In summary, deletions of chromosome 22q11 play an important causative role in conotruncal cardiac defects. The phenotype observed in patients with these deletions is widely variable, ranging from isolated cardiac defects to DiGeorge syndrome. All aspects of the CATCH syndrome can be observed singly or jointly with these deletions. There appears to be conservation of deletion size within families despite significant variability in the phenotype. This variable expressivity does not correlate with deletion size or result from genetic imprinting. Candidate genes for the various abnormalities in CATCH syndrome have been identified and their potential is being actively evaluated.

ATRIOVENTRICULAR SEPTAL DEFECTS: TRISOMY
21-RELATED AND FAMILIAL FORMS

Atrioventricular septal defects (AVSD), also known as atrioventricular canal defects or endocardial cushion defects, are the most common cardiac malformations encountered in Down's syndrome (trisomy 21) (27) and Down's syndrome accounts for approximately 60% of AVSDs (28). While the vast majority of individuals with the clinical features of Down's syndrome have complete trisomy 21, a minority of patients have small duplications of chromosome 21. Molecular and cytogenetic mapping of these small duplications has permitted the definition of regions of chromosome associated with various aspects of the Down syndrome phenotype including AVSDs (29, 30). In this manner, the AVSD critical region has been assigned to chromosome 22q22.1-qter, which is a 9 Mb interval (29, 30) (Fig. 3).

Two collagen VI genes, COL6A1 and COL6A2, are clustered in the AVSD critical region on chromosome 21. Since collagen VI is expressed in fetal heart, (31) these two genes have been considered candidates for the AVSD in Down's syndrome. Davies and co-workers initially described RFLPs for these two genes and then assessed children with Down's syndrome and their parents (32, 33). While they found some haplotypes that were unique in families with offspring with Down's syndrome with an AVSD, there was no single haplotype that predicted AVSDs and these results could be explained by small sample size or linkage disequilibrium. Therefore, no firm conclusions can be drawn at this time about the role of collagen VI in the causes of AVSDs in Down's syndrome.

Although the majority of AVSDs occur as part of a syndrome such as Down's syndrome, isolated AVSDs can be recurrent in families. Studies suggest that offspring born to affected adults have a 10% risk of CHD including AVSD and TOF (34, 35). In addition, several large pedigrees have been reported in which isolated AVSDs were inherited as an autosomal dominant trait with reduced penetrance (36–38). Linkage studies performed with these large families have excluded the critical region on chromosome 21 defined with microduplications but have not yet established the familial AVSD locus (36–38).

FAMILIAL SUPRAVALVULAR AORTIC STENOSIS
AND WILLIAMS SYNDROME

Supravalvular aortic stenosis (SVAS) is an unusual form of CHD presenting in three ways: (a) an autosomal dominant familial arteriopathy with SVAS, main and branch pulmonary artery stenoses, and obstructions of various large and small systemic arteries; (b) a sporadic arteriopathy indistinguishable from the inherited form (which presumptively represents de novo mutations); and (c)

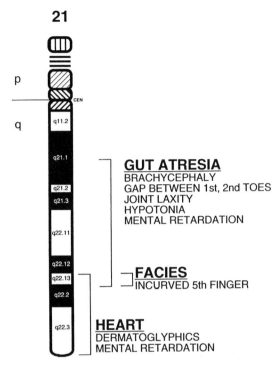

Figure 3 Down's syndrome phenotypic map resulting from molecular analysis of two patients with microduplications of portions of 21q. (From Ref. 29.)

Williams syndrome, which includes the same arteriopathy accompanied by hypersocial personality, developmental delay, characteristic dysmorphic facial features, and infantile hypercalcemia (39). Williams syndrome is generally sporadic but has been transmitted from affected parent to child.

A series of molecular genetic investigations, principally by Mark Keating's group at the University of Utah, have revealed that the SVAS arteriopathy most probably results from elastin gene defects. First, genetic linkage analyses of three families with autosomal dominant SVAS localized the SVAS gene to the long arm of chromosome 7 (40, 41). The elastin gene was known to lie in the SVAS critical region and became the leading candidate gene. Subsequently, another family with autosomal dominant SVAS was found to have a balanced translocation between chromosomes 7 and 6, which cosegregated with the SVAS (42) (Fig. 4). DNA sequencing at the breakpoint revealed that the translocation disrupted the elastin gene (43). Molecular analysis of a family with autosomal dominant SVAS demonstrated a 100 kb deletion at the 3' end of the

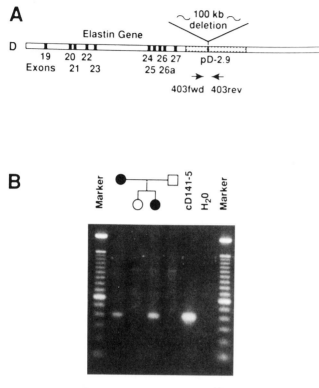

Figure 4 PCR analyses showing a deletion allele from a patient with familial SVAS. (A) Map of a genomic clone shows the deletion breakpoint in the elastin gene and the location of the oligonucleotide primers (403fwd and 403rev). (B) Oligonucleotide primers directed across the deletion breakpoint (403fwd and 403rev) yield a PCR product of the predicted size (403 bp) in affected members of the SVAS family and in the genomic clone (cD141-5), but not in unaffected family members. These data show that the deletion allele disrupts the elastin gene. (From Ref. 44.)

elastin gene, including the terminal nine exons (44). Although these molecular studies strongly implicated elastin abnormalities in SVAS, the mechanism underlying the arteriopathy remained unclear. That is, it was possible to propose that the arteriopathy resulted from a dominant negative effect of abnormal elastin generated from truncated transcripts or that inadequate quantities of elastin were incorporated into the extracellular matrix, resulting in the vascular abnormalities. Analysis of the elastin gene in Williams syndrome patients resolved this issue.

Since the arteriopathy associated with Williams syndrome is both clinically and histologically indistinguishable from that found in the familial SVAS, investigators probed for elastin gene defects in patients with Williams syndrome. Ewart and co-workers demonstrated haploinsufficiency at the elastin locus by FISH in nine individuals with Williams syndrome, including two rare pairs of affected parent and child (45). Moreover, gene dosage data using cosmids flanking the two ends of the elastin gene revealed that the entire gene was deleted. Subsequent FISH studies using an elastin probe revealed submicroscopic deletions in 96% of patients with classic Williams syndrome (n = 114) (46). The full extent of the submicroscopic deletions in Williams syndrome have not been established. Current efforts are underway to map the region physically in order to clone additional genes, which, when deleted, result in other aspects of the Williams syndrome phenotype (47).

Since deletions of the entire elastin gene cause SVAS in Williams syndrome, it follows that incorporation of insufficient elastin protein into the extracellular matrix underlies the arteriopathy. Presumably, the same mechanism applies in familial SVAS. What remains uncertain is precisely how insufficient elastin incorporation results in this arteriopathy, an issue of substantial importance and possible clinical relevance. Development of a elastin-deficient mouse model through transgenesis, which is in progress, will permit the experimental approach to this issue (47).

HOLT-ORAM SYNDROME

The heart-hand syndrome was first described in 1960 by Hold and Oram in four generations of a family with atrial septal defects (ASDs) and thumb anomalies (48).This syndrome is an autosomal dominant trait with a high degree of penetrance but variable expressivity. While secundum ASDs are the most commonly observed heart anomaly in Holt-Oram syndrome (HOS), a range of cardiac phenotypes include normal, first-degree atrioventricular block, ostium primum ASDs, isolated ventricular septal defects, and hypoplastic left heart syndrome (49). The limb abnormalities also vary to include structures derived from the embryonic radial ray (radius, carpal, and thenar bones), unilaterally or bilaterally, with severity ranging from triphalangeal thumb to phocomelia. Cytogenetic abnormalities have been described with HOS including partial deletion of the long arm of a B chromosome (either chromosome 4 or 5) (50), deletions at chromosome 14q23-24. (51), and a pericentric inversions of chromosome 20 with breakpoints at p13 and q13.2 (52).

Several linkage studies have been recently reported for HOS. Ruiz and co-workers excluded linkage of HOS to chromosome 14q23–24 in a Belgian family with five affected individuals (53). Terrett and co-workers genotyped 30 affected persons from seven families with HOS, linking it with one family to a region on chromosome 12q. Four of the other smaller families also provided positive lod scores for markers from 12q but HOS in one family was excluded from this region (one family was uninformative). For the five families with HOS linked to 12q, the maximal lod score was 7.76 with D12S79 at $\Theta = 0.00$ and the HOS region was defined to a 21 cM region between D12S78 and D12S86. Bonnet and co-workers reported definition of the same HOS critical region on 12q from analysis of nine families but failed to detect any genetic heterogeneity (54). Basson and co-workers analyzed two large HOS families, finding linkage with both to 12q2 (55). Observed recombinant events refined the HOS critical region to 6 cM between D12S84 and D12S79. Despite linkage to the same region, one family had mild cardiac involvement (10 affected persons with normal hearts; five with an ASD; one with an ASD and a conduction defect) while the other had more severe cardiac defects (all 19 affected persons with an ASD, VSD, or both and a high percentage with conduction defects). In contrast, the skeletal abnormalities were more severe in the former family. Thus, while genetic heterogeneity does exist in HOS, the variable expressivity appears to be attributable, at least to some extent, to allelism.

NOONAN SYNDROME

In 1968, Noonan reported 19 patients with dysmorphic features similar to Turner-Ullrich syndrome (45,XO) and cardiac abnormalities including pulmonary valve dysplasia, aortic coarctation, patent ductus arteriosus, and hypertrophic cardiomyopathy (56). Noonan syndrome is inherited as an autosomal dominant trait. Linkage analysis in a large Dutch family with eight affected members mapped the gene for Noonan syndrome to 12q in a 14 cM region between D12S84 and D12S366 (57). It is interesting that the Noonan critical region includes the Holt-Oram syndrome critical region, although it seems unlikely that the two diseases are allelic. Subsequent analysis of an additional 21 small families with Noonan syndrome demonstrated genetic heterogeneity in at least one family.

WATSON SYNDROME

Watson described a syndrome consisting of pulmonic stenosis, café-au-lait spots, and mental retardation with autosomal dominant inheritance (58). Subsequent reports included patients with neurofibromata (59, 60). Hence, Watson syndrome has been called Noonan–neurofibromatosis syndrome. Linkage studies have, therefore, focused on the NF1 locus (the gene for neurofibromatosis type 1) on chromosome 17. Two studies with three Watson syndrome families established linkage to markers flanking NF1 (61, 62). To resolve the issue of whether the gene defect in Watson syndrome was allelic to NF1, tightly linked to NF1, or a microdeletion syndrome, the NF1 gene was examined. Molecular studies of NF1 in two families with Watson syndrome demonstrated an intragenic 80 kb deletion (63) and an in-frame 42 bp insertion-duplication (64), convincingly proving that this syndrome is allelic with neurofibromatosis type 1.

The NF1 gene product, neurofibromin, has been shown to play a role in cardiac morphogenesis. Two strains of NF1 knockout mice were produced by Brannan and co-workers (65) and Jacks and co-workers (66). Mice heterozygous for the mutation did not have neurofibromatosis and had no cardiac disease. In the homozygous state, the mutations were lethal to the fetuses due to hydrops fetalis. In one study, examination of the hearts from homozygotes revealed truncus arteriosus, hypoplastic myocardium, and decreased endothelial density at the endocardial cushions of the atrioventricular canal (which had properly septated) (65). Several other tissues including skeletal muscle were also hypoplastic. In the other study, the hearts from homozygous animals showed double outlet right ventricle and a hypoplastic myocardium (66). Thus, two NF1 gene mutations resulted in conotruncal heart defects. It is unclear whether the differences in the cardiac phenotype (i.e., truncus arteriosus vs. double outlet right ventricle) derive from the slight differences in the NF1 mutations or from the varying genetic background.

Aside from potential cardiogenic effects of NF1 via expression in neural crest tissue, which is a well-established contributor to conotruncal development (67), the NF1 gene is expressed directly in the developing fetal heart in a developmentally controlled fashion (68, 69). One isoform of neurofibromin shows peak expression at 12 days after conception, which is precisely the stage at which the homozygous mutant mice demonstrate the cardiac abnormalities (65, 68). A second alternatively spliced form of the NF1 gene has also been detected in fetal and adult heart (69).

FAMILIAL TOTAL ANOMALOUS PULMONARY VENOUS RETURN

Total anomalous pulmonary venous return (TAPVR) as an isolated cardiac anomaly is usually sporadic but has rarely reported to be familial (70, 71). Inheritance of the familial form is believed to be autosomal dominant with decreased penetrance and variable expressivity (70–72). Linkage analysis using a large Utah–Idaho family with seven affected individuals and 17 obligate carriers (presumed instances of nonpenetrance) mapped the TAPVR gene to chromosome 4p13–q12, achieving a maximal two-point lod score of 6.51 using D4S174 at $\Theta = 0.00$ (72). The investigators were unable to detect any trinucleotide repeat expansions in the affected persons as a potential genetic mechanism for TAPVR in this family. In addition, they were only able to localize the TAPVR to 30 cM. Future efforts toward identifying the TAPVR gene will utilize the candidate gene approach, since opportunities to refine the critical region using additional meioses are limited by the extreme rarity of familial TAPVR (72).

LATERALITY DEFECTS: CONNEXIN43 GENE DEFECTS, X-LINKED HETEROTAXY SYNDROME, KARTAGENER SYNDROME, AND MOUSE MODELS

Heterotaxy syndromes are defects in laterality manifesting with visceroatrial situs abnormalities that are often accompanied by complex CHD. They occur both sporadically and familially with autosomal recessive, autosomal dominant, or X-linked inheritance. Discussed below are the connexin43 gene defects that cause autosomal recessive heterotaxy, linkage for X-linked heterotaxy, defects in cilia-related genes in Kartagener syndrome, and two mouse models of autosomal recessive heterotaxy unrelated to connexin43.

Recent evidence has implicated the connexins in embryonic morphogenesis, adding to their known function as the intercellular membrane channels of gap junctions. Based on the knowledge that connexin43 is the primary connexin in heart, Britz-Cunningham and co-workers analyzed patients with CHD for mutations in a small region of the connexin43 gene that encodes the carboxyl terminal signal with predicted phosphorylation sites (73). They found missense mutations in all six patients with heterotaxy syndrome whom they analyzed, identifying two mutant alleles in four of these six by sequencing only 400 bp of the approximately 1300 bp coding region. In contrast, no mutations were found in analysis of DNA from 25 control individuals. Among 24 patients with a variety of other forms of CHD, one mutation was found in a patient with a familial atrial septal defect. The authors then transfected connexin-defective L929 cells with a plasmid encoding connexin43 with the most common mutation (Ser364Pro). Subsequent study of dye transfer kinetics after microinjection revealed functional abnormalities in the mutant connexin43 compared to wild type protein (73). These fascinating studies provide solid evidence for the role of connexin43 mutations, acting in an autosomal recessive manner, in the genesis of heterotaxy. The finding of a mutation associated with a familial ASD provides impetus for analyzing patients with a wider variety of CHD.

Further proof of an important role for connexin43 mutations in CHD comes from the connexin43-deficient mouse model. Reaume and co-workers produced a mouse with a disrupted connexin43 gene (74). Examination of homozygote animals with the null mutation revealed enlargement of the right ventricular outflow region that was filled with intraventricular septate, resulting in pulmonary atresia (Fig. 5). No other abnormalities were found in these mice. This phenotype differs from that seen in the patients with connexin43 defects.

Whether this results from the nature of the molecular defect (i.e., null mutation vs. missense mutations affecting phosphorylation) or from differences between murine and human cardiac development remains to be addressed. Production of transgenic animals with connexin43 missense mutations and further patient studies may resolve this issue.

Casey and co-workers mapped a gene for X-linked heterotaxy syndrome in a large family to Xq24-q27.1 (75). Penetrance was complete but variable expressivity was present. Affected males in this family manifested either asplenia or polysplenia, complex CHD consistent with heterotaxy, and various midline defects. Using a 1-lod-unit support interval, a 16 cM critical region was defined. A portion of this region can probably be excluded since interstitial deletions at Xq25 in males do not result in heterotaxy.

Kartagener syndrome, also known as primary ciliary dyskinesia, consists of dextrocardia with situs inversus, bronchiectasis, and sinusitis. Affected males are infertile due to immobile sperm. This syndrome is usually inherited as an autosomal recessive trait, although families with patterns consistent with X-linked and autosomal dominant inheritance have been reported (76). Among families with the autosomal recessive form of Kartagener syndrome, the decreased numbers of affecteds with situs inversus compared to the expected numbers have led to the hypothesis that the homozygous state results in indifferent lateralization (i.e., one-half of homozygotes are situs solitus and one-half are situs inversus).

The primary defects in Kartagener syndrome are axonemal, including absence of dynein arms or radii. Specific Kartagener syndrome genes have not been mapped nor have gene mutations been identified. The human cytoplasmic dynein heavy-chain gene was localized to chromosome 14qter by FISH, (77) making this a candidate locus for Kartagener syndrome. In the mouse, the homologous region is on chromosome 12 in the region containing the *iv* locus (see below) (78).

The *iv/iv* mouse is a naturally occurring mouse strain inheriting sidedness abnormalities as an autosomal recessive trait. Approximately 40% of the inbred mice have CHD consistent with heterotaxy syndrome, while half of the remainder are situs inversus or situs solitus (79). The *iv* gene was linked to mouse chromosome 12 near the immunoglobulin heavy-chain gene complex at the telomere (80, 81). Subsequently, McGrath and co-workers refined the localization of *iv* using duplication/deficiency mapping, showing that the gene lies telomeric to the immunoglobulin heavy-chain gene complex (82). Further efforts to isolate the *iv* gene are in progress. An allelic *iv* mutant called *legless* was produced by insertional mutagenesis and exhibits a more complex phenotype including heterotaxy (83).

The second murine locus associated with laterality defects is *inv*, discovered in a transgenic mouse produced by insertional mutagenesis (84). Mice that

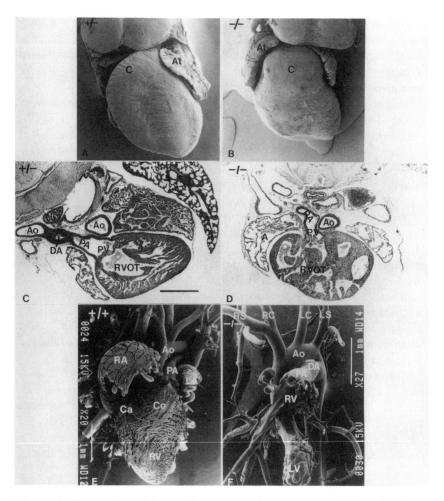

Figure 5 Comparison of the cardiac anatomy between *connexin43* null and control mice. Scanning electron micrographs of the ventral views of hearts from (A) a newborn heterozygote and (B) a homozygote. Heterozygotes exhibited normal cardiac morphology. In homozygotes, the right ventricular conus was enlarged. Co, conus region; At, atrium. Transverse histological sections through the hearts of (C) a heterozygote and (D) a homozygote mouse at the level of the right ventricular outflow tract. Histologic characteristics of the heterozygotes were normal. In homozygotes, the right ventricular cavity was divided by septa into numerous interconnected subcavities that frequently were blind-ended. Ao, aorta; PA, pulmonary artery; DA, ductus arteriosus; PV, pulmonary valve; RVOT, right ventricular overflow tract; and A, atrium. Grid bar, 1 mm.

are homozygous for the *inv* mutation have situs inversus of the abdominal viscera and, with one exception, of the heart. Six of eight homozygotes had l-looping of the ventricles. Mating with *iv* homozygous mice demonstrated that *inv* is not allelic with *iv*. Using an interspecific backcross, the *inv* gene was mapped to mouse chromosome 4 near the *v-mos, Tsha,* and *Hxb* loci.

MOUSE MODELS OF CONGENITAL HEART DISEASE

An increasing number of transgenic mouse models are being generated with disruption of one or more genes. While the purpose of these studies has not been to generate CHD in the mouse, a variety of cardiac phenotypes have emerged. In a few instances, naturally occurring mouse mutants will also be discussed. It is anticipated that the observations made in these animals will ultimately prove relevant to the pathogenesis of CHD in humans. The discussion below is grouped by gene class: *trans*-acting factors, growth factors, and extracellular matrix proteins. Gene mutations in the mouse with CHD, both spontaneous and induced, which have direct correlates to human disease are discussed above.

Trans-Acting Factors

Homeobox Gene Knockouts

Hox-1.5. Chisaka and Capecchi produced *hox-1.5* gene disruption in a mouse (85). *Hox-1.5* is a homeobox gene that is expressed in presomitic mesoderm and ectoderm early in development (7.5–8.0 days after conception) and in a variety of tissues including the aortic trunk later in development (12.5 days after conception). Animals homozygous for the disrupted *hox-1.5* gene die at or shortly after birth and have multiple anomalies resembling DiGeorge syndrome. These include craniofacial abnormalities, thymic aplasia, lack of parathyroid glands, and a hypoplastic thyroid. The cardiac defects were not cono-

---

Corrosion casts prepared by retrograde perfusion of methyl methacrylate casting compound into the aorta of (E) normal and (F) homozygous mice. This compound consistently back-filled the right ventricular chamber (RV) of normal mice (E) despite the presence of pulmonary valves. However, only very small amounts of casting compound entered either the right ventricular cavity (RV) or left ventricular cavity (LV) of homozygotes (F). RA, right atrium; Ao, aorta; PA, pulmonary artery; Ca, coronary artery; Co, conus; RV, right ventricle; RS, right subclavian artery; RC, right carotid artery; LC, left carotid artery; LS, left subclavian artery; LV, left ventricle; DA, ductus arteriosus. (From Ref. 74.)

truncal but included defective semilunar valves, absent right carotid artery, and ventricular wall abnormalities, especially a thin right ventricular wall. This mouse model fulfills the predicted importance of homeobox genes in mammalian development generally and neural crest structures in cardiac development specifically (86).

Nkx2-5/Csx. A homeobox gene named *Nkx2-5* (87) and, alternatively, *Csx* (88) was cloned from the mouse by homology with the *Drosophila* homeobox gene *tinman*. Flies with *tinman* mutations develop no visceral or cardiac mesoderm, resulting in an absence of heart formation (89, 90). In the mouse, *Nkx2-5* is expressed in early cardiac progenitor cells preceding myogenesis and continues to be expressed into adulthood. Recently, Lyons and co-workers produced mice with gene disruptions in *Nkx2-5* (91). Homozygous embryos developed a beating heart tube but cardiac looping did not occur. The heart did develop myocardial and endocardial layers separated by cardiac jelly, as is normal, but failed to form endocardial cushions in the cleft demarcating the primitive atrium from the ventricle. Analysis of the expression of several myofilaments genes demonstrated that most were normal (*myosin heavy chains α* and *β; α-cardiac actin; myosin light chains 1A, 1V,* and *2A*) but *myosin light chain 2V* expression was markedly reduced. These studies provide novel insights into cardiac organogenesis and myogenesis. Although severe gene defects in the human *Nkx2-5* homolog would likely prove lethal, missense mutations in noncritical portions of the gene might create survivable CHD.

Pax-3. Pax-3 is a member of the *Pax* gene family which contain a domain homologous to the *Drosphila* paired box. *Pax-3*, which also contains a homeobox, is expressed in neural crest cell derivatives and in the neuroepithelium. Gene defects in *Pax-3* are responsible for Waardenburg syndrome in humans (92) and the *splotch* phenotype in mice (93). The *splotch* phenotype, which varies with the particular mutation, can include a white splotch on the abdomen, exencephaly, spina bifada, meningocele, and CHD. Examination of the hearts from sp^{1H}/sp^{1H} mice revealed truncus arteriosus (94) while sp^d/sp^d mutation animals had double-outlet right ventricle (95). The sp^{1H}/sp^d heterozygote hearts showed an equal proportion of truncus arteriosus and double outlet right ventricle. The sp^{1H} mutation, associated with more severe neural tube defects, was induced by x-irradiation and is therefore likely due to result from a *splotch* gene deletion. The sp^d mutation, which is associated with milder neural tube defects, arose spontaneously and is due to a point mutation within the paired box domain (96). In order to understand the abnormal neural crest cell migration and neural tube closure, studies have been performed examining neural cell adhesion molecule (N-CAM) in *splotch* mice (97, 98). Although N-CAM protein is present in an appropriate spatiotemporal distribution, heavier isoforms are present on Western blots on day 9 after conception, which normally appear on day 11. These heavier isoforms result from premature sialylation of N-CAM. This work suggests that *Pax-3* protein mediates the posttranslational sialylation of N-CAM, which, in turn, affects migration of neural crest cells through the extracellular matrix.

Other Trans-Acting Genes

Retinoic Acid Receptors. Retinoic acid and vitamin A derivatives are important in modulating morphogenesis of several organs. Reinoids act through two families of nuclear retinoic acid receptors: the retinoic acid receptors (RARs) and the retinoic X receptors (RXRs). RXRs can bind DNA as homodimers or form heterodimers with RARs, which also then bind DNA. Two groups recently produced RXRα null mice with similar phenotype (99, 100). The mutation is an embryonic lethal that resulted in distinctive myocardial abnormalities as well as optic malformations. Examination of the fetal mouse hearts revealed marked hypoplasia of the compact layer of the myocardium of both free walls and septum resulting in some muscular VSDs (99, 100) (Fig. 6). The mitotic index and DNA synthesis were normal in the myocardium, as was expression of the appropriate cardiac myocyte-specific genes (99). When RXRα$^{-/-}$/RARα$^{-/-}$ and RXRα$^{-/-}$/RARγ$^{-/-}$ mice were generated, persistent truncus arteriosus and a variety of aortic arch anomalies were noted (99). These studies reinforce the recognized role of reinoids and their receptors in cardiac morphogenesis.

WT-1. WT-1 is a zinc finger protein that binds DNA. It plays an important role in the differentiation of the urogenital system. Individuals who are heterozygous for null mutations of WT-1 may have cryptorchidism and hypospadias, whereas those inheriting dominant point mutations have streak gonads and ambiguous genitalia. Both sets of patients are predisposed to Wilms' tumors due to loss of heterozygosity of WT-1. In order to study WT-1 further, Kreidberg and co-workers produced a transgenic mouse with a WT-1 null mutation (101). Heterozygote animals were normal up to 10 months of age but homozygotes died at day 13-15 after conception. As expected, examination of the homozygotes revealed a variety of urogenital abnormalities. In addition, there was thinning of the myocardium similar to the myocardial abnormalities identified in the RXRα-deficient mice.

N-myc. *N-myc* belongs to the myc family of protooncogenes that are basic helix–loop–helix DNA-binding proteins. *N-myc* plays a role in embryogenesis and is expressed in several developing tissues including the heart and visceral arches (102). Several transgenic mice with *N-myc* mutations have been produced (103-106). Homozygous null mutations are lethal in the mouse at midgestation,

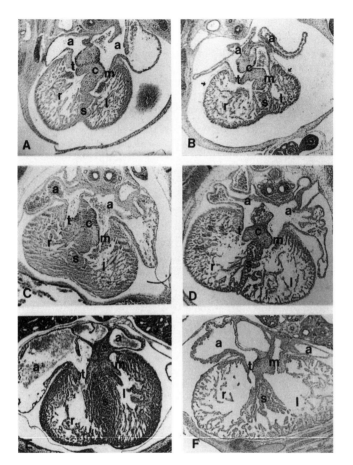

Figure 6 Comparison of the cardiac anatomy between RXRα null and wild-type mouse embryos. Transverse sections at the level of the atrioventricular valves. A,C, and E are from a wild-type embryo; B, D, and F are from a homozygous littermate. Embryos were isolated at E12.5 (A,B), E13.5 (C,D), and E14.5 (E,F) of development. A, atria; C, endocardial cushion; l, left ventricle; m, mitral valve; r, right ventricle; s, interventricular septum; t, tricuspid valve. Arrows in B point to the loosely attached pericardial layer; arrow in F indicates a VSD. (From Ref. 100.)

with abnormalities found in the urogenital system, central nervous system, and heart (105, 106). The cardiac abnormality appears to be arrested development with a thin myocardium and inadequate septation. A leaky mutation results in abnormal lung development in homozygotes but no apparent cardiac phenotype (104). Compound heterozygote fetuses with one null and one leaky *N-myc* al-

lele die at approximately day 12.5 after conception (103). Examination of fetal hearts revealed hypoplasia of the compact layer of the myocardium without other structural cardiac defects. Lung development was also disturbed.

Transcriptional Enhancer Factor 1

Transcriptional enhancer factor 1 (TEF-1) is a transcriptional factor belonging
to the class containing a DNA-binding motif, TEA. In humans, it activates
transcription through SV40 and papillomavirus-16 virus enhancers (107). TEF-
1 may be identical to the M-CAT binding factor that binds M-CAT motifs in
several myofilament genes. When the gene was disrupted using a retroviral gene
trap, homozygous embryos died at day 11–12 after conception from cardiac
dysfunction (107). Histological examination showed thin ventricular wall with
minimal trabeculae. On ultrastructural examination, the myofibers were normal.
Analysis of four myofibrillar mRNAs and proteins revealed normal gene expression and protein levels. These studies show that TEF-1 plays a role in
myocardial development, but the precise mechanism resulting in this cardiac
phenotype has not been elucidated. The myocardial abnormalities in TEF-1$^{-/-}$
fetuses resemble closely that found in homozygotes with other transcriptional-
related gene disruptions. Thus, this final cardiac phenotype apparently can result
from perturbations in the expression of a variety of genes active in cardio-
myogenesis.

Growth Factor Receptors

Platelet-Derived Growth Factor Receptors

Platelet-derived growth factors (PDGFs) make up a family of mitogens that play
a role in cell differentiation and growth in a variety of tissues. There are three
PDGF dimers (AA, BB, and AB) constituted by PDGF A and/or B polypeptide chains. There are two PDGF receptors (PDGFRs): PDGFRα and
PDGFRβ. PDGFRα binds both PDGF A and B chains while PDGFRβ binds
only PDGF B. The PDGFRα gene is deleted in the *Patch* mouse (108). *Patch*
is an autosomal recessive lethal with effects on nonneuronal, neural-crest-de-
rived cells, overlapping the PDGFRα expression pattern (109). *Patch* homozygote fetuses have craniofacial abnormalities, thymic aplasia, or hypoplasia, and
90% have truncus arteriosus. Abnormalities were found in the extracellular
matrix through which the neural crest cells migrate, with larger than normal
proteoglycan-containing granules (108). These matrix abnormalities are present
prior to the onset of neural crest cell migration, suggesting a causal role.

Transgenic mice homozygous for a PDGFRβ gene disruption have been
produced, resulting in kidney and hematological abnormalities but no cardiac

phenotype (110). In contrast, mice deficient for PDGF B have cardiac pathology in addition to similar kidney and hematological phenotypes (111). The right ventricular walls lacked a myocardial compact layer, showing exuberant thin trabeculae. Since a lack of PDGFRβ, which binds PDGF dimers BB and AB, does not affect cardiac development, the myocardial abnormalities form the PDGF B deficiency would seem to result from the absence of PDGF BB and AB dimers to bind to PDGFRα. The substantial difference in the cardiac phenotype seen in the PDGFRα-deficient mice highlights the complexity of this system and the need for further studies.

Insulin-Like Growth Factor II Receptor

Insulin-like growth factor II receptor (IGF2R) also known as IGF2/cation-independent mannose 6-phosphate receptor, is a paternally imprinted gene that binds IGF2. Lau and co-workers created a transgenic mouse with targeted disruption of IGF2R (112). As expected, heterozygous mice inheriting the mutant allele from their fathers had a normal phenotype since transcription occurs from only the maternal allele. Mice with maternally inherited IGF2R mutations died shortly after birth. These animals were larger than wild-type siblings and had a tail kink. Examination of their hearts revealed three-times normal size, myocardial hyperplasia, and large sinusoids in the ventricular septum.

Extracellular Matrix Genes

Vascular Cell Adhesion Molecule

Vascular cell adhesion molecule (VCAM-1) is a transmembrane protein belonging to the immunoglobulin superfamily. Its extracellular portion comprises seven Ig-like domains. Domains I and IV interact with the α4 integrins. While VCAM-1 is recognized for its role in inflammatory responses, it also plays a role in embryological development. In the developing heart, VCAM-1 is expressed in the myocardium, especially in the outflow tract and atrioventricular septum.

VCAM-1 knockout mice were recently produced by targeted homologous recombination by two groups (113, 114). Generally, homozygous mutant animals did not survive beyond day 13.5 after conception. The cardiac abnormalities included a hemorrhagic pericardial effusion of uncertain cause (without a generalized bleeding diathesis), a lack of epicardium, incomplete ventricular septation, and a myocardial compact layer that was reduced in thickness (Fig. 7). This range of defects exceeds the cardiac abnormalities found the in α4 integrin knockout mouse (discussed below) and the spatial expression pattern of the α4 integrins, suggesting that VCAM-1 may interact with an additional receptor during cardiac development.

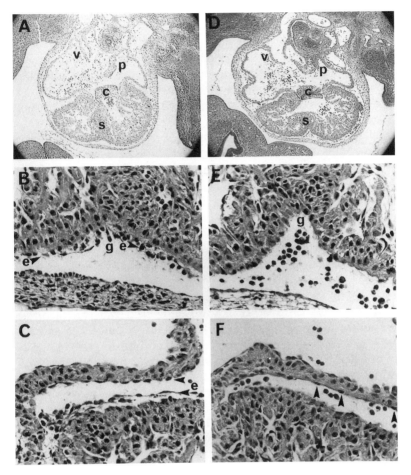

Figure 7 Comparison of the cardiac anatomy between VCAM-1 null and wild-type mouse embryos. Histological sections of hearts from wild-type embryos (A, B, and C) and VCAM-1 −/− embryos (D, E, and F) at E11.5. v, atrial valve leaflets; p, septum primum; c, endocardial cushions; s, intraventricular septum; g, ventricular groove; e, epicardium; and avs, atrial ventricular sulcus. Note the large amount of blood below the ventricular groove within the pericardial space (E). The micrographs in C and F are of the atrial/ventricular junction and avs located immediately to the right of the endocardial cushions and immediately below the septum primum. Note the pocket of cells in the avs of the wild-type heart (indicated with the curved arrow in C) that is absent in the VCAM-1 −/− heart. The rows of epicardial cells from wild-type hearts are indicated by horizonal arrowheads. The locations of scattered epicardial cells present on the atrial wall of the VCAM-1 −/− embryo are indicated by vertical arrowheads. (A, D: 80x; B, C, E, F: 320x). (From Ref. 113.)

α4 *Integrins*

Integrins are cell surface receptors that mediate cell–intracellular matrix and cell–cell interactions. They are heterodimeric glycoproteins, made up of an α and a β subunit. The α4 integrins include an α4 subunit associated with either β1 or β7 subunit. Both α4β1 α4β7 bind VCAM-1 and fibronectin (115). The α4 integrins are expressed in the epicardium and in the endocardial cushions during cardiac development (113).

An α4 knockout mouse was generated recently by targeted homologous recombination (115). Like the VCAM-1 deficient mouse embryos, embryos with the α4 integrin deficiency also lacked an epicardium and had blood in the pericardial space. In contrast, myocardial compact layer formation and ventricular septation were normal in the α4 integrin-deficient mouse.

Fibronectin

Fibronectins are glycoproteins transcribed by a single gene with alternative splicing. As a constituent of extracellular matrix, they play a role in cell adhesion and migration (116). In the developing heart, fibronectins are believed to be important for the migration of endocardial cells through the cardiac jelly to form the endocardial cushions (117), as well as in the migration of precardiac mesoderm to the future site of the heart tubes (118). A fibronectin knockout mouse was produced by targeted homologous recombination (119). Homozygous animals died before day 14.5 after conception with numerous abnormalities. When examined at day 8.5 after conception, 7 of 20 homozygous embryos had no visible primitive heart. In these embryos, microscopic analysis showed that the cardiac primordia had failed to fuse. Cardiac morphology was also abnormal in the animals with cardiac structures, manifesting as thickened myocardium, deficient cardiac jelly, and abnormal or absent endocardium.

ACKNOWLEDGMENTS

The author thanks Drs. Tim McQuinn and Ira Parness for their thoughtful reviews of the manuscript.

REFERENCES

1. Wilson DI, Burn J, Scambler P, Goodship J. DiGeorge syndrome: part of CATCH-22. J Med Genet 1993; 30:852–856.
2. DiGeorge, AM. Discussion on a new concept of the cellular basis of immunology. J Pediatr 1965; 67:907–908.
3. Van Mierop LHS, and Kusche LM. Cardiovascular anomalies in DiGeorge syndrome and importance of neural crest as a possible pathogenetic factor. Am J Cardiol 1986; 58:133–137.

4. de la Chapelle AR, Herva R, Koivisto M, Aula O. A deletion in chromosome 22 can cause DiGeorge syndrome. Hum Genet 1981; 57:253–256.

5. Greenberg F, Elder FFB, Haffner P, Northrup H, Ledbetter DH. Cytogenetic findings in a prospective series of patients with DiGeorge anomaly. Am J Hum Genet 1988; 43:605–611.

6. Shapira M, Borochowitz Z, Bar-El H, Dar H, Etzioni A, Lorber A. Deletion of the short arm of chromosome 10 (10p13): report of a patient and review. Am J Med Genet 1994; 52:34–38.

7. Driscoll DA, Budarf ML, Emanuel BS. A genetic etiology for DiGeorge syndrome: consistent deletions and microdeletions of 22q11. Am J Hum Genet 1992; 50:924–933.

8. Driscoll DA, Salvin J, Sellinger B, Budarf ML, McDonald-McGinn DM, Zackai EH, and Emanuel BS. Prevalence of 22q11 microdeletions in DiGeorge and velocardiofacial syndromes: implications for genetic counselling and prenatal diagnosis. J Med Genet 1993; 30:813–817.

9. Carey AH, Kelly D, Halford S, Wadey R, Wilson, D, Goodship J, Burn J, Paul T, Sharkey A, Dumanski J, Nordenskjold M, Williamson R, Scambler PJ. Molecular genetic study of the frequency of monosomy 22q11 in DiGeorge syndrome. Am J Hum Genet 1992; 51:964–970.

10. Demczuk S, Desmaze C, Aikem M, Prieur M, Ledeist F, Sanson, M, Rouleau G, Thomas G, Aurias A. Molecular cytogenetic analysis of a series of 23 DiGeorge syndrome patients by fluorescence in situ hybridization. Ann Genet 1994; 37:60–65.

11. Desmaze C, Prieu, M, Amblard F, Aikem M, LeDeist F, Demczuk S, Zucman J, Plougastel B, Delattre O, Croquette M-F, Breviere G-M, Huon C, Le Merrer M, Mathieu M, Sidi D, Stephan J-L, Aurias A. Physical mapping by FISH of the DiGeorge critical region (DGCR): involvement of the region in familial cases. Am J Hum Genet 1993; 53:1239–1249.

12. Augusseau S, Jouk S, Jalber, P, Prieur, M. (1986). DiGeorge syndrome and 22q11 rearrangements. Hum Genet 1986; 74:206.

13. Budarf ML, Collins J, Gong W, Roe B, Wang Z, Bailey LC, Sellinger B, Michaud D, Driscoll DA, Emanual BS. Cloning a balanced translocation associated with DiGeorge syndrome and identification of a disrupted candidate gene. Nature Genet 1995; 10:269–278.

14. Demczuk S, Aledo R, Zucman J, Delattre O, Desmaze C, Dauphinot L, Jalbert P, Rouleau GA, Thomas G, Aurias A. Cloning of a balanced translocation breakpoint in the DiGeorge syndrome critical region and isolation of a novel potential adhesion receptor gene in its vicinity. Hum Mol Genet 1995; 4:451–458.

15. Shprintzen RJ, Goldberg RB, Lewin ML, Sidoti EJ, Berkman MD, Argamaso, RV, Young, D. A new syndrome involving cleft palate, cardiac anomalies, typical facies, and learning disabilities: velo-cardio-facial syndrome. Cleft Palate J 1978; 15:56–62.

16. Goldberg, R, Motzkin B, Marion R, Scambler PJ, Shprintzen RJ. Velo-cardio-facial syndrome: a review of 120 patients. Am J Med Genet 1993; 45:313–319.

17. Young D, Shprintzen RJ, and Goldberg RB. Cardiac malformations in the velo-cardio-facial syndrome. Am J Cardio 1980; 46:43–48.

18. Driscoll DA, Spinner, NB, Budarf ML, Mcdonald-McGinn DM, Zackai EH, Goldberg RB, Shprintzen RJ, Sall HM, Zonana J, Jones MC, Mascarello, JT, Emanuel BS. Deletions and microdeletions of 22q11.2 in velo-cardio-facial syndrome. Am J Med Genet 1992; 44:261–268.

19. Kelly D, Goldberg R, Wilson D, Lindsay E, Carey A, Goodship J, Burn J, Cross I, Shprintzen RJ, Scambler PJ. Confirmation that the velo-cardio-facial syndrome is associated with haplo-insufficiency of genes at chromosome 22q11. Am J Med Genet 1993; 45:308–312.

20. Scambler PJ, Kelley D, Lindsay E, Williamson R, Goldberg R, Shprintzen R, Wilson DI, Goodship JA, Cross IE, Burn, J. Velo-cardio-facial syndrome associated with chromosome 22 deletions encompassing the DiGeorge locus. Lancet 1992; 339:1138–1139.

21. Holder SE, Winter RM, Kamath S, Scambler PJ. Velocardiofacial syndrome in a mother and daughter: variability of the clinical phenotype. J Med Genet 1993; 30:825–827.

22. Wilson DI, Goodship JA, Burn J, Cross IE, Scambler PJ. Deletions within chromosome 22q11 in familial congenital heart disease. Lancet 1992; 340:573–575.

23. Goldmuntz E, Driscoll D, Budarf ML, Zackai EH, McDonald-McGinn DM, Biegel JA, Emanuel BS. Microdeletions of chromosomal region 22q11 in patients with congenital conotruncal cardiac defects. J Med Genet 1993; 30:807–812.

24. Johnson MC, Watson MS, Strauss AW. Deletions in chromosome 22: a common cause of conotruncal and aortic arch defects. J Am Coll Cardiol 1995; 351A.

25. Webber SA, Hatchwell E, Barber JCK, Crolla JA, Salmon AP, Keeton BR, Dennis NR, Temple IK. Importance of microdeletions of chromosomal region 22q11 in the etiology of congenital conotruncal malformations: a 2 year prospective study. J Am Coll Cardiol 1995; 271A.

26. Morrow B, Goldberg R, Carlson C, Gupta RD, Sirotkin H, Collins J, Dunham I, O'Donnell H, Scambler P, Shprintzen R, Kucherlapati R. Molecular definition of the 22q11 deletions in velo-cardiac-facial syndrome. Am J Hum Genet 1995; 56:1391–1403.

27. Tandon R, and Edwards JE. Cardiac malformation associated with Down's syndrome. Circulation 1973; 47:1349–1355.

28. Carmi R, Boughman JA, Ferencz C. Endocardial cushion defect: further studies of 'isolated' versus 'syndromic' occurrence. Am J Med Genet 1992; 43:569–575.

29. Korenberg JR, Bradley C, Disteche CM. Down syndrome: molecular mapping of the congenital heart disease and duodenal stenosis. Am J Hum Genet 1992; 50:294–302.

30. Korenberg JR, Chen X-N, Schipper R, Sun Z, Gonsky R, Gerwehr S, Carpenter N, Daumer C, Dignan P, Distech C, Graham JMJ, Hugdins L, McGillivray B, Miyazaki K, Ogasawara N, Park JP, Pagon R, Pueschel S, Sack G, Say B, Schuffenhauer S, Soukup S, Yamanaka T. Down syndrome phenotypes: the consequences of chromosomal imbalance. Proc Natl Acad Sci USA 1994; 91:4997–5001.

31. Duff K, Williamson R, Richards SJ. Expression of genes encoding 2 chains of

the collagen type VI molecule during human fetal heart development. Int J Cardiol 1990; 27:128–129.

32. Davies GE, Howard CM, Gorman LM, Farrer MJ, Holland AJ, Williamson R, Kessling AM. Polymorphisms and linkage disequilibrium in the COL6A1 and COL6A2 gene cluster: novel DNA polymorphisms in the region of a candidate gene for congenital heart defects in Down's syndrome. Hum Genet 1993; 90:521–525.

33. Davies GE, Howard CM, Farrer MJ, Coleman MM, Cullen LM, Williamson R, Wyse RKH, Kessling AM. Unusual genotypes in the COL6A1 gene in parents of children with trisomy 21 and major congenital heart defects. Hum Genet 1994; 93:443–446.

34. Emanuel R, Somerville J, Inns A, Withers A. Evidence of congenital heart disease in the ofspring of parents with atrioventricular defects. Br Heart J 1983; 49:144–147.

35. Burn J, Coffey R, Little J, Pembrey M, Somerville J, Dennis N, Keeton B. Recurrence risks in the offspring of adults born with major heart defects: first results of a British collaborative study. Am J Hum Genet 1990; 47:A121.

36. Wilson L, Curtis A, Korenberg JR, Schipper RD, Allan L, Chenevix-Trench G, Stephenson A, Goodship J, Burn J. A large, dominant pedigree of atrioventricular septal defect (AVSD): exclusion from the Down sydnrome critical region on chromosome 21. Am J Hum Genet 1993; 53:1262–1268.

37. Cousineau AJ, Lauer RM, Pierpont ME, Burns TL, Ardinger RH, Patil ER, Sheffield VC. Linkage analysis of autosomal dominant atrioventricular canal defects: exclusion of chromosome 21. Hum Genet 1994; 93:103–108.

38. Gennarelli M, Novelli G, Digilio MC, Giannotti A, Marino B, Dallapiccola B. Exclusion of linkage with chromosome 21 in families with recurrence of non-Down's atrioventricular canal. (Letter) Hum Genet 1994; 94:708–710.

39. Williams JC, Baratt-Boyes BG, Lowe JB. Supravalvular aortic stenosis. Circulation 1961; 24:1311–1318.

40. Ewart AK, Morris CA, Ensing GJ, Loker J, Moore C, Leppert M, Keating M. A human vascular disorder, supravalvular aortic stenosis, maps to chromosome 7. Proc Natl Acad Sci USA 1993; 90:3226–3230.

41. Olson TM, Michels VV, Lindor N, Pastores G, Weber J, Schaid D, Driscoll D, Feldt R, Thibodeau S. Autosomal dominant supravalvular aortic stenosis: localization to chromosome 7. Hum Mol Genet 1993; 2:869–873.

42. Morris CA, Loker J, Ensing G, Stock AD. Supravalvular aortic stenosis cosegregates with a familial 6;7 translocation which disrupts the elastin gene. Am J Med Genet 1993; 46:737–744.

43. Curran ME, Atkinson DL, Ewart AK, Morris CA, Leppert MF, Keating MT. The elastin gene is disrupted by a translocation associated with supravalvular aortic stenosis. Cell 1993; 73:159–168.

44. Ewart AK, Jin W, Atkinson D, Morris CA, Keating MT. Supravalvular aortic stenosis associated with a deletion disrupting the elastin gene. J Clin Invest 1994; 93:1071–1077.

45. Ewart AK, Morris CA, Atkinson D, Jin W, Sternes K, Spallone P, Stock AD, Leppert M, Keating MT. Hemizygosity at the elastin locus in a developmental disorder, Williams syndrome. Nature Genet 1993; 5:11–16.

46. Lowery MC, Morris CA, Ewart A, Brothman LJ, Zhu XL, Leonard CO, Carey JC, Keating M, Brothman AR. Strong correlation of elastin deletions, detected by FISH, with Williams syndrome: evaluation of 235 patients. Am J Hum Genet 1995; 57:49–53.

47. Keating MT. Genetic approaches to cardiovascular disease: supravalvular aortic stenosis, Williams syndrome, and long-QT syndrome. Circulation 1995; 92:142–147.

48. Holt M, Oram S. Familial heart disease with skeletal malformations. Br Heart J 1960; 22:236–242.

49. Hurst JA, Hall CM, Baraitser M. The Holt-Oram syndrome. J Med Genet 1991; 28:406–410.

50. Rybak M, Kozlowski K, Kleczkowsha A, Lewandowska J, Sololowski J, Soltysik-Wilk E. Holt-Oram syndrome associated with ectromelia and chromosomal aberrations. Am J Dis Child 1971; 121:490–495.

51. Turleau C, de Grouchy J, Chavin-Colin F, Dore F, Seger J, Dautzenberg M-D, Arthuis M, Jeanson C. Two patients with interstitial del (14q), one with features of Holt-Oram syndrome: exclusion mapping of PI (alpha-1-antitrypsin). Ann Genet 1984; 27:237–240.

52. Yang SP, Sherman S, Derstine JB, Schonberg SA. Holt-Oram syndrome gene may be on chromosome 20. Pediatr Res 1990; 27:137A.

53. Ruiz JC, Legius E, Cuppens H, Moens P, Marynen P, Cassiman J-J. Exclusion of linkage to 14q23-24 in a family with Holt-Oram syndrome. Clin Genet 1995; 46:257–259.

54. Bonnet D, Pelet A, Legeai-Mallet L, Sidi D, Mathieu M, Parnet P, Plauchu H, Serville F, Schinzel A, Weissenbach J, Kachaner J, Munnich A, Lyonnet S. A gene for Holt-Oram syndrome maps to the distal long arm of chromosome 12. Nature Genet 1994; 6:405–408.

55. Basson CT, Cowley GS, Solomon SD, Weissman B, Poznanski AK, Traill TA, Seidman JG, Seidman CE. The clinical and genetic spectrum of the Holt-Oram syndrome (heart-hand syndrome). N Engl J Med 1994; 330:885–891.

56. Noonan JA. Hypertelorism with Turner phenotype. A new syndrome with associated congenital heart disease. Am J Dis Child, 1968; 116:373–380.

57. Jamieson CR, van der Burgt I, Brady AF, van Reen M, Elsawi MM, Hol F, Jeffrey S, Patton MA, Mariman E. Mapping a gene for Noonan syndrome to the long arm of chromosome 12. Nature Genet 1994; 8:357–360.

58. Watson GH. Pulmonary stenosis, cafe-au-lait spots, and dull intelligence. Arch Dis Child 1967; 42:303–307.

59. Allanson JE, Hall JG, Van Allen MI. Noonan phenotype associated with neurofibromatosis. Am J Med Genet 1985; 21:457–462.

60. Opitz JM, Weaver DD. The neurofibromatosis-Noonan syndrome. Am J Med Genet 1985; 21:477–490.

61. Allanson JE, Upadhyaya M, Watson GH, Partington M, MacKenzie A, Lahey

D, MacLeod H, Sarfarazi M, Broadhead W, Harper PS, Huson SM. Watson syndrome: is it a subtype of type 1 neurofibromatosis. J Med Genet 1991; 28:752–756.

62. Upadhyaya M, Sarfarazi M, Huson S, Broadhead W, Allanson J, Fryer A, Harper PS. Linkage of Watson's syndrome to chromosome 17 markers. J Med Genet 1990; 27:209.

63. Upadhyaya M, Shen M, Cherryson A, Farnham J, Maynard J, Huson SM, Harper P. Analysis of mutations at the neurofibromatosis 1 (NF1) locus. Hum Mol Genet 1992; 1:735–740.

64. Tassabehji M, Strachan T, Sharland M, Colley A, Donnai D, Harris R, Thakker N. Tandem duplication within a neurofibromatosis I (NF1) gene exon in a family with features of Watson syndrome and Noonan syndrome. Am J Hum Genet 1993; 53:90–95.

65. Brannan CI, Perkins AS, Vogel KS, Ratner N, Nordlund ML, Reid S, Buchberg AM, Jenkins NA, Parada LF, Copeland NG. Targeted disruption of the neurofibromatosis type-1 gne leads to developmental abnormalities in heart and various neural crest-derived tissues. Genes Dev 1994; 8:1019–1029.

66. Jacks T, Shih TS, Schmitt EM, Bronson RT, Bernards A, Weinberg RA. Tumour predisposition in mice heterozygous for a targeted mutation in Nf1. Nature Genet. 1994; 7:353–361.

67. Kirby ML, Gale TF, Stewart DE. Neural crest cells contribute to normal aorticopulmonary septation. Science 1983; 220:1059–1061.

68. Huynh DP, Nechiporuk T, Pulst SM. Differential expression and tissue distribution of type I and type II neurofibromins during mouse fetal development. Dev Biol 1994; 161:538–551.

69. Gutmann DH, Andersen LB, Cole JL, Swaroop M, Collins FS. An alternatively-spliced mRNA in the coarboxy terminus of the neurofibromatosis type 1 (NF1) gene is expressed in muscle. Hum Mol Genet 1993; 2:989–992.

70. Bleyl S, Ruttenberg HD, Carey JC, Ward K. Familial total anomalous pulmonary venous return: a large Utah-Idaho family. Am J Med Genet 1994; 54:462–466.

71. Raisher BD, Dowton SB, Grant SW. Father and two children with total anomalous pulmonary venous return. Am J Med Genet 1991; 40:105–106.

72. Bleyl S, Nelson L, Odelberg SJ, Ruttenberg HD, Otterud B, Leppert M, Ward K. A gene for familial total anomalous pulmonary venous return maps to chromosome 4p13-q12. Am J Hum Genet 1995; 56:408–415.

73. Britz-Cunningham SH, Maithili BS, Shah MM, Zuppan CW, Fletcher WH. Mutations of the Onnexin43 gap-junction gene in patients with heart malformations and defects of laterality. N Engl J Med 1995; 332:1323–1329.

74. Reaume AG, de Sousa PA, Kulkarni S, Langille BL, Zhu D, Davies TC, Juneja SC, Kidder GM, Rossant J. Cardiac malformation in neonatal mice lacking connexin43. Science 1995; 267:1831–1834.

75. Casey B, Devoto M, Jones KL, Ballabio A. Mapping a gene for familial situs abnormalities to human chromosome Xq24-q27.1. Nature Genet 1993; 5:403–407.

76. Narayan D, Krishnan SN, Upender M, Ravikumar TS, Mahoney MJ, Dolan TF,

Teebi AS, Haddad GG. Unusual ineritance of primary ciliary dyskinesia (Kartagener's syndrome). J Med Genet 1994; 31:493–496.

77. Narayan D, Desai T, Banks A, Patanjali SR, Ravikumar TS, Ward DC. Localization of the human cytoplasmic dynein heavy chain (DNECL) to 14qter by fluorescence in situ hybridization. Genomics 1994; 22:660–661.

78. Mikami A, Paschal BM, Mazumdar M, Vallee RB. Molecular cloning of the retrograde transport motor cytoplasmic dynein (MAP 1C). Neuron 1993; 10:787–796.

79. Icardo JM, Sanchez de Vega MJ. Spectrum of heart malformations in mice with situs solitus, situs inversus, and associated visceral heterotaxy. Circulation 1991; 84:2547–2558.

80. Brueckner M, D'Eustachio P, Horwich AL. Linkage mapping of a mouse gene, iv, that controls left-right asymmetry of the heart and viscera. Proc Natl Acad Sci USA 1989; 86:5035–5038.

81. Hanzlik AJ, Binder M, Layton WM, Rowe L, Layton M, Taylor BA, Osemlak MM, Richards JE, Kurnit DM, Stewart GD. The murine *situs inversus viscerum* (iv) gene responsible for visceral asymmetry is linked tightly to the Igh-C cluster on chromosome 12. Genomics 1990; 7:389–393.

82. McGrath J, Horwich AL, Brueckner M. Duplication/deficiency mapping of *situs inversus viscerum* (iv), a gene that determines left-right asymmetry in the mouse. Genomics 192; 14:643–648.

83. Singh G, Supp DM, Schreiner C, McNeish J, Merker H-J, Copeland NG, Jenkins NA, Potter SS, Scott W. *Legless* insertional mutation: morphological, molecular, and genetic characterization. Genes Dev 1991; 5:2245–2255.

84. Yokoyama T, Copeland NG, Jenkins NA, Montgomery CA, Elder FFB, Overbeek PA. Reversal of left-right asymmetry: a situs inversus mutation. Science 1993; 260:679–682.

85. Chisaka O, Capecchi MR. Regionally restricted developmental defects resulting from targeted disruption of the mouse homeobox gene *hox*-1.5. Nature 1991; 350:473–483.

86. Kirby ML, Waldo KL. Role of neural crest in CHD. Circulation 1990; 82:332–340.

87. Lints TJ, Parsons LM, Hartley L, Lyons I, Harvey P. Nkx-2.5: a novel murine homeobox gene expressed in early heart progenitor cells and their myogenic descendants. Development 1993; 119:419–431.

88. Komuro I, Izumo S. Csx: a murine homeobox-containing gene specifically expressed in the developing heart. Proc Natl Acad Sci USA 1993; 90:8145–8149.

89. Azpiazu N, Frasch M. *tinman* and *bagpipe*: two homeobox genes that determine cell fates in the dorsal mesoderm of *Drosophila*. Genes Dev 1993; 7:1325–1340.

90. Bodmer R. The gene *tinman* is required for specification of the heart and visceral muscles in *Drosophila*. Development 1993; 118:719–729.

91. Lyons I, Parsons LM, Hartley L, Li R, Andrews JE, Robb L, Harvey RP. Myogenic and morphogenetic defects in the heart tubes of murine embryos lacking the homeobox gene Nkx2-5. Genes Dev 1995; In press.

92. Tassabehji M, Read AP, Newton VE, Patton M, Gruss P, Harris R, Strachen T.

Mutations in PAX3 gene causing Waardenburg syndrome type 1 and type 2. Nature Genet 1993; 3:26–30.

93. Epstein DJ, Vekemans M, Gros P. splotch (Sp2h), a mutation affecting development of the mouse neural tube, shows a deletion within the paired homeodomain of Pax-3. Cell 1991; 67:767–774.

94. Franz T. Persistent truncus arteriosus in the Splotch mutant mouse. Anat Embryol 1989; 180:457–474.

95. Franz T. The splotch (SP1H) and Splotch-delyated (Spd) alleles: differential phenotypic effects on neural crest and limb musculature. Anat. Embryol 1993; 187:371–377.

96. Vogan KJ, Epstein DJ, Trasler DG, Gros P. The splotch-delayed (Spd) mouse mutant carries a point mutation within the paired box of the Pax-3 gene. Genomics 1993; 17:364–369.

97. Moase CE, Trasler DG. N-CAM alterations in splotch neural tube defect mouse embryos. Development 1991; 113:1049–1058.

98. Neale SA, Trasler DG. Early sialylation on N-CAM in splotch neural tube defect mouse embryos. Teratology 1994; 50:118–124.

99. Kastner P, Grondona JM, Mark M, Gansmuller A, LeMeur M, Decimo D, Vonesch J-L, Dolle P, Chambon P. Genetic analysis of RXRa developmental function: convergence of RXR and RAR signaling pathways in heart and eye morphogenesis. Cell 1994; 8:987–1003.

100. Sucov HM, Dyson E, Gumeringer CL, Price J, Chien KR, Evans RM. RXRa mutant mice establish a genetic basis for vitamin A signaling in heart morphogenesis. Genes Dev 1994; 8:1007–1018.

101. Kreidberg JA, Sariola H, Loring JM, Maeda M, Pelletier J, Housman D, Jaenisch R. WT-1 is required for early kidney development. Cell 1993; 74:679–691.

102. Kato K, Kanamori A, Wakamatsu Y, Sawai S, Kondos H. Tissue distribution of N-myc expression in the early organogenesis period of the mouse embryo. Dev Growth Differ 1991; 33:29–36.

103. Moens CB, Stanton BR, Parada LF, Rossant J. Defects in heart and lung development in compound heterozygotes for two different targeted mutations at the N-myc locus. Development 1993; 119:485–499.

104. Moens CB, Auerbach AB, Conlon RA, Joyner AL, Rossant J. A targeted mutation reveals a role for N-myc in branching morphogenesis in the embryonic mouse lung. Genes Dev 1992; 6:691–704.

105. Sawai S, Shimono A, Wakamatsu Y, Palmes C, Hanaoka K, Kondoh H. Defects of embryonic organogenesis resulting from targeted disruption of the N-myc gene in the mouse. Development 1993; 117:1445–1455.

106. Charron J, Malynn BA, Fisher P, Stewart V, Jeannotte L, Goff SP, Robertson EJ, Alt FW. Embryonic lethality in mice homozygous for a targeted disruption of the N-myc gene. Genes Dev 1992; 6:2248–2257.

107. Chen Z, Friedrich GA, Soriano P. Trascriptional enhancer factor 1 disruption by a retroviral gene trap leads to heart defects and embryonic lethality in mice. Genes Dev 1994; 8:2293–2301.

108. Stephenson DA, Mercola M, Anderson E, Wang C, Stiles CD, Bowen-Pope DF,

Chapman VM. The platelet-derived growth factor receptor alpha subunit gene is deleted in the mouse mutation patch (PH). Proc Natl Acad Sci USA 1991; 88:6–10.

109. Schatteman GC, Morrison-Graham K, Weston JA, Bowen-Pope DF. PDGF receptor alpha-subunit expression during mouse development: pattern of expression and consequences of gene disruption. Development 1992; 115:123–131.

110. Soriano P. Abnormal kidney development and hematological disorders in PDGF beta-receptor mutant mice. Genes Develop 1994; 8:

111. Leveen P, Pekny M, Gebre-Medhin S, Swolin B, Larsson E, Betsholtz C. Mice deficient for PDGF B show renal, cardiovascular, and hematological abnormalities. Genes Dev 1994; 8:1875–1887.

112. Lau MMH, Stewart CEH, Liu Z, Bhatt H, Rotwein P, Stewart CL. Loss of the imprinted IFG2/cation-independent mannose 6-phosphate receptor results in fetal overgrowth and perinatal lethality. Genes Dev 1994; 8:2953–2963.

113. Kwee L, Baldwin HS, Shen HM, Stewart CL, Buck C, Buck CA, Labow MA. Defective development of the embryonic and extraembryonic circulatory systems in vascular cell adhesion molecule (VCAM-1) deficient mice. Development 1995; 121:489–503.

114. Gurtner GC, Davis V, Li H, McCoy MJ, Sharpe A, and Cybulsky MI. Targeted disrution of the murine *VCAM1* gene: essential role of VCAM-1 in chorioallantoic fusion and placentation. Genes Dev 1995; 9:1–14.

115. Yang JT, Rayburn H, Hynes RO. Cell adhesion events mediated by alpha4 integrins are essential in placental and cardiac development. Development 1995; 121:549–560.

116. Hynes RO. Fibronectins. New York: Springer-Verlag, 1990.

117. Ffrench-Constant C, Hynes RO. Patterns of fibronectin gene expression and splicing during cell migration in chicken embryos. Development 1988; 104:369–382.

118. Linask KK, Lash JW. A role for fibronectin in the migration of avian precardiac cell. I. Dose-dependent effects of fibronectin antibody. Dev Biol 1988; 129:315–323.

119. George EL, Georges-Labouesse EN, Patel-King RS, Rayburn H, Hynes RO. Defects in mesoderm, neural tube and vascular development in mouse embryos lacking fibronectin. Development 1993; 119:1079–1091.

7

Molecular Biology of Nitric Oxide Synthases

Thomas Michel and Kazuhiro Sase
Brigham and Women's Hospital and Harvard Medical School
Boston, Massachusetts

Santiago Lamas
Center for Biological Investigations
Madrid, Spain

Organic nitrate vasodilator drugs have been in clinical use for more than a century. these drugs, which include such important cardiovascular agents as nitroglycerin, isosorbide dinitrate, and sodium nitroprusside, are metabolized to form nitric oxide (NO) by poorly understood enzymatic and nonenzymatic pathways. NO is a free radical gas, highly lipophilic and chemically reactive, and can form stable adducts with diverse chemical moieties (reviewed in ref. 34). For example, NO can interact with reduced thiol groups to form nitrosothiol compounds with distinct biological properties (79), or may react with superoxide to form the highly reactive peroxynitrite anion (7). The NO formed from organic nitrate vasodilators leads to characteristic pharmacological effects in diverse target tissues (reviewed in ref. 56). An important molecular target of NO is the soluble isoform of guanylate cyclase, a heterodimeric hemoprotein expressed in many tissues, including vascular smooth muscle cells, blood platelets, and cardiac myocytes. In vascular smooth muscle cells, guanylate cyclase activation, and the consequent rise in intracellular cyclic GMP, leads to vasorelaxation. Nonvascular smooth muscle, including smooth muscle cells in the gut and lung, also relaxes in response to NO formed from organic nitrate vasodilator drugs. In blood platelets, guanylate cyclase activation leads to an inhibition of platelet aggregation. The organic nitrate vasodilator drugs elicit important pharmacological responses in diverse tissues.

The presence in numerous tissues of molecular targets responding to NO metabolized from exogenously administered drugs suggested that endogenous pathways might exist that are modulated by NO-dependent signaling. However, only in the past decade was the endogenous synthesis of nitric oxide documented in mammalian cells (reviewed in 59, 60). Over the past 5 years, a family of mammalian nitric oxide synthases was purified, cloned, and characterized at the molecular level. This chapter will review recent advances in understanding the structural and regulatory features of the NO synthase isoforms.

NO SYNTHASE ISOFORMS

In mammalian cells, NO production is catalyzed by a ubiquitous family of nitric oxide synthases that share similar calmodulin-dependent catalytic mechanisms to oxidize the amino acid L-arginine to form NO and citrulline (34, 45, 49, 59, 60). Three distinct isoforms of NOS have been identified by protein purification and molecular cloning approaches: the neural (nNOS or NOS1), inducible (iNOS or NOS2), and endothelial (eNOS or NOS3) isozymes. The NOS isoforms share significant sequence similarity and contain conserved putative cofactor binding sites, yet there are important differences between the isoforms in their cellular and molecular regulation. These isoforms, each products of distinct genes located on different human chromosomes, demonstrate a characteristics pattern of tissue-specific expression (see Table 1). The nNOS was originally purified from cerebellum and cloned from a brain cDNA library (12), but subsequently was found to be expressed also in skeletal muscle (58) and pulmonary epithelium (3). The iNOS, originally purified and cloned (44, 47, 94) from a macrophage cell line, is expressed following immunoactivation of a wide variety of cells and tissues (cf. 5, 19, 27, 60). The eNOS was originally purified (64) and cloned (35, 39, 61, 74) from vascular endothelium, but has since been discovered in renal (81) and pulmonary epithelium (76), cardiac myocytes (6), brain (26), and blood platelets (71).

The roles of all three NOS isoforms in cardiovascular regulation have been explored, using a variety of experimental approaches; this chapter will focus on the transcriptional, translational and postranslational control mechanisms involved in NOS regulation. The isolation and characterization of cDNA and genomic clones encoding these three archetypal NOS isoforms have led to development of reagents and experimental approaches that have uncovered novel structural and regulatory features of this gene family.

Table 1 Tissue Distribution of NOS Isoforms

Neuronal NOS (nNOS, NOS1)	Inducible NOS (iNOS, NOS2)	Endothelial NOS (eNOS, NOS3)
Brain	Macrophages	Vascular endothelium
Peripheral nerves	Microvascular endothelium	Brain (hippocampus)
Skeletal muscle	Epithelial cells	Blood platelets
Pulmonary epithelium	Mesangial cells	Cardiac myocytes
	Vascular smooth muscle	Renal epithelium
	Hepatocytes	Pulmonary epithelium
	Cardiac myocytes	
	Glial cells	
	Others	

TRANSCRIPTIONAL REGULATION OF NO SYNTHASES

All three NOS isoforms undergo transcriptional regulation, but there are important differences in modulation of transcription between the different isoforms. Original formulations contrasted the different NOS isoforms isolated in brain (or endothelium) vs. macrophage as being "constitutive" or "inducible," but it is now clear that the cellular synthesis of all three archetypal enzyme isoforms may be dynamically regulated. Furthermore, for a given NOS isoform, there may be important differences in transcriptional regulation among the different tissues in which the isoform is expressed.

Neuronal NOS (nNOS, NOS1)

A detailed understanding of nNOS transcriptional regulation has been hampered by the complexity of its promoter organization (28, 87, 93), and is further stymied by the challenges of studying cell-specific gene expression in neuronal tissues. At least two closely linked but distinct nNOS promoter regions have been identified (93), each of which is coupled to distinct upstream transcription start sites spliced to a common exon 2 (see Table 2). Recently, additional nNOS upstream exons were identified in an analysis of cDNAs isolated from human hippocampus (Sase and Michel, unpublished observations). Studies of the structural organization of the human gene for neuronal nitric oxide synthase gene (NOS1) show that the gene spans a region over 200 kilobases (kb), and the putative promoter regions contain consensus sequences encoding functional domains that may be involved in the binding of several transcription factors (28, 93). Transcriptional heterogeneity might form the basis for differential tissue-

Table 2   Organization of Human NOS Genes

	Neural (nnOS, NOS1)	Macrophage (iNOS, NOS2)	Endothelial (eNOS, NOS3)
Human chromosome	12	17	7
Promoter features			
TATA box	? (multiple transcription start sites)	yes	no
Upstream intron: (putative) cis-reg-	yes	yes	no
ulatory sequences:	(numerous)	NF-κB (AP-1) (TNF-RE) IRF-1 others	SP-1 (GATA) (SSRE) (hp-ERE) (NF-1)

specific and developmental expression patterns, as a consequence of alternative promoter usage coupled with cell-specific *trans*-acting transcription factors.

Inducible NOS (iNOS, NOS2)

Transcriptional control mechanisms form an important basis for cellular regulation of iNOS (44, 47,94). Recent evidence suggests the existence of several highly similar and closely linked human iNOS genes (9,53), but it remains to be established that these iNOS-like genes are expressed; further details of the transcriptional regulation of these closely linked genes are not yet available. Analysis of the promoter region of the mouse iNOS gene promoter (46,96) led to the characterization of two major 5' flanking regulatory regions, one LPS-sensitive and the other IFN-γ sensitive, the latter possessing functional characteristics of an enhancer. The LPS-sensitive region contains a binding site for the transcription factor NF-κB, a factor implicated in the activation of diverse genes activated in the inflammatory response. Xie et al. have shown that NF-κB/rel participates in the transcriptional regulation of iNOS in macrophages (95). Analysis of the corresponding 5' flanking regulatory region in the human iNOS gene has not yet been reported, although there is significant nucleotide sequence similarity of the human and mouse promoters (20). A large and growing number of cell types are being discovered to express iNOS under different conditions of gene induction (see Table 1). It has recently been found that iNOS may be expressed in tissues or cells under physiological conditions, without any known exposure to immunoactivating stimuli (54), suggesting that iNOS may be subserving a physiological role in some tissues. As for nNOS,

transcription of the iNOS gene appears to involve several alternative first exons (22); Sase and Michel, unpublished observations), which may play a role
in the tissue-specific expression of iNOS.

As new roles for previously identified cytokines are being identified, and
new cytokines are isolated, it is increasingly clear that cytokine regulation of
iNOS is complexly determined. For example, interleukins 4, 8, and 10, transforming growth factors, epidermal growth factor, fibroblast growth factors,
insulinlike growth factor-1, macrophage deactivating factor, macrophage stimulating protein, platelet-derived growth factor, osteopontin, and dexamethasone
have been found to inhibit NO synthesis induced in different species and cell
types. (10,41). Few studies have addressed the mechanisms responsible for
negative modulation of the abundance of the iNOS transcript. Vodovotz et al.
showed that TGF-β suppresses iNOS mRNA and protein abundance in a macrophage cell line by posttranscriptional mechanisms (84). However, in vascular smooth muscle cells, iNOS induction may be suppressed at a transcriptional
level (63). In addition to regulation by cytokines, it is becoming increasingly
clear that certain antioxidant molecules, such as pirrolidine dithiocarbamate
(PDTC), as well as the lymphokine, interleukin-13, also inhibit expression of
the iNOS gene in mesangial cells (40,72), quite possibly by inhibiting the activation of NF-κB. The use of alternative first noncoding exons, documented
for iNOS transcripts, may also represent another level of complexity in iNOS
transcriptional regulation (22). Mechanistic insight into these observations will
likely derive from characterizations of the iNOS promoter in different cell types
now underway.

Endothelial NOS (eNOS, NOS3)

Characterization of the 5' flanking regulatory region of human eNOS (50,67)
revealed the presence of a TATA-less promoter together with the identification
of consensus sequences that could serve as potential sites of binding to a significant number of transcription factors, including SP-1 and GATA sites (see
Table 2). However, detailed functional characterizations of this region have not
yet been published. Hemodynamic shear-stress and chronic exercise are among
the stimuli associated with an increased abundance of the eNOS transcript
(4,61,75), but the mechanisms remain obscure. Consensus sequences present
in the eNOS 5' flanking region may represent cis-regulatory elements responsive to shear stress (shear stress response elements [SSRE]. Acute phase reac-
tants, AP-1, AP-2, and NF-1 among others (50,67,83) may provide the means
for transcriptional regulation of the eNOS gene in response to physiological or
pathophysiological perturbations. eNOS transcript abundance in endothelial cells
does not appear to be importantly regulated by cyclic GMP, NOS inhibitors,
NO donor drugs, or reduced thiols (Lamas and Michel, unpublished observa-

tions). However, cytokines such as TNF-α are associated with a decrease in eNOS message and protein abundance in aortic endothelial cells while, paradoxically, NO synthesis increases (38,39). The TNF-α-induced decrease in the abundance of the eNOS mRNA in bovine aortic endothelial cells appears to be secondary to a decrease in eNOS mRNA stability (98), yet there is no evidence for induction of iNOS under these conditions. Alternative use of polyadenylation sites located in the 3' untranslated region of the eNOS mRNA (Sase and Michel, unpublished observations) may influence the differential stability or targeting of eNOS transcripts.

The TNF-α-induced increase in cellular NO production may reflect the activation by TNF-α of pathways for the increased cellular synthesis of tetrahydrobiopterin, a key cofactor for enzymatic production of NO (70,98). several groups have documented iNOS induction upon cytokine exposure in microvascular endothelial cells or in rat aortic endothelial cells (5,8,80), thereby showing the differential expression of NOS isoforms in endothelial cells depending upon cell source and species of origin.

The availability of eNOS cDNA probes has facilitated numerous, occasionally contradictory, lines of investigation into the influence of diverse experimental conditions on the abundance of the eNOS transcript. For example, hypoxia may be a determinant of eNOS expression in cultured endothelial cells, causing a decrease in steady-state eNOS transcript levels associated with a decease in eNOS mRNA stability (51). By contrast, chronic hypoxia in animal models is associated with an increase in eNOS expression (78). An important recent observation is that the expression of eNOS in cultured endothelial cells is profoundly influenced by cell proliferation: transcript and protein abundance diminishes significantly when cells reach confluence (2). Thus, any factors that secondarily influence endothelial cell growth rate may confound the interpretation of primary effects on eNOS gene expression. Among many other perturbations, sex steroids (30, 92) or lipoproteins (cf. 42) may also influence the abundance of the eNOS transcript; the former effects may reflect the presence in the human eNOS gene of several half-palindromic estrogen response elements (hpERE). The nature, magnitude, and physiological relevance of these and other manipulations on eNOS transcript abundance continue to be actively investigated. Certainly, any extrapolation from cultured cells to animal models, much less to clinical pathology, must be made with caution.

COVALENT MODIFICATIONS OF NITRIC OXIDE SYNTHASES

Although the regulation of NOS transcript abundance may represent an important determinant of NOS protein abundance, posttranslational regulation is clearly an important point for regulation of NOS function, and serves to identify the different NOS isoforms. As discussed above, the iNOS appears to be regulated primarily at the level of transcription. Once the iNOS protein is synthesized, its enzymatic activity appears to be persistently activated by calmodulin, which remains bound to the enzyme and is fully effective in stimulating iNOS even at low levels of intracellular calcium (21). Although capable of being regulated at the transcriptional level, the endothelial (eNOS) and neural (nNOS) isoforms are usually constitutively expressed in their cells of origin, but are only transiently activated by receptor-mediated increases in intracellular calcium. The transient activation of NOS may thereby integrate signals that affect cellular calcium homeostasis as well as cyclic nucleotide signaling (through guanylate cyclase activation), thereby leading to the transduction of both inter- and intracellular signals (34). All three NOS isoforms thus undergo some form of posttranslational modulation, the role and regulation of which remain under active investigation.

The endothelial nitric oxide synthase (eNOS) is regulated by a complex pattern of covalent modifications, including phosphorylation (52), myristoylation (15,43,65), and palmitoylation (68). All three NOS isoforms have now been shown to be phosphorylated in cell culture (60), yet the nature and functional consequences of phosphorylation remain incompletely understood. N-terminal myristoylation, a key determinant for membrane targeting of eNOS (15,16), is unlikely to take place in either iNOS or nNOS, since the obligate N-terminal consensus sequence (66) is not present in these two isoforms. Palmitoylation, which plays a role in the reversible association of eNOS with cell membranes, has not yet been reported for the other isoforms; other covalent posttranslational modifications of NOS isoforms remain unexplored. The interrelationships among eNOS phosphorylation, palmitoylation, and myristoylation are likely to be important determinants coordinating the NO signaling pathway with other signal transduction systems in the endothelium.

Phosphorylation of NO Synthases

Phosphorylation is an important mechanism for the posttranslational regulation of many key proteins, including hormone receptors, metabolic enzymes, transcription factors, as well as diverse intracellular effector molecules (for review see 37). NOS phosphorylation has been explored in several studies, yet the biological significance of this pathway is not yet well characterized. For example, although the neural isoform of NOS (nNOS) has been shown to be an excellent substrate for a variety of protein kinases in vitro (13,57), the effects of nNOS phosphorylation on enzyme activity remain controversial, and, to date, phosphorylation of nNOS in neurons has not been definitively demonstrated. Phosphorylation of iNOS has been reported (60), but the cellular consequences of this modification have not yet been characterized. Phosphorylation of the NOS isoforms is of particular interest since it would permit crosstalk between NO and other signaling pathways, and may also serve as a modulator of other posttranslational modifications of the nitric oxide synthases.

In intact endothelial cells, the eNOS is reversibly phosphorylated in response to agonists (52), and there is a correlation between enzyme phosphorylation and cytosolic localization, suggesting that eNOS signaling may be regulated by phosphorylation. Treatment of endothelial cells with phorbol esters has also been shown to diminish NO production, suggesting that phosphorylation may inhibit eNOS activity (82); hemodynamic shear stress may also influence eNOS phosphorylation (23). An important clinical correlation may be derived from recent studies by Craven et al., who correlated increased protein kinase C activity with decreased NO production in glomeruli isolated from diabetic rats (24). These investigators further demonstrated that inhibition of PKC restored normal NO production. These findings raise the possibility that changes in eNOS phosphorylation could underlie the alterations in NO signaling observed in diabetic vascular disease, underscoring the importance of investigating this mechanism for eNOS regulation.

Subcellular Localization of Nitric Oxide Synthases

All three NOS isoforms have been found to undergo targeting to specific subcellular organelles. For example, nNOS is targeted to the cytoskeleton of skeletal muscle, and this localization appears to be mediated by protein–protein interactions between nNOS and dystrophin (14). In tissue macrophages, iNOS can be found in a particulate subcellular fraction, but the mechanisms by which this localization is achieved have not yet been clearly delineated (85). The eNOS is predominantly membrane associated (64), but in response to agonists, such as bradykinin, the enzyme undergoes partial redistribution from membrane to cytosol (52). For many signaling proteins, the dynamic regulation of their subcellular distribution represents an important mechanism for cellular regulation (reviewed in 18,66,73,90). For example, in response to specific agonists, protein kinases might migrate from cytosol to plasma membrane or cell nucleus; cell surface receptors may internalize; G proteins can translocate to the cell cytosol. These migrations may serve either to activate or attenuate the cellular signals mediated by these proteins, and, in several instances, are modulated by specific posttranslational modifications, including phosphorylation and acylation. Thus, like other important signaling molecules, including hormone receptors and cellular oncogenes, eNOS shows dynamic regulation of its subcellular localization. The biochemical mechanisms and biological consequences of eNOS translocation are incompletely understood. However, features of eNOS posttranslational modifications show striking parallels with other signaling molecules that similarly undergo subcellular translocations. The subcellular targeting of all three NOS isoforms may play an important role in the biochemical consequences of NO synthesis; for eNOS, this targeting is importantly regulated by enzyme acylation.

Acylation of Nitric Oxide Synthases

eNOS is unique among the NOS isoforms in being modified by N-terminal myristoylation; the cotranslational addition of this 14-carbon saturated fatty acid is necessary for eNOS targeting to the endothelial cell membrane (15,16,43). However, translocation of the enzyme from membrane to cytosol does not result from loss of the myristate moiety: this modification is cotranslational and typically irreversible, precluding its dynamic regulation by agonists (66,73). In addition, the stable membrane association of myristoylated proteins often requires additional hydrophobic or electrostatic interactions in addition to those between myristate and membrane lipids. Reversible posttranslational modifications, such as phosphorylation or palmitoylation, may determine the subcellular localization of myristoylated proteins and provide a mechanism for their regulation.

The observations that eNOS undergoes phosphorylation, and that its phosphorylation is enhanced by agonists that also stimulate dissociation of the enzyme from cell membranes, raised the possibility that phosphorylation of eNOS at the cell membrane triggers its translocation to the cytosol (52). However, a myristoylation-deficient mutant eNOS undergoes phosphorylation despite restriction to the cytosol, suggesting that phosphorylation may be a consequence rather than a cause of eNOS translocation (16). It was subsequently found that eNOS is reversibly palmitoylated (68). Because palmitoylation, unlike myristoylation, is a reversible posttranslational modification (66), it provides a potential mechanism for agonist regulation of eNOS subcellular localization.

Agonist regulation of protein palmitoylation has previously been described for G protein-coupled receptors, such as the β-adrenergic receptor (62). For some peripheral membrane proteins, the loss of palmitate may correlate with protein redistribution to the cytosolic subcellular fraction. Agonists activating G protein α_s appear to stimulate α_s palmitate turnover, specifically accelerating depalmitoylation (55,89,90). There are striking parallels for eNOS: pulse-chase experiments in endothelial cells biosynthethically labeled with [3H]palmitate show that bradykinin treatment promotes eNOS depalmitoylation (68). Loss of the 16-carbon saturated fatty acid palmitate, and its hydrophobic interactions with cell membranes, could be the mechanism for release of eNOS from the membrane and translocation to the cytosol in response to bradykinin.

The palmitoylation of several signaling proteins has been shown to influence their signaling activities as well as their subcellular localization (55,66,88,89). However, important differences have been noted in the regulatory roles of palmitoylation, even among closely related proteins. For example, the β_2 and α_2 adrenergic receptors both undergo palmitoylation, but only for the β_2 receptor was a clear role for palmitoylation in receptor-effector coupling documented to date (36,62). The receptor-mediated processes that regulate reversible palmitoylation of signaling proteins are not well understood, and few enzymes involved in the formation or hydrolysis of palmitoyl–protein thioesters have been extensively characterized. A protein palmitoylthioesterase was recently isolated and cloned from bovine brain (17). This palmitoylthioesterase is expressed in diverse cell types (17) including vascular endothelial cells (Michel and Michel, unpublished observations), but its regulatory characteristics are not fully defined, and its relationship to eNOS palmitoylation is completely unknown. Perhaps eNOS activation itself could influence depalmitoylation by a variety of plausible mechanisms: conformational changes in eNOS associated with calmodulin binding may alter the access or affinity of the thioesterase, or NO production itself may play a role. It has recently been shown that nitric oxide reduces [^{3}H]palmitate labeling of two nerve growth cone-associated proteins (29). NO might regulate palmitoyl thioesterase activity or directly influence eNOS palmitoylation via nitrosothiol formation at the site(s) of palmitoylation; these possibilities represent novel mechanisms for product regulation of an enzyme, and could even be germane to mechanisms of pharmacological nitrate tolerance.

No general consensus sequence for protein palmitoylation has been identified (55,66,90), although some dually acylated G protein a subunits and members of the Src family of tyrosine kinases are palmitoylated at a cysteine residue within a conserved N-terminal sequence: MGCXXS. However, this cysteine-containing N-terminal sequence is not found in any of the currently known NOS isoforms. Palmitoylation of eNOS takes place on two cysteine residues near the protein's N-terminus (Cys-15 and Cys-26) that define a novel motif for protein palmitoylation (69). The two palmitoylated cysteines flank an unusual Gly-Leu repeat ([Gly-Leu]$_5$) not previously described in the molecular biology/protein sequence database; the specific structural determinants of eNOS palmitoylation remain to be defined within this sequence motif. Mutagenesis of the palmitoylation site cysteine residues (to alanine) markedly attenuates the association of eNOS with the particulate subcellular fraction, documenting a key role for this post-translational modification in eNOS targeting (69). The myristoylation-deficient mutant eNOS also fails to undergo palmitoylation (68), plausibly because the mutant is not targeted to the plasma membrane, the presumed site for protein palmitoylation (66). The myristoylation-deficient eNOS is thus de facto an acylation-deficient enzyme, undergoing neither of the fatty acid modifications characteristic of the wild-type eNOS; this acylation-deficient enzyme is entirely cytosolic. The palmitoylation-deficient mutant eNOS still undergoes myristoylation, and, as noted above, its membrane targeting is reduced but not completely abrogated. Dual acylation of eNOS is thus required for efficient membrane localization, with cotranslational N-myristoylation and posttranslational thiopalmitoylation playing key roles in enzyme targeting.

Determining the specific particulate subcellular fraction to which the eNOS is targeted was an elusive goal until recent investigations documented the localization of eNOS in plasmalemmal caveolae (77). Caveolae are small invaginations in the plasma membrane characterized by a distinct lipid composition and by the presence of the transmembrane protein caveolin (reviewed in 1). Caveolae are a prominent feature of the endothelial cell plasma membrane, and may serve as sites for the sequestration of signaling molecules such as receptors, G proteins, and protein kinases. The targeting of eNOS to plasmalemmal caveolae is dependent upon palmitoylation of the protein: the palmitoylation-deficient enzyme, which shows a reduced affinity for the membrane fraction overall, fails entirely to be targeted to caveolae (77). It is plausible that agonist-induced depalmitoylation of eNOS promotes the dissociation of the enzyme from proximity to activating molecules (or substrate or cofactors?) localized in caveolae, and may serve as a feedback mechanism for eNOS activation.

The regulation of eNOS subcellular localization, which is likely to be achieved by the integrated control of palmitoylation and phosphorylation, will probably have important functional consequences. Since NO activates molecular targets outside the endothelial cell, such as the guanylate cyclase in platelets or in vascular smooth muscle, it further seems likely that the intracellular localization of the eNOS could affect the signaling roles of its product. Depalmitoylation and translocation of eNOS could also influence NO signaling in the vasculature by removing the enzyme from proximity to caveolae-localized receptors and/or intracellular effectors, and thereby modulate the response to extracellular signals. Palmitoylation of eNOS may thus represent an important control point for the regulation of NO biological activities in the vascular wall. eNOS expressed in nonendothelial tissues may undergo distinct patterns of covalent modification and subcellular targeting, and it will be important to determine whether similar regulatory pathways maintain for eNOS expression in these tissues. Future experiments to delineate the roles of palmitoylation (if any) and phosphorylation in the regulation of the other NOS isoforms may provide insights into the common and distinct regulatory features of these key enzymes.

Polymorphisms in Human NOS Genes

The central role of nitric oxide in blood pressure homeostasis led to studies testing the hypothesis that polymorphisms in NOS gene expression or abnormalities in NOS cellular regulation may be associated with hypertension. To date, there have been no compelling experimental or population-based studies in support of this hypothesis. Indeed, the eNOS gene fails to show genetic linkage with human hypertension (11); the iNOS gene maps to a region in the rat genome linked to hypertension in SHR rats (25), but disease association, and/ or the relevance of this finding to human disease, has yet to be established. A recent study found an association between polymorphisms in noncoding regions of the human eNOS gene and atherosclerosis in cigarette smokers (86); the significance of this association remains to be established. A polymorphism in the eNOS cDNA sequence, predictive of a conservative amino acid change, was found with higher frequency in a cohort of patients with vasospastic angina than in control patients (97), but the functional consequences of this genetic polymorphism have yet to be clarified. By contrast, the inactivation of specific NOS genes has significant consequences in gene-targeted mice (see below).

Cardiovascular Phenotype of NO Synthase Gene Knockout Mice

All three mammalian NOS isoforms have been inactivated by homologous recombination in mouse embryo-derived stem cells, and stable homozygote mice have been bred in which expression of the individual NOS isoforms is attenuated (31,48,91,32). Detailed characterizations of cardiovascular physiology or cardiac development have not yet been reported for these NOS "knockout" mice, but studies to date have not detected any gross structural changes in the cardiovascular system. The nNOS-deficient mouse (31) shows no evident cardiac abnormalities and has a normal resting blood pressure; these mice were found to have smaller cerebral infarcts after experimental stroke (33) suggesting a role for nNOS in pathophysiology of stroke. The iNOS-deficient mouse (48,91) likewise shows no gross cardiac abnormalities and has a normal resting blood pressure and heart rate. However, after injection with endotoxin, the iNOS-deficient mice show an attenuated hypotensive response, most likely due to the lack of iNOS induction in these animals. The most striking cardiovascular phenotype is seen in the eNOS-deficient mice (32), who demonstrate an elevated resting blood pressure; the resting heart rate is normal and, like the other NOS knockout mice, there are no gross cardiac abnormalities. More detailed pharmacological analyses of the NOS knockout mice are being performed, and may lead to the recognition of novel roles and interactions of the NO pathway in control of cardiovascular function.

REFERENCES

1. Anderson RG. Caveolae: where incoming and outgoing messengers meet. Proc Natl Acad Sci USA 1993; 90:10909-10913.
2. Arnal JF, Yamin J, Dockery S, Harrison DG. Regulation of endothelial nitric oxide synthase mRNA, protein, and activity during cell growth. Am J Physiol 1994; 267:C1381-C1388.
3. Asano K, Chee CBE, Gaston M, Lilly CM, Gerard C, Drazen JM, Stamler JS. Constitutive and inducibe nitric oxide gene expression, regulation and activity in human lung epithelial cells. Proc Natl Acad Sci USA 1994; 91:10089-10093.
4. Awolesi MA, Widmann MD, Sessa WC, Sumpio BE. Cyclic strain increases endothelial nitric oxide synthase activity. Surgery 1994; 116:439-44.
5. Balligand J-L, Ungureanu-Longrois D, Simmons WW, et al. Induction of NO synthase in rat cardiac microvascular endothelial cells by IL-1β and IFN-γ. Am J Physiol 1995; 268:H1293-H1303.
6. Balligand J-L, Kobzick L, Han X, Kaye DM, Belhassen L, O'Hara DS, Kelly RA, Smith TW, Michel T. Nitric oxide-dependent parasympathetic signaling is due to activation of constitutive endothelial nitric oxide synthase (NOS3) in cardiac myocytes. J Biol Chem 1995; 270:14582-14586.
7. Beckman JS, Beckman TW, Chen J, Marshall PA, Freeman BA. Apparent hydroxyl radical production by peroxynitrite: implications for endothelial injury from nitric oxide and superoxide. Proc Natl Acad Sci USA 1990; 87:1620-1624.
8. Bereta M, Bereta J, Georgoff I, Coffman FD, Cohen S, Cohen MC. Methylxanthines and calcium-mobilizing agents inhibit the expression of cytokine-inducible nitric oxide synthase and vascular cell adhesion-molecule-1 in murine microvascular endothelial cells. Exp Cell Res 1994; 212:230-242.
9. Bloch KD, Wolfram JR, Roberts JD, Zapol DG, Lepore JJ, Filippov G, Thomas JE, Brown D, Jacob HJ, Bloch DB. Three members of the nitric oxide synthase II gene family co-localize to human chromosome 17. Genomics 1995; 27:526-530.
10. Bogden C, Röllinghoff M, Vodovotz Y, Xie Q-W, Nathan C. Regulation of inducible nitric oxide synthase in macrophages by cytokines and microbial products. In: Mashihi N, ed. Immunotherapy of Infections. New York: Marcel Dekker, 1994:37-54.
11. Bonnardeaux A, Nadaud S, Charru A, Jeunemaitre X, Corvol P, Soubrief F. Lack of evidence for linkage of the encothelial cell nitric oxide synthase gene to essential hypertension. Circulation 1995; 91:96-102.
12. Bredt DS, Hwang PW, Glatt CE, Lowenstein C, Reed RR, Snyder SH. Cloned and expressed nitric oxide synthase structurally resembles cytochrome P-450 reductase. Nature 1991; 351:714-718.
13. Bredt DS, Ferris CD, Snyder SH. Nitric oxide synthase regulatory sites. J Biol Chem 1992; 267:10976-10981.
14. Brenman JE, Chao DS, Xia H, Aldape K, Bredt DS. Nitric oxide synthase complexed with dystrophin and absent from skeletal muscle sarcolemma in Duchenne muscular dystrophy. Cell 1995; 82: 743-752.
15. Busconi L, Michel T. Endothelial nitric oxide synthase: N-terminal myristoylation determines subcellular localization. J Biol Chem 1993; 268:8410-8413.

16. Busconi L, Michel T. Endothelial nitric oxide synthase membrane targeting: evidence against involvement of a specific myristate receptor. J Biol Chem 1994; 269:25016–25020.

17. Camp LA, Verkruyse LA, Afendis SJ, Slaughter CA, Hofmann SL. Molecular cloning and expression of palmitoyl-protein thioesterase. J Biol Chem 1994; 269:23212–23219.

18. Casey PJ. Lipid modifications of G-proteins. Curr Opin Cell Biol 1994; 6:219–225.

19. Charles IG, Palmer RMJ, Hickery MS, Bayliss MT, Chubb AP, Hall VS, Moss DW, Moncada S. Cloning, characterization and expression of a cDNA encoding an inducible nitric oxide synthase from the human chondrocyte. Proc Natl Acad Sci USA 1993; 90:11419–11423.

20. Chartrain NA, Geller DA, Koty PP, et al. Molecular cloning, structure, and chromosomal localization of the human inducible nitric oxide synthase gene. J Biol Chem 1994; 269:6765–6772.

21. Cho HJ, Xie QW, Calayca J, Mumford RA, Swiderek KM, Lee TD, Nathan C. Calmodulin is a subunit of nitric oxide synthase from macrophages. J Exp Med 1992; 176:599–604.

22. Chu SC, Wu H-P, Banks TC, Eissa T, Moss J. Structural diversity in the 5′-untranslated region of cytokine-stimulated human inducible nitric oxide synthase mRNA. J Biol Chem 1995; 270:10625–10630.

23. Corson MA, Berk BC, Navas J-P, Harrison DG. Phosphorylation of endothelial nitric oxide synthase in response to shear stress. Circulation (Supplement) 1993; 88:A0977.

24. Craven PA, Studer RK, DeRubertis FR. Impaired nitric oxide-dependent cyclic guanosine monophosphate generation in glomeruli from diabetic rats. J Clin Invest 1994; 93:311–320.

25. Deng AY, Rapp JP. Locus for inducible, but not a constitutive, nitric oxide synthase cosegregates with blood pressure in the Dahl salt-sensitive rat. J Clin Invest 1995; 95:2170–2177.

26. Dinerman JL, Dawson TM, Schell MJ, Snowman A, Snyder SH. Endothelial nitric oxide synthase localized to hippocampal pyramidal cells: implications for synaptic plasticity. Proc Natl Acad Sci USA 1994; 91:4214–4218.

27. Geller DA, Lowenstein CH, Shapiro RA, Nussler AK, Di Silvio M. Wang SC, Nakayama Dk, Simmons RL, Snyder SH, Billiar TR. Molecular cloning and expression of inducible nitric oxide synthase from human hepatocytes. Proc Natl Acad Sci USA 1993; 90:3491–3495.

28. Hall AV, Antoniou H, Wang Y, et al. Structural organization of the human neuronal nitric oxide synthase gene (NOS1). J Biol Chem 1995; 269:33082–33090.

29. Hess DT, Patterson SI, Smith DS, Pate Skene JH. Neuronal growth cone collapse and inhibition of protein fatty acylation by nitric oxide. Nature. 1993; 366:562–565.

30. Hishikawa K, Nakaki T, Marumo T, Suzuki H, Kato R, Saruta T. Up-regulation of nitric oxide synthase by estradiol in human aortic endothelial cells. FEBS Lett. 1995; 369:291–93.

31. Huang PL, Dawson TM, Bredt DS, Snyder SH, Fishman MC. Targeted disruption of the neuronal nitric oxide synthase gene. Cell 1993; 75:1273–1286.

32. Huang PL, Huang Z, Mashimo H, et al. Hypertension in mice lacking the gene for endothelial nitric oxide synthase. Nature 1995; 377:239–242.

33. Huang Z, Huang PL, Panahian N, Dalkara T, Fishman MC. Effects of cerebral ischemia in mice deficient in neuronal nitric oxide synthase gene. Science 1994; 265:1883–1885.

34. Ignarro LJ. Biosynthesis and metabolism of endothelium-derived nitric oxide. Annu Rev Pharmacol Toxicol 1990; 30:535–560.

35. Janssens SP, Shimouchi A, Quertermous T, Bloch DB, Bloch KD. Cloning and expression of a cDNA encoding human endothelium-derived relaxing factor/nitric oxide synthase. J Biol Chem 1992; 267:14519–14522.

36. Kennedy ME, Limbird LE. Mutations of the α2A-adrenergic receptor that eliminate detectable palmitoylation do not perturb receptor-G-protein coupling. J Biol Chem 1993; 268:8003–8011.

37. Krebs E. Phosphorylation-dephosphorylation of enzymes. Annu Rev Biochem 1979; 48:923–59.

38. Lamas S, Michel T, Brenner B, Marsden P. Nitric oxide synthesis in endothelial cells: evidence for a pathway inducible by tumor necrosis factor-α. Am J Physiol 1991; 261:C634–641.

39. Lamas S, Marsden PA, Li GK, Tempst P, Michel T. Endothelial nitric oxide synthase: molecular cloning and characterization of a distinct constitutive enzyme isoform. Proc Natl Acad Sci USA 1992; 89:6348–6352.

40. Lamas S, Saura M, Martínex-Dalmau R, Rodríguez-Puyol M, Rodriguez-Puyol D. Human recombinant interleukin-13 (rHuIL-13) inhibits the expression and activity of inducible nitric oxide synthase (iNOS) in human mesangial cells (HMC). J Am Soc Nephrol 1994; 5:585.

41. Laskin JD, Heck DE, Laskin DL. Multifunctional role of nitric oxide in inflammation. Trends Endocrinol Metab 1994; 5:377–382.

42. Liao JK, Shin WS, Lee WY, Clark SL. Oxidized low-density lipoprotein decreases the expression of endothelial nitric oxide synthase. J Biol Chem 1995; 270:319–324.

43. Liu J, Sessa WC. Identification of a covalently bound amino-terminal myristic acid in endothelial nitric oxide synthase. J Biol Chem 1994; 269:11691–11694.

44. Lowenstein CJ, Glatt CS, Bredt DS, Snyder SH. Cloned and expressed macrophage nitric oxide synthase contrasts with the brain enzyme. Proc Natl Acad Sci USA 1992; 89:6711–6715.

45. Lowenstein CJ, Snyder SH. Nitric oxide, a novel biologic messenger. Cell 1992; 70:705–707.

46. Lowenstein CJ, Alley EW, Raval P, et al. Macrophage nitric oxide synthase gene: two upstream regions mediate the induction by interferon γ and lipopolysaccharide. Proc Natl Acad Sci USA 1993; 90:9730–9734.

47. Lyons CR, Orloff GJ, Cunningham JM. Molecular cloning and functional expression of an inducible nitric oxide synthase from a murine macrophage cell line. J Biol Chem 1992; 267:6370–6374.

48. MacMicking JD, Nathan C, Hom G, et al. Altered responses to bacterial infection and endotoxic shock in mice lacking inducible nitric oxide synthase. Cell 1995; 81:641–650.

49. Marletta MA. Nitric oxide synthase: aspects concerning structure and catalysis. Cell 1994; 78:927–930.

50. Marsden PA, Heng HHQ, Scherer SW, et al. Structure and chromosomal localization of the human constitutive endothelial nitric oxide synthase gene. J Biol Chem 1993; 268:17478–17488.

51. McQuillan LP, Leung GK, Marsden PA, Kostyk SK, Kourembanas S. Hypoxia inhibits expression of eNOS via transcriptional and posttranscriptional mechanisms. Am J Physiol 1994; 267:H1921–H1927.

52. Michel T, Li GK, Busconi L. Phosphorylation and subcellular translocation of endothelial nitric oxide synthase. Proc Natl Acad Sci USA 1993; 90:6252–6256.

53. Mohaupt MG, Elzie JL, Ahn KY, Clapp WL, Wilcox CS, and Kone BC. Differential expression and induction of mRNAs encoding two inducible nitric oxide synthases in rat kidney. Kidney Int 1994; 46:653–665.

54. Morrissey JJ, McCraken R, Kaneto H, Vehaskari M, Montani D, Klahr S. Location of an inducible nitric oxide synthase mRNA in the normal kidney. Kidney Int. 1994; 45:998–1005.

55. Mumby SM, Kleuss C, Gilman AG. Receptor regulation of G-protein palmitoylation. Proc Natl Acad Sci USA. 1994; 91:2800–2804.

56. Murad F. Cyclic guanosine monophosphate as a mediator of vasodilation. J Clin Invest 1986; 78:1–5.

57. Nakane M, Mitchell J, Forstermann U, Murad F. Phosphorylation by calcium calmodulin-dependent protein kinase II and protein kinase C modulates the activity of nitric oxide synthase. Biochem Biophys Res Commun 1991; 180:1396–1402.

58. Nakane M, Schmidt HHW, Pollock J, Forstermann U and Murad F. Cloned human brain nitric oxide synthase is highly expressed in skeletal muscle. FEBS Lett. 1993; 316:175–180.

59. Nathan C. Nitric oxide as a secretory product of mammalian cells. FASEB J 1992; 6:3051–3064.

60. Nathan C and Xie Q-W. Regulation of biosynthesis of nitric oxide. J Biol Chem 1994; 269:13725–13728.

61. Nishida K, Harrison DG, Navas JP, Fisher AA, Dockery SP, Uematsu M, Nerem RM, Alexander RW, Murphy TJ. Molecular cloning and characterization of the constitutive bovine aortic endothelial cell nitric oxide synthase. J Clin Invest 1992; 90:2092–2096.

62. O'Dowd BF, Hnatowich M, Caron MG, Lefkowitz RJ, Bouvier M. Palmitoylation of the human beta 2-adrenergic receptor. Mutation of Cys341 in the carboxyl tail leads to an uncoupled nonpalmitoylated form of the receptor. J Biol Chem 1989; 264:7564–7569.

63. Perrella MA, Yoshizumi M, Fen Z, et al. Transforming growth factor-β1, but not dexamethasone, down-regulates nitric-oxide synthase mRNA after its induction by interleukin-1β in rat smooth muscle cells. J Biol Chem 1994; 269:14595–14600.

64. Pollock JS, Forstermann U, Mitchell JA, Warner TD, Schmidt HHW, Nakane M,

Murad F. Purification and characterization of particulate endothelium-derived relaxing factor synthase from cultured and native bovine aortic endothelial cells. Proc Natl Acad Sci USA 1991; 88:10480–10484.

65. Pollock JS, Klinghofer V, Forstermann U, Murad F. Endothelial nitric oxide synthase is myristylated. FEBS Lett. 1992; 309:402–404.

66. Resh MD. Myristylation and palmitylation of Src family members: the fats of the matter. Cell 1994; 76:411–413.

67. Robinson LJ, Weremowicz S, Morton CC, Michel T. Isolation and chromosomal localization of the human endothelial nitrix oxide synthase (NOS3) gene. Genomics 1994; 19:350–357.

68. Robinson LJ, Busconi L, Michel T. Agonist-modulated palmitoylation of endothelial nitric oxide synthase. J Biol Chem 1995; 270:995–998.

69. Robinson LJ, Michel T. Mutagenesis of palmitoylation sites in endothelial nitric oxide synthase identifies a novel motif for dual acylation and subcellular targeting. Proc Natl Acad Sci USA 1995; 92:11776–11780.

70. Rosenkranz-Weiss P, Sessa WC, Milstien S, Kaufman S, Watson CA, Pober JS. Regulation of nitric oxide synthesis by proinflammatory cytokines in human umbilical vein endothelial cells. J Clin Invest 1994; 93:2236–2243.

71. Sase K and Michel T. Expression of constitutive endothelial nitric oxide synthase in human blood platelets. Life Sci 1995; 57:2049–2055.

72. Saura M, López S, Rodríguez Puyol M, Rodríguez Puyol D, Lamas S. Regulation of inducible nitric oxide synthase expression in rat mesangial cells and isolated glomeruli. Kidney Int 1995; 47:500–509.

73. Sefton BM and Buss JE. The covalent modification of eukaryotic proteins with lipid. J Cell Biol 1987; 104:1449–1453.

74. Sessa WC, Harrison JK, Barber CM, Zeng D, Durieux MD, D'Angelo DD, Lynch KR, Peach MJ. Molecular cloning and expression of a cDNA encoding endothelial cell nitric oxide synthase. J Biol Chem 1992; 267:15274–15276.

75. Sessa WC, Pritchard K, Seyedi N, Wang J, Hintze TH. Chronic exercise in dogs increases coronary vascular nitric oxide production and endothelial cell nitric oxide synthase gene expression. Circ Res 1994; 74(2):349–53.

76. Shaul PW, North AJ, Wu LC, Wells LB, Trannon TS, Lau KS, Michel T, Marstraf LR, Star RA. Endothelial nitric oxide synthase is expressed in cultured human bronchiolar epithelium. J Clin Invest 1994; 94:2231–2236.

77. Shaul PW, Smart EJ, Robinson LJ, German Z, Yuhanna IS, Ying Y, Anderson RGW, Michel T. Acylation targets endothelial nitric-oxide synthase to plasmalemmal caveolae. J Biol Chem 1996; :in press.

78. Shaul PW, North AJ, Brannon TS, Ujiie K, Wells LB, Nisen PA, Lowenstein CJ Snyder SH and Star RA. Prolonged in vivo hypoxia enhances nitric oxide synthase type I and type III gene expression in adult rat lung. Am J Respir Cell Mol Biol 1995; 13:167–174.

79. Stamler JS, Singel DJ, Loscalzo J. Biochemistry of nitric oxide and its redox-activated forms. Science 1992; 258:1898–1902.

80. Suschek C, Rothe H, Fehsel K, Enczmann J, Kolb-Bachofen V. Induction of a macrophage-like nitric oxide synthase in cultured rat aortic endothelial cells. J Immunol 1993; 151:3283–3291.

81. Tracey WR, Pollock JS, Murad F, Nakane M, Forstermann U. Identificiation of an endothelial-like type III NO synthase in LLC-PK1 kidney epithelial cells. Am J Physiol 1994; 266:C22–C28.

82. Tsukahara H, Gordienko DV, Goligorsky MS. Continuous monitoring of nitric oxide release from human umbilical vein endothelial cells. Biochem Biophys Res Commun 1993; 193:722–729.

83. Venema RC, Nishida K, Alexander RW, Harrison DG, Murphy TJ. Organization of the bovine gene encoding the endothelial nitric oxide synthase. Biochim Biophys Acta 1994; 1218:413–420.

84. Vodovotz Y, Bogdan C, Paik J, Xie Q-W, Nathan C. Mechanisms of suppression of macrophage nitric oxide release by transforming growth factor beta. J Exp Med 1993; 178:605–613.

85. Vodovotz Y, Russel D, Xie Q-W, Bogdan C, Nathan C. Vesicle membrane association of nitric oxide synthase in primary mouse macrophages. J Immunol 1995; 154:2914–2925.

86. Wang XL, Sim AS, Badenhop RF, McCedie RM, Wilcken DEL. A smoking dependent risk of coronary artery disease associated with a polymorphism of the endothelial nitric oxide synthase gene. Nature Med 1996; 2:41–45.

87. Wang Y and Marsden PA. Nitric oxide synthases: biochemical and molecular regulation. Curr Opin Nephrol Hypertens 1995; 4:12–22.

88. Wedegaertner PB, Chu DH, Wilson PT, Levis MJ, Bourne HR. Palmitoylation is required for signaling functions and membrane attachment of Gqα and Gsα. J Biol Chem 1993; 268:25001–25008.

89. Wedegaertner PB, Bourne HR. Activation and depalmitoylation of Gsα. Cell 1994; 77:1063–1070.

90. Wedegaertner PB, Wilson PT, Bourne HR. Lipid modifications of trimeric G-proteins. J Biol Chem 1995; 270:503–506.

91. Wei X-q, Charles IG, Smich A, et al. Altered immune responses in mice lacking inducible nitric oxide synthase gene. Nature 1995; 375:408–411.

92. Weiner WP, Lizasoian I, Baylis SA, Knowles RG, CHarles IG and Moncada S. Induction of calcium-dependent nitric oxide synthases by sex hormones. Proc Natl Acad Sci USA 1994; 91:5212–5216.

93. Xie J, Roddy P, File TK, Murad F, Young AP. Two closely linked but separable promoters for human neuronal nitric oxide synthase gene trancription. Proc Natl Acad Sci USA 1995; 92:1242–1246.

94. Xie Q-W, Cho HJ, Calaycay J, et al. Cloning and characterization of inducible nitric oxide synthase from mouse macrophages. Science 1992; 256:225–228.

95. Xie Q-W, Whisnant R, Nathan C. Promoter of the mouse gene encoding calcium-independent nitric oxide synthase confers inducibility by interferon γ and bacterial lipopolysaccharide. J Exp Med 1993; 177:1779–1784.

96. Xie Q-W, Kashiwabara Y, Nathan C. Role of the transcription factor NF-κB/Rel in induction of nitric oxide synthase. J Biol Chem 1994; 269:4705–4708.

97. Yasue H, Yoshimura M, Sugiyama S, Sumida H, Okumura K, Ogawa H, Kugiyama K, Ogawa Y, Nakao K. Association of a point mutation of the endot-

helial cell nitric oxide synthase (eNOS) gene with coronay spasm. Circulation (Suppl) 1995; 92:1-363.

98. Yoshizumi M, Perrella MA, Burnett JC, Lee M-E. Tumor necrosis factor downregulates an endothelial nitric oxide synthase mRNA by shortening its half-life. Circ Res 1993; 73:205–209.

8

Signaling Through Heterotrimeric G Proteins

**Yibang Chen, Anya Harry,
and Ravi Iyengar**
*Mount Sinai School of Medicine
New York, New York*

Complex organisms coordinate the functions of their various organs to achieve balance that sustains and propagates life. Such coordination is required for both normal acute and long-term functions, as well as for responses to changes in the environment of the organism. In mammals one of the key systems subject to such regulation is the cardiovascular system. Many hormones and neurotransmitters regulate the cardiovascular system. These include epinephrine, acetylcholine, and angiotensin. These neurotransmitters and hormones function as extracellular messengers that are recognized at the surface of the target cell. Then the information they carry is transferred into the cell. A multicomponent system in the plasma membrane is used for signal transduction (1). The component that specifically recognizes the external signal is the receptor. Upon receiving the signal, the receptor activates the signal transducer, the heterotrimeric guanine nucleotide binding protein (G protein). Receptor activation of the G protein results in dissociation of the G protein into Gα and Gβγ subunits. Both components of the activated G protein can independently regulate effectors. Typical G protein effectors are intracellular (second) messenger-generating enzymes or ion channels. Generation of the intracellular messages and/or direct regulation of channel activity allows the cell to mount a response to the extracellular signal. Recent experiments suggest that in addition to regulating second messenger-producing enzymes and ion channels, G protein subunits may, by currently unknown mechanisms, regulate protein kinase cascades involved in proliferation and growth.

G PROTEIN-COUPLED RECEPTORS

The conversion of a biological stimulus to a physiological response often begins with recognition of the signal by a specific receptor either within the cell or at the cell surface membrane in the target tissue. Cell surface receptors span the membrane and trigger a cellular response by a cascade of protein–protein interactions, or by stimulating the generation of cytoplasmic, diffusible second messengers, leading to the initiation of a cascade of phosphorylation, and/or dephosphorylation reactions resulting in biochemical or physiological responses. One large class of cell surface receptors couple to heterotrimeric G proteins. These receptors are single chain transmembrane glycoproteins. All G protein-coupled receptors are thought to share a common secondary structure. Over the last decade the complementary DNA for more than 100 G protein-coupled receptors have been cloned. Although from the deduced amino acid sequence the overall homology between G protein coupled receptors is low, the predicted secondary structure is remarkably conserved through evolution. Hydrophobicity analysis of the receptor protein indicates seven putative transmembrane-spanning segments with an extracellular amino terminus and an intracellular carboxyl terminus. Without exception, all known G protein-coupled receptors are thought to have such a structure (2). Direct physical evidence for this structure remains to be obtained.

Site-directed mutagenesis and construction of chimeric receptors have allowed for the identification of regions within the receptor involved in binding extracellular ligands and in interacting with the G protein. For most small molecules such as biogenic amines the ligand binding site is located within the hydrophobic transmembrane regions (2). For larger extracellular molecules such as the glycoprotein hormones, some of the determinants for binding are on the external surface of the receptor. One feature of the binding site is that the receptor specifically recognizes two classes of ligands: agonists, which, upon binding promote interactions between the receptor and cognate G protein; and antagonists, which specifically bind to the receptors but do not initiate interactions of the liganded receptors with G proteins.

For all receptors, the regions that interact with the G proteins are located in the cytoplasmic loops that connect the different putative transmembrane regions and in the carboxy-terminal tail. Most often the third cytoplasmic loop is involved in G protein interactions. These regions specify which G protein the receptor interacts with. Thus, the primary structure of the receptor encodes bidirectional specificity: signal recognition and the capability to transmit the signal to a specific intracellular response pathway. A schematic representation of a prototypic G protein coupled receptor is shown in Figure 1. In mammalian systems, G protein-coupled receptors can be functionally classified into three large groups according to which G protein family they interact with. Specificity of coupling is not absolute: there are many examples of a receptor capable of coupling to more than one G protein receptor in its native environment. An early example is the angiontensin receptor in the liver, which couples to two different classes of G proteins (3).

HETEROTRIMERIC G PROTEINS

Upon occupancy by agonist, the receptor activates the G proteins. To understand how receptors activate G proteins it is necessary to understand how G proteins oscillate between inactive and active states. The G protein is a heterotrimer. The α-subunit of the G protein is a 39–52 kDa protein containing a guanine nucleotide binding site that has intrinsic GTPase activity. The α-subunit belongs to a large superfamily of GTPases that function in many cellular processes such as protein synthesis, vesicle transport and docking, and, of

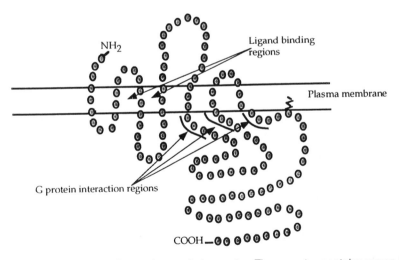

Figure 1 A typical G protein-coupled receptor. The receptor contains seven hydrophobic stretches that are depicted as membrane-spanning regions. Domains within the receptor involved in ligand binding and in G protein interactions are indicated. These regions are most often implicated for these functions in many G protein-coupled receptors. However, there are known exceptions where other regions of the receptors are also involved in both ligand binding and G protein interactions.

course, in signal transduction. The heterotrimeric G proteins also contain β and γ subunits. The β and γ subunits are very tightly associated with each other and do not dissociate from each other in nondenaturing conditions. Hence for all practical purposes the heterotrimeric G protein functions as a dimer of α and βγ subunits.

In its inactive state the G protein is a heterotrimer with GDP bound to the guanine nucleotide-binding site. This is the result of the αγ subunits increasing the affinity of the α subunit for GDP and the GDP increasing the affinity of the α subunit for βγ subunits. Interaction of the agonist occupied receptor with the GDP-bound heterotrimeric G-protein triggers the release of GDP and the binding of GTP. Although the affinities of Gα for GDP and GTP are similar within the cell, GTP binding to the vacant site predominates because there is 10 times more GTP than GDP in the cytoplasm. In concomitant fashion, the Gα subunits separate from the Gβγ subunits (4). An important feature of receptor activation of G proteins is that for a single agonist binding and dissociation step the receptor can activate several G proteins. This allows for considerable amplification of the signal at this stage.

Both the GTP liganded Gα and Gβγ subunits are independently able to transmit the signal further downstream by stimulating effectors. Often effectors are enzymes that produce second messengers such as 3′,5′ cyclic adenosine monophosphate (cAMP), inositol 1,4,5 triphosphate (IP$_3$), or diacylglycerol (DAG). Certain types of channels such as one class of K$^+$ channels also function as effectors for G proteins (5). Typical α- and βγ-regulated effector processes are described in detail below. The cell surface signal transduction process is terminated by two control mechanisms: (a) hydrolysis of the gamma phosphate of the GTP molecule bound to the Gα-subunit into GDP and (b) dissociation of the agonist from the receptor. The GTPase activity is thought to be very important in regulating transmembrane signal transduction because it functions independently of the receptor signal (4). In some G protein pathways, such as the cAMP pathway, the catalytic rate of the GTPase is independent of the Gα subunit interaction with any other component and thus the G protein serves as a clock that defines the temporal window during which signal transmission may occur. In other G protein pathways, most notably in the phospholipase C system, the catalytic rate of the GTPase is stimulated by the effector, which in effect allows the G protein to "hold" the signal until it has been transmitted to the effector (6). Upon hydrolysis of the bound GTP to GDP, the Gα subunit dissociates from the effector and reassociates with Gβγ subunits resulting in a return of the G protein to the inactive state. This GTPase cycle is depicted in Figure 2.

G proteins are classified by their capability to interact specifically with certain classes of receptors and effectors. Like receptors, the G proteins exhibit bidirectional specificity. This specificity determines the routing of signal flow

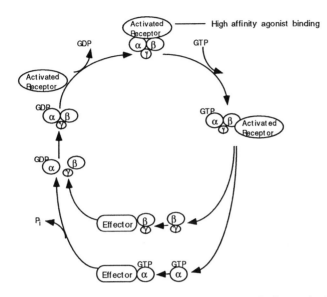

Figure 2 The GTPase cycle of the heterotrimeric G protein. In the resting state the G protein is a heterotrimer with GDP bound to the Gα-subunit. The agonist-occupied (activated) receptor associates with the G protein to promote the dissociation of GDP. This results in a transient complex between the agonist-occupied receptor and vacant G protein. This complex represents the GTP sensitive "high-affinity state" of the receptor. The receptor also promotes the association of GTP with the G protein. GTP occupancy results in the activation of the G protein and the concomitant production of GTP-liganded Gα subunit and βγ subunits. Both subunits regulate effectors. Upon hydrolysis of GTP by the intrinsic GTPase activity of the Gα subunit, the Gα subunit dissociates from the effector and associates with the Gβγ subunits, thus terminating the Gβγ regulation of effectors. The GDP-bound Gα subunit has high affinity for the Gβγ subunits and the Gβγ subunits in turn stabilize GDP binding to the Gα subunit, thus returning the G protein and the system to the inactive state.

across the membrane. Early classification of G proteins was based on their capability to regulate the effector adenylyl cyclase, since this was the system in which G proteins were discovered. G_s was the G protein that stimulated adenylyl cyclase and G_i inhibited adenylyl cyclase. When the heterotrimeric nature of the G protein became known, and with the subsequent cloning of the complementary DNAs for the different subunits, the classification was then based on the identity of the α subunit (7). Thus, G_s indicates a heterotrimeric G protein whose α subunit is $α_s$. Four classes of G protein α subunits are now known: $α_s$, $α_q$, $α_i$, and $α_{12}$. Each class has several members. This classification is strongly supported by experimental evidence that the α subunit of the G protein specifies which receptor is coupled to which effector. The effector specificity of α subunits is close to absolute. Thus, all members of the α_s family stimulate adenylyl cyclase and all members of the α_q family stimulate phospholipase C. The α_i family, however, is somewhat more diverse. Within the α_i family there are three distinct subfamilies. The α_t subfamily functions in the visual system where it couples the photoreceptor, rhodopsin, to the effector cGMP-phosphodiesterase, converting light into chemical signals. In addition, there is the α_o subfamily whose direct effectors are unknown and there is the α_i subfamily that inhibits adenylyl cyclase. One characteristic of most members of the G_i family is their susceptibility to be ADP-ribosylated by pertussis toxin. The acceptor site for ADP-ribosylation is a cysteine in the carboxy-terminus region involved in receptor contact. Hence ADP-ribosylation of α_i results in uncoupling the G protein from the receptor and inhibiting receptor regulation of effectors. The fourth family, consisting of α_{12} and α_{14}, was recently discovered and their cognate receptors and effectors remain as yet unknown. The known routing pathways of the various $G\alpha$ subunits are summarized in Figure 3.

The $G\beta\gamma$ heterodimers are tightly (noncovalently) associated with each other. They can be functionally exchanged with $G\alpha_s$, $G\alpha_q$, or $G\alpha_i$ subunits.

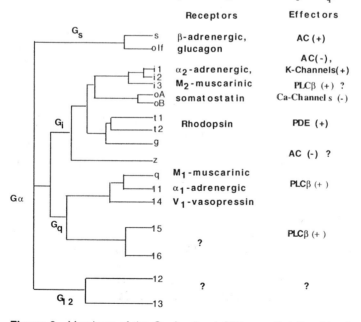

Figure 3 Members of the $G\alpha$ family of GTPases. Relationships between the α-subunits are represented as a phylogenetic tree. Typical receptors and effectors that interact with each class of $G\alpha$ subunit in native environment are shown. AC, adenylyl cyclase; PDE, cGMP phosphodiesterase; PLCβ, phospholipase Cβ.

Five mammalian Gβ subunits have been cloned sharing 50–90% sequence homology and six mammalian Gγ subunits have been cloned showing greater diversity with 27–75% sequence homology. For the most part, the various Gβ and Gγ subunits form heterodimers in vitro that have similar functional capabilities (8). However, not all combinations of β and γ subunits are naturally found. The Gβ subunit has a molecular mass of 35–36 kDa. The Gγ subunit has a molecular mass of 7.3–8.5 kDa. It is possible that the γ subunit may have a determining role in Gβγ function, but at the current time there is little evidence to support this notion. In spite of their structural diversity, most combinations of Gβγ subunits that have been tested show similar functions. They preferentially interact with and stabilize the GDP bound forms of Gα subunits. They are required for the Gα subunit interaction with the receptor, since only the heterotrimer interacts with the receptor. Free Gβγ subunits are also capable of regulating certain subtypes of effectors. Currently known effectors regulated by Gβγ are listed in Table 1.

G PROTEIN EFFECTORS

Adenylyl Cyclase

Adenylyl cyclases produce the intracellular messenger cAMP in response to signals from G proteins. In most mammalian systems adenylyl cyclase is stimulated by the α_s subunit. The only exception is an adenylyl cyclase from testis, which is not stimulated by α_s. However, in lower organisms such as bacteria and yeast adenylyl cyclase is a constitutive enzyme and is not generally regulated by extracellular signals. Recent studies have revealed considerable molecular heterogeneity in mammalian adenylyl cyclases. Eight distinct adenylyl cyclases have been cloned and characterized (9,10). All of these isoforms are single polypeptides that are intrinsic membrane proteins. They share a complex membrane-spanning structure similar to those of transporters. The presumed secondary structure of a mmamalian adenylyl cyclase is shown in Figure 4. All

Table 1   Signaling by Gβγ Subunits

Receptor	Effector	Effect
M2-Muscarinic	K$^+$ channels	Stimulation
α2-Adrenergic	Adenylyl cyclase 2	Conditional
D2-dopamine		Stimulation
α-Adrenergic	Adenylyl cyclase 1,8	Inhibition
D2-Dopamine		
FMLP receptors	Phospholipase C-β	Stimulation
Somatostatin	Ca^{2+} channels	Inhibition

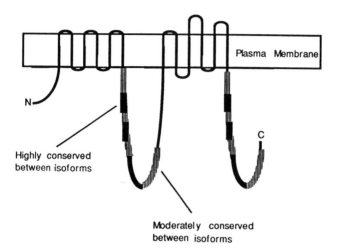

Figure 4   Schematic representation of a mammalian adenylyl cyclase. The two sets of six hydrophophic regions are depicted as transmembrane regions. The central cytoplasmic loop and C-terminal contain regions that are conserved between the two halves as well as between the different adenylyl cyclases. The highly conserved regions (>80% homology) are depicted as solid bars; the moderately (>60% homology) conserved regions are shown as hatched regions. These regions are thought to be involved in both catalytic activity and in interactions with G protein subunits.

of the cloned mammalian adenylyl cyclases are stimulated by α_s. In addition to the basic capability of receiving signals from α_s, the different adenylyl cyclases are stimulated by other mechanisms. Adenylyl cyclases 1 and 8 are stimulated by Ca^{2+}/calmodulin. Adenylyl cyclases 2 and 4 are extensively stimulated by $G\beta\gamma$ subunits in the presence of α_s. Adenylyl cyclases 2 and 7 are stimulated by protein kinase C. Thus, depending on which adenylyl cyclase form is present in the cell, cAMP levels can be altered by a variety of signals.

Phospholipase C

Four mammalian isozymes of phospholipase C (PLC)-β have been cloned (11). All isoforms are stimulated by G protein subunits. Like the different G protein-regulated mammalian adenylyl cyclases, the G protein-regulated phospholipases C have a conserved structure. The PLC-βs are single-chain polypeptides but are not intrinsic membrane proteins, as are adenylyl cyclases. All members of the PLC-β family are stimulated by members of the α_q family, although there is some difference in potencies. In addition, PLC-$\beta2$ and $\beta3$ are also stimulated by $G\beta\gamma$ subunits. Thus like the adenylyl cyclase system, the phospholipase C system is also capable of receiving signals from both the α and βγ subunits of G proteins.

K+ Channels

In addition to enzymes, ion channels are thought to be directly regulated by G protein subunits. The best studied of these is the inward-rectifying K+ channels in the atria. One class of inward rectifiers is regulated by muscarinic receptors through pertussis toxin-sensitive G proteins. Molecular cloning and reconstitution studies show that the channel is composed of two types of proteins that are related to each other and belong to the family of K+ channel proteins (12,13). Current evidence indicates that this channel is opened by direct interactions with Gβγ subunits (14,15). This pathway is one of the best characterized for Gβγ subunit-mediated signaling from receptor to effector.

MAP–Kinase Pathway

Many growth factors transmit their signals through the MAP–kinase pathway. Receptors for growth factors are tyrosine kinases, which upon autophosphorylation, bind adaptor proteins that allow the receptors to promote GTP for GDP exchange and thus activate the monomeric G protein Ras. Activated Ras then transmits the signal to the Ser-Thr kinase Raf. This results in activation of the MAP-kinase cascade. Upon activation the MAP-kinases (also called ERK1 and ERK2) translocate to the nucleus, where it regulates gene expression (16). Components of this pathway are summarized in Figure 5. This pathway is thought to be very important for proliferative signaling. In addition to receptor–tyrosine kinases many G protein-coupled receptors such as thrombin, bradykinin, and angiotensin receptors stimulate the MAP-kinase pathway. The mechanism by which heterotrimeric G proteins activate the MAP-kinase pathway is not known. It has been suggested that the Gβγ subunits are responsible for activation of the MAP-kinase pathway (17). Although this may be the case in experimentally designed conditions, it appears that in native systems, receptors such as α_2-adrenergic receptors or D2-dopamine receptors that activate the more abundant G proteins such as G_i and G_o and thus produce many Gβγ subunits do not generally activate the MAP-kinase cascade, even though components of the cascade are ubiquitously expressed. Thus at the current time the mechanisms by which heterotrimeric G proteins regulate the MAP-kinase cascade have not been fully elucidated.

G PROTEIN PATHWAYS IN CARDIOVASCULAR FUNCTION

Many hormones and neurotransmitters that signal through heterotrimeric G proteins regulate both cardiac and vascular functions. Among the best studied

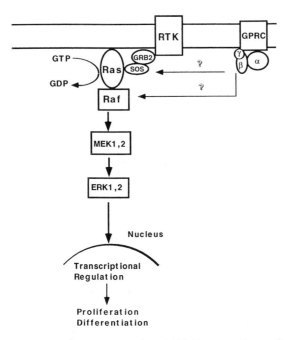

Figure 5   Components of the MAP-kinase pathway. Growth-factor binding to recep-
tor-tyrosine kinase results in autophosphorylation and recruitment of the adaptor
protein GRB2 to the cell surface by interactions between the SH2 domains of GRB2
and the phosphotyrosine on the receptor. GRB2 in turn recruits the guanine nucleotide exchange protein SOS that activates Ras by promoting exchange of GDP for
GTP. Activated Ras then recruits and activates the serine-threonine kinase Raf, which
in turn activates the dual-specificity kinase MEK, which then phosphorylates and
activates MAP-kinase (ERK1 and 2). Activated MAP-kinase translocates to the
nucleus where it regulates gene expression. At the present time it is not known how
G protein-coupled receptors (GPRC) feed into the MAP-kinase pathway. It has been
suggested that G proteins regulate Ras activity. It is also known that protein kinase
C, which is downstream of phospholipase-Cβ, can activate Raf.

of these are epinephrine and norepinephrine, which are known to increase
cardiac contractility by elevation of cAMP. Increased secretion of catecholamines and their effects on cardiac β-adrenergic receptors are thought to constitute an important component of the response system required for cardiac
function during stress. In chronic congestive heart failure there is a decreased
β-adrenergic response (18). In the failing human ventricular myocardium the
density of β-adrenergic receptors is about half of what is found in the normal
heart. The locus of the decreased β-adrenergic response appears to be the re-

ceptor itself. Stimulation of cAMP downstream of the β-adrenergic receptor appears to be normal in failing myocardial tissue and regulation of cardiac contractility by other extracellular agents such as histamine appears normal (19). Recent studies by Lefkowitz and co-workers have provided compelling evidence that the density of β-adrenergic receptors can affect cardiac function (20). Transgenic mice were created that overexpress β-adrenergic receptors in myocardial tissue. A several- (10–40) fold increase in β-adrenergic receptor substantially altered cardiac function. In isolated atria from transgenic animal with elevated levels of β-adrenergic receptors, basal isometeric tension was increased, indicating an increased inotropy. In vivo cardiac catheterization provided additional evidence that increased density of β-adrenergic receptors results in conversion of the left ventricle to a maximal inotropic state (20). These findings provide clear evidence that density of the β-adrenergic receptor is a crucial factor in myocardial function. An interesting aspect of these experiments is that they provide the first evidence that the relative ratios of the receptors to other components of the signaling system are important in regulating the responsiveness of the system in vivo. In transgenic animals with greatly increased β-adrenergic receptors in the myocardium, the basal increase in physiological responses is not further increased by β-adrenergic receptor agonists. This indicates that receptor has intrinsic signaling capability and that the rest of the signal transduction system is capable of limiting the receptor response. These experiments suggest that there is an optimum value for relative ratios of the signaling components in the construction of a responsive system. This latter conclusion has implications for therapeutic interventions. In cases where there is a decrease in a component of the signal transduction system or a loss of coupling, an optimal response may still be obtained by altering the ratios of the components. With the availability of methods that allow for gene transfer in a tissue-selective manner, this may be possible. Expression of signaling components could be one therapeutic approach for cardiovascular disorders.

REFERENCES

1. Iyengar R, Birnbaumer L. Overview in G proteins. San Diego: Academic Press, 1990, 1–17.
2. Dohlman HG, Thorner J, Caron MG, Lefkowitz RJ. Model systems for the study of seven transmembrane segment receptors. Annu Rev Biochem 1991; 60:653–689.
3. Pobiner BF, Hewlett EL, Garrison JC. Role of N_i in coupling angiotensin receptors to inhibition of adenylate cyclase in hepatocytes. J Biol Chem 1985; 260:6200–6209.
4. Gilman AG. G proteins: transducers of receptor generated signals. Annu Rev Biochem 1987; 56:615–650.
5. Neer EJ. Heterotrimeric G proteins: organizer of transmembrane signals. Cell 1995; 80:249–257.

6. Berstein G, Blank JL, Jhon D-Y, Exton JH, Rhee SG, Ross EM. Phospholipase
    Cβ1 is a GTPase activating protein for Gq/11 its physiological effectors. 1992; Cell
    70:411–418.

7. Simon MI, Strathmann MP, Gautam N. Diversity of G proteins in signal trans-
    duction. 1991; Science 252:802–808.

8. Smrcka AV, Sternweis PC. Regulation of purified subtypes of phosphatidylinositol-
    specific phospholipase C-β by G protein α and βγ subunits. 1993; J Biol Chem
    268:9667–9674.

9. Iyengar R. Molecular and functional diversity of mammalian G_s stimulated adenylyl
    cyclases. FASEB J 1993; 7:768–775.

10. Taussig R, Gilman AG. Mammalian membrane bound adenylyl cyclases. J Biol
    Chem 1995; 270:1–5.

11. Lee C-W, Lee K-H, Lee SB, Park D, Rhee SG. Regulation of Phospholipase C-
    β4 by ribonucleotides and the α-subunit of Gq. J Biol Chem 1994; 269:25335–
    25338.

12. Krapivinsky G, Gordon E, Wickman K, Velimirovic B, Krapivinsky L, Clapham
    DE. The G protein gated atrial K^+ channel I_{KACh} is a heteromultimer of two in-
    wardly rectifying K^+ -channel proteins. Nature 1995; 374:135–141.

13. Kofuji P, Davidson N, Lester HA. Evidence that neuronal G-protein gated inwardly
    rectifying K^+ channels are activated by Gβγ subunits and function as hetero-
    multimers. Proc Natl Acad Sci USA 1995; 92:6542–6546.

14. Wickman KD, Iniguez-Lluhi JA, Davenport PA, Taussig R, Kravinsky GB, Linder
    ME, Gilman AG, Clapham DE. Recombinant G-protein βγ-subunits activate the
    muscarinic gated atrial potassium channel. Nature 1995; 368:255–257.

15. Krapivinsky G, Krapivinsky L, Wickman K, Clapham DE. Gβγ directly bind to
    the G protein gated K^+ -channel I_{KACh}. J Biol Chem 1995; 270:29059–29062.

16. Avruch J, Zhang X-H, Kyriakis JM. Raf mets Ras: completing the framework of
    a signal transducing pathway. TIBS 1994; 19:279–283.

17. Crespo P, Xu N, Simonds WF, Gutkind JS. Ras dependent activation of MAP-
    kinase pathway mediated by G-protein βγ subunits. Nature 1994; 369:418–420.

18. Bristow MR, Ginsburg R, Minobe W, Cubicciotti RS, Sagemam WS, Lurie K,
    Billingham ME, Harrison DC, Stinson EB. Decreased catecholamine sensitivity and
    β-adrenergic density in failing human hearts. N Eng J Med 1982; 307:205–211.

19. Bristow MR, Kantrowitz NE, Ginsburg R, Fowler MB. β-Adrenergic receptors in
    heart muscle disease and heart failure. J Mol Cell Cardiol 1985; 17:(Supplement)
    41–52.

20. Milano CA, Allen LF, Rockman HA, Dolber PC, McMinn TR, Chien KR,
    Johnson TD, Bond RA, Lefkowitz RJ. Enhanced myocardial function in transgenic
    mice overexpressing the β2-adrenergic receptor. Science 1994; 264:583–585.

9

Molecular Physiology of Cardiac Sodium Channels

Sarah K. England and Michael M. Tamkun
Vanderbilt University School of Medicine
Nashville, Tennessee

INTRODUCTION

The electrically excitable cells of the heart each display a complex and unique action potential. Ventricular, atrial, and Purkinje cell action potentials are composed of five similar phases that vary in duration and shape. The depolarizing phase (phase 0), which is a determinant of action potential propagation through the myocardium, is mediated by a rapid influx of Na^+ ions via voltage-sensitive Na^+ channels. These Na^+ channels play the greatest role in cardiac regions where depolarization is rapid. Phase 0 is followed by a rapid but incomplete repolarization due to Na^+ channel inactivation and K^+ efflux through transiently active K^+ channels (phase 1). The plateau phase (phase 2) follows and is composed of a K^+ efflux and an inactivating Ca^{2+} influx that is the stimulus for myocyte contraction. This delicate balance of inward and outward current determines both the magnitude and duration of the plateau. The action potential is terminated by a rise in K^+ permeability (phase 3) that ultimately repolarizes the cell back to the resting membrane potential (phase 4).

Modification of any ionic current in the heart is a potential mode of therapeutic intervention for regulating both the strength and frequency of contrac-

173

tion. Antiarrhythmic drugs presently used, as well as agents under development, modify action potential characteristics primarily by slowing the rate of phase 0 depolarization or lengthening action potential duration, which are alterations that should make problems such as reentrant arrhythmias less likely. Since the voltage-gated channels of the cardiac sarcolemma are the pharmacological targets of these agents, ion channel proteins are of great clinical importance. Increased knowledge of the structure, function, regulation, and molecular pharmacology of these channels should be acquired. This chapter will review the progress that numerous laboratories have made in understanding the structure and function of the voltage-gated Na^+ channels in mammalian myocardium.

Although this chapter will focus on the voltage-gated Na^+ channel producing the rapid depolarization in phase 0 of ventricular and Purkinje cell action potentials, the diversity of voltage-gated Na^+ current in heart suggests the existence of multiple cardiac Na^+ channel isoforms. As a specific example, a class of cardiac Na^+ channels that exhibit activation and inactivation kinetics significantly slower than those responsible for the fast Na^+ current of phase 0 have been described (1–5). These currents are masked by the larger inward and outward currents discussed above (1,6), which probably explains why we know so little about these atypical cardiac Na^+ channels. While their physiological relevance remains unknown, these currents may contribute to phase 2 of the action potential. One group has described a slow Na^+ channel in the myocardial membranes of genetically cardiomyopathic hamsters (7) and in skeletal muscle fibers excised from patients with Duchenne muscular dystrophy (8). The functional attributes of this type of Na^+ channel are also quite distinct from the phase 0 Na^+ channel, and from other cloned channels that have been expressed from cDNA, and indicate the existence of distinct cardiac Na^+ channel isoforms that may be disease related. In addition to these functional studies, two structurally defined Na^+ channel isoforms have been found in heart based on molecular cloning techniques. There is evidence that an isoform designated $Na_v2.1$ in humans and $Na_v2.3$ in mice (9,10), and another isoform represented by an incomplete Na^+ channel cDNA sequence (11), are present in heart. However, these channels may be of nonmyocyte origin since endothelial, glial, and vascular smooth muscle cells represent a significant percentage of the cells that exist in heart. Nevertheless, these observations suggest the existence of Na^+ conducting channels that exhibit very distinct functional and structural properties from the predominant cardiac Na^+ channel involved in phase 0 depolarization.

PHARMACOLOGY OF CARDIAC Na^+ CHANNELS

The pharmacological characterization of Na^+ channels has employed two toxins that have high affinity (K_d values in the low nM range) for most Na^+ channel isoforms. Tetrodotoxin (TTX) is a toxin first isolated from the Japanese puffer fish that physically blocks inward Na+ current through the channel by binding near or in the ion pore (12). Saxitoxin (STX) is synthesized by marine dinoflagellates and is often concentrated in shellfish during red tide blooms. It is structurally similar to TTX and binds to the same site on the channel. [^{3}H]STX is the ligand of choice for binding studies since its affinity for the channel is somewhat greater than that of TTX. In contrast, TTX is preferred for block of ionic current since TTX is much easier to obtain than unlabeled STX.

Studies using STX and TTX have simplified the characterization of Na+ channel isoforms and provided the first direct evidence that distinct cardiac and neuronal isoforms existed. The predominant Na+ current observed in mammalian cardiac myocytes is TTX-resistant (K_D = 1–5 μM), distinct from the predominant Na+ current in nerve and skeletal muscle, which is sensitive to nanomolar concentrations of TTX and STX (K_D = 5–30 nM) (13). Skeletal muscle expresses the TTX-resistant cardiac Na+ channel during early development and following denervation (14), but little of this isoform exists in adult tissue. The presence of Na+ channels in heart other than the TTX-resistant form is supported by TTX/STX-binding studies. Approximately 20% of the binding sites for STX in rat heart homogenates exhibit high affinity (14,15), suggesting the presence of a Na+ channel isoform other than the predominant TTX/STX-resistant channel. Some of these high affinity sites are associated with peripheral nerve since chemical destruction of sympathetic innervation during development decreases the number of high-affinity binding sites (15). However, the remaining high-affinity sites, along with the unusual inward currents described previously, suggest that additional cardiac myocyte channels exist.

Na+ channels have been the target of antiarrhythmic drug development since they play an essential role in cardiac action potential generation and propagation. Many of the class I agents display use-dependent block, suggesting that they would be more effective against an arrhythmia. Such use-dependent compounds (which include quinidine and lidocaine) bind with greater affinity to the open state of the channel, meaning that the greater the number of action potentials the greater the drug binding. A large effort has gone into development of class I agents, with two of the best examples being encainide and flecainide. These drugs, along with others, went into full clinical trial during the Cardiac Arrhythmia Suppression Trial (CAST) studies. In this study, designed to test whether suppression of ventricular ectopy after a myocardial infarction reduces the incidence of sudden death, Na+ channel block by encainide and flecainide was shown to increase mortality unexpectedly compared to a group receiving placebo alone. The majority of the group died from arrhythmia or other cardiac causes (16). Although the mechanisms underlying the excess mortality remain unknown at the present time, the CAST study emphasizes the need for increased understanding of cardiac Na^+ channel physiology and pharmacology. The results of CAST are one reason why there has been a large shift in thinking away from class I drugs and toward class III agents, which usually prolong the action potential by inhibition of repolarizing currents. These agents, however, have their own set of problems, perhaps the most notable being the development of torsade de pointes (17).

OVERVIEW OF Na^+ CHANNEL MOLECULAR BIOLOGY

One important finding that initiated interest in cloning cardiac Na^+ channels was the observation that Na^+ channels in various tissues had distinct properties, suggesting that multiple isoforms encoded by distinct genes were present in different tissues. For example, not only are cardiac Na^+ channels less sensitive to TTX but these cardiac Na^+ channels may also be more sensitive to inhibition by the antiarrhythmic agent lidocaine than the brain channels (18). Thus, it was originally thought that comparison of neuronal and cardiac channel cDNA clones would reveal the TTX and lidocaine-binding sites and lay the foundation for rational antiarrhythmic drug design. The goal of identifying the TTX receptor site on the channel has been realized using this approach. The cloning efforts described below have, within a 10 year period, led to a revolution in our understanding of voltage-gated Na^+ channel structure, function, pharmacology, regulation, and pathology. We now know that specific types of human skeletal muscle myotonias are due to point mutations in the skeletal muscle Na^+ channel isoform gene (19–20), which suggests that gene therapy approaches that target defective Na^+ channel genes can be attempted in the near future. While to date we have no hard evidence that defective cardiac Na^+ channel genes are responsible for human disease, the precedence set with skeletal muscle suggests that susceptibility to some cardiac arrhythmias may be due to such a molecular genetic defect.

Two things made the cloning of the first voltage-sensitive Na^+ channel possible: the relative abundance of channel protein in eel electroplax tissue, and the STX/TTX binding methodology described above. The eel channel was detergent-solubilized from its native membrane and purified by following STX binding activity through various purification procedures. The purified eel channel is composed of a single heavily glycosylated polypeptide of approximately 240,000 daltons in molecular weight (21). Using both antibodies and amino acid sequence derived from the purified eel channel, Numa and colleagues cloned and sequenced the eel NaCh cDNA, thereby obtaining the first complete amino acid sequence of a voltage-sensitive ion channel (22). The eel channel is composed of four homologous regions (I–IV) that can be further subdivided into 6 potential membrane-spanning domains: domain I2 is homologous to domain IV2 (see Fig. 5). The fourth membrane-spanning domain (S4) in each region contains a concentration of positive charge, with each third amino acid being either an arginine or lysine. This S4 domain has become a candidate for the voltage-sensing structure of the channel, since one expects the voltage sensor to be a region of concentrated charge within the transmembrane electric field (i.e., in the middle of the protein). Using the eel cDNA as a probe, the Numa group isolated cDNA molecules from rat brain libraries that code for three Na⁺ channel isoforms derived from separate genes (23,24). These isoforms are very similar to each other and to the eel channel, although regions of nonhomology exist. The brain Na⁺ channels were expressed and functionally assayed in *Xenopus* oocytes microinjected with mRNA produced from cloned channel cDNA (25), demonstrating that only the large cloned protein is necessary for voltage-dependent ion transport activity. Thus, the eel and rat brain channels are large (1800–2100 amino acids) transmembrane proteins (24 membrane spanning domains) with a fourfold symmetry. Within this structure lies the voltage-sensor, gating apparatus, ion pore, selectivity filter, TTX binding site, and the binding sites for drugs such as lidocaine, quinidine, and encainide. Functional expression of the eel channel from the cloned cDNA has not been possible.

At the present time, a total of six full-length mammalian Na⁺ channel cDNA sequences have been characterized by the molecular cloning approach: three isoforms from rat brain (23,24), one from rat heart (26), one from skeletal muscle (27), and one from mouse heart and uterus (10). All but the last of these reported mammalian cDNA sequences predict proteins that exhibit striking similarity to one another (>80% overall amino acid sequence identity) and appear to comprise a single multigene family. The human homologs to these six rodent channels have been cloned and show 68–93% amino acid sequence identity with the rodent channels (9,28–32). The human $Na_v2.1$ and mouse $Na_v2.3$ Na⁺ channels cloned from heart and uterus appear to represent a second gene subfamily, with only 40–45% sequence identity to the previously mentioned mammalian clones. This channel has been placed in subfamily Na_v2 while the others are designated to be in the Na_v1 subfamily. The cloned, full-length mammalian channels and their tissue-specific expression are summarized in Table 1.

There is evidence from molecular cloning that the eel and mammalian Na⁺ channels have related members in such diverse species as *Drosophila* (33,34), squid (35), and jellyfish (36). The amino acid sequence similarity between all these channels is shown in Figure 1. The invertebrate channels are least related to the mammalian proteins. The jellyfish channel is least similar to the others, as may be expected, since the jellyfish is evolutionarily the oldest animal with a nervous system. Na⁺ channels are thought to have a common ancestry with other voltage-dependent ion channels and appear to have evolved from potassium channels via two rounds of gene duplication (12). Potassium channels are

Table 1 Summary of Cloned Mammalian Sodium Channel Alpha Subunits

Rat Clone	Human Homolog	Primary Tissue Distribution	Heterologous Expression In
Rat brain I	SCN1	Brain	Oocytes
Rat brain II	HBA	Brain	Oocytes, CHO cells
Rat brain III	SCN3	Brain	Oocytes
Rat heart 1	hH 1	Atrium, ventricle	Oocytes, CHO cells
Rat SkM 1	hSkM1	Skeletal muscle	HEK 293 cells, oocytes
—	Nav2.1	Atrium, ventricle, uterus	Not successful to date

Only full-length cDNA clones are listed.

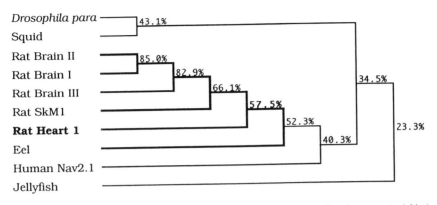

Figure 1 Possible phylogenetic relationship among cloned voltage-gated Na+ channels. Amino acid sequence similarity scores are indicated. Human homologs to the rat proteins are not listed since the sequence similarity is greater than 90% when one compares the rat and human brain and muscle NaChs.

composed of four separate protein subunits, each having six membrane-spanning domains. In view of the extensive structural diversity that exists among members of the voltage-dependent potassium channel family (with greater than 25 genes cloned in the rat) (37), it is predicted that additional mammalian Na+ channel isoforms will be identified by molecular cloning.

CLONING OF VOLTAGE-GATED Na+ CHANNELS FROM RAT AND HUMAN MYOCARDIUM

Molecular cloning of the predominant TTX-R Na+ channel in newborn rat heart was first accomplished by Rogart and co-workers (26). Screening a newborn rat heart cDNA library with cRNA fragments encoding the amino- and carboxyl-termini of the previously cloned rat brain II Na+ channel (23) yielded cDNA clones that showed strong cardiac RNA-specific hybridization. Three overlapping clones were identified that spanned the entire newborn rat heart Na+ channel sequence. The channel represented by this clone was named rat heart I (rHI). Prediction of transmembrane topology by hydropathy analysis revealed high similarity with the eel Na+ channel, with four large (229–280 residues each) hydrophobic domains each composed of six potential membrane-spanning segments including a positively charged amphipathic segment designated S4. The total amino acid sequence similarity between rH1 and the eel channel, rat brain II, or rat skeletal muscle isoform is 65%, 77%, and 60%, respectively. The regions of greatest conservation (61–91%) are the sequences within the four homologous repeats, especially in the transmembrane-spanning regions of repeats III and IV, while little sequence conservation (12–40%) is observed in the cytoplasmic sequence linking these repeats. An exception here is the linking sequence between repeats III and IV, in which the conservation is greater than 90% between these clones. Figure 2 shows the primary sequence of rat heart 1 aligned with the rat skeletal muscle and brain type II channels and the human $Na_v2.1$ channel. As will be discussed, the highly conserved sequences illustrated in Figure 2 are in functionally important regions and the few sequence differences that do exist in these regions impart isoform-specific properties such as TTX resistance.

While the Rogart group pursued the molecular cloning of rh1, identification of the human cardiac TTX-resistant voltage-dependent Na^+ channel was undertaken by Kallen and collaborators (28). In this case, probes derived from rH1 were used to screen an adult human cardiac cDNA library. Ninety positive clones were identified and 23 partial and overlapping clones were isolated and sequenced. Sequence analysis produced a 8491 base pair (bp) cDNA designated as hHl for human heart 1. This human cardiac Na^+ channel showed striking identity with rH1 (93%, with 2016 amino acids as compared to 2019 amino acids in rat heart 1), indicating these two proteins represent species homologs of the same isoform.

HETEROLOGOUS EXPRESSION AND STRUCTURE–FUNCTION STUDIES

To study the relationships between channel amino acid sequence and function, and to confirm that the rat and human cardiac Na^+ channel clones do encode proteins that function as the native cardiac Na^+ current, it was necessary to express these channels in heterologous systems and characterize the current electrophysiologically. The principle expression system used for the cloned heart Na^+ channels has been the *Xenopus* oocyte, which does not contain endogenous Na^+ currents. Expression work in mammalian tissue culture cells (38,39) has

---

Figure 2 Comparison of rat heart 1 to other cloned Na^+ channels. The rat heart I (rH1) channel sequence, deduced from its cloned cDNA (26), is compared to the sequences of rat skeletal muscle 1 (rSkM) (27), rat brain II (rBII) (23), and human $Na_v2.1$ (h$Na_v2.1$) (9). The dashed lines represent gaps inserted to maximize the alignment. The suggested locations of the 24 putative membrane spanning regions are indicated with bold lines above the sequence. The proposed pore-forming sequence is indicated by the line labeled with a P. The arrow in the P region between IS5 and IS6 indicates the cysteine residue that is responsible for the TTX-resistance of the cardiac isoform. The boxed residues in the P region of repeats III and IV are involved in determining ion selectivity.

```
rH I    MANL----LL PRGTSSFRRF TRESLAAIEK RMAEKQARGG SATSQESREG LQEEEAPRPQ LDLQASKKLP DLYGNPPREL IGEPLEDLDP FYSTQK-TFI
rSkM    MASSSLPNLV PPGPHCLRPF TPESLAAIEQ RAVEEEA--- --RLQRNKQM EIEEPERKPR SDLEAGKNLP LIYGDPPPEV IGIPLEDLDP YYSDKK-TFI
rBII    MARSVL---V PPGPDSFRFF TRESLAAIEQ RIAEEKAK-- --RPKQERKD EODDENGPKPN SDLEAGKSLP FIYGDIPPEM VSEPLEDLDP YYINKK-TFI
hNav2.I M-------LA SPEPKGLVPF TKESFELIKQ HIA-------- ----KTHNE DHEEEDLKPN PDLEVGKKLP FIYGNLSQGM VSEPLEDVDP YYYKKKNTFI
                                                                                        II S1              II S2
        VLNKGKTIFR FSATNALYVL SPFHPVRRAA VKILVHSLFS MLIMCTILTN CVFMAQHDPP PWTKYVEYTF TAIYTFESLV KILARGFCLH AFTFLRDPWN
        VLNKGKAIFR FSATPALYIL SPFSIVRRVA IKVLIHALFS MFIMITILTN CVFMTMSNPP SWSKHVEYTF TGIYTFESLI KILARGFCID DFTFLRDPWN
        VLNKGKAISR FSATSALYIL TPFNPIRKLA IKILVHSLFN VLIMCTILTN CVFMTMSNPP DWTKNVEYTF TGIYTFESLI KILARGFCLE DFTFLRNPWN
        VLNKNRTIFR FNAASILCTL SPFNCIRRTT IKVLVHPFFQ LFILISVLID CVFMSLTNLP KWRPVLENTL LGIYTFEILV KLFARGVWAG SFSFLGDPWN
        II S3               II S4               II S5
        WLDFSVIVMA YYTTEFVDLGN VSALRTFRVL RALKTISVIS GLKTIVGALI QSVKKLADVM VLTVFCLSVF ALIGLQLFMG NLRHKCVRNF TELNGTNGS-
        WLDFSVITMA YVTEFVDLGN ISALRTFRVL RALKTIVIP GLKTIVGALI QSVKKLSDVM ILTVFCLSVF ALVGLQLFMG NLRQKCVRWP PPMNDTNTTW
        WLDFIVITFA YVTEFVDLGN VSALRTFRVL RALKTISVIP GLKTIVGALI QSVKKLSDVM ILTVFCLSVF ALIGLQLFMG NLRNKCLQWP P---------
        WLDFSVTVFE VIIRYSPLDF IPTLQTARTL RILKIIPLNQ GLKSLVGVLI HCLKQLIGVI ILTLFFLSIF SLIGMGLFMG NLKHKCFRWP QENE------
                                                                                                              P
        ---------- --VEADGL-- --VWNSL--- -------DV YLNDPANYLL KNGTTDVLLC GNSSDAGTCP EGYRCLKAGE NPDHGYTSFD SFAWAFLALF
        YGNDTWYSND TWYGNDTWYI NDTWNSQESW AGNSTFDWEA YINDEGNYFF LEGSNDALLC GNSSDAGHCP EGYECIKAGR NPNYGYTSYD TFSWAFLSLF
        -DNSTFEINI TSFFNNSL-- --DWNGTAFN RTVNMFNWDE YIEDKSHFYF LEGQNDALLC GNSSDAGQCP EGYICVKAGR NPNYGYTSFD TFSWAFLSLF
        ---------- ----NETLH- -------N RTGNPY---- YIRETENFYY LEGERYALLC GNRTDAGQCP EGYMGPPNVL GNLGVKKAGI NPQGFTNFD SFGWALFALF
                 ▼                        II S6
        RLMTQDCWER LYQQTLRSAG KIYMIFFMLV IFLGSFYLVN LILAVVAMAY EEQNQATIAE TEEKEKRFQE AMEMLKKEHE ALTIR------ -----
        RLMTQDYWEN LFQLTLRAAG KTYMIFFVVI IFLGSFYLIN LILAVVAMAY AEQNEATLAE AEQKEAEFQQ MLEQLKKQQE EAQAAAAAAS AESRDFSGAG
        RLMTQDFWEN LYQLTLRAAG KTYMIFFVLV SFLFSFYMAS LFLGILAMAY EEEKQRVGEI SKKIEPKFQQ TGKELQEGNE T---------- -----
        RLMAQDYPEV LYHLILYASG KVYMIFFVVV SFLFSFYMAS LFLGILAMAY EEEKQRVGEI SKKIEPKFQQ TGKELQEGNE T---------- -----
        GVDTVSRSSL EMSPLAPVTN HERKSKRRKR LSS--GTEDG GODRLPKSDS EDGPRA---- -LNQLSLT-- -------HG L--SRTSM-- RPRSSRGSIF
        ---------- ---------- ---------- -------GEEA DGDPTHNKDC NGSLDASG-- ---------- EK-------- ---------- ----------
        GIGVFSESSS VASKLSSKSE KELKNRRKKK KQKEQAGEEE KEDAVRKSAS EDSIRKKGFQ FSLEGSRLTY EKRFSSPHQS LLSIRGSLFS PRRNSRASLF
        TF--RRRDQG SEADFADDEN STAGESESHR TSLLVPWPL- -RHPSAQGQP GPGASA-PGY VLNGKRNSTV DCNGVVSLLG AGDAEATSPG SYLLRPMVLD
        ---------- ---------- ---------- ---------G PPRPS----- ---------- ---CSA---- ---------- ---------- ----------
        NFKGRVKDIG SENDFADDEH STFEDNDSRR DSLFVPWVRHG ERRPSNVSQA SRASRGIPTL PNNGKMHSAV DCNGVVSLVG -GPSALTSPV GQLL------
        ---------- ------DEA KTIQIEMKKR SPI-------- ---------- ---------- ---------- ---------- ---------- ----------
        RPPDTTTPSE EPGGPQMLTP QAPCADGFEE PGARQRALSA VSVLTSALEE LEESHRKCPP CWNRFAQHYL IWECCPLWMS IKQKVKFVVM DPFALDTITM
        ---------- ---------- ---------- ----DSAISDAMEE LEEANDKCPP WNYKCANHYL IWNCCAPWVK FKHIIYLIVM DPFVDLGITI
        -PEGTTTETE IR--KRRSSS YHVSMDLLED PS-RQRAMSM ASILTNTMEE LEESRQKCPP CWYKFANMCL IWDCCKPWLK VKHVVNLVVM DPFVDLAITI
        ---------- ---------- ---------- ----S TDTSLDVLED ATLRHK---- ------- CE LEKSKKICPL YWYFAKSTFL IWNCCAPWLK LKEFVHRIIM APFTDLFLII
        II S2                                                II S3               II S4
        CIVLNTLFMA LEHYNMTAEF EEMLQVGNLV FTGIFTAEMT FKIIALDPYY YFQQGWNIFD SIIVILSLME LGLSRMGNLS VLRSFRLLRV FKLAKSWPTL
        CIVLNTLFMA MEHYPMTEHF DNVLSVGNLV FTGIFTAEWV LKLIAMDPYY YFQQGWNIFD SFIVTLSLVE LGLANVQGLS VLRSFRLLRV FKLAKSWPTL
        CIVLNTLFMA MEHYPMTEQF SSVLSVGNLV FTGIFTAEWV FKIIALDPYY YFQEGWNIFD GFIVSLSLME LGLANVGGLS VLRSFRLLRV FKLAKSWPTL
        CIILNVCFLT LEHYPMSKQT NTLLNIGNLV FTGIFTAEMT FKIIAMHPYG YFQVGWNIFD SFIVSLSLME LSLANVAGMA LLRFRMLRI FKLGKYWPTF
        II S5                                                II S6
        NTLIKIIGNS VGALGNLTLV LAIIVFIFAV VGMQLFGKNY SELRHRISDS GLLPRWHWMD FFHAFLIIFR ILCGEWIETM WDCMEVSGQS LCLLVFLLVM
        NMLIKIIGNS VGALGNLTLV LAIIVFIFAV VGMQLFGKSY KECVCKIASD CNLPRWHWMD FFHSFLIVFR ILCGEWIETM WDCMEVAGQA MCLTVFMWVM
        NMLIKIIGNS VGALGNLTLV LAIIVFIFAV VGMQLFGKSY KECVCKISND CELPRWHWMD FFHSFLIVFR ILCGEWIETM WDCMEVAGQS WCIPFYLMVI
        QILMWSLSNS MVALKDLVLL LFTFIFFSAA FGMKLFGKNY EEFVCHIDKD CQLPRWHHMH FFHSFLNVFR ILCGEWIETM WDCMEVAGQS WCIPFYLMVI
        II S6
        VIGNLVVLNL FLALLLSSFS ADNLTAPDED GEMNNLQLAL ARIQRGLRFV KRTTWDFCCG ILRRRPKKKA ALATHSQLPS CITAPRSPPP PEVEKVPPAR
        VIGNLVVLNL FLALLLSSFS ADSLAASDED GEMNNLQIAI GRIKWGIGFA KTFLLGLLRG KILSPKEIIL SLGEPGGAGE ----NAEEST PEDEKKEPPP
        VIGNLVVLNL FLALLLSSFS SDNLAATDDD WEMNNLQIAI GRIKWGIGFA KFVRKQKALD EIKPLEDLNN ----KKDSCI SNHITIEIGK
        LIGNLLVLYL FLALV-SSFS SCKDVTAEEN NEAKNLQLAV ARIKKGINYV ---LLKILCK TQNVPKDTMD HVNE------ --VYVKED--I SDHTLSELSN
        KETRFEEDKR PCGQTPGDSE PVCVPIAVAE SDTEDQEEDE ENSLGTEEES SKQESQVVSG GHEPYQEPRA WSQVSETTSS EAGASTSQAD WQQEQKTEPQ
        EDKELKD--- -NH-ILNHVG TTDGPRSSIE LD--HLNFIN NPYLTIQVPI ASEESDL--- ---------- --EMPTEEET DAFSEPEDIK KPLQPLYDGN
        DLNYLKD--- -GNGTTSGIG SSVEKYVVDE SD--YMSFIN NPSLTVTVPI ALGESDF--- ---------- ---ENLDN KEIQSKSGDG GSKEKIKQSS
        TQDFLKDKEK SSGTEKNAT- ---------- -ENESQSLIP SPSVSETVPI ASGSDF-- ---------- ---ENLDN RKTCCKIVEH NWFKCFIGLV TLLSTGTLAF
        III S1
        APGCGETPED SYSEGSTADM TNTADLLEQI PDLGDKVKDP EDCFTEGCVR RCPCCMVDTT QSPGKVWWRL RKTCYRIVEH SWFETFIIFM ILLSSGALAF
        SSVCSTADYK PPEEDPE--- -------EQA EENEQGE-QP EECFTEACVK RCPCLYVDIS QGRGKMWWTL RRACFKIVEH NWFETFIVFM ILLSSGALAF
        SSEGSTVDIG APAEG----- ------EQP EAEPEESLEP EACFTEDCVR KFKCCQISIE EGKGKLWWNL RKTCYKIVEH NWFETFIVFM ILLSSGALAF
        SSECSTVDIA ISEEE----EM FYGGERSKH- ---------- ---LKNGCRRG SSLSGGQSA SKKGKINQNI RKTCCKIVEN NWFKCFIGLV TLLSTGTLAF
        III S2                              III S3                  III S4
        EDIYLEERKT IKVLLEYADK MFTYVFVLEM LLKWVAYGFK KYFTNAWCWL DFLIVDVSLV SLVANTLGFA EMGPIKSLRT LRALRPLRAL SRFEGMRVVV
        EDIYIEQRRV IRTILEYADK VFTYIFILEM LLKWVAYGFK VYFTNAWCWL DFLIVDVSII SLVANWLGYS ELGPIKSLRT LRALRPLRAL SRFEGMRVVV
        EDIYIEQRKT IKTMLEYADK VFTYIFILEM LLKWVAYGFQ KYFTNAWCWL DFLIVDVSLV SLTANALGYS ELGAIKSLRT LRALRPLRAL SRFEGMRVVV
        EDIYIDQRKT IKILLEYADK IFTYIFILEM LLKWVAYGFK AYFSNGWYRL DFVVVIVFCL SLIGKT---- --REELKPLIS MKFLRPLRAL SQFERMRVVV
        III S5                                                          P
        NALVGAIPSI MNVLLVCLIF WLIFSIMGVN LFAGKFGRCI NQTEGDLPLN YTIVNNKSEC ESMVTGELY --WTKVKVNFD NVGAGYLALL QVATFKGWMD
        NALLGAIPSI MNVLLVCLIF WLIFSIMGVD LFAGKFYYCV NTTTSER-FD ISVVNNKSEC ESLMYTGQV- RWHNVKVNYD NVGLGYLSLL QVATFKGWMD
        NALLGAIPSI MNVLLVCLIF WLIFSIMGVN LFAGKFYHCI NYTTGEM-FD VSVVNNYSEC QALIESNQTA RWKNVKINFD NVGLGYLSLL QVATFKGWMD
        RALIKTTLPT LNVFLVCLNI WLIFSIMGVG LFAGRFYECI DPTSGER-FP SSEVNNKSRC ESLLWENAKM NFD NVGNGFLSLL QVATFNGWMIT
        IMYAAVDSRG YEEQPQWEDN LYNNYVFVVF IIFGSFFTLN LFIGVIIDNF NQQKKKLGGQ DIFMTEEQKK YYNAMKKLGS KKPQKPIPRP LNKYQGFIFD
        IMYAAVDSRE KEEQPHVEVN LYMYLYFVIF IIFGSFFTLN LFIGVIIDNF NQQKKKFGGK DIFMTEEQKK YYNAMKKLGS KKPQKPIPRP ANKFQGNVFD
        IMYAAVDSRN VELQPKYEDN LYMYLYFVIF IIFGSFFTLN LFIGVIIDNF NQQKKKLGGQ DIFMTEEQKK YYNAMKKLGS KKPQKPIPRP ANKFQGMVFD
        INNSAIDSVA VNIGPHFEVN IYFLYFLPLS MLITVIIDNF NKHKIKLGGS KIFITVKKQRK QDYQKLKKLMY EDSQRPVPRP LSCLIFD
        IV S1                                   IV S2                  IV S3
        IVTKQAFDVT IMFLICLNMV TMMVETDDQS PEKVNILAKI NLLFVAIFTG ECIVKMAALR HYYFTIGWNI FDFVVVILSI VGTVLSDIIQ KYFFSPTLFR
        FVTKQVFDIS IMILICLNMV TMMVETDDQS QLKVDILYNI NMVFIIIFTG ECVLKMFALR HYYFTIGWNI FDFVVVILSI VGLALSDLIQ KYFVSPTLFR
        FVTKQVFDIS IMILICLNMV TMMVETDDQS QEMTNILYWI NLVTFIIFTG ECVLKLISLR HYYYFTIGWNI FDFVVVILSI VGMFLAELIE KYFVSPTLFR
        VVTSQAFNVI VMVLICFQAI AWMIDTDVQS LQMSIALYWI NSIFVMLYTM ECILKLIAFR CFYFTIAWNI FDFMVVIFSI LGLILGCLPNTVG SYLVPPSLVQ
        IV S4                                   IV S5                  IV S6
        VIRLARIGRI LRLIRGAKGI RTLLFALMMS LPALFNIGLL LFLVMFIYSI FGMANFAYVK KESGIDDMFN FQTFANSMLL LFQITTSAGW DGLLSPILNT
        VIRLARIGRV LRLIRGAKGI RTLLFALMMS LPALFNIGLL LFLVMFIYSI FGMSNFAYVK REGGIDDMFN FETFGNSILC LFEITTSAGW DGLLAPILNS
        VIRLARIGRI LRLIRGAKGI RTLLFALMMS LPALFNIGLL LFLVMFIYAI FGMANFAYVK REVGIDDMFN FETFGNSMIC LFQITTSAGW DGLLAPILNT
        LILLSRIIHM LRLGKGPKVF HNLMLPLMLS LPALNIILL IFLVMFIYAV FGMANFAYVK KEAGINDVSN FETFGNSMLC LFQVAIFKGW DGMLDAIFNS
        GPPYCDPN-L PNSNGSRGNC GSPAVGILFF TTYIIISFLI VVNMYIAIIL ENFSVATEES TEPLSEDDFD MFYEIWEKFD PEATQFIEYL ALSDFADALS
        GPPDCDPTLE NPGTNVRGDC GNPSIGICFF CSYIIISFLI VVNMYIAVIL ENFSVATEES SEPLSEDDFE MFYEVWEKFD PDATQFIDYS KLSDFAAALD
        GPPDCDPEKD HPGSSVKGDC GNPSVGIFFF VSYIIISFLV VVNMYIAVIL ENFSVATEES AEPLSEDDFE MFYEVWEKFD PDATQFIEFC KLSDFAAALD
        KWSDCDPDNL NPGTPVDGDC GNPSVGIFFF VSYIIISFLI VVNMYIVVVM EFINIASKK NFKIITCEFI LTNQFHKKLV LKKNKRSPQ
        EPLRIAKPNQ ISLINMDLPM VSGDRIHCMD ILFAFTKRVL GESGEMDALK IQMEEKFMAA NPSKISYEPI TTLRRKHEE VSATVIQRAF RRHLLQRSVK
        EPLKIAKPNK IKLITLDLPM VPGDKIHCLD ILFALTKRVL GESGEMDALK IQMEEKFMAS NPSKVSYEPI TTLRKRQEE VCAIKIQRAY RRHLLQRSVK
        PPLLIAKPNK VQLIADLPM VPGDKIHCLD ILFALTKEVL GDSGEMDALR IQMEERFMAS NPSKVSYEPI TTLRKRQEE VSAIVIQRAY RRYLLKQKVK
        PPLFMAKPNK GQLIALDLPM AVGDRIHCLD ILLAFTKRVW GQDVRMEKVV SIESGFLLA NPFKITCEPI TTTLRKRQEE VSATIIQRAY RRHLLKRDMK
        HASFLFRQQA GGSGLSDEDA PEREGLIAYM MNGNFSR--- ---------- --RSAPLSSS ISSTSFPPSY DSVTRATSON LPVRASDYSR SEDLADFPPS
        QASYMYRHSQ DG---NDDGA PEKEGLLANT MNKMYGHEKE GDGVQSQGEE EKASTEDAGP TVEPEPTSSS DTALTPSPPP LPPSSSP--- ----PQGQTV
        KVSSIYKKDK GK----DEGT PIKEDIITDK L---------- ---------- ---ENSTPEKTDV TPSTTSPPSY DSVTKPEKEK FEKDKSE----- ----KEDKG-
        NTSDIHMIDG DR-----DVH ATKEGAY--- ---FDKAKE KSPIQSQ--- ---------- ---------- ---------- ---------- ----------
        PDRDRESIV
        RPGVKESLV
        -KDIRESKK
        -------T
```

served to confirm that the oocyte is faithful in terms of synthesizing a channel protein with wild-type properties. When the *Xenopus* oocytes were injected with cRNA transcribed from either the rH1 or hH1 cDNA clones, and resulting Na^+ currents measured using two electrode voltage-clamp, channel kinetics consistent with the native cardiac Na^+ current were observed (Fig. 4B)(40,41). Both the rat and human cardiac Na^+ channels expressed in the oocytes showed about a 100-fold lower sensitivity to block by TTX ($K_d = 2$ µM) than the cloned skeletal muscle or brain channels, consistent with the native Na^+ channels found in mammalian cardiac myocytes. Although cofactors and other posttranslational modifications may modulate this cardiac Na^+ channel function, these results directly indicated that the low sensitivity for TTX resides in the primary structure of the rH1 protein. In addition, these data indicated that only the cloned protein is required for functional cardiac Na^+ current.

Most of the structure–function information that exists on voltage-gated Na^+ channels has been collected using site-directed mutagenesis of the rat brain II channel expressed in the oocyte system. The functional consequences of replacing arginine residues with glutamine in the S4 segment of domain 1 were examined by Stühmer et al. by site-directed mutagenesis of the rat brain II Na^+ channel (42). Neutralizations of S4 segment-positive charge in domain 1 results in decreased steepness in the voltage dependence of activation and caused a shift in the current–voltage relationship toward more positive potentials. These experiments have supported the idea that the S4 domains are involved in voltage sensing. However, such interpretations may be questioned. If S4 plays primarily a structural role in terms of holding the transmembrane helices in the proper orientation, any alteration to S4 could indirectly affect voltage-sensing without S4 being the true sensor itself. The identification of regions involved in Na^+ channel inactivation and ion permeation has been more straightforward.

Whereas voltage-dependent activation appears to involve S4, the inactivation has been localized to interdomain 3–4 (ID3–4). The first indication that the cytoplasmic sequence between repeats III and IV was involved in channel inactivation was that inactivation was inhibited by an antibody directed against this region (43–45). Subsequent site-directed mutagenesis experiments have confirmed that this cytoplasmic sequence, specifically the three residues, isoleucine, phenylalanine, and methionine, probably represents the "inactivation gate" (46,47). Removal of these three amino acids or substitution with glutamine slows or completely abolishes Na^+ channel inactivation. The current working hypothesis is that these amino acids move into the open pore of the channel after it opens, thereby blocking the ion conduction through the pore and resulting in the inactivated state of the channel. The substitution of highly conserved positive and negative amino acids in this region has little effect on inactivation. While these studies have been primarily done with the rat brain type II channel, this role of the III–IV linker has been confirmed with mutagenesis studies of the rat heart channel (48).

The highest degree of amino acid sequence identity among Na$^+$ channels is found within the S5-S6 interhelical region that is believed to form membrane-penetrating hairpin structures that contribute to the formation of the ion pore (see Fig. 5) (49). An important study that revolutionized the Na$^+$ channel field was the discovery that two amino acid substitutions in the voltage-dependent Na$^+$ channel protein alter the ion selectivity (50). Replacement of the highly conserved lysine at position 1422 in the third domain and alanine at 1714 in the fourth domain with glutamic acids altered the ion selectivity of the rat brain II Na$^+$ channel now to favor Ca^{2+} over Na$^+$. This result emphasizes how major functional differences between Na$^+$ and Ca^{2+} channels can be determined by only 2 of the approximately 2000 amino acids. Additional experiments supporting the role of these sequences in forming the pore involve alteration of TTX sensitivity. If well-conserved glutamic acid residues in the rat brain type II pore are mutated to uncharged amino acids, the affinity for TTX is drastically reduced (51). It appears that the aspartic and glutamic acid residues in domains 1, 2, and 4 provide fixed negative charge within the pore that is required of high-affinity TTX binding.

The mutagenesis studies with the cardiac Na$^+$ channel isoform that have attracted the most attention are those that have focused on why the cardiac isoform shows resistance to TTX and high sensitivity to Cd^{2+} block while the opposite sensitivities are true for the skeletal muscle and brain isoforms. Since these agents are believed to bind within the pore, defining amino acids involved in TTX and Cd^{2+} block advances our knowledge of the pore. Comparison of potential pore sequence between the TTX-resistant cardiac isoform and the TTX-sensitive forms from brain and skeletal muscle are illustrated in Figure 2 (see regions identified with a P). The negatively charged amino acids such as glutamic acid, which are required for TTX sensitivity, are conserved between the cardiac and brain isoforms. However, one difference that does exist is within the sequence between S5 and S6 in repeat I. In this region TTX-sensitive channels have either a tyrosine or a phenylalanine while the heart isoform has a cysteine in this position (see arrow, Fig. 2). Mutation of this single cysteine residue to a tyrosine renders the cardiac channel sensitive to TTX, with the K$_d$ going from 950 nM to 1.32 nM (52). In addition, the Cd^{2+} sensitivity of the mutant decreased about 30-fold. When the tyrosine found in the skeletal muscle form was changed to a cysteine, this mutant was now TTX resistant and Cd^{2+} sensitive (53). These data again illustrate how a single amino acid change in a very large protein can have major effects on channel properties.

ROLE OF THE BETA SUBUNIT IN Na$^+$ CHANNEL FUNCTION

The eel Na$^+$ channel is composed of a single heavily glycosylated polypeptide of approximately 240,000 daltons in molecular weight (21), again emphasizing that the α subunit alone is sufficient for function. In contrast, the rat brain channel has two small subunits, designated β1 and β2, in addition to the large α subunit (54). The rat skeletal muscle Na⁺ channel α subunit isoform, and probably the cardiac isoform as well, are assembled with only the β1 subunit (55). Catterall and co-workers (56) were the first to purify enough β1 subunit protein for amino acid sequence determination, allowing the design of oligo-nucleotide probes for library screening and eventual cloning. The translated nucleotide sequence of the cDNA (Fig. 3) predicts a protein with molecular mass of 23 kDa, a size agreeing well with the deglycosylated mature β1 sub-unit (57). An N-terminal signal sequence is present in addition to four sites for N-linked glycosylation. Biochemical analysis indicates that the fully glycosylated protein has an apparent molecular weight of 36 kDa. The predicted structure from sequence analysis is a single transmembrane-spanning region with an extracellular N-terminus and an intracellular C-terminus as diagrammed in Fig-ure 5. Three of the four putative N-linked glycosylation sites are located in the predicted extracellular domain. Northern blot analysis of β1 subunit expression indicates the gene is expressed primarily in rat brain, skeletal muscle, and spinal cord (56), while multiple β subunits have been detected in rat brain, skeletal muscle, sciatic nerve, and heart using subunit-specific antibodies (58). The human homolog of the rat β1 has been cloned and expressed by George and co-workers (59). While the human clone is nearly identical to the rat protein, the steady-state tissue distribution of the mRNA differs from the rat. While expression is greatest in human brain and skeletal muscle, significant mRNA expression was found in both atrium and ventricle. Whether this hybridization represents the β1 isoform or a related species is unknown. It is interesting that mRNA expression was significantly reduced in cardiomyopathic left ventricle as compared to normal tissue (59). This difference could be due to either the replacement of myocytes with fibrous tissue or an actual downregulation in the diseased state. The β2 subunit has also been cloned by the Catterall group and it is similar in size and transmembrane topology to the β1 protein (55).

MGRLLALVVGAALVSSACG GCVEVDSETEAVYGMTFKILCISCKRRSE

TNAETFTEWTFRQKGTEEFVKILRYENEVLQLEEDERFEGRVVWNGSR

GTKDLQDLSIFITNVTYNHSGDYECHVYRLLFFENYEHNTSVVKKIHI

EVVDKANRDMASIVSEIMMYVLIVVLTIWLVAEMIYCYKKIAAATETA

AQENASEYLAITSESKENCTGVQVAE

Figure 3 Structure of the human beta 1 subunit. Amino acid sequence of the cloned human beta 1 subunit (59). The boxed N-terminal sequence represents the signal peptide and the potential N-linked glycosylation sites are marked with a (●). The bar highlights a single putative membrane-spanning domain.

The β1 subunit is somewhat isoform-specific in terms of its functional effects. For example, coexpression of the β1 subunit with the rat brain II α subunit in the *Xenopus* oocyte system increases inactivation rate, shifts the voltage dependence of steady-state inactivation to the left , and increases the rate of recovery from inactivation (55,56). An additional effect is a twofold increase in channel expression compared to when the subunit is expressed alone. As shown in Figure 4A similar effects on inactivation rate are observed when the human skeletal muscle isoform is coexpressed in oocytes with the human β1 subunit. However, as shown in Figure 4B, coexpression of the human β subunit with the human cardiac Na$^+$ channel does not have a significant effect on inactivation kinetics. This lack of effect disagrees with the finding that β1 mRNA is abundant in both human atrium and ventricle. Perhaps the β1 in heart is associated with Na$^+$ isoforms other than the TTX-resistant cardiac channel. An an alternative, it may be assembled with the cardiac channel in native tissue but we simply have yet to discover the functional role β1 plays with this isoform. It should be emphasized that some investigators have reported an effect of the β1 subunit on cardiac Na$^+$ channel inactivation. When Marban and co-workers expressed the rat β1 subunit with the human cardiac Na$^+$ channel, a 1.5-3 fold increase in inactivation was observed (60). At the present time, there does not appear to be any indication that the β subunits are responsible for drug binding sites. However, at this early stage in their discovery, much work remains to be done. The functional effects of coexpression of various alpha isoforms with β2 with or without β1 have not yet been reported.

TISSUE AND CELLULAR EXPRESSION OF THE CARDIAC Na$^+$ CHANNEL

Northern blot analysis and RNase protection assays have shown that rH1 is abundantly expressed in heart and denervated skeletal muscle but is not detectable in brain, kidney, spleen, liver, uterus, or adult skeletal muscle (26,28,61). Thus, the tissue-specificity of rH1 expression seems well confined to cardiac tissue. Analysis of mRNA in whole tissue, while an important first step, provides little information with respect to the specific cell types within the heart that express the channel. Nonmyocyte cells make a significant contribution to the total mRNA isolated from this organ. Conversely, undetectable mRNA levels may lead to the interpretation that the channel is not expressed in, or physiologically important to, a given tissue. However, mRNA could be expressed at high levels in cells that represent a small percentage of the tissue.

Western blot analysis and immunoprecipitation are used to detect proteins within a given tissue and have provided insight into rH1 protein expression. Three separate antibodies were generated against peptides corresponding to diverse portions of rH1 and used in Western blot analysis of partially purified

A

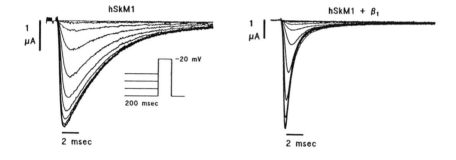

B

Human Cardiac Na⁺ Channel (hH1)

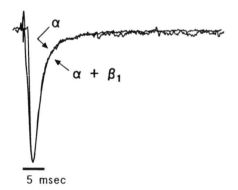

5 msec

Figure 4 Functional effects of the β1 Na⁺ channel subunit. A. Coexpression in *Xenopus* oocytes of the skeletal muscle with the cloned human β1 subunit. The left panel shows the expression of the skeletal muscle α subunit alone, the right panel shows the currents obtained after co-expression with β1. Note the differences in inactivation rate. B. Coexpression β1 with the cardiac alpha subunit. In this case coexpression with β1 had little effect on inactivation rate. (Data kindly provided by Dr. Paul Bennett, Departments of Pharmacology and Medicine, Vanderbilt Medical School.)

cat cardiac membranes (62). All antibodies recognized an identical 240 kD band corresponding to rH1, supporting the Northern blot data that rHl is found abundantly in the heart. Immunoprecipitation of rH1 with these antibodies did not detect β subunit association with rH1, however, technical difficulties cited by the authors may make the β subunit undetectable. Although these studies provide insight into protein characterization and confirm that rH1 protein is located in cardiac membranes, they do not specify the location of rH1 to the various structures of the heart. To determine the precise localization of rH1 within cardiac tissue, immunocytochemical studies using antibodies generated against this channel were performed. The antibodies previously mentioned localized rH1 to surface and t-tubular membranes of atrial and ventricular muscle cells and to the intercalated discs between adjacent ventricular muscle cells (61,62). While these studies have aided our understanding of Na$^+$ channel localization, it is amazing how little we know with respect to the distribution of the cardiac isoform in heart. Questions dealing with its distribution within the pacemaker and conduction systems remain to be answered. Equally interesting are the questions dealing with cell-specific Na$^+$ channel expression and distribution in diseased myocardium.

CARDIAC Na$^+$ CHANNEL REGULATION

Antiarrhythmic drug therapy, especially with Na$^+$ channel blockers, has yet to make significant clinical progress. Perhaps some of the mortality found in the CAST study was due to changes in cell surface Na$^+$ channel levels induced by the actual drug treatment. Alteration of Na$^+$ channel current levels can occur at multiple steps along the DNA to protein pathway. Drug therapy could affect the transcriptional activity of the gene, the half-life of its mRNA, the transcriptional efficiency of the mRNA, or the transport of nascent channels to the cell surface. Modification of any of these steps could alter Na$^+$ channel current density, the rate of action potential propagation, excitation conduction, and susceptibility to some arrhythmias. While there is no evidence to suggest that such mechanisms were operating in the CAST study, the experiments reviewed below suggest that such drug-induced modulation of cardiac Na$^+$ channel number does occur.

One important effect of the class I antiarrhythmic therapy may occur at the level of Na$^+$ channel transcription. Chronic in vitro treatment of adult rats with the class I drug mexiletine increased cardiac Na$^+$ channel number by 3.6-fold as shown by [^{3}H]batrachotoxin ([^{3}H]BTX) binding experiments (63). [^{3}H]BTX is a neurotoxin ligand that binds to a specific site on most Na$^+$ channels and is used in place of saxitoxin/tetrodotoxin binding to quantitate cardiac channel density, since [^{3}H]BTX binds the cardiac isoform with much greater affinity than either STX or TTX. Animals treated with mexiletine showed a threefold increase in cardiac Na^+ channel mRNA (64), suggesting that drug-induced channel upregulation is due to an increase in gene transcription. The increase in mRNA was mimicked by treatment with the class IV antiarrhythmic drug verapamil. Perhaps the increase in Na^+ channel number is a compensatory mechanism by the cardiac muscle cells in response to decreased electrical activity. Intracellular Ca^{2+} is greatly influenced by activity in muscle, making cytoplasmic Ca^{2+} a candidate second messenger for the upregulation. Cultured neonatal myocytes were treated with verapamil or the calcium ionophore A23187 to examine further the relationship between cytoplasmic Ca^{2+} and channel mRNA (64). Although verapamil did not produce a significant increase in mRNA encoding the cardiac Na^+ channel, A23187 strongly reduced mRNA levels. If one assumes that asynchronous action potentials and contraction of these cultured myocytes were the reason for the insignificant rise in mRNA levels with verapamil, these data are consistent with calcium mediating the regulation of Na^+ channel mRNA. Similar regulatory mechanisms probably exist in rat skeletal muscle. Saxitoxin-binding experiments measured increased Na^+ channel number in cultured skeletal muscle cells following chronic treatment with bupivacaine (65,66). Similar to the mexiletine studies, mRNA levels increased in response to channel block. As with the cultured cardiac myocytes, A23187 strongly reduced mRNA levels.

Modulation of Na^+ channels can be accomplished also at the protein level. Phosphorylation by both protein kinase A (cAMP-dependent protein kinase) and protein kinase C have been demonstrated to modulate the behavior of the rat brain type II Na^+ channel. This channel contains numerous consensus sites for PKA phosphorylation in the intracellular domain between homologous repeats I and II and a well-conserved PKC site (serine 1506) is found in the cytoplasmic III–IV linker. This PKC site has been implicated in regulating inactivation (45) and is found in *Drosophila*, eel, and all but one mammalian Na^+ channel isoform (9). Phosphorylation of this site by PKC leads to a slowing of inactivation with no effect on the voltage-dependence of inactivation (67,68). Phosphorylation of the PKA sites (serines 623, 573, 610, and 687; serine 610 can also be phosphorylated by PKC) (see Fig. 5) results in a decrease in peak current amplitude (69). PKC phosphorylation of serine 554 appears to also decrease peak current (70). These decreases in current are due to a failure of the channels to activate in response to depolarization with no change in the rate of inactivation of the channels that do open. A highly significant finding by the Catterall group is that the PKA-induced decrease is seen only if the PKC site at serine 1506 is phosphorylated (71). Mutating the PKC serine to an alanine blocks functional effects of PKA phosphorylation while replacing the serine with a negative glutamic acid mimics phosphorylation and allows PKA modification of channel function. Hence phosphorylation by these two parallel signalling systems is one way in which neuronal signals may be integrated.

Summary of Structure Function Studies on the Na+ Channel

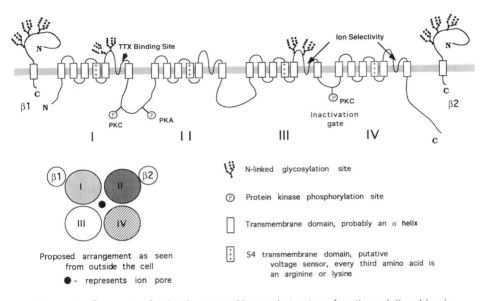

Figure 5 Summary of subunit composition and structure–function relationships in voltage-gated Na+ channels. Indicated are the regions implicated by site-directed mutagenesis in voltage-sensing, inactivation, ion selectivity, and tetrodotoxin (TTX) binding. The four homologous domains are proposed to form a structure with four-fold symmetry around the actual ion pore. The sequence between each S5 and S6 domain "hairpinning" into the membrane is proposed to form one-quarter of the lining of the ion pore.

Na+ channel phosphorylation by both PKA and PKC pathways is likely also to play an important role in the cardiac myocyte. As with the rat brain type II channel, PKA phosphorylation prevents Na+ channel opening. Isoprenaline depresses the cardiac action potential maximum upstroke velocity, presumably by decreasing the inward Na+ current (72). This effect is blocked by beta receptor blockade and mimicked by phosphodiesterase inhibitors. Using canine, guinea pig, and rabbit ventricular myocytes with on-cell macropatch voltage clamp to maintain the myocyte cytoplasmic composition, Ono et. al. (73) showed the cAMP analogs shifted the midpoints for voltage-dependent availability and conductance in the hyperpolarizing direction. These effects were inhibited by PKA blockers. The direct inhibition of Na+ current by beta receptor-activated G-proteins has been proposed by Schubert and co-workers in addition to the indirect cAMP action (74). The role of PKC in cardiac Na channel regulation has been implicated in studies examining the effect of angiotensin II on Na^+ current. Angiotensin II increased current amplitude and accelerated the rate of current inactivation in rat neonatal myocytes (75,76). These effects were mimicked by phorbol esters and diacylglycerol analogs, both of which are activators of PKC. Since PKC activation leads to a decrease in peak current produced by the rat brain type II channel as described above, the Catterall group performed experiments with the cloned rat heart Na^+ channel similar to those with the rat brain type II channel (39). Following expression of the rat cardiac Na^+ channel in Chinese hamster lung cells, PKC activation decreased current, which was in part caused by an 8–14 mV leftward shift in the steady-state inactivation curve. Channel activation was unchanged. Similar effects were observed in neonatal rat myocytes, except that the time course of inactivation was slowed.

In summary, PKA activation appears to decrease Na^+ current in cardiac cells as it does in brain while PKC activation has been reported to both increase and decrease peak current in cardiac myocytes. Given the number of potential phosphorylation sites and their ability to influence each other, as demonstrated by the fact that PKA effects in the rat brain II channel are dependent on PKC phosphorylation of serine 1506, is not surprising that different groups report differing results with respect to PKC inhibition of cardiac Na^+ current. What is clear is that phosphorylation of the cardiac Na^+ channel protein can affect channel function. Therefore, it is likely that both cardiac disease and modulation of sympathetic tone affect the cardiac Na^+ channel via the protein kinase systems. The relationship between autonomic tone and sudden death has been documented (77) and increased vagal stimulation started shortly after the onset of an acute ischemic episode in conscious dogs has an antifibrillatory effect (77). Channel modulation could explain also the difficulties observed with antiarrhythmic drugs, since the channels upon which these drugs are acting are likely to vary kinetically as a function of time and cellular localization. When this issue is placed upon that of altered channel gene regulation, antiarrhythmic drug therapy is truly aiming at a "moving target" (78).

SUMMARY

Molecular cloning technology has greatly expanded our knowledge of voltage-gated Na^+ channel diversity. The combination of molecular cloning, heterologous expression, and site-directed mutagenesis work described in this chapter has dramatically expanded our understanding of rapid depolarization in phase 0 of the cardiac action potential. As summarized in Figure 5, we now have a good idea of the Na^+ channel structures involved in voltage-sensing, inactivation, ion permeation/selectivity, and protein kinase regulation. However, it is also apparent that we have only scratched the surface of this field. Recent advances in chromosomal mapping and analysis and disease linkage will determine whether the cardiac Na^+ channel is responsible for human cardiac disease. The functional and molecular cloning data reviewed here suggest that additional, structurally distinct, Na^+ channels are present in the heart. Further efforts in cloning, functional expression, linkage to human disease, and correlation of these channels with cardiac currents will provide both the basic scientist and clinician with greater knowledge of cardiac physiology and the potential treatment of cardiac pathology.

ACKNOWLEDGMENT

MMT is an Established Investigator of the American Heart Association and was supported by NIH grants HL 49330 and HL 46681 and a grant from the Muscular Dystrophy Association. SKE is supported by NSF fellowship BIR-9406860.

REFERENCES

1. Saint DA, Ju YK, Gage PW. A persistent Na^+ current in rat ventricular myocytes. J Physiol (London) 1992; 453:219–231.
2. Bkaily G, Jacques D, Yamamoto T, Sculptoreanu A, Payet MD. Three types of slow inward currents as distinguished by melittin in 3-day old embryonic heart. Can J Physiol Pharmacol 1988; 66:1017–1022.
3. Coraboeuf E. Voltage clamp studies of the slow inward current. In: Zipes DP, Bailey JC, Elharrar V, eds. The Slow Inward Current and Cardiac Arrhythmias. The Hague, The Netherlands: Martinus Nijhoff Publishers, 1980:25–95.
4. Bkaily G, Jacques D, Sculptoreanu A, Yamamoto T, Carrier D, Vigneault D, Sperelakis N. Apamin, a highly potent blocker of the TTX -and Mn^{2+}-insensitive fast transient Na^+ current in young embryonic heart. J Mol Cell Cardiol 1991; 23:25–39.
5. Lee KS. A novel slow inward Na^+ current at the plateau potential of guinea pig and monkey ventricular cell action potentials. J Mol Cell Cardiol 1990; 22 (Supp I):S.15.
6. Zilberter YI, Starmer CF, Starobin J, Grant AO. Late Na channels in cardiac cells: the physiological role of background Na channels. Biophys J 1994; 67(1):153–160.
7. Jacques D, Bkaily G. Presence of early embryonic slow Na^+ channels in cardiomyopathic hamster. Biophy J 1991; 59:259a.
8. Bkaily G, Jasmin G, Tautu C, Prochek L, Yamamoto T, Sculptoreanu A, Peyrow M, Jacques D. A tetrodotoxin and Mn^{2+}-insensitive Na^+ current in Duchenne muscular dystrophy. Muscle Nerve 1990; 13:939–948.
9. George AL, Knittle TJ, Tamkun MM. Molecular cloning of an atypical voltage-gated Na^+ channel expressed in human heart and uterus: evidence for a distinct gene family. Proc Natl Acad Sci USA 1992; 89:4893–4897.

10. Felipe A, Knittle TJ, Doyle KL, Tamkun MM. Primary structure and differential expression during development and pregnancy of a novel voltage-gated Na+ channel in the mouse. J Biol Chem 1994; 269(48):30125–30131.

11. Sills MN, Xu YC, Baracchini E, Goodman RH, Cooperman SS, Mandel G, Chien KR. Expression of diverse Na+ channel messenger RNAs in rat myocardium. Evidence for a cardiac specific Na+ channel. J Clin Invest 1989; 84:331–336.

12. Hille B. Ionic Channels of Excitable Membranes. Sunderland, MA: Sinauer Associates, 1992.

13. Brown AM, Lee KS, Powell T. Voltage clamp and internal perfusion of single rat heart muscle cells. J Physiol (London) 1981; 318:455–477.

14. Rogart RB. High STX affinity vs. low STX affinity Na+ channel subtypes in nerve, heart, and skeletal muscle. Ann NY Acad Sci 1986; 479:402–430.

15. Catterall WA, Coppersmith J. High-affinity saxitoxin receptor sites in vertebrate heart. Evidence for sites associated with autonomic nerve endings. Mol Phamacol 1981; 20:526–532.

16. Echt DS, Liebson PR, Mitchell LB, Peters RW, Obias-Manno D, Barker AH, Arensberg D, Baker A, Friedman L, Greene HL, Huther ML, Richardson DW, and the CAST Investigators. Mortality and morbidity in patients receiving encainide, flecainide, or placebo. The Cardiac Arrhythmia Suppression Trial. N Engl J Med 1991; 324:781–788.

17. Roden DM. Current status of class III antiarrhythmic drug therapy. Am J Cardiol 1993; 72:44B–49B.

18. Bean BP, Cohen CT, Tsien RW. Lidocaine block of cardiac Na+ channels. J Gen Physiol 1983; 81:613–642.

19. Rojas CV, Wang J, Schwartz LS, Hoffmann EP, Powell BR, Brown RH. A Met-to-Val mutation in the skeletal muscle Na+ channel alpha-subunit in hyperkalemic periodic paralysis. Nature (London) 1991; 354:387–389.

20. Ptacek LJ, Johnson KJ, Griggs RC. Genetics and physiology of the myotonic muscle disorders. N Engl J Med 1993; 328:482–489.

21. Agnew WS, Levinson SR, Brabson JS, Raftery MA. Purification of the tetrodotoxin-binding component associated with the voltage-sensitive Na+ channel from *Electrophorus electricus* electroplax membranes. Proc Natl Acad Sci USA 1978; 75:2606–2610.

22. Noda M, Shimizu S, Tanabe T, Takai T, Kayano T, Ikeda T, Takahashi H, Nakayama H, Kaknaoka Y, Minamino N, Kkangawa K, Matsuo H, Raftery MA, Hirose T, Inayama S, Hayashida H, Miyata T, Numa S. Primary structure of *Electrophorus electricus* Na+ channel deduced from cDNA sequence. Nature (London) 1984; 312:121–127.

23. Noda M, Ikeda T, Kayano T, Suzuki H, Takeshima H, Kurasaki M, Takahashi H, Numa S. Existence of distinct Na+ channel messenger RNAs in rat brain. Nature (London) 1986; 320:188–192.

24. Kayano T, Noda M, Flockerzi V, Takahashi H, Numa S. Primary structure of rat brain Na+ channel III deduced from the cDNA sequence. FEBS Lett 1988; 228:187–194.

25. Goldin AL, et al. Messenger RNA coding for the α subunit of the rat brain Na

channel is sufficient for expression of functional channels in *Xenopus* oocytes. Proc Natl Acad Sci USA 1986; 83:7503–7507.

26. Rogart RB, Cribbs LL, Muglia LK, Kephart DD, Kaiser MW. Molecular cloning of a putative tetrodotoxin-resistant rat heart Na+ channel isoform. Proc Natl Acad Sci USA 1989; 86:8170–8174.

27. Trimmer JS, Cooperman SS, Tomiko SA, Zhou J, Crean SM, Boyle MB, Kallen RG, Sheng Z, Barchi RL, Sigworth FJ, Goodman RH, Agnew WS, Mandel G. Primary structure and functional expression of a mammalian skeletal muscle Na+ channel. Neuron 1989; 3:33–49.

28. Gellens ME, George AL, Chen L, Chahine M, Horn R, Barchi RL, Kallen RG. Primary structure and functional expression of the human cardiac tetrodotoxin-insensitive voltage-dependent Na+ channel. Proc Natl Acad Sci USA 1992; 89:554–558.

29. George AL, Komisarof J, Kallen RG, Barchi RL. Primary structure of the adult human skeletal muscle voltage-dependent Na+ channel. Ann Neurol 1992; 31:131–137.

30. Ahmed CMI, Ware DH, Lee SC, Patten CD, Ferrer-Montiel AV, Schinder AF, McPherson JD, Wagner-McPherson CB, Wasmuth JJ, Evans GA and Montal M. Primary structure, chromosomal localization, and functional expression of a voltage-gated Na+ channel from human brain. Proc Natl Acad Sci USA 1992; 89:8220–8224.

31. Malo MS, Blanchard BJ, Andresen JM, Srivastava K, Chen XN, Li X, Jabs EW, Korenberg JR, Ingram VM. Localization of a putative human brain Na+ channel gene (SCN1A) to chromosome band 2q24. Cytogen Cell Genet 1994; 67:178–186.

32. Malo M, Srivastava K, Andresen JM, Chen XN, Korenberg JR, Ingram VM. Targeted gene walking by low stringency polymerase chain reaction: Assignment of a putative human brain Na+ channel gene (SCH3A) to chromosome 2q24-31. Proc Natl Acad Sci USA 1994; 91:2975–2979.

33. Salkoff L, Butler A, Wei A, Scavarda N, Giffen K, Ifune C, Goodman R and Mandel G. Genomic organization and deduced amino acid sequence of a putative Na+ channel gene in *Drosophila*. Science 1987; 237:744–749.

34. Loughney K, Kreber R, Ganetzky B. Molecular analysis of the para locus, Na+ channel gene in *Drosophila*. Cell 1989; 58:1143–1154.

35. Rosenthal JJC, Gilly WF. Amino acid sequence of a putative Na+ channel expressed in the giant axon of the squid *Loligo opalescens*. Proc Natl Acad Sci USA 1993; 90:10026–10030.

36. Anderson PAV, Holman MA, Greenberg RM. Deduced amino acid sequence of a putative Na+ channel from the scyphozoan jellyfish *Cyanea capillata*. Proc Natl Acad Sci USA 1993; 90:7419–7423.

37. Roberds SL, Knoth KM, Po S, Blair TA, Bennett PB, Hartshorne RP, Snyders DJ and Tamkun MM. Molecular biology of the voltage-gated potassium channels of the cardiovascular system. J Cardiovasc Electrophysiol 1993; 4:68–80.

38. Lalik PH, Krafte DS, Volberg WA, Ciccarelli RB. Characterization of endogenous Na+ channel gene expressed in Chinese hamster ovary cells. Am J Physiol 1993; 264:C803–809.

39. Qu Y, Rogers J, Tanada T, Scheuer T, Catterall WA. Modulation of cardiac Na^+ channels expressed in a mammalian cell line and in ventricular myocytes by protein kinase C. Proc Natl Acad Sci USA 1994; 91:3289-3293.

40. Cribbs LL, Satin J, Fozzard HA, Rogart RB. Functional expression of the rat heart I Na^+ channel isoform; demonstration of properties characteristic of native cardiac Na^+ channels. FEBS 1990; 275(1,2):195-200.

41. Krafte DS, Davison K, Dugrenier, Estep K, Josef K, Barchi RL, Kallen RG, Silver PJ, Ezrin AM. Pharmacological modulation of human cardiac Na^+ channels. Eur J Pharmacol 1994; 266:245-254.

42. Stühmer W, Conti F, Suzuki H, Wang X, Noda M, Yahagi N, Kubo H, Numa S. Structural parts involved in activation and inactivation of the Na^+ channel. Nature (London) 1989; 339:597-693.

43. Vessilev P, Scheuer T, Catterall WA. Identification of an intracellular peptide segment involved in Na^+ channel inactivation. Science 1988; 241:1658-1661.

44. Vessilev P, Scheuer T, Catterall WA. Inhibition of inactivation of single Na^+ channels by a site-directed antibody. Proc Natl Acad Sci USA 1989; 86:817-8151.

45. Catterall, WA. 1988 Structure and function of voltage-sensitive ion channels. *Science* 242, 50-61.

46. West JW, Patton DE, Scheuer T, Wang Y-L, Goldin AL, Catterall WA. A cluster of hydrophobic amino acid residues required for fast Na^+ channel inactivation. Proc Natl Acad Sci USA 1992; 89:10910-10914.

47. Patton DE, West JW, Catterall WA, Goldin AL. Amino acid residues required for fast Na^+ channel inactivation. Charge neutralizations and deletions in the III-IV linker. Proc Natl Acad Sci USA. 1992; 89:10905-10909.

48. Hartman HA, Tiedeman AA, Chen SF, Brown AM, Kirsch GE. Effects of III-IV linker mutations on human heart Na^+ channel inactivation gating. Circ Res 1994; 75:114-122.

49. Guy HR, Conti F. Pursuing the structure and function of voltage-gated channels. Trends Neurosci 1990; 13:201-206.

50. Heinemann SH, Terlau H, Stuhmer W, Imoto K, Numa S. Calcium channel characteristics conferred on the Na^+ channel by single mutations Nature (London) 1992; 356:441-443.

51. Terlau H, Heinemann SH, Stühmer W, Pusch M, Conti F, Imoto K, Numa S. Mapping the site of block by tetrodotoxin and saxitoxin of Na^+ channel II. FEBS Lett 1991; 293:93-96.

52. Satin J, Kyle JW, Chen M, Bell P, Cribbs LL, Fozzard HA, Rogart RB. A mutant of TTX-resistant cardiac Na^+ channels with TTX-sensitive properties. Science 1992; 256:1202-1205.

53. Backx PH, Yue DT, Lawrence JH, Marban E, Tomaselli GF. Molecular localization of an ion binding site within the pore of mammalian Na^+ channels. Science 1992; 257:248-251.

54. Tamkun MM, Talvenheimo JA, Catterall WA. The Na^+ channel from rat brain. Reconstitution of neurotoxin-activated ion flux and scorpion toxin binding from purified components. J Biol Chem 1984; 259:1676-1688.

55. Isom LL, De Jongh K, Catterall WA. Auxiliary subunits of voltage-gated ion channels. Neuron 1994; 12:1183-94.

56. Isom LL, DeJongh KS, Patton DE, Reber BF, Offord J, Charbonneau H, Walsh K, Goldin AL, Catterall WA. Primary structure and functional expression of the beta$_1$ subunit of the rat brain Na⁺ channel. Science 1992; 256:839–842.

57. Messner DJ, Catterall WA. The Na⁺ channel from rat brain. Separation and characterization of subunits. J Biol Chem 1985; 260:10597–10604.

58. McHugh-Sutkowski E, Catterall WA. Beta$_1$ subunits of Na⁺ channels. Studies with subunit-specific antibodies. J Biol Chem 1990; 265:12393–12399.

59. Makita N, Bennett PB, George AL. Voltage-gated Na⁺ channel β1 subunit mRNA expresssed in adult human skeletal muscle, heart, and brain is encoded by a single gene. J Biol Chem 1994; 269:7571–7578.

60. Nuss HB, Marban E. Functional association of α and β1 subunits of human heart (hH1) and rat skeletal muscle (μ1) sodium channels expressed in *Xenopus* oocytes. Circulation 1994; 90:I197.

61. Cohen SA. Immunocytochemical characterization of the rat cardiac Na⁺ channel (abstr). Circulation 1991:84 (Suppl 2):II–182.

62. Cohen SA, Levitt LK. Partial characterization of the rH1 Na⁺ channel protein from the rat heart using subtype-specific antibodies. Circ Res 1993; 73:735–742.

63. Taouis M, Sheldon RS, and Duff HJ. Up-regulation of the rat cardiac Na⁺ channel by in vivo treatment with a class I antiarrhythmic drug. J Clin Invest 1991; 88:375–378.

64. Duff HJ, Offord J, West J, Catterall WA. Class I and IV antiarrhythmic drugs and cytosolic calcium regulate mRNA encoding the Na⁺ channel alpha subunit in rat cardiac muscle. Mol Pharmacol 1992; 42:570–574.

65. Sherman SJ, Catterall WA. Electrical activity and cytosolic calcium regulate levels of tetrodotoxin-sensitive Na⁺ channels in cultured rat muscle cells. Proc Natl Acad Sci USA 1984; 81:262–266.

66. Sherman SJ, Chrivia J, Catterall WA. Cyclic 3′:5′ monophosphate and cytosolic calcium exert opposing effects on biosynthesis of tetrodotoxin-sensitive Na⁺ channels in rat muscle cells. J Neurosci 1985; 5:1570–1576.

67. Numann R, Catterall WA, Scheuer T. Functional modulation of brain Na⁺ channels by protein kinase C phosphorylation. Science 1991; 254:115–118.

68. West JW, Numann R, Murphy BM, Scheuer T, Catterall WA. Identification of a phosphorylation site in a conserved intracellular loop that is required or modulation of Na⁺ channels by protein kinase C. Science 1991; 254:866–868.

69. Murphy BJ, Rossie S, DeJongh KS, Catterall WA. Identification of the sites of selective phosphorylation and dephosphorylation of the rat brain Na⁺ channel α subunit by cAMP-dependent protein kinase and phosphoprotein phosphatases. J Biol Chem 1993; 268:27355–27362.

70. Catterall WA, Scheuer T, West JW, Numann R, Patton DE, Duff HJ, Goldin AL. Structure and Modulation of Voltage-Gated Na⁺ Channels. In: Spooner PM, Brown AM, Catterall WA, Kaczorowski GJ, Strauss HC, eds. Ion Channels in the Cardiovascular System. New York: Futura, 1994:317–339.

71. Li M, West JW, Numann R, Murphy BJ, Scheuer T, Catterall WA. Convergent regulation of sodium channels by protein kinase C and cAMP-dependent protein kinase. Science 1993; 261:1439–1442.

72. Grant AO, Wendt DJ. Block and modulation of cardiac Na⁺ channels by antiar-

rhythmic drugs, neurotransmitters and hormones. Trends Pharmacol Sci 1992; 13:352–358.

73. Ono K, Fozzard HA, Hanck DA. Mechanism of cAMP-dependent modulation of cardiac sodium channel current kinetics. Circ Res 1993; 72:807–815.

74. Schubert B, VanDongen AM, Kirsch GE and Brown AM. Beta-adrenergic inhibition of cardiac sodium channels by dual G-protein pathways. Science 1989; 245:516–9.

75. Moorman JR, Kirsch GE, Lacerda AE and Brown AM. xAngiotensin II modulates cardiac Na$^+$ channels in neonatal rat. Circ Res 1989; 65:1804–189.

76. Nilius B, Tytgat, J, Albitz R. Modulation of cardiac Na channels by angiotensin II. Biochim Biophys Acta 1989; 1014:2592–62.

77. Schwartz PJ. Autonomic markers for sudden cardiac death. In: Spooner PM, Brown AM, Catterall WA, Kaczorowski GJ, Strauss HC, eds. Ion Channels in the Cardiovascular System. New York: Futura, 1994:35–60.

78. Roden DM, Tamkun MM. Toward a molecular view of cardiac arrhythmogenesis. Trrends Cardiovasc Med 1994; 4:278–286.

10

Molecular Properties of Cardiac Potassium Channels in Health and Disease

**Marie-Noelle S. Langan and
Diomedes E. Logothetis**
Mount Sinai School of Medicine
New York, New York

GENERATION AND CONDUCTION OF CARDIAC ACTION POTENTIALS

The heart is a complex organ comprised of many different cell types, the overall task of which is the efficient and coordinate propulsion of blood to the brain and systemic circulations. Electrical signals spreading among the excitable heart cells control the frequency, strength, duration, and synchrony of the cardiac contraction. These electrical signals, or action potentials, of distinct cardiac cell types display complex and unique characteristics. In most cardiac cells, the resting membrane potential (E_r) is maintained close to the equilibrium potential for potassium (E_K), ~ -90 mV. In general, inward current (inward movement of the positive ions Na^+ or Ca^{2+}) depolarizes (membrane potential becomes more positive relative to E_r) while outward current (outward flow of K^+ or inward flow of Cl^-) repolarizes (membrane potential returns toward E_r) cardiac cell membranes. The shape of the action potentials of different cardiac cell types vary due to the distinct ion channels involved.

Figure 1 shows in schematic form cardiac action potentials that can be described generally by five phases. Phase 0, the upstroke or rapid depolarization phase, is mainly caused by inward Na^+ current (I_{Na}) through voltage-activated Na^+ channels (Fig. 1A), except in the sinoatrial (SA) and atrioventricular (AV) nodal cells where it is due to Ca^{2+} entry (I_{Ca}) through voltage-activated Ca^{2+} channels (Fig. 1B). Phase 1, the early rapid repolarization phase (appears as a notch in the action potential waveform), is partly due to inactivation of the Na^+ current, and partly due to transient outward currents (I_{to}) that can be carried by Cl^- and/or K^+. Phase 2, the plateau phase, a near balance of small inward and outward currents, maintains the cell membrane voltage at a depolarized level for a few hundred milliseconds, thus determining the strength and duration of the myocardial contraction. Phase 3, the final rapid repolarization phase, is caused by an increasing predominance of outward (I_K) currents over inactivating inward currents. Phase 4, the resting membrane potential and diastolic depolarization phase, is dominated by I_K currents that maintain the membrane potential stably near E_K (the equilibrium potential for K^+), except in certain cardiac cells (e.g., SA node, parts of the atria, the distal portion of the AV node, the His-Purkinje fibers), where the membrane potential gradually depolarizes (diastolic depolarization) due to a net slow inward current generated by several ions.

Normal excitation in heart muscle depends on the sequential transmission of such action potentials. The normal sequence of excitation in the heart consists of de novo spontaneous depolarization of the sinus node, the spread of excitation to the atrium followed by conduction over the atrioventricular node and the His-Purkinje system, which finally leads to the almost synchronous depolarization of the ventricle. Loss of coordination of electrical activity as a function of time can result in arrhythmias that in turn can seriously compromise the contractile efficiency of the heart. Cardiac arrhythmias may arise from disturbances of impulse initiation (abnormal automaticity or triggered rhythms), conduction (reentrant rhythms), or both. All cells in the major conducting pathway share the ability of de novo impulse generation with the sinus node,

---

Figure 1   Currents and channels in typical cardiac action potentials in (A) atrial and ventricular cells and (B) sinoatrial cells. Approximate time courses of the currents associated with the channels or pumps are shown symbolically without representing their magnitudes relative to each other. I_{Na}, inward excitatory current carried by sodium ions; I_{Ca-L}, L-type calcium channels current; I_{Ca-T}, T-type calcium channels current; $I_{Na/Ca}$, current generated by the Na/Ca countertransport system; I_{K1}, inward rectifier K^+ current; I_K, delayed rectifier K^+ current; I_{to}, transient outward K^+ current; I_{KACh}, acetylcholine-sensitive K^+ current; I_{KATP}, ATP-sensitive K^+ current; I_f, net inward current, "pacemaker current." (Adapted from Ref. 1.)

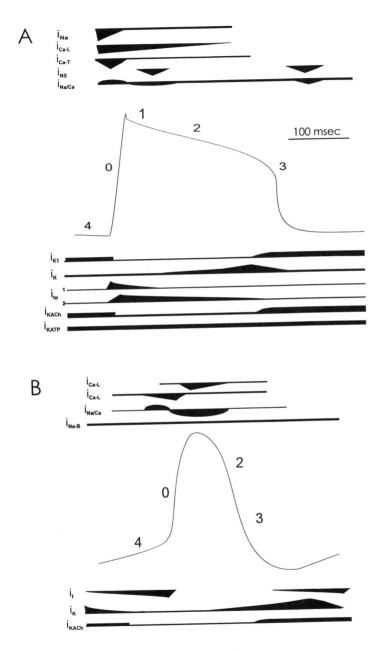

and are thus subsidiary pacemaker cells. They become important sites of impulse generation when the sinus node fails to initiate the cardiac cycle or when their automaticity is enhanced. Depolarization in diastole implies that inward currents predominate over outward currents, resulting in a net inward current (phase 4 of the action potential). Automatic rhythms occur spontaneously as a result of a change in the balance of phase 4 currents, requiring no previous trigger. A net increase in outward currents will decrease automaticity while the opposite will occur with a net decrease in outward currents.

The triggered rhythms are a group of arrhythmias that result from abnormal impulse initiation that depends on a preceding membrane depolarization. These arrhythmias are the result of afterdepolarizations occurring during phase 3 or 4. If these after-depolarizations reach a threshold value, an action potential may ensue. Repetitive depolarizations may arise during the plateau of the initiating or triggering action potential. In the ventricle this produces the classic example of a triggered arrhythmia, torsade de Pointes (a ventricular tachycardia with a classic shifting axis about the electrocardiographic baseline). Because the triggered action potentials arise from a positive level of membrane potential (where Na^+ channels have not fully recovered from inactivation), they have upstrokes that are primarily dependent on the inward calcium current. However, their genesis is linked to conditions that cause action potential prolongation, particularly by drugs that block the outward repolarizing potassium currents.

The homogeneity of repolarization typical of healthy cardiac tissue is important in the coherent propagation of the electrical impulse. When dispersion of repolarization occurs (for example, in ischemia, when a group of cells repolarize more rapidly than the others) the electrical impulse may form reentrant circuits by reexcitation of cells that have repolarized more rapidly than their neighbors. Such circuits have been well described in animal models of ischemia and infarction (2). In cardiac tissue scarred by old trauma, changes in the anatomical structure of the myocardium (anisotropy) lead to patches of slowly conducting tissues and to areas of unidirectional block. This disparity of conduction between adjacent cells again predisposes to reentry (3). Reentrant ventricular tachycardias are the most common arrhythmia following a myocardial infarction (4,5).

PRESENCE OF K⁺ CHANNELS IN HEART

In this chapter our objective will be to review our current understanding of the major cardiac potassium channels thought to participate in the various phases of the cardiac action potential, along with their presumed recombinant representatives, their potential roles in clinical arrhythmias, and their modulation by antiarrhythmic drugs. We will refer to the channel protein as K_x (where X will denote the specific type of K^+ channel), and to the current carried by channel K_x as I_{Kx}. Block of K^+ channels active at a given phase of the action potential would be expected to either produce membrane depolarization (membrane potential more positive than E_K) or, if the membrane is already depolarized, to delay the normal repolarization process. Activation of K^+ channels from either the closed or a low probability of opening states would be expected to produce membrane repolarization (membrane potential toward E_K).

Patch-clamp studies (6) have revealed that often there are several functionally distinct channels (even for those passing the same ion), that give rise to a given macroscopic current implicated at a specific phase of the cardiac action potential. Moreover, variations in channel characteristics that are dependent on both cardiac tissue type and species have been appreciated.

Cloning and heterologous functional expression of ion channels have surpassed predictions from patch-clamp studies as to the existence of multiple isoforms within a given subfamily. Further functional diversity has been demonstrated by examples of heterologous assembly of certain subfamily members. Cardiac K^+ channels cloned thus far can be classified within four distinct structural modes proposed for recombinant potassium channels at large (Fig. 2).

Although rapid progress has been made in the cloning of ion channels, we are only at the beginning of establishing strategies and criteria for successful assignment of recombinant channels to endogenous cardiac currents (8). Moreover, even though structure–function studies have identified regions involved in channel gating, permeation, and inactivation, a higher-order appreciation of ion channel structure–function, needed for efficient drug design, remains poor.

K^+ CHANNELS IN THE EARLY RAPID REPOLARIZATION PHASE

The phase of early repolarization (phase 1) returns the membrane potential from its peak value to the region of $+10 \pm 10$ mV that sets the early plateau voltage. Changes in the currents underlying phase 1 will alter the level of the early plateau voltage, which in turn could influence other voltage-dependent plateau currents and therefore the action potential duration (APD). Several distinct current components have been implicated as participants during this phase such as the voltage-dependent inactivation of I_{Na}, a Ca^{2+}-activated I_{Cl} (9,10), a Ca^{2+}-activated K^+ current, $I_{to,2}$ (11–15), or an Na^+-activated K^+ current I_{K-Na} (16). We shall limit our discussion to the transient voltage-dependent outward K^+ current, $I_{to,1}$ (17–20), the only K_{to} channel for which recombinant candidates have been proposed. $I_{to,1}$ not only modulates phase 1 but also contributes to the plateau and early part of phase 3 repolarization. As shown in Figure 3, $I_{to,1}$ currents show rapid voltage-dependent activation (reported times to peak are on

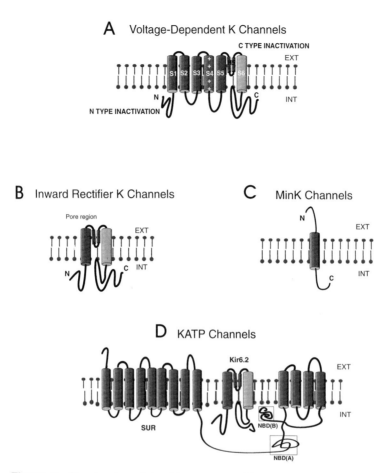

Figure 2 Structural models of known recombinant potassium channels. N = N-terminus; C = C-terminus. A. Voltage-dependent K^+ channels. These channels have six putative transmembrane domains (labeled S_1–S_6). The pore is located between S_5 and S_6 (labeled H_5). Extracellular (EXT); C type, inactivation is denoted and found to be in the region near the pore and the sixth transmembrane domain. The rapid, N type, inactivation is intracellular (INT) and has been localized to the N terminus (N). Voltage gating has been ascribed to the S_4 transmembrane domain (denoted by positive charges). B. Inward rectifier K channels. These channels have two putative transmembrane domains that resemble the S_5 and S_6 domains of the voltage-dependent K^+ channels. The pore region resembling the H_5 region of voltage-gated K^+ channels is denoted. C. MinK Channels. These channels have a single transmembrane domain with no resemblance to the inward rectifier or voltage-dependent K^+ channels. D. K_{ATP} channels. The Kir 6.2 channel is a two-transmembrane domain structure similar to the inward rectifiers. The sulfonylurea receptor (SUR) couples with this (and possibly other inward rectifiers). It is likely that the SUR provides the nucleotide-binding domains (NDB) that are capable of interacting with the channel to influence gating, as depicted in the K_{ATP} model (See Fig. 9). C, C=terminus. (Adapted from Ref. 7.)

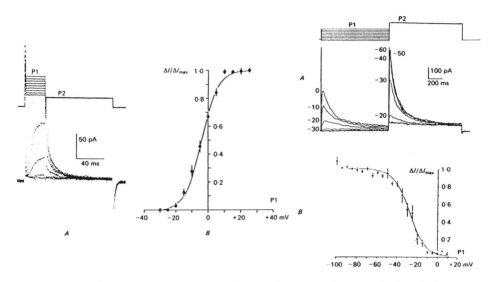

Figure 3 Steady-state activation and inactivation properties of native $I_{to,1}$. Left. A. Steady-state activation experiments, using a conventional two-pulse protocol. The test pulse, P2 (–40 mV), gave the relative amplitude of the outward tail current that had been previously activated by brief (30 ms) depolarizing pulses (P1) from –40 to +20 mV (before the inactivation process became involved). The holding potential was – 60 mV. B. Normalized amplitudes ($\Delta I/\Delta I_{max}$) were plotted as a function of the P1 potential yielding the activation curve shown. The threshold for activation of this current was near –30 mV and full activation was accomplished by +10 mV. The data denote mean values (± SEM) from four experiments. Right. A. Steady-state inactivation experiments, using a conventional two-pulse protocol. The test pulse, P2, depolarized the cell from –60 to +20 mV for 1 s. The inactivating prepulse, P1, had the same duration and displaced the membrane potential in the range of –100 to +20 mV in 10 mV steps. B. Inactivation was measured as the ratio of $\Delta I/\Delta I_{max}$ during P2 and plotted as a function of the P1 potential yielding the inactivation curve shown. Inactivation was fully removed at –70 mV and was virtually complete at approximately –10 mV. The data are plotted as mean ± SEM (n = 7). (Adapted from Ref. 18.)

the order of milliseconds to tens of milliseconds; ref. 21), and inactivation kinetics that are either monoexponential (on the order of tens of milliseconds; ref. 18,22,23) or biexponential (with a slow time constant on the order of hundreds of milliseconds; ref. 24,25). These transient outward K^+ currents also show sensitivity to block by 4-aminopyridine (4-AP; ref. 18).

$I_{to,1}$ is a nearly universal current in the mammalian myocardium. In human tissues it has been described in atrium (12,26,27) and ventricle (23,28–30). $I_{to,1}$ shows prominent species and regional variations (e.g., 17,31, see below) and functional heterogeneity, as evidenced by differences in properties such as single-channel conductance, activation and inactivation kinetics, suggesting the presence of more than one $K_{to,1}$ channel protein. Modulation by α_1-adrenergic stimulation through a pertussis toxin (PTX)-insensitive pathway has been demonstrated but great species-dependent variability was obtained when control of $I_{to,1}$ by protein kinase C (PKC) or protein kinase A (PKA) was tested (21,32).

I_{to} has only recently been implicated in clinical arrhythmias. Regional differences have been shown in the density of I_{to} channels in various parts of the atrium (33) as well as in the epicardium vs. the endocardium of the ventricle (26,34–37). It has been suggested that in pathological conditions or when certain antiarrhythmics are given (e.g., Flecainide) these regional inhomogeneities may exert an arrhythmogenic effect by providing an area of conduction block (33,38). Patch-clamp studies of isolated cells have been used to characterize the changes in ionic currents during exposure to ischemia-mimicking conditions. Action potential recordings from cells in a 5-day infarcted heart model usually showed either no presence of phase 1 or reduced phase 1, suggesting a loss in the voltage-dependent transient outward current (39). Studies designed to determine the kinetics and magnitude of I_{to} demonstrated that the loss in the notch was accompanied by changes in I_{to} density. In addition, the small I_{to} currents recorded in some cells from the infarcted heat displayed a slowed recovery from inactivation (40). Furthermore, tedisamil has been shown to have an antifibrillatory action in hearts of only those animals showing prominent $I_{to,1}$ currents (41). Thus, inhibition of $I_{to,1}$ may provide a beneficial effect in species or areas of the heart where this channel has a dominant role in action potential repolarization.

Candidate recombinant representatives of $I_{to,1}$ have been reported. Cardiac Kv1.4 (8,42,43) and Kv4.2 (43) channels display rapidly inactivating currents when heterologously expressed in *Xenopus* oocytes (42,44). Although Kv1.4 has the predicted voltage-dependence for activation and the expected sensitivity of 4-AP, its recovery from inactivation (restitution) is 50-fold slower than $I_{to,1}$ (45). In contrast, Kv4.2 expressed in mammalian cell lines shows restitution time constants closer to those of native ones (46) but compromised 4-AP sensitivity (44). It has been suggested that although these channels do not faithfully represent native $I_{to,1}$ as homomeric complexes, perhaps they do so as heteromeric ones (46). In support of this hypothesis, it was shown that coexpression of Kv1.4 with another cardiac channel Kv1.2 (43,47) which shows little inactivation with rapid restitution, gave rise to a hybrid channel with fast "Kv1.4-like" inactivation kinetics and rapid "Kv1.2-like" restitution kinetics. Such heteromerization has not been shown yet for native $I_{to,1}$ channels, but were it true, a differential expression of heteromeric subunits would be consistent with species- and regional-dependent variations in the density of $I_{to,1}$ channels as well as their functional heterogeneity.

K+ CHANNELS IN THE PLATEAU PHASE

The plateau phase (phase 2) reflects a delicate balance between inward and outward currents. As a result, relatively small changes in the net ionic current can significantly change the membrane potential. In several species, the K^+ current at the plateau phase consists predominantly of two components with characteristically different kinetic properties: one that activates rapidly but then spontaneously inactivates with depolarization (I_{Kr}), and a second, I_{Ks}, severalfold larger component that shows much slower kinetics of activation and no inactivation (48). There are considerable interspecies differences in the relative abundance of I_{Kr} and I_{Ks}.

I_{Kr} shows strong inward rectification (the channel passes inward current more readily than outward current) and is selectively blocked by the newer class III antiarrhythmic drugs E-4031 and dofetilide (48,49) (Table 1). This chan-

Table 1 Class III Antiarrhythmic Drugs

Drug	I_{Kr}	I_{Ks}	I_{k1}	I_{to}	I_{KATP}	References
Blockers						
Class 1						
Quinidine	++	+	+/-	+/++	++	206–215
Disopyramide	+	–	+/-	–	+	207,215
Procainamide	+	–	–	–	+	207,215
Flecainide	++	–	–	++	+	208,216–8
Propafenone	+++	++	–	++	+	208,215,219
Class 111						
Sotalol	+	–	–	–	–	207,220-3
Amiodarone	++	+	+	–	+	204,209,224–6
Clofilium	++	+	+	+++	+	207,227–30
Tedisamil	+	++	–	++	–	231
Dofetilide	+++	–	–	–	–	207,227
Azimilide	+++	++	–	–	–	232
Sematilide	+	–	–	–	–	221
Tolbutamide	–	–	–	–	+++	233
Glibenclamide	–	–	–	–	+	233
Openers						
Pinacidil	–	–	–	–	+++	233
Cromakalim	–	–	–	–	++	233,234

+, $IC_{50} > 10\mu M$;
++, $1\mu M < IC_{50} < 10\mu M$;
+++, $IC_{50} < 1\mu M$;
–, no effect.
NB IC_{50} is subject to variations as influenced by experimental conditions and voltage clamp protocols.

nel has been described in human atrial (50) and ventricular myocytes (30,51). Shibasaki identified a 1.6 pS delayed rectifier channel in rabbit SA node (under physiological solutions), the macroscopic averaged currents of which inactivated, resembling I_{Kr} (52). Block of I_{Kr} prolongs the APD (45). Blockers of I_{Kr} have been shown to prolong the QT interval in the electrocardiogram and occasionally to produce ventricular arrhythmias and sudden death.

The occurrence of triggered arrhythmias, not provoked by exogenous drug intake, is the curse of the long QT syndrome (LQTS). This is an inherited cardiac disorder that causes syncope and sudden death from ventricular tachy-arrhythmias, specifically torsade de pointes and ventricular fibrillation, usually in otherwise healthy young individuals. The recent discoveries regarding this disease are a prime example of the potential power of applying molecular techniques in arrhythmias secondary to congenital causes. In 1991, a tight linkage was discovered between autosomal dominant LQT and a polymorphism at H-RAS (53). This discovery localized an LQT gene (LQT1) to chromosome 11p15.5 and made genetic testing possible in some families. In 1993, however, different laboratories identified families that were not linked to this chromosome (54,55). In 1994, two additional loci were identified: LQT2 on chromosome 7q35-36 and LQT3 on chromosome 3p21-24 (56,57). Around the same time a novel human cDNA was cloned from a hippocampal cDNA library (58). This human ether-a-go-go-related gene (HERG) was localized to human chromosome 7, which had a predicted amino acid sequence homology to K^+ channels and was shown to be strongly expressed in the heart (59). Curran and colleagues provided evidence that HERG is LQT2 and that mutations in HERG cause the chromosome 7-linked forms of LQTS.

Expression and characterization of HERG into oocytes showed that this recombinant K^+ channel behaved as I_{Kr} (Fig. 4) in all respects except in the block by class III antiarrhythmics (60), a difference that is currently under further characterization (61).

Moreover, the inward rectification of HERG has been accounted for by the inactivation process exhibited by these channels (60,62). In an elegant mechanistic study, using tetraethylammonium (TEA) ions to block the channel pore, Smith and colleagues demonstrated that only in the presence of external TEA was there a change in the HERG current kinetics. This result suggested competition for block by TEA with a C-type activation process (63–65), further evidence for which was presented by a double mutant of two residues in the general region where C-type inactivation is controlled (62).

The kinetics of the HERG activation indicated that this channel could be important in suppression of arrhythmias, particularly early afterdepolarizations. Such a role of I_{Kr} would be consistent with the sudden death seen in patients with long QT syndrome or those treated with antiarrhythmic channel-blocking I_{Kr} (62,66).

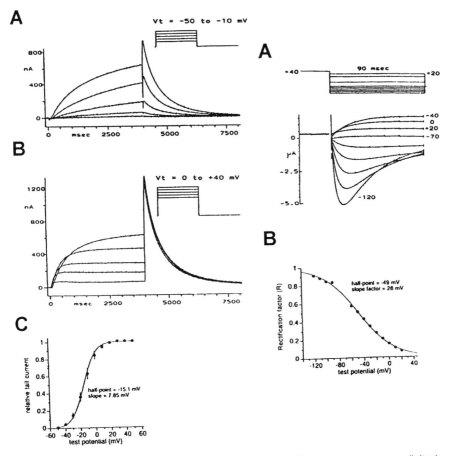

Figure 4   Steady-state activation and inactivation experiments from currents elicited by depolarizing voltage steps in *Xenopus* oocytes injected with HERG cRNA. Left. A. Currents activated by 4 s pulses, applied in 10 mV increments from −50 to −10 mV. Current during the pulse progressively increased wth voltage, as did tail current upon return to the holding potential (−70 mV). B. Currents activated by 4 s pulses, applied in 10 mV increments from 0 to +40 mV. Current magnitude during the pulse progressively decreased with voltage, whereas the tail current saturated at +10 mV. C. Voltage dependence of HERG channel activation. Amplitude of tail currents was measured at −70 mV following 4 s pulses and then normalized relative to the largest current. Right. A. Currents recorded at test potentials of +20, 0, −40, and −70 to −120 mV (in 10 mV steps) following activation with a 260 ms pulse to +40 mV ([K$^+$]$_o$ = 10 mM). Only the final 30 ms of the activating pulse is shown, followed by the 90 ms tail current. B. Voltage dependence of "rapid" inactivation of HERG current. The rectification factor, R, is the normalized current amplitude (with respect to the maximal) at each potential. (Adapted from Ref. 60.)

I_{Ks} shows a small channel conductance that is sensitive to β-adrenergic stimulation. Its characteristic slow kinetics (it takes seconds to approach a steady state) mean that during an action potential only a small fraction of I_{Ks} channels are activated. With increased heart rates, however, its deactivation is incomplete, and therefore its additive activation contributes a larger current amplitude. It is prominent in guinea pig (48) and dog ventricle (67), but not in rat (68), cat (69), or rabbit (70). Its presence in human heart is not clear (30,50). Single-channel properties have not been characterized for this channel, presumably due to its small conductance.

I_{Ks} is about 50-fold less sensitive to the antiarrhythmic drug clofilium than I_{Kr}, and is not at all sensitive to E-4031 or dofetilide (45). It is most sensitive to acute exposures of amiodarone (71). It is not clear whether the class III activity of amiodarone can be attributed to block of I_{Ks}. The most likely recombinant candidate for I_{Ks} is minK, a channel cloned originally from rat kidney and human genomic DNA (72) but also cloned from rat uterus (73) and neonatal mouse hearts (74). MinK codes for a single transmembrane protein (~ 130 amino acid long) that bears no homology to other cloned channels (see Fig. 2). When expressed in oocytes or mammalian cells, minK gives rise to currents similar to I_{Ks} (75) (Fig. 5) that are sensitive to block by clofilium, external Ba^{2+} and TEA.

Although I_{Ks} native currents are clearly modulated by PKA and PKC (reviewed in 76), minK modulation studies have produced conflicting results (74,77,78). Moreover, minK shows no consensus or alternative PKA phosphorylation sites. These differences remain to be resolved.

Multiple other K^+ currents can also be active during the plateau phase of the cardiac action potentials. A delayed rectifier current (passes outward current more readily than inward current), faster than I_{Kr}, has been detected in rat (79) and human atrial myocytes (50). A similar current had been previously reported in embryonic chick ventricular cells (80). The recombinant equivalent of this delayed rectifier channel appears to be the Kv1.5 channel cloned from rat (43) mouse (81) or human ventricle (8). In the rat it is expressed equally well in atrium as it is in ventricle (43). Yet human Kv1.5 mRNA expression seems to be confined to the atrium (8). Another background current that is active at plateau potentials has also been described in guinea pig ventricular myocytes and has been termed I_{Kp} (82,83). No recombinant representative of this current has been reported yet. A Ca^{2+}- activated maxi K^+ channel has likewise been observed in chick embryonic ventricular myocytes (Logothetis and Clapham, 1985, unpublished data). Figure 6 shows whole-cell currents of a chick embryonic ventricular cell, obtained from depolarizations from a holding potential of –65 mV to a test potential of +65 mV. Small whole-cell delayed rectifier currents can be recorded as previously shown (80). It is inter-

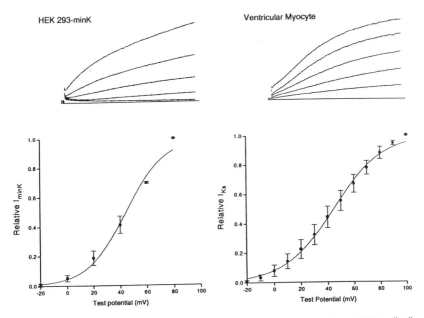

Figure 5 Minimal K⁺ channel current expressed in transfected HEK 293 cells (I_{minK}) resembles native delayed rectifier K⁺ current (I_{Ks}) recorded from guinea pig heart. Left. Top. The current tracings illustrate whole-cell I_{minK} recorded from a transfected HEK 293 cell (calibration: 60 pA, 250 ms) during successive 2 s depolarizing pulses from a holding potential of –40 mV to test potentials between +20 and +100 mV. Bottom. Isochronal activation curve for I_{minK} (mean values ± SEM, n = 11). Relative K⁺ current amplitudes are expressed as the fraction of time-dependent current activated at the most positive test potential. Right. Top. The current tracings illustrate whole-cell I_{Ks} recorded from a guinea pig ventricular myocyte (calibration: 500 pA, 250 ms) during successive 2 s depolarizing pulses from a holding potential of –40 mV to test potentials between +20 and +100 mV. Bottom. Isochronal activation curve for I_{Ks} (mean values ± SEM, n = 7). Relative K⁺ current amplitudes are expressed as the fraction of time-dependent current activated at the most positive test potential. (Adapted from Ref. 75.)

esting that superimposed on the macroscopic delayed rectifier K⁺ currents, unitary events could also be resolved. Under physiological solutions the single-channel conductance of these maxi K⁺ channels was estimated to be ~ 180 pS. A subsequent whole-cell recording on the same cell (delayed rectifier currents have run down), but now with the free Ca²⁺ concentration 10-fold greater in the pipette than in the previous recording, revealed an increased frequency of single-channel openings. Application of 50 nM charybdotoxin in the bathing solution greatly reduced the frequency of channel openings.

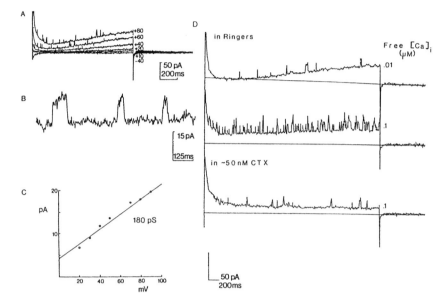

Figure 6 Noninactivating Ca^{2+}-activated maxi K^+ channels in chick embryonic ventricular cells. A. Maxi K^+ channels resolved during a whole-cell recording with step voltages at the indicated levels from a holding potential of -65 mv ($C = 11.0$ pF). Cells were bathed in Ringer's solution with $[K]_o = 4$ mM and $[K]_i = 145$ mM, and 1 mM cobalt replacing extracellular calcium. The voltage pulses were 1 s in duration. B. Unitary current events shown at an expanded time scale and higher current gain. C. The slope conductance of the maxi K^+ channels was approximately 180 pS in same solutions as in (A). D. A cell ($C = 14.8$ pF) patch-clamped twice with pipettes containing different free Ca^{2+} concentrations. In the top recording the pipette contained 0.01 μM free Ca^{2+} (11 mM EGTA and 1mM $CaCl_2$). In the middle recording the pipette contained 0.1 μM free Ca^{2+} (0.1 mM EGTA, 0.1 mM $CaCl_2$). The bottom record is from the same recording as in the middle panel but with 50 nM charybdotoxin in the bathing solution.

These channels are distinct from the transient Ca^{2+}-activated currents, previously described (e.g., 11). The frequency of encountering these maxi K^+ channels in excised patches was less than 1:20 patches. This rarity of I_{K-Ca} may explain why this conductance has not been previously described.

One important generalization that can be made about plateau currents described here is that they all conduct small K^+ currents in order to offset the correspondingly small Ca^{2+} currents. As we have seen, this can be accomplished by a number of mechanisms, including an intrinsically small conductance with slow activation kinetics (I_{Ks}), by limiting the unitary conductance by inactivation at plateau voltages (I_{Kr}), by partial inactivation at depolarized potentials ($I_{to,1}$) or finally by limiting the level of channel density ($I_{K(Ca)}$).

K$^+$ CHANNELS IN THE REPOLARIZATION PHASE AND RESTING PHASES

Progressive decay of I_{Ca} (due to inactivation) in combination with increases in outward I_K terminates the plateau phase and initiates the late rapid phase of repolarization (phase 3). The early phase of repolarization involves currents we have already considered (e.g. I_{Ks}, I_{Kr} and to a less extent $I_{to,1}$).

K$_1$ CHANNELS

As repolarization proceeds, K_1 channels, which were closed during the plateau phase, are progressively reactivated. I_{K1}, as well as other related inwardly rectifying K$^+$ currents (e.g., frog skeletal muscle as well as starfish and tunicate eggs), exhibit three unique properties when compared to other known channels (84). First, they open with a moderate to steep voltage dependence on hyperpolarization. They show an e-fold decrease in conductance for each 5–10 mV of depolarization, which corresponds to movement of an equivalent gating charge of 2.5–5 electronic charges (contrast this value with similar measurements of the dependence of activation of voltage-gated Na$^+$ and K$^+$ channels giving a gating valence of 5 to 6 electronic charges). Second, the voltage dependence of their gating depends on the extracellular K$^+$ concentration. Thus, changes in the external K$^+$ concentration shift both E_K and the steepness of the activation curve (85–87), suggesting that extracellular K$^+$ ions bound to or passing through these channels interact with the gating mechanism (84,88). In contrast, changes in the intracellular concentration of K$^+$, do not have similar effects on the voltage dependence of channel gating (85,89,90). Third, their steep inward rectification arises from a steeply voltage-dependent gating process (91), with (92) or without (93) a superimposed block by Mg^{2+}. Physiological levels of intracellular Mg^{2+} have resulted in voltage-dependent block of I_{K1}, while reductions in intracellular Mg^{2+} have allowed recording of outward currents (94,95). Yet depolarizations positive to E_K in the absence of Mg^{2+} cause I_{K1} channels to close in a time-and voltage-dependent manner (87). Figure 7 shows I_{K1} currents, their current–voltage, and voltage-activation curves.

At physiological extracellular K$^+$ concentrations, the outward current through K_1 channels is limited to the voltage range between the resting potential and $\sim$ –30 mV. Thus I_{K1} contributes to the repolarization of the action potential in precisely this voltage range. The density of K_1 channels seems to be greater in ventricle than in atrium, which may partially account for the slower phase 3 repolarization in atrial vs. ventricular action potentials (96). At

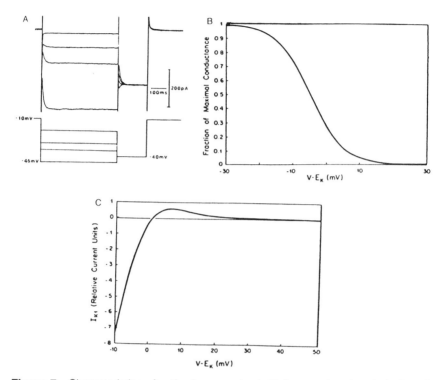

Figure 7 Characteristics of native I_{K1} currents. A. Voltage protocol and whole-cell currents obtained from a ventricular cell bathed in 40 mM K$^+$ (E_K = –25 mV). The membrane potential was held at a level 15 mV positive to E_K (–10 mV) where there was little steady-state activation of I_{K1}. It was then stopped to various potentials for 500 ms, to allow activation of I_{K1} and then to –40 mV where the relative currents (tails) were measured. B. Activation curve of normalized I_{K1} currents to the maximal currents measured under symmetrical K$^+$. For all levels of external K$^+$ tested, I_{K1} currents were half maximally activated 5 mV negative to E_K. C. Current-voltage relationship predicted from the activation curve shown in (B). (Adapted from Ref. 88.)

rest, a significant fraction of K$_1$ channels is activated and as such I_{K1} is often referred to as a background current (86). Very low density of K$_1$ channels in nodal cells may account in part for the relatively depolarized levels of phase 4 compared to the phase 4 of ventricular cells (97). Blocking I_{K1} can cause a limited prolongation of APD and induce membrane depolarization (45).

A recombinant equivalent of K$_1$ channel appears to be IRK1, which was first isolated from a mouse macrophage cell line (J774), and is also expressed in mouse forebrain, cerebellum, heart, and skeletal muscle, but not in kidney (98). This channel (Kir2.1) belongs to a family of inwardly rectifying K$^+$ channels (Kir), containing two putative segments per subunit (see Fig. 2).

K_{ACH} CHANNELS

Another K^+ channel, activated by acetylcholine (ACh) or adenosine via m2-muscarinic or A1-purinergic receptors respectively, is K_{ACh}. This channel is thought to be abundant in atria and pacemaking cells and to be mainly responsible for the membrane hyperpolarization observed during vagal stimulation (99). Vagal stimulation produces a net increase in outward K_{ACh} currents during phase 4 depolarization, thereby decreasing automaticity. K_{ACh} activation was shown to involve second messengers confined to the plasma membrane (100), specifically the heterotrimeric, pertussis toxin-sensitive GTP-binding (G) proteins (101,102). Several studies have focused on the mechanism of K_{ACh} gating and have identified direct actions of specific G-protein subunits (103–107). Following several years of debate, at present it is generally accepted that the $\beta\gamma$ subunits of G-proteins ($G_{\beta\gamma}$) are primarily responsible for gating this channel. K_{ACh} was the first effector shown to be directly affected by the $G_{\beta\gamma}$ subunits (103). Since then, numerous other proteins have been shown to be affected by $G_{\beta\gamma}$ subunits, including the N-type and P/Q-type Ca^{2+} channels (108,109). More important, however, regarding the debate, is that recombinant channels (Kir3.0 subfamily), members of the inwardly rectifying K^+ channel family, have been shown to couple to G-protein-linked receptors and to bind and respond directly to $G_{\beta\gamma}$ subunits.

K_{ACh} was recently shown to be composed of two subunits, GIRK1 (or Kir3.1; ref. 110,111) and CIR (or Kir3.4; ref. 112), which could be coprecipitated from atrial membranes by antibodies directed specifically against GIRK1 (112). Moreover, heterologous coexpression of the two subunits in *Xenopus* oocytes or mammalian cell lines gave large currents with biophysical properties identical to those of K_{ACh} (112). Heterologous coexpression of two corresponding highly related human subunits (hGIRK1 and KGP) in oocytes resulted in their heteromeric assembly, as evidenced by their coprecipitation, regardless of the subunit targeted by the antibody used (113). Homomeric assembly of either subunit alone is not sufficient to produce K_{ACh} currents. On the one hand, homomeric assembly of CIR or CIR homologs has produced channels with distinct single-channel properties from those of K_{ACh} (112,113). On the other hand, homomeric assembly of GIRK1 in mammalian cells has failed to produce functional channels altogether (112,113). *Xenopus* oocytes have been shown to express an endogenous "CIR-like" protein that allows functional expression of GIRK1 in oocytes (114), and that appears to coprecipitate with heterologously expressed GIRK1 (113), thus explaining the "K_{ACh}-like" characteristics of expression of GIRK1 alone in this system (110,111). Both subunits have been shown to bind $G_{\beta\gamma}$ subunits directly (115). C-terminal hydrophilic segments of GIRK1 have likewise been shown to bind $G_{\beta\gamma}$ subunits (116–118), while the N-terminus of GIRK1 can bind, albeit weakly, the heterotrimeric form of the G protein as well (118). Application or coexpression of $G_{\beta\gamma}$ with the GIRK1 and CIR subunits resulted in stimulation of channel activity (112). Figure 8 shows that coexpression of the CIR homolog, KGP, with $G_{\beta\gamma}$ subunits in *Xenopus* oocytes produced over a threefold stimulation of background currents (unpublished results, Logothetis, et al.).

Even though heteromeric assembly of the two subunits in oocytes reproduced the single-channel characteristics of K_{ACh} and its proper response to $G_{\beta\gamma}$ subunits, it failed to reproduce the desensitization kinetics seen with native activation of K_{ACh} by ACh applications (e.g. by 10 μM ACh; ref. 110). It is possible that additional elements are required to reconstitute fully in oocytes the behavior seen in atrial cells. Recently, Sui and colleagues (120) identified cytosolic components which, when applied to inside-out patches from either native atrial membranes or from oocytes heterologously expressing the recombinant K_{ACh} subunits, activate K_{ACh} independently of direct G-protein gating. The cytosolic components are used in a two-step process. The first step involves

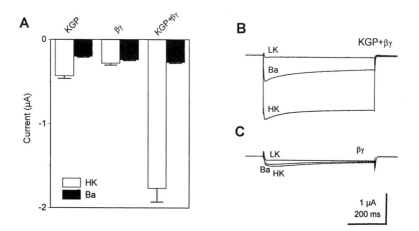

Figure 8 $G_{\beta\gamma}$ subunits stimulate KGP channel currents when coexpressed in *Xenopus* oocytes. KGP channel expression in *Xenopus* oocytes gave inwardly rectifying currents that were blocked by 200 μM Ba^{2+}. A. Oocytes expressed $G_{\beta2-\gamma2}$ subunits (cDNAs were kindly provided by Dr. Melvin Simon) showed smaller currents and no significant block by 200 μM Ba^{2+}. When KGP and Gβγ subunits were coexpressed in oocytes there was more than threefold stimulation of KGP currents that were blocked by 200 μM Ba^{2+}. Current amplitudes at –80 mV were plotted in bar graph form to indicate the effect of $G_{\beta\gamma}$ subunits on the magnitude of the current. Each pair of bars is the mean ± SEM of 6 oocytes. KGP currents were measured using two-electrode voltage clamp as previously described (113). HK, high K^+ solutions (96 mM K^+ in the bath); Ba, 200 μM $BaCl_2$; LK, low K^+ solutions (2 mM K^+ in the bath). B, C. Representative current traces.

channel modification to a distinct functional state, which requires intracellular ATP hydrolysis, is Mg^{2+}-dependent, and occurs in the minutes time scale. Such modification of native rat K_{ACh} has previously been presented (121) but has proven difficult to reproduce in other species (122). The second step utilizes physiological intracellular Na^+ to gate the ATP-modified channels. K_{ACh} is thus a Na^+-activated K^+ channel, the first shown to require prior modification in order to allow channel gating by physiological concentrations of intracellular Na^+. Possible interactions of these two distinct gating mechanisms of K_{ACh} (i.e. direct G-protein gating vs. Na^+ gating of ATP-modified channels) and the physiological consequences of such interactions remain to be elucidated.

The role of this channel in arrhythmias can so far only be suspected based on circumstantial evidence. The most likely mechanism would be automaticity since K_{ACh} function is thought to be most important in phase 4. Interestingly, Sui and colleagues showed that block of the Na^+/K^+ pump (by cardiac glycosides or zero external K^+) activated K_{ACh} in a manner indistinguishable from that of intracellular Na^+. Atrial myocytes isolated from failing human hearts have exhibited a lower resting membrane potential than healthy atrial cells (123), suggesting that changes in automaticity may play an important role in the well-documented increases in arrhythmias seen in patients with heart failure. Furthermore, whole-cell and single-channel recordings of cells from heart failure patients demonstrated reduced I_{KACh} current density (as well as I_{K1}) and reduced sensitivity to ACh, suggesting that changes in these channels or their modulation may more specifically be the mechanism responsible for these arrhythmias. It has recently been appreciated that adenosine can terminate many atrial tachycardias thought to be automatic by their responses to pacing. This might suggest an important role for K_{ACh} in these arrhythmias as well.

K_{ATP} CHANNELS

ATP-sensitive K^+ channels are closed by intracellular ATP and are likely to couple metabolism to the excitable state of the cell (124). These channels are prevalent in insulin-secreting β cells of the pancreas, widely distributed in the cardiovascular and central nervous systems, and are of great importance in hypoxic and ischemic situations since they serve as metabolic sensors (125–127). In cardiac myocytes K_{ATP} channels possess a larger unitary conductance than both K_1 and K_{ACh} channels ($\sim$ 80 pS under symmetrical 150 mM K^+) and a characteristic bursting pattern of activity with brief intraburst open durations. I_{K-ATP} shows moderate inward rectification (as compared to the strong rectification of I_{K1} and I_{K-ACh}), which is similarly due to voltage-dependent block by internal cations such as Mg^{2+} and Na^+ (126,128,129). K_{ATP} channels have been classified according to their ATP sensitivity (127): type I channels are blocked by micromolar concentrations of intracellular ATP, such as those in cardiac (124), skeletal (130), and smooth muscle (131) and pancreatic β cells (132–

134); type II channels are blocked by millimolar concentrations of ATP and were originally described in neurons (135); type III channels (e.g., tracheal smooth muscle, epithelial cells) show similar sensitivity to ATP as type II channels but differ in their ability to be activated by micromolar concentrations of Ca^{2+} (136,137). Other nucleotides mimic the inhibitory action of ATP but with less potency (order of potency: ATP > ADP > AMP > CTP > GTP > UTP > ITP; ref. 138,139). ADP, for example, antagonizes the ATP inhibition of channel opening to produce a rightward shift in the current inhibition as a function of ATP concentration curve. At concentrations higher than 250 μM, ADP can itself inhibit K_{ATP} channel activity in the absence of ATP. Thus it is thought that some nucleoside diphosphates, like ADP, compete with ATP for the same inhibitory binding site. The inhibitory actions at this site are Mg^{2+}-independent.

A second distinct action of nucleoside diphosphates (NDPs) is that, in an Mg^{2+}-dependent manner and in the absence of ATP, they can stimulate K_{ATP} channels, such as following rundown of channel activity. UDP is the most effective among nucleoside diphosphates in inducing K_{ATP} channel openings in ventricular cardiac cells (140). Terzic and colleagues have proposed a model (141) in which the channel is depicted to possess two nucleotide-binding sites (Fig. 9). When the channel can open spontaneously (i.e., is phosphorylated or in the spontaneous operative condition), ATP binds to site 1 and blocks the channel but at this state NDPs can antagonize ATP binding and relieve some of the block. Following rundown of spontaneous channel activity, NDPs can restore channel openings by binding to site 2 (i.e., channel is in the dephosphorylated state or NDP-induced operative condition) but now ATP binding to site 1 blocks activity, not allowing NDPs to antagonize the binding. Thus, this putative channel modification (i.e., phosphorylation) controls the affinity of site 1 to NDPs.

It is now well established that sulfonylureas are specific blockers of K_{ATP} channels in insulin-secreting cells, neuronal tissues, cardiac and skeletal muscles (142–145). Sulfonylureas do not seem to affect other K^+ channel types. A

Figure 9   Hypothetical model of the K_{ATP} channel. A. If neither the P_1 nor the P_2 sites are phosphorylated, the K_{ATP} channel would be closed and unable to respond to NDP or ATP. B. To open spontaneously, K_{ATP} channels would have to be phosphorylated at site P_1. Binding of ATP to the site 1 inhibits spontaneous channel openings. C. When the P_1 site is dephosphorylated (rundown of spontaneous opening), NDPs induce channels to open provided that the P_2 site is phosphorylated. ATP inhibits NDPs-induced channel openings as potently and effectively as spontaneous openings. D. When the P_1 and P_2 sites are phosphorylated, NDPs require the property to antagonize the ATP-induced inhibitory gating. A, ATP-binding inhibitory site; N, NDP-binding site; P_1, P_2, phosphorylation sites (Adapted from Ref. 141.)

A
                                     Extracellular

                                     Intracellular

B

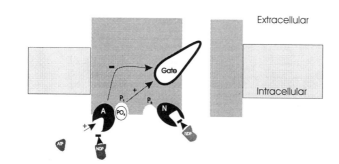

C

D

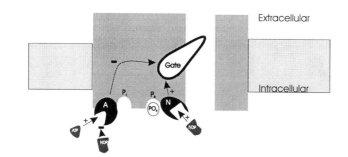

second generation of sulfonylurea drug derivatives (e.g,. glyburide) has shown highly selective binding affinity and potency in both electrophysiological and secretory studies (125). Such derivatives have proven extremely useful for type II diabetic patients by causing K_{ATP} channel block and insulin secretion. There are several chemically distinct classes of channel activator ligands (125). The effective concentrations of pinacidil, for example, one of the most effective K^+ channel openers in cardiac myocytes, are several orders of magnitude higher than those evoking vasodilation (146–148). Channel activation depends critically on intracellular ATP levels and involves an apparent competition with ATP (149–151), such that at levels less than 500 μM internal ATP pinacidil is effective but at levels between 1 and 3 mM it is ineffective (151,152).

Cardiac K_{ATP} channels, just like K_{ACh} channels, can be activated by adenosine or ACh (106,122,153). In contrast with K_{ACh} application of the activated form of G_α subunits (of the pertussis toxin sensitive kind), but not $G_{\beta\gamma}$ could directly activate K_{ATP} channels (122,153). The G-protein-dependent actions on K_{ATP} were shown to work by antagonizing the ATP-dependent gating (154).

The sulfonylurea receptor (SUR) was recently cloned and shown to be a member of the ATP-binding cassette superfamily, with multiple transmembrane-spanning domains and two potential nucleotide-binding folds (155). Expression of SUR alone reproduced high-affinity binding of sulfonylureas but not K^+ currents. Cloning of another member of the inward rectifier family, BIR ($K_{ir}6.2$), and coexpression with SUR, produced K_{ATP} channel activity that showed proper ATP inhibition, proper sulfonylurea block, and activation by channel openers (156). Both SUR and BIR are highly expressed in insulin-secreting pancreatic β cells and islets. Cardiac equivalents may also have been isolated (157). Since BIR expression alone produced no I_{K-ATP}, a model was proposed in which SUR and BIR formed a complex with unknown stoichiometry (see Fig. 2). In such a model, the sulfonylurea effects and presumably the two nucleotide-binding sites would be contributed to the complex by SUR, while the channel characteristics and possibly its modulation by phosphorylation, channel openers, and pH (158) could be contributed by BIR or BIR-like channels.

In heart, activation of K_{ATP} channels has been implicated as a cause for both the shortening of the APD (151, 159–162) and the marked cellular K^+ loss that occurs under conditions of low intracellular ATP levels, such as during hypoxia and ischemia. The resultant hyperpolarization and shortening of the action potential would limit contractile activity, thus reducing energy use. The accumulation of extracellular K^+ may be important in the development of lethal ventricular arrhythmias, which are the leading cause of death at the time of myocardial infarction. In smooth muscle cells, K_{ATP} channels control tone by modulating the activity of voltage-dependent Ca^{2+} channels. K_{ATP} channel openers have been mostly used as antihypertensives (pinacidil, minoxidil, and diazoxide). The K_{ATP} channels have been also implicated in the reduction of coronary vascular resistance induced by ischemia (163).

All of these actions have been linked to the clinical phenomenon known as "preconditioning" (repeated brief coronary artery ischemia–reperfusion cycles conferring protection to the heart from irreversible ischemic damage during subsequent longer episodes of ischemia) and have stimulated enormous interest. Establishing the role of K_{ATP} channels in this and related phenomena (e.g., "stunned myocardium") has, however, been controversial. Conflicting results may have arisen because of inconsistencies in the methods used to establish the occurrence of preconditioning in a variety of models.

The manifestations of "preconditioning" have been measured in several ways, including direct observation of the reduction in or prevention of shortening of APD (164), quantification of changes in the amount and time to recovery of myocardial contractile function, documentation of the occurrence or absence of various arrhythmias, and the pathological determination of the amount of myocardial cell necrosis (165). The sublethal ischemia protocols used to precondition have also been variable (both with regard to the duration and the number of sublethal ischemic episodes, as well as in terms of the timing of the measurement of the resulting functional changes). The animal models have included many species with differing coronary anatomical characteristics (particularly with regard to collateral flow; ref. 166–170) and different experimental preparations (particularly with regard to the anesthetic used). Finally, evidence for the involvement of the K_{ATP} channel in this phenomenon has thus far been indirect, making use of pharmacological modulators of this channel (e.g., openers) or of the adenosine receptor. The importance of the adenosine A_1 receptor in preconditioning has provided the strongest evidence. Adenosine and R-PIA, a selective A_1 receptor agonist, have been shown to mimic preconditioning. A selective A_1-receptor antagonist (DPCPX) was shown to prevent preconditioning. Activation of the A_1 receptor was then shown to lead to an increase in K_{ATP} channel activity via PTX-sensitive G proteins (106,153,171). In preconditioning protocols or with A_1 receptor activation, blockade of the K_{ATP} channel (with glibenclamide) would counter the beneficial effects (172,173).

K_{ATP} channel openers have also been shown to mimic preconditioning. Cromakalim and pinacidil were shown to reduce ischemic damage, an effect that could be reversed by the administration of glyburide (174–176). Nicorandil, a nicotinamide potassium channel opener was found to improve postischemic contractile function (stunning) and to diminish infarct size in irreversible ischemia (177,178). It should be noted that the effects of these pharmaceutical agents on the occurrence of peri-ischemic arrhythmias has been variable, since lower doses have seemed to diminish them (179) whereas higher doses have been associated in an increase in ventricular fibrillation (180,181). Furthermore, each of these drugs has been found not to give the expected results by at least one laboratory (182–186), although often in different models than in the positive studies. The lack of efficacy has been postulated to be related to the potent vasodilator activity of the K_{ATP} openers. Future work on K_{ATP} openers focusing on the determination of the molecular mechanism of action of these agents may allow more specific targeting of the beneficial effects. Electrophysiological as well as pharmacological evidence has suggested that K_{ATP} channels make up a diverse class of ion channels (127). The recent cloning of the first known K_{ATP} channel provides the means for investigation of tissue-specific isoforms and their structural determinants with the hope of addressing the channel diversity and allowing development of tissue selective blockers.

K$^+$ CHANNELS AND ANTIARRHYTHMIC DRUGS

Prolonging repolarization to minimize disparity between cells is often the goal of antiarrhythmic medications. To date, the class of drugs that predominantly block potassium channels (class III) have had the most promising effects clinically. Rendering the development of antiarrhythmic drugs difficult, however, is the fact that prolongation of the repolarization in an attempt to inhibit arrhythmias can contradictorily be arrhythmogenic (e.g., producing torsade de pointes). However, other drugs (non-class III) that result in similar degrees of action-potential prolongation (but through the blockade of different channels) do not have the same likelihood of producing such triggered arrhythmias. In fact, the antiarrhythmic with the lowest incidence of such proarrhythmia (amiodarone) is the most potent prolonger of APD (187,188). This paradox remains to be understood but demonstrates the need for better understanding of the mechanisms of drug actions.

For two decades the approach to antiarrhythmic drug development and administration focused on the Vaughan Williams classification, which originated at a time when knowledge of the electrophysiological mechanisms involved was less extensive than at present (189). This classification was mainly based on the most prominent ion blocked (class 1: Na^+ channel blockers; class 2: beta blockers; class 3: K^+ channel blockers; class 4: Ca^{2+} channel blockers). A new classification has been proposed (coined the "Sicilian Gambit") incorporating some of the recent knowledge of the molecular targets for drug actions. In this classification drugs were tabulated with regards to all the ionic channels they blocked and/or receptors they modulated (1). Many of the class 1 antiarrhythmics were shown to also block K^+ channels. However, this panel did not address the specific K^+ channels that were blocked and also left out K^+ channel openers.

POTASSIUM CHANNEL BLOCKERS

Studies demonstrating increases in the mortality of certain patients treated with class 1 antiarrhythmics (190) and better survival in those treated with amiodarone (191,192), predominantly a K^+ channel blocker, have added excitement to the development of new K^+ channel blockers. As discussed above, their potential in prolonging repolarization and thus homogenizing the refractory period of anisotropic tissue should theoretically diminish the frequency of reentrant rhythms (the most common cause of arrhythmias), especially with concomitant ischemia. Furthermore, unlike Na^+ channel blockers, K^+ blockers leave contractility unchanged or slightly increased (193,194), allowing their use in patients with heart failure, commonly associated with arrhythmias. The small inotropic effect is attributable to prolongation of the APD, resulting in increased Ca^{2+} influx during the plateau phase and enhancement of release of Ca^{2+} from the sarcoplasmic reticulum (195).

The current most commonly targeted for antiarrhythmic drug action is I_{Kr}, since it is critical in repolarization, terminating the plateau phase and initiating phase 3. The current-voltage relationship of I_{Kr} predicts that block should be enhanced in partially depolarized (e.g., ischemic) tissue (49). Many compounds are in various stages of development and are more or less specific to this current (Table 1). However, the first clinical trials are once again plagued by the occurrence of torsade de pointes. Their efficacy seems to be disappointingly less than the old standard amiodarone, demonstrating the need for far more sophisticated understanding of the mechanism of clinical arrhythmias.

Information about the desired properties of K^+ channel blockers as antiarrhythmics (e.g., their selectivity among tissues and their kinetics of binding) relies thus far on data from in vitro and in vivo studies. Drug–channel interactions have been studied in myocytes isolated from various animals and more recently from human hearts. A major problem in such studies is posed by the lack of specific blockers to eliminate multiple overlapping ionic conductances. Heterologous expression of cloned channels can be used to circumvent this problem. Recent work with stably transfected cell lines lacking such multiplicity of K^+ conductances provides evidence of the power of this approach. The electrostatic and hydrophobic components of antiarrhythmic block of the human cardiac hKv1.5 have been described in this manner (205). Drug effects have been recorded in oocytes injected with several of the cloned K^+ channels, allowing one to see the importance of voltage dependence. Having established the various characteristics of blockade of the different channels, the structural basis for these effects could be explored by site-directed mutagenesis experiments.

POTASSIUM CHANNEL ACTIVATORS

Activation of potassium channels has been essentially limited to the ATP sensitive K^+ channel (pinacidil, cromakalim, and nicorandil). Their use has been studied in view of the potential of producing "preconditioning-like" effects or in the treatment of hypertension. However, the concomitant induction of arrhythmias in many studies has hampered their use. It is interesting, however, that they have been shown to prevent arrhythmias in dog models normally producing torsade de pointes. This has not been extended to human trials. The recently cloned inward rectifier representing a K_{ATP} channel will certainly trigger studies on the actions and the development of K_{ATP} openers acting in a tissue specific manner.

ACKNOWLEDGMENTS

We thank Drs. Neil Castle, David Clapham, Yoshihisa Kurachi, and Nabil ElSheriff for reading the manuscript. We also thank Millie Tolson and Ibet Irizarry for secretarial assistance. DEL is supported through grants from the National Institutes of Health (HL54185) and American Heart Assosiation: National Center (96011620) and New York City Affiliate.

REFERENCES

1. Task Force of the Working Group on Arrhythmias of the European society of Cardiology. The Sicilian Gambit: a new approach to the classification of antiarrhythmic drugs based on their actions on arrhythmogenic mechanisms. Circulation 1991; 84:1831–1851.
2. Dilon S, et al. Influence of anisotropic tissue structure on reentrant circuits in the subepicardial border zone of subacute infarcts. Circ Res 1988; 63:182–206.
3. Downar E, et al. Endocardial mapping of ventricular tachycardia in the intact human ventricle. J Am Coll Cardiol 1988; 11:782–791.
4. Janse MJ, et al. Electrophysiological mechanisms of ventricular arrhythmias resulting from myocardial ischemia and infarction. Physiol Rev 1989; 69:1049–1169.
5. Josephson ME, et al: Mechanisms of ventricular tachycardia. Circulation 1987; 75:41.
6. Hamill OP, et al. Improved patch-clamp techniques for high-resolution current recording from cells and cell-free membrane patches. Pflügers Arch 1981; 391:85–100.
7. Phillipson LH. ATP-sensitive K^+ channels. Paradigm lost, paradigm regained. Science 1995; 270:1159.
8. Tamkun MM, et al. Cloning and expression of human cardiac potassium channels. In Zipes and Jalife, eds. Cardiac Electrophysiology: From Cell to Bedside. Philadelphia: WB Saunders, 1995.

9. Zygmunt AC, Gibbons WR. Calcium-activated chloride current in rabbit ventricular myocytes. Circ Res 1991; 68:424–437.
10. Zygmunt AC, Gibbons WR. Properties of the calcium-activated chloride current in heart. J Gen Physiol 1992; 99:391–414.
11. Callewaert G, et al. Existence of a calcium-dependent potassium channel in the membrane of cow cardiac Purkinje cells. Pflügers Arch 1986; 406:424–426.
12. Escande D, et al. Two types of transient outward currents in adult human atrial cells. Am J Physiol 1987; 252:H142–H148.
13. Giles W, Imaizumi Y. Comparison of potassium currents in rabbit atrial and ventricular cells. J Physiol 1988; 405:123–145.
14. Hiraoka M, Kawano S. Calcium-sensitive and insensitive transient outward current in rabbit ventricular myocytes. J Physiol 1989; 410:187–212.
15. Tseng GN, Hoffman BF. Two components of transient outward current in canine ventricular myocytes. Circ Res 1989; 64:633–647.
16. Kameyama M, et al. Intracellular Na$^+$ activates a K$^+$ channel in mammalian cardiac cells. Nature 1984; 309:354–356.
17. Josephson IR, et al. Early outward current in rat ventricular cells. Circ Res 1984; 54:157–162.
18. Giles W, van Ginneken A. A transient outward current in isolated cells from the crista terminalis of rabbit heart. J Physiol 1985; 368:243–264.
19. Nakayama T, Irisawa H. Transient outward current carried by potassium and sodium in quiescent atrioventricular node cells of rabbits. Circ Res 1985; 57:65–73.
20. Callewaert G, et al. Identification of a transient outward K$^+$-channel in single cardiac Purkinje cells. Arch Int Physiol Biochem 1985; 93:P16–P17.
21. Campbell DL, et al. The cardiac calcium-independent transient outward potassium current: kinetics, molecular properties, and role in ventricular repolarization. In: Zipes, Jalife eds. Cardiac Electrophysiology: From Cell to Bedside. Philadelphia: WB Saunders, 1995.
22. Campbell DL, et al. The calcium-independent transient outward potassium current in isolated ferret right ventricular myocytes. I. Basic characterization and kinetic analysis. J Gen Physiol 1993; 101:571–601.
23. Näbauer M, et al. Characteristics of transient outward current in human ventricular myocytes from patients with terminal heart failure. Circ Res 1993; 73:386–394.
24. Clark RB, et al. Properties of the transient outward current in rabbit atrial and ventricular cells. J Physiol 1988; 405:147–168.
25. Castle NA. Identification of two distinct K$^+$ currents activated by depolarization in rat ventricular myocytes. Biophys J 1992; 61:A307.
26. Shibata EF, et al. Contributions of a transient outward current to repolarization in human atrium. Am J Physiol 1988; 257:H1773–H1781.
27. Gross GJ, et al. Characterisation of transient outward current in young human atrial myocytes. Cardiovasc Res 1995; 29:112–117.
28. Näbauer M, et al. Presence of large transient outward current in human ventricular myocytes. Circulation 1992; 86:1–67.

29. Wettwer E, et al. Transient outward current in human and rat ventricular cardiomyocytes. Circulation 1992; 86:1–617.

30. Beuckelmann DJ, et al. Alterations of potassium currents in isolated human ventricular myocytes from patients with terminal heart failure. Circ Res 1993; 73:379–385.

31. Antzelevitch C, et al. Heterogeneity within the ventricular wall: electrophysiology and pharmacology of epicardial, endocardial, and M-cells. Circ Res 1991; 69:1427–1449.

32. Braun AP, et al. Intracellular mechanisms for α_1-adrenergic regulation of the transient outward current in rabbit atrial myocytes. J Physiol 1990; 431:689–712.

33. Yamashiti T, et al. Regional differences in transient outward current density and inhomogeneities of repolarization in rabbit right atrium. Circulation 1995; 92:3061–3069.

34. Litovsky SH, Antzelevitch C. Transient outward current prominent in canine ventricular epicardium but not endocardium. Circ Res 1988; 62:166–126.

35. Furukawa T, et al. Differences in transient outward currents in feline endocardial and epicardial myocytes. Circ Res 1990; 67:1287–1291.

36. Fedida D, Giles WR. Regional variations in action potentials and transient outward current in myocytes isolated from rabbit left ventricle. J Physiol (Lond) 1991; 442:191–209.

37. Lukas A, Antzelevitch C. Differences in electrophysiological response of canine ventricular epicardium and endocardium to ischemia. Circulation. 1993; 88:2903–2915.

38. Krishnan SC, Antzelevitch C. Flecainide-induced arrhythmia in canine ventricular epicardium. Phase 2 reentry? Circulation 1993; 87:562–572.

39. Lue W-M, Boyden PA. Abnormal electrical properties of myocytes from chronically infarcted canine heart. Alterations in V_{max} and the transient outward current. Circulation 1992; 85:1175–1188.

40. Jeck C, et al. Transient outward current in subendocardial Purkinje myocytes surviving in the infarcted heart. Circulation 1995; 92(3): 465–473.

41. Tsuchihashi K, Curtis MJ. Influence of tedisamil on the initiation and maintenance of ventricular fibrillation: chemical defibrillation by I_{to} blockade? J Cardiovasc Pharmacol 1991; 18:445–456.

42. Tseng-Crank J, et al. Molecular cloning and functional expression of a potassium channel cDNA isolated from a rat cardiac library. FEBS Lett 1990; 268:63–68.

43. Roberds SL, Tamkun MM. Cloning and tissue-specific expression of five voltage-gated potassium cDNAs expressed in rat heart. Proc Natl Acad Sci USA 1991; 88:1798–1802.

44. Baldwin TJ, et al. Characterization of a mammalian cDNA for an inactivating voltage-sensitive K$^+$ channel. Neuron 1991; 7:471–483.

45. Tseng G-N. Potassium channels: their modulation by drugs. In: Zipes, Jalife, eds. Cardiac Electrophysiology: From Cell to Bedside. Philadelphia: WB Saunders, 1995.

46. Roberds SL, et al. Molecular biology of the voltage-gated potassium channels of the cardiovascular system. J Cardiovasc Electrophysiol 1993; 4:68–80.

47. Paulmichl M, et al. Cloning and expression of a rat cardiac delayed rectifier potassium channel. Proc Natl Acad Sci USA 1991; 88:7892-7895.

48. Sanguinetti MC, Jurkiewicz NK. Two components of cardiac delayed rectifier K+ current. Differential sensitivity to block by class III antiarrhythmic agents. J Gen Physiol 1990; 96:195-215.

49. Colatsky TJ, et al. Channel specificity in antiarrhythmic drug action. Mechanism of potassium channel block and its role in suppressing and aggravating cardiac arrhythmias. Circulation 1990; 82:2235-2242.

50. Wang Z, et al. Delayed rectifier outward current and repolarization in human atrial myocytes. Circ Res 1993; 73:276-285.

51. Veldkamp MW, et al. Delayed rectifier channels in human ventricular myocytes. Circulation 1995; 92:3497-3504.

52. Shibasaki T. Conductance and kinetics of delayed rectifier potassium channels in nodal cells of the rabbit heart. J Physiol 1987; 387:227-250.

53. Keating M, et al. Linkage of a cardiac arrhythmia, the long QT syndrome and the Harvey ras-1 gene. Science 1991; 252:704-706.

54. Curran M, et al. Locus heterogeneity of autosomal dominant long QT syndrome. J Clin Invest 1993; 92:799-803.

55. Benhorin J, et al. Evidence of genetic heterogeneity in the long QT syndrome. Science 1993; 260:1960-1962.

56. Jiang C, et al. Two long QT syndrome loci map to chromosomes 3 and 7 with evidence for further heterogeneity. Nature Genet 1994; 8:141-147.

57. Towbin JA, et al. Evidence of genetic heterogeneity in Romano-Ward long QT syndrome: analysis of 23 families. Circulation 1994; 90:2635-2644.

58. Warmke JW, Ganetsky B. A family of potassium channel genes related to eag in Drosophila and mammals. Proc Natl Acad Sci USA 1994; 91:3438-3442.

59. Curran M, et al. A molecular basis of cardiac arrhythmias: HERG mutations cause long QT syndrome. Cell 1995; 80:795-803.

60. Sanguinetti MC, et al. A mechanistic link between an inherited and an acquired cardiac arrhythmia: HERG encodes the I_{Kr} potassium channel. Cell 1995; 81:299-307.

61. Kiehn J, et al. Single-channel properties of HERG, the channel encoding I_{K4}. Biophys J 1996; 70:A361.

62. Smith PL, et al. The inward rectification mechanism of the HERG cardiac potassium channel. Nature 1996; 379:833-836.

63. Hoshi T, et al. Two types of inactivation in Shaker K+ channels: effects of alterations in the carboxy-terminal region. Neuron 1991; 7:547-556.

64. López-Barneo J, et al. Effects of external cations and mutations in the pore region of C-type inactivation of Shaker potassium channels. Recept Chan 1993; 1:61-71.

65. Yellen G, et al. An engineered cysteine in the external mouth of a K+ channel allows inactivation to be modulated by metal binding. Biophys J 1994; 66:1068-1075.

66. Miller C. The inconstancy of the human heart. Nature 1996; 379:767-768.

67. Tseng GN, et al. Passive properties and membrane currents of canine ventricular myocytes. J Gen Physiol 1987; 90:671-701.
68. Apkon M, Nerbonne JM. Characterization of two distinct depolarization activated K^+ currents in isolated adult rat ventricular myocytes. J Gen Physiol 1991; 97:973-1011.
69. Follmer CH, et al. Modulation of the delayed rectifier, I_K, by cadmium in cat ventricular myocytes. Am J Physiol 1987b; 262:C75-C83.
70. Carmeliet E. Voltage- and time-dependent block of the delayed K^+ current in cardiac myocytes by dofetilide. J Pharmacol Exp Ther 1992; 262:809-817.
71. Balser JR, et al. Suppression of time-dependent outward current in guinea pig ventricular myocytes. Actions of quinidine and amiodarone. Circ Res 1991; 69:519-529.
72. Murai T, et al. Molecular cloning and sequence analysis of human genomic DNA encoding a novel membrane protein which exhibits a slowly activating potassium channel activity. Biochem Biophys Res Commun 1989; 161: 176-181.
73. Pragnell M, et al. Estrogen induction of a small putative K channel mRNA in rat uterus. Neuron 1990; 4:807-812.
74. Honoré E, et al. Cloning, expression, pharmacology, and regulation of a delayed rectifier K channel in mouse heart. EMBO J 1991; 10:2805-2811.
75. Freeman LC, and Kass RS. Expression of a minimal K^+ channel protein in mammalian cells and immunolocalization in guinea pig heart. Circ Res 1993; 73:968-973.
76. Kass RS. Delayed potassium channels in the heart: cellular, molecular, and regulatory properties. In: Zipes, Jalife, eds. Cardiac Electrophysiology: From Cell to Bedside. Philadelphia: WB Saunders, 1995.
77. Blumenthal EM, Kaczmarek LK. Modulation by cAMP of a slowly activating potassium channel expressed by *Xenopus* oocytes. J Neurosci 1992; 12:290-296.
78. Busch AE, et al. Regulation by second messengers of the slowly activating, voltage-dependent potassium current expressed in *Xenopus* oocytes. J Physiol 1992; 450:491-502.
79. Boyle WA, Nerbonne JM. A novel type of depolarization-activated K^+ current in isolated adult rat atrial myocytes. Am J Physiol 1991; 260:H1236-1247.
80. Clapham DE, Logothetis DE. Delayed rectifier potassium current in embryonic chick heart ventricle. Am J Physiol 1988; 254:H192-H197.
81. London B, et al. Cloning and expression of the gene encoding the murine delayed rectifier potassium channel Kv1.5. Biophy J 1994; 66:A106.
82. Yue DT, Marban E. A novel cardiac potassium channel that is active and conductive at depolarized potentials. Pflügers Arch 1988; 413:127-133.
83. Backx PH, Marban E. Background potassium conductance active during the plateau of the action potential in guinea pig ventricular myocytes. Circ Res 1992; 72:890-900.
84. Hille B. Ionic Channels of Excitable Membranes. Sunderland, MA: Sinauer Associates, 1992: 607.
85. Pennefather P, et al. Effects of external and internal K^+ on activation and deactivation of the inwardly rectifying background K^+ current (I_{K1}) in isolated canine Purkinje myocytes. Biophys J 1987; 51:256a.

86. Harvey RD, Ten Eick, RE. Characterization of the inward-rectifying potassium current in cat ventricular myocytes. J Gen Physiol 1988; 91:593–615.

87. Saigusa A, Matsuda H. Outward currents through the inwardly rectifying potassium channel of guinea-pig ventricular cells. Jpn J Physiol 1988; 38:77–91.

88. Pennefather P, Cohen IS. Molecular mechanisms of cardiac K^+-channel regulation. In: Zipes, Jalife, eds. Cardiac Electrophysiology: From Cell to Bedside. Philadelphia: WB Saunders, 1990.

89. Hagiwara S, Yoshii M. Effects of internal potassium and sodium on the anomalous rectification of the starfish egg as examined by internal perfusion. J Physiol 1979; 292:251–265.

90. Leech CA, Stanfield PR. Inward rectification in frog skeletal muscle fibres and its dependence on membrane potential and external potassium. J Physiol 1981; 319:295–309.

91. Kurachi Y. Voltage-dependent activation of the inward-rectifier potassium channel in the ventricular cell membrane of guinea-pig heart. J Physiol 1985; 366:365–385.

92. Burton FL, Hutter OF. Selectivity to flow of intrinsic gating in inwardly rectifying potassium channel from mammalian skeletal muscle. J Physiol 1990; 424:253–261.

93. Silver MR, DeCoursey TE. Intrinsic gating of inward rectifier in bovine pulmonary artery endothelial cells in the presence or absence of internal Mg^{2+}. J Gen Physiol 1990; 96:109–133.

94. Matsuda H, et al. Ohmic conductance through the inwardly rectifying K channel and blocking by internal Mg^{2+}. Nature 1987; 325:156–159.

95. Vandenberg CA. Inward rectification of a potassium channel in cardiac ventricular cells depends on internal magnesium ions. Proc Natl Acad Sci USA 1987; 84:2560–2564.

96. Hume JR, Uehara A. Ionic basis of the different action potential configurations of single guinea pig atrial and ventricular myocytes. J Physiol 1985; 368:525–544.

97. Noma A, et al. Resting K conductances in pacemaker and non-pacemaker heart cells of the rabbit. Jpn J Physiol 1984; 34:245–254.

98. Kubo Y, et al. Primary structure and functional expression of a mouse inward rectifier potassium channel. Nature 1993; 362:127–133.

99. Trautwein W, Dudel J. Zum mechanismus der membranwirkung des acetylcholin an der herzmuskelfaser. Pflügers Arch 1958; 266:324–334.

100. Soejima M, Noma A. Mode of regulation of the ACh-sensitive K-channel by the muscarinic receptor in rabbit atrial cells. Pflügers Arch 1984; 400:424–431.

101. Pfaffinger PJ, et al. GTP- binding proteins couple cardiac muscarinic receptors to a K channel. Nature 1985; 317:536–538.

102. Breitwiser GE, Szabo G. Uncoupling of cardiac muscarinic and β-adrenergic receptors from ion channels by a guanine nucleotide analogue. Nature 1985; 317:538–540.

103. Logothetis DE, et al. The βγ subunits of GTP-binding proteins activate the muscarinic K^+ channel in heart. Nature 1987; 325:321–326.

104. Codina J, et al. The α subunit of the GTP binding protein G_K opens atrial potassium channels. Science 1987; 236:442–445.

105. Logothetis DE, et al. Specificity of action of guanine nucleotide-binding regulatory protein subunits on the cardiac muscarinic K^+ channel. Proc Natl Acad Sci USA 1988; 85:5814–5818.

106. Ito H, et al. On the mechanism of G protein βγ subunit activation of the muscarinic K^+ channel in guinea pig atrial cell membrane. J Gen Physiol 1992; 99:961–983.

107. Wickman KD, et al. Recombinant G-protein βγ subunits activate the muscarinic-gated atrial potassium channel. Nature 1994; 368:255–257.

108. Ikeda SR. Voltage-dependent modulation of N-type calcium channels by G-protein βγ subunits. Nature 1996; 380:255–258.

109. Herlitze S, et al. Modulation of Ca^{2+} channels by G-protein βγ subunits. Nature 1996; 380:258–262.

110. Kubo Y, et al. Primary structure and functional expression of a rat G-protein-coupled muscarinic potassium channel. Nature 1993; 364:802–806.

111. Dascal N, et al. Atrial G protein-activated K^+ channel: expression cloning and molecular properties. Proc Natl Acad Sci USA 1993; 90:10235–10239.

112. Krapivinsky G, et al. The G-protein-gated atrial K^+ channel I_{KACh} is a heteromultimer of two inwardly rectifying K^+-channel proteins. Nature 1995; 374:135–141.

113. Chan KW, et al. A recombinant inwardly rectifying potassium channel coupled to GTP-binding proteins. J Gen Physiol 1996; 107:381–397.

114. Hedin KE, et al. Cloning of a *Xenopus laevis* inwardly rectifying K^+ channel subunit that permits GIRK1 expression of I_{KACh} currents in oocytes. Neuron 1996; 16:423–429.

115. Krapivinsky G, et al. $G_{βγ}$ binds directly to the G-protein-gated K^+ channel, I_{KACh}. J Biol Chem 1995; 270:29059–29062.

116. Inanobe A, et al. $G_{βγ}$ directly binds to the carboxyl terminus of the G protein-gated muscarinic K^+ channel, GIRK1. Biochem Biophys Res Commun 1995; 212:1022–1028.

117. Kunkel MT, Peralta EG. Identification of domains conferring G protein regulation of inward rectifier potassium channels. Cell 1995; 83:443–449.

118. Huang C-L, et al. Evidence that direct binding of $G_{βγ}$ to the GIRK1 G protein-gated inwardly rectifying K^+ channel is important for channel activation. Neuron 1995; 15:1133–1143.

119. Kurachi Y, et al. Short-term desensitization of muscarinic K^+ channel current in isolated atrial myocytes and possible role of GTP-binding proteins. Pflügers Arch 1987; 410:227–233.

120. Sui JL, et al. Activation of the muscarinic K^+ channel by a G-protein-independent mechanism. 1996; Submitted for publication.

121. Kim D. Modulation of acetylcholine-activated K^+ channel function in rat atrial cells by phosphorylation. J Physiol 1991; 437:133–155.

122. Kurachi Y, et al. G protein activation of cardiac muscarinic K^+ channels. Prog Neurobiol 1992; 39:229–246.

123. Koumi S, et al. Alterations in muscarinic K$^+$ channel response to acetylcholine and to G protein-mediated activation in atrial myocytes isolated from failing human hearts. Circulation 1994; 90:2213-2224.

124. Noma A. ATP-regulated K$^+$ channels in cardiac muscle. Nature 1983; 305:147-148.

125. Gopalakrishnan M, et al. ATP-sensitive K$^+$ channels: pharmacologic properties, regulation, and therapeutic potential. Drug Dev Res 1993; 28:95-127.

126. Terzic A, et al. Nucleotide regulation of ATP sensitive potassium channels. Cardiovascular Res 1994; 28:746-753.

127. Ashcroft SJH, Ashcroft FM. Properties and function of ATP-sensitive K$^+$ channels. Cell Signal 1990; 2:197-214.

128. Findlay I. The effects of magnesium upon adenosine triphosphate-sensitive potassium channels in a rat insulin-secreting cell line. J Physiol 1987; 391:611-629.

129. Findlay I. ATP-sensitive K$^+$ channels in rat ventricular myocytes are blocked and inactivated by internal divalent cations. Pflügers Arch. 1987; 410:313-320.

130. Spruce AE, et al. Voltage-dependent ATP-sensitive potassium channels of skeletal muscle membrane. Nature 1985; 316:736-738.

131. Standen NB, et al. Hyperpolarizing vasodilators activate ATP-sensitive K$^+$ channels in arterial smooth muscle. Science 1989; 245:177-180.

132. Cook DL, Hales CN. Intracellular ATP directly blocks K$^+$ channels in pancreatic beta-cells. Nature 1984; 311:271-273.

133. Sturgess NC, et al. The sulfonylurea receptor may be an ATP-sensitive potassium channel. Lancet 1985; 1:474-475.

134. Rorsman P, Trube G. Glucose-dependent K$^+$ channels in pancreatic beta cells are regulated by intracellular ATP. Pflügers Arch 1985; 405:305-309.

135. Ashford MLJ, et al. Glucose-induced excitation of cat hypothalamic neurons in vitro is mediated by ATP-sensitive K$^+$ channels. Pflügers Arch 1989; 415:31P.

136. Kunzelmann K, et al. Characterization of potassium channels in respiratory cells. I. General properties. Pflügers Arch 1989; 414:291-296.

137. Groschner K, et al. Ca^{2+}-activated K$^+$ channels in airway smooth muscle are inhibited by cytoplasmic adenosine triphosphate. Pflügers Arch 1991; 417:517-522.

138. Davies N, et al. ATP-dependent potassium channels of muscle cells: their properties, regulation, and possible functions. J Bioenerg Biomembr 1991; 23:509-535.

139. Lederer WJ, Nichols CJ. Nucleotide modulation of the activity of rat heart ATP-sensitive K$^+$ channels in isolated membrane patches. J Physiol 1989; 419:193-211.

140. Tung RT, Kurachi Y. On the mechanism of nucleotide diphosphate activation of the ATP-sensitive K$^+$ channel in ventricular cell of guinea-pig. J Physiol 1991; 437:239-256.

141. Terzic A, et al. Dualistic behavior of ATP-sensitive K$^+$ channels toward intracellular nucleoside diphosphates. Neuron 1994; 12:1049-1058.

142. Schmid-Antomarchi H, et al. The antidiabetic sulfonylurea glibenclamide is a

potent blocker of the ATP-sensitive K$^+$ channels in insulin-secreting cells. Biochem Biophys Res Commun 1987a; 146:21–25.

143. Schmid-Antomarchi H, et al. The receptor for antidiabetic sulfonylureas controls the activity of the ATP-modulated K$^+$ channel in insulin-secreting cells. J Biol Chem 1987; 262:15840–15844.

144. Zünkler BJ, et al. Concentration-dependent effects of tolbutamide, meglitinide, glipizide, glibenclamide, and diazoxide on ATP-regulated K$^+$ currents in pancreatic beta cells. Naunyn Schmiedebergs Arch Pharmacol 1988; 337:225–230.

145. Miller RJ. Glucose-regulated potassium channels are sweet news for neurobiologists. Trends Neurosci 1990; 13:197–199.

146. Hamilton TC, Weston AH. Cromakalim, nicorandil and pinacidil: novel drugs which open potassium channels in smooth muscle. Gen Pharmacol 1989; 20:1–9.

147. Edwards G. Weston AH. Potassium channel openers and vascular smooth relaxation. Pharmacol Ther 1990; 48:237–258.

148. Longman SD, Hamilton TC. Potassium channel activator drugs: mechanism of action, pharmacological properties, and therapeutic potential. Med Res Rev 1992; 12:73–148.

149. Thuringer D, Escande D. Apparent competition between ATP and the potassium channel opener RP 49356 on ATP-sensitive K$^+$ channels of cardiac myocytes. Mol Pharmacol 1989; 36:897–902.

150. Ripoll C, et al. Modulation of ATP-sensitive K$^+$ channel activity and contractile behavior in mammalian ventricle by the potassium channel openers cromakalim and RP 49356. J Pharmacol Exp Ther 1990; 255:429–435.

151. Arena JP, Kass RA. Activation of ATP-sensitive K$^+$ channels in heart cells by pinacidil: dependence of ATP. Am J Physiol 1989; 257:H2092–2096.

152. Tseng GN, Hoffman BF. Actions of pinacidil on membrane currents by intracellular ATP and cAMP. Pflügers Arch 1990; 415:414–424.

153. Kirsch GE, et al. Coupling of ATP sensitive K$^+$ channels to A$_1$ receptors by G proteins in rat ventricular myocytes. Am J Physiol 1990; 259:H820–H826.

154. Terzic A, et al. G proteins activate ATP-sensitive K$^+$ channels by antagonizing ATP-dependent gating. Neuron, 1994; 12:885–893.

155. Aguilar-Bryan L, et al. Cloning of the β cell high-affinity sulfonylurea receptor: a regulator of insulin secretion. Science 1995; 268:423–426.

156. Inagaki N, et al. Reconstitution of I$_{KATP}$: an inward rectifier subunit plus the sulfonylurea receptor. Science 1995; 270:1166–1170.

157. Inagaki N, et al. Cloning and functional characterization of a novel ATP-sensitive potassium channel ubiquitously expressed in rat tissues, includingpancreatic islets, pituitary, skeletal muscle, and heart. J Biol Chem 1995; 270:5691–5694.

158. Forestier C, et al. Mechanism of action of K-channel-openers on frog skeletal muscle K$_{ATP}$ channels: interactions with nucleotides and protons. J Gen Physiol 1996; in press.

159. Escande D, et al. The potassium channel opener cromakalim (BRL34915) activates ATP-dependent K$^+$ channels in isolated cardiac myocytes. Biochem Biophys Res Commun 1988; 154:620–625.

160. Sanguinetti MC, et al. BRL34915 (cromakalim) activates ATP-sensitive K^+ current in cardiac muscle. Proc Natl Acad Sci USA 1988; 85:8360-8364.

161. McCullough JR, et al. Electrophysiological actions of BRL34915 in isolated guinea-pig ventricular myocytes. Drug Dev Res 1990; 19:141-151.

162. Martin CL, Chin K. Pinacidil opens ATP-dependent K^+ channels in cardiac myocytes in an ATP- and temperature-dependent manner. J Cardiovasc Pharmacol 1990; 15:510-514.

163. Weiss JN, Venkatesh N. Metabolic regulation of cardiac ATP-sensitive K^+ channels. Cardiovasc Drugs Ther 1993; 7:499-505.

164. Surawicz B. Role of potassium channels in cycle length dependent regulation of action potential duration in mammalian cardiac Purkinje and ventricular muscle fibres. Cardiovasc Res 1992; 26:1021-1029.

165. Gross GJ, Auchampach JA: Blockade of ATP-sensitive potassium channels prevents myocardial preconditioning in dogs. Circ Res 1992; 70:223-233.

166. Liu GS, et al. Protection against infarction afforded by preconditioning is mediated by A_1 adenosine receptors in the rabbit heart. Circulation 1991; 84:350-356.

167. Thornton JD, et al. Intravenous pretreatment with A_1-selective adenosine analogues protects the heart against infarction. Circulation 1992; 85:659-665.

168. Fralix TA, et al. Evaluating the protective effects of adenosine in the isolated perfused rat heart: changes in metabolism and intracellular ion homeostasis. Am J Physiol 1993; 264:C986-C994.

169. Sack S, et al. Ischaemic preconditioning- time course of renewal in the pig. Cardiovasc Res 1993; 27(4):551-555.

170. Auchampach JA, Gross GJ. Blockade of adenosine A_1 receptors prevents preconditioning in dogs. FASEB J 1992; 6:1812.

171. Thornton JD, et al. Pretreatment with pertussis toxin blocks the protective effects of preconditioning: evidence for G_i-protein mechanism. J Mol Cell Cardiol 1993; 25:311-320.

172. Yao Z, Gross GJ. A comparison of adenosine-induced cardioprotection and ischemic preconditioning in dogs. Circulation 1994; 89:1229-1236.

173. Gross GJ, Auchampach JA. Role of ATP dependent potassium channels in myocardial ischemia. Cardiovasc Res 1992; 26:1011-1016.

174. Grover GJ, et al. Anti-ischemic effects of the potassium channel activators pinacidil and cromakalim and the reversal of these effects with the potassium channel blocker, glyburide. J Pharmacol Exp Ther 1989; 251:98-104.

175. Grover GJ, et al. Reduction of ischemic damage in isolated rat hearts by the potassium channel opener RP 52891. Eur J Pharmacol 1990; 191:11-18.

176. Cole W, et al. ATP-regulated K^+ channels protect the myocardium against ischemia-reperfusion damage. J Mol Cell Cardiol 1991; 23(Suppl III):III-465.

177. Grover GJ, et al. Nicorandil improves post-ischemic contractile function independently of direct myocardial effects. J Cardiovasc Pharmacol 1990b; 15(5):698-705.

178. Auchampach JA, Gross GJ. Anti-ischaemic actions of potassium channel openers in experimental myocardial ischaemia/reperfusion injury in dogs. Eur Heart J 1993; 14:10-15.

179. Yao Z, Gross GJ. Effects of the K_{ATP} channel opener bimakalim on coronary blood flow, monophasic action potential duration and infarct size in dogs. Circulation 1994; 89:1769–1775.

180. Chi L, et al. Profibrillatory actions of pinacidil in a conscious canine model of sudden coronary death. J Cardiovasc Pharmacol 1990; 452–464.

181. Wolleben C, et al. Influence of ATP-sensitive potassium channel modulators on ischemia-induced fibrillation in isolated rat hearts. J Mol Cell Cardiol 1989; 21(8):783–788.

182. Thornton JD, et al. Blockade of ATP-sensitive potassium channels increases infarct size but does not prevent preconditioning in rabbit hearts. Circ Res 1993b; 72:44–49.

183. Auchampach JA, et al. The new K^+ channel opener RP 52891 reduces experimental infarct size in dogs in the absence of systemic hemodynamic changes. J Pharmacol Exp Ther 1991; 259:961–967.

184. Sakamato S, et al. Effects of pinacidil on myocardial blood flow and infarct size after acute left anterior descending coronary artery occlusion and reperfusion in awake dogs with and without a coexisting left circumflex coronary artery stenosis. J Cardiovasc Pharmacol 1989; 14:747–755.

185. Kitzen J, et al. Potassium channel activators cromakalin and celikalim (WAY-120-491) fail to decrease myocardial infarct size in the anaesthetized canine. Pharmacology 1992; 45:71–82.

186. Downey JM: An explanation for the reported observation that ATP-dependent potassium channel openers mimic preconditioning. Cardiovasc Res 1993; 27:1565.

187. Burkart F, et al. Effect of antiarrhythmic therapy on mortality in survivors of myocardial infarction with asymptomatic complex ventricular arrhythmias. J Am Coll Cardiol 1990; 16:1711–1718.

188. Hii JT, et al. Precordial QT interval dispersion as a marker of torsade de pointes. Disparate effects of class la antiarrhythmic drugs and amiodarone. Circulation 1992; 86:137601382.

189. Vaughan Williams EM. Classification of antiarrhythmic drugs. In: Sandoe E, Flensted-Jensen E, Olesen EH, eds. Symposium on Cardiac Arrhythmias. Astr, Denmark: Elsevier, 1970:449–541.

190. The Cardiac Arrhythmia Suppression Trial Investigators. Effect of encainide and flecainide on mortality in a randomized trial of arrhythmia suppression after myocardial infarction (CAST-1). N Engl J Med 1989; 406–412.

191. Pfisterer M, et al. Long-term benefit of 1-year amiodarone treatment for persistent complex ventricular arrhythmias after myocardial infarction. Circulation 1993; 87:309–311.

192. Mason JW. A comparison of seven antiarrhythmic drugs in patients with ventricular tachyarrhythmias. N Engl J Med 1993; 329:452–458.

193. Carlsson L, et al. QTU prolongation and torsades de pointes induded by putative Class III antiarrhythmic agents in the rabbit: etiology and interventions. J Cardiovasc Pharmacol 1990; 16:276–285.

194. Josephson MA, Singh BS. Hemodynamic effects of class III antiarrhythmic

agents. In: N. SB, ed. Control of Cardiac Arrhythmias by Lengthening Repolarization. Mount Kisco, NY: Futura, 1988:153–174.

195. Tande PM, et al. Rate-dependent class III antiarrhythmic action, negative chronotropy and positive inotropy of a novel I_K blocking drug, UK68,798; Potent in guinea pig but no effect in rat myocardium. J Cardiovasc Pharmacol 1990; 16:401–410.

196. Black SC, Lucchesi BR. UK-68798, A class III antiarrhythmic drug with antifibrillatory properties. Cardiovasc Drug Rev 1992; 10:170–181.

197. Chadwick CC, et al. Identification of a specific radioligand for the cardiac rapidly activating delayed rectifier K^+ channel. Circ Res 1993; 72:707–714.

198. Duan D, et al. Potassium channel properties of propafenone in rabbit atrial myocytes. J Pharmacol Exp Ther 1993; 264:1113–1123.

199. Dukes ID, et al. Tedisamil blocks the transient delayed rectifier K^+ current in mammalian cardiac and glial cells. J Phamacol Exp Ther 1990; 254:560–569.

200. Furukawa T, et al. Time- and voltage-dependent block of the delayed K^+ current by quinidine in rabbit sinoatrial and atrioventricular nodes. J Pharmacol Exp Ther 1989; 251:756–763.

201. Hiraoka M, et al. Effects of quinidine on plateau currents of guinea pig ventricular myocytes. J Mol Cell Cardiol 1986; 18:1097–1106.

202. Imaizumi Y, Giles WR. Quinidine induced inhibition of transient outward current in cardiac muscle. Am J Physiol 1987; 253:H704–H708.

203. Roden DM, et al. Quinidine delays I_K activation in guinea pig ventricular myocytes. Circ Res 1988; 62:1055–1058.

204. Salata JJ, Wasserstrom JA. Effects of quinidine on action potentials and ionic current in guinea pig ventricular myocytes. Circ Res 1988; 62:324–337.

205. Snyders DJ, Yeola SW. Determinants of antiarrhythmic drug action: electrostatic and hydrophobic components of block of the human cardiac hKv1.5 channel. Circ Res 1995; 77:575–583.

206. Furukawa T, et al. Time- and voltage-dependent block of the delayed K^+ current by quinidine in rabbit sinoatrial and atrioventricular nodes. J Pharmacol Exp Ther 1989; 251:756–763.

207. Duff HJ, et al. High and low- affinity sites for [^{3}H] dofetilide binding to guinea pig myocytes. Circ Res 1995; 77:718–725.

208. Slawsky MT, Castle NA. K^+ channel blocking actions of flecainide compared with those of propafenone and quinidine in adult ventricular myocytes. J Pharmacol Exp Ther 1994; 269:66–74.

209. Balser JR, et al. Suppression of time-dependent outward current in guinea pig ventricular myocytes. Actions of quinidine and amiodarone. Circ Res 1991; 69:519–529.

210. Roden DM, et al. Quinidine delays I_K activation in guinea pig ventricular myocytes. Circ Res 1988; 62:1055–1058.

211. Salata JJ, Wasserstrom JA. Effects of quinidine on action potentials and ionic currents in isolated canine ventricular myocytes. Circ Res 1988; 62:324–337.

212. Balser JR, et al. Suppression of time-dependent outward current in guinea pig

ventricular myocytes. Actions of quinidine and amiodarone. Circ Res 1991; 69:519–529.

213. Hiraoka M, et al. Effects of quinidine on plateau currents of guinea pig ventricular myocytes. J Mol Cell Cardiol 1986; 18:1097–1106.

214. Haworth RA, et al. Inhibition of ATP-sensitive potassium channels of adult rat heart cells by antiarrhythmic drugs. Circ Res 1989; 65:1157–1160.

215. Sakuta H, et al. Blockade of antiarrhythmic drugs of glibenclamide-sensitive K$^+$ channels in *Xenopus* oocytes. Br J Pharmacol 1992; 107:1061–1067.

216. Follmer CH, Colatsky TJ. Block of delayed rectifier potassium current, I$_K$, by flecaininde and E4031 in cat ventricular myocytes. Circulation 1990; 82:289–293.

217. Follmer CH, et al. Differential block of cardiac delayed rectifier current by class 1c antiarrhythmic drugs: evidence for open channel block. Cardiovasc Res 1992; 26:1121–1130.

218. Wang DW, et al. Voltage dependent inhibition of ATP-sensitive potassium channels by flecainide in guinea pig ventricular cells. Cardiovasc Res 1995; 29:520–525.

219. Duan D, et al. Potassium channel properties of propafenone in rabbit atrial myocytes. J Pharmacol Exp Ther 1993; 264:1113–1123.

220. Nakaya H, et al. Effects of MS-551, A new class III antiarrhythmic drug on action potential and membrane currents in rabbit ventricular myocytes. Br J Pharmacol 1993; 109:157–163.

221. Lynch JJ, et al. Comparison of binding to rapidly activating delayed rectifier K$^+$ channel, I$_{Kr}$, and effects on myocardial refractoriness for class III antiarrhythmic agents. J Cardiovasc Pharmacol 1995; 25:336–340.

222. Vanoli E, et al. Sympathetic activation, ventricular repolarization and I$_{Kr}$ blockade: implications for the antifibrillatory efficacy of potassium channel blocking drugs. J Am Coll Cardiol 1995; 25:1609–1614.

223. Yao Z, et al. Activation of cardiac K$_{ATP}$ channels: an endogenous protective mechanism during repetitive ischemia. Am J Physiol 1993; 264:H495–504.

224. Carmeliet E. Use-dependent block of the delayed K$^+$ current in rabbit ventricular myocytes. Cardiovasc Drugs Ther 1993; 7:599–604.

225. Sato R, et al. Amiodarone blocks the inward rectifier potassium channel in isolated guinea pig ventricular cells. J Pharmacol Exp Ther 1994; 269:1213–1219.

226. Funck-Brentano C. Canaux potassiques et arythmies. Arch Mal Coeur 1992; 85:9–13.

227. Chadwick CC, et al. Identification of a specific radioligand for the cardiac rapidly activating delayed rectifier K$^+$ channel. Circ Res 1993; 72:707–714.

228. Arena JP, Kass RS. Block of heart potassium channels by clofilium and its tertiary analogs: relationship between drug structure and type of channel blocked. Mol Pharmacol 1988; 34:60–66.

229. Castle NA. Selective inhibition of potassium currents in rat ventricle by clofilium and its tertiary homolog. J Pharmacol Exp Ther 1991; 257:342–350.

230. Friedrichs GS, et al. Antifibrillatory effects of clofilium in the rabbit isolated heart. Br J Pharmacol 1994; 113:209–215.

231. Dukes ID, et al. Tedisamil blocks the transient delayed rectifier K^+ current in mammalian cardiac and glial cells. J Phamacol Exp Ther 1990; 254:560–569.

232. Fermini B, et al. Use-dependent effects of the class III antiarrhythmic agent NE-10064 (azimilide) on cardiac repolarization: block of delayed rectifier potassium and L-type calcium currents. J Cardiovasc Pharmacol 1995; 26:259–271.

233. Quayle JM, et al. Pharmacology of ATP-sensitive K^+ current in smooth muscle cells from rabbit mesenteric artery. Am J Physiol 1995; 269:C1112–1118.

234. Heath BM, Terrar DA. Effect of glibenclamide, forskolin and isoprenaline on the parallel activation of K_{ATP} and reduction of I_K by cromakalim in cardiac myocytes. Cardiovasc Res 1994; 28:818–822.

11

Plasma Membrane Calcium Channels

Andrew R. Marks
Mount Sinai School of Medicine
New York, New York

The development of the patch-clamp technique for the study of ion channels approximately 20 years ago (19, 42) permitted detailed examination of the physiological properties of the voltage-dependent calcium channels (VDCC) that regulate muscle contraction in the cardiovascular system. Organic calcium channel blockers were discovered and characterized (54). These compounds have become mainstays in the pharmacotherapy of cardiovascular diseases. Meanwhile, evidence accumulated indicating that calcium ions could act as intracellular messengers in many critically important signal transduction pathways. With the realization of the importance of calcium as a second messenger in cellular processes, attention was directed towards the molecules mediating calcium fluxes, and the mechanisms by which calcium fluxes were regulated.

In 1984, using [^{3}H]nitrendipine (a calcium channel antagonist), the dihydropyridine-receptor (DHPR) was isolated from skeletal muscle transverse tubules (7). In 1987, the primary structure of a VDCC was elucidated from cDNA cloning (52). Since 1987, cDNAs encoding the α_1 subunits of calcium channels from cardiac and smooth muscles and brain have been cloned by several laboratories (23, 28, 29, 31, 34). Calcium channels, together with other calcium regulatory proteins including calcium pumps (both plasma membrane and sarcoplasmic reticulum forms) and calcium/Na$^+$ exchangers, are distributed on the plasma membrane as well as the membranes of intracellular organelles. Table 1 illustrates different pathways in which calcium fluxes are mediated. The development in Roger Tsien's laboratory of experimental techniques allowing calcium measurements using fluorescent calcium indicators, quin2, fura2 (17), and fluo-3 (35), the refinement of biochemical approaches to studying calcium channels, and the application of recombinant DNA techniques, have led to the elucidation of the structure and/or function of a variety of calcium channels from nerve, muscle, and other excitable cells.

CALCIUM AND CALCIUM REGULATORS

Calcium acts as a ubiquitous second messenger in diverse signaling systems. At steady state, calcium is distributed unevenly throughout the cell, with the lowest concentration in the cytoplasm. In normal resting cells the cytoplasmic free calcium concentration is low (10^{-7} M), but extracellular and organellar (e.g., ER) [Ca^{2+}] are approximately four orders of magnitude higher. The steady-state intracellular calcium concentration ([Ca^{2+}]$_i$) may be altered by changes in membrane potential or by agonist stimulation that results in increased calcium flux into the cytoplasm.

In excitable cells, cytoplasmic free calcium concentration is regulated by calcium influx through VDCCs on the plasma membrane and calcium release into the cytoplasm via intracellular calcium release channels that include members of the inositol 1,4,5-trisphosphate (IP$_3$) receptor and ryanodine receptor (RyR) families (see Chapter 12). In the cytoplasm, calcium ions bind to calcium-binding proteins that contain multiple EF hand structures, including troponin and calmodulin. They, in turn, activate enzymes participating in downstream cellular events. A rise to ~ 1 μM in free cytosolic calcium triggers cellular responses, including muscle contraction, fertilization, hormone secretion, and T-cell activation. In response to increasing [Ca^{2+}]$_i$, calcium-ATPases are activated to pump calcium ions back across the plasma membrane to the extracellular

Table 1 Ca Transporting Systems of Cell Membranes

Transporting Mode	Membrane	Ca Affinity
Channels	Plasma membranes	
	Endo (sarco) plasmic reticulum	Low
ATPases	Plasma membranes	
	Endo (sarco) plasmic reticulum	High
Exchangers (Na/Ca)	Plasma membranes	
	Inner mitochondrial membrane	Low
Electrophoretic uniporters	Inner mitochondrial membrane	Low

space or into the lumen of endoplasmic reticulum (ER) or other intracellular vesicles that store calcium, thus maintaining normal $[Ca^{2+}]_i$.

CALCIUM CHANNELS AND EXCITATION–CONTRACTION COUPLING IN THE HEART

Excitation-contraction coupling (Fig. 2) in the heart requires the activation of the calcium-release channel in the sarcoplasmic reticulum (SR) (8). Calcium influx via the voltage-gated calcium channel of the transverse tubule triggers the release of calcium from the SR into the cytosol via the Ryr/calcium-release channel. This phenomenon is referred to as calcium-induced calcium release (15). Cytosolic calcium binding to troponin C activates the contractile apparatus (3).

Thus, calcium signaling during striated muscle contraction is mediated by the cooperative activation of both VDCCs and intracellular calcium release channels (8). The VDCCs in both cardiac and skeletal muscles are comprised of five subunits encoded by four separate genes (Fig. 1). Skeletal and cardiac muscle likewise contain distinct isoforms of homotetrameric Ryr/intracellular calcium release channels encoded by separate genes (see Chapter 12). Thus, in each type of striated muscle, at least five separate genes encode the major channels forming the pathways for calcium signaling during muscle contraction. The primary structures of these calcium channels have been deduced from cDNA cloning, and their critical roles in E-C coupling are well established (8). We have shown that the four genes encoding the five subunits of the DHPR are also coordinately regulated during myogenic development (5). Important functional differences exist between fetal and mature hearts in terms of calcium

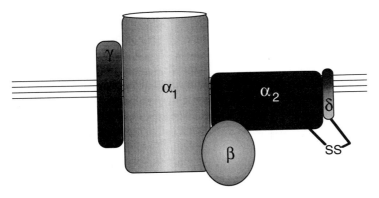

Figure 1   Subunit structure of the VDCC. The voltage-dependent calcium channel (VDCC) is comprised of five subunits, α_1 (which forms the channel pore), α_2, β, γ, and δ. The γ subunit is only expressed in skeletal muscle (see text for details).

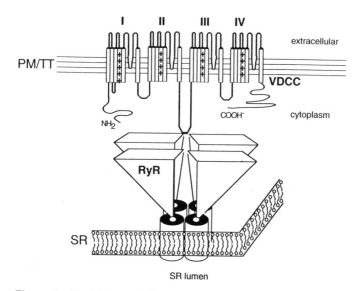

Figure 2 Model for excitation–contraction coupling. In cardiac and skeletal muscles the voltage-dependent calcium channel (VDCC) on the specialized region of the plasmamembrane known as the transverse tubule (PM/TT) serves either as a calcium influx channel (cardiac muscle) or as a voltage-sensor (skeletal muscle). In cardiac muscle, calcium influx via the VDCC activates the ryanodine receptor (RyR2), which then releases calcium from the sarcoplasmic reticulum (SR). This phenomenon is referred as calcium-induced calcium release. This release of calcium raises cytoplasmic calcium from 10^{-9} M to $\sim 10^{-7}$ M and activates muscle contraction. In skeletal muscle the intracellular loop between domains II and III of the skeletal muscle α_1 subunit of the VDCC is believed to interact physically with RyR1 to activate it. This interaction is though to be triggered by a voltage-dependent conformational change in the VDCC (see text for detailed discussion) mediated by charge movement involving the positively charged amino acid residues (denoted +) in the fourth transmembrane segment of each motif of the VDCC.

handling (1, 2, 11, 24, 27, 57). Newborn hearts require higher extracellular calcium to optimize contractility and a "deficiency" in sarcoplasmic reticulum development has been proposed (25, 32, 43, 53). Furthermore, it has been shown that the neonatal heart is highly sensitive to calcium channel blockers (44).

In addition to developmental regulation, VDCC expression is regulated during heart failure. Abnormal calcium homeostasis has been demonstrated in failing human myocardium (36). Our laboratory (6, 16, 48) and others (33) have demonstrated that mRNA levels of the SR calcium-ATPase and DHPR are decreased in end-stage human heart failure.

STRUCTURE OF VOLTAGE-DEPENDENT CALCIUM CHANNELS

The best-characterized VDCC is the L-type calcium channel from skeletal muscle, which is a complex comprised of five subunits: α_1, β, γ, α_2, and δ (9). The primary structure of each of these five subunits has been determined by cDNA cloning (26, 41, 52). The cDNA encoding the α_1 subunit of the cardiac DHPR has been isolated from rabbit (34) and encodes a polypeptide of 2171 amino acids that is 66% homologous to the skeletal muscle DHPR. The α_1 subunit has predicted sizes of 175 kDa in skeletal (52) and 210 kDa in cardiac muscle (34). About 10% of the skeletal α_1 subunits found in muscle tissue have a molecular weight (MW) of 212 kDa, which is thought to be a precursor of the smaller form that is a product of specific proteolysis (9). The α_2 subunit is a glycoprotein (143 kDa with glycosylation and 105 kDa without glycosylation) (9). The 20 kDa δ subunit is encoded by the same mRNA as the α_2 (12, 13). Four genes encoding β subunits have been identified, three with multiple splicing products. The MW of the β subunit is ~58 kDa (41). The 25 kDa γ subunit (20 kDa without glycosylation) contains three predicted N-glycosylation sites (26). Coimmunoprecipitation with specific antibodies against the subunits and cosedimentation on sucrose gradients has demonstrated the association of the five subunits forming the calcium channel complex (7). However, the α_1 subunit itself can form a functional calcium channel as demonstrated by expression in L-cells (39). The structure of the cardiac L-type calcium channel of the transverse tubule is similar to that of the skeletal muscle form with the exception that the γ subunit has not been detected in the cardiac muscle calcium channel complex. The proteins making up the VDCCs include transmembrane domains, calcium flux pores, and electrical sensing domains. The VDCCs also serve as pharmacological receptors, with specific sites for activator and antagonist ligands linked to channel function.

On the basis of distinct biophysical and pharmacological properties, VDCCs have been further classified into L type, T type, N type, and P type (21). The L-type VDCCs form a gene family that is related to other ion channels by virtue of highly conserved primary structures consisting of four internally repeated motifs comprising 24 putative transmembrane segments (Fig. 3). Each motif has six putative transmembrane segments. The fourth transmembrane segment in each motif contains positively charged amino acids, arginine or lysine, at every third or fourth residue. Mutational studies have demonstrated that these regions contribute to the voltage-sensor function of sodium (47) and potassium channels (38). By analogy, the S4 region has been called the voltage-sensor in calcium channels. The intracellular regions also contain putative protein kinase phosphorylation sties, suggesting the involvement of the channel in a regula-

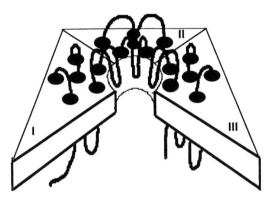

Figure 3 Model of proposed channel pore of the VDCC. An exploded view of the possible transmembrane topography of the VDCC allows visualization of the channel pore by removal of one-quarter of the channel (motif IV). The H5 domains, which are believed to dip into the membrane and form the pore of the channel, are shown lining the pore. The remaining six transmembrane segments are depicted as clustered around the pore. (Courtesy of Dr. Yong-sheng Ma.)

tory function. The VDCCs bind to dihydropyridines (DHP) with μM affinity and are specifically inhibited by DHP calcium-channel antagonists.

A common feature among membrane proteins is the presence of 16–30 amino acid residues on their N-terminals serving as signals for translocating to membranes that are characteristically hydrophobic and contain one or more positively charged amino acids. However, the NH_2-terminal region of the α_1 subunits of L-type calcium channels shows no hydrophobic segment when analyzed by the hydropathy plots. Thus, a leader signal sequence has not been identified.

DIVERSITY AMONG CALCIUM CHANNELS

Calcium channels are a diverse class of molecules found in all excitable cells. Although they share an overall structural similarity, multiple isoforms can be expressed within a single cell. Diversity within the calcium channel gene family is due in part to the expression of distinct α_1 subunit genes as well as to alternative splicing (31, 40). cDNA sequence comparison between the cardiac and smooth muscle α_1 subunits reveals that they are encoded by a single gene that is distinct from the gene encoding the skeletal muscle α_1 subunit (4, 40). In rat brain, at least four different calcium channels are expressed, each encoded by a distinct gene as demonstrated by Southern blot and DNA sequencing analysis (45). These molecules have been named class A, B, C, and D. The molecule of the class C type shares 90–97% identity with that found in cardiac muscle, rabbit lung, and rat aorta. Polymerase chain reaction and cDNA cloning studies have provided evidence that the diversity is derived from the alternate use of equally sized exons encoding the IVS3 transmembrane region (31, 40). Using genomic sequence analysis and S1 nuclease protection assays, two groups have demonstrated that the rat brain class C calcium channel variability arises from developmentally regulated, mutually exclusive splicing of a single primary transcript (14, 46). Human fibroblasts contain only the cardiac calcium channel subtype, which exhibits at least four sites of molecular diversity due to alternative splicing at the IIS6, IIIS2, IVS3, and C-terminal regions.

FUNCTIONAL PROPERTIES AND MODULATION OF THE L-TYPE CALCIUM CHANNEL

L-type calcium channels are activated by membrane depolarization and transduce electrical signals into chemical signals. Functional similarities among L-type calcium channels include slow, long-lasting currents and unitary conductance with mono- and divalent charge carriers; high affinity for DHPs and sensitivities to both inorganic and organic calcium channel blockers and a stereotypic response to organic calcium channel agonists; regulation by cyclic AMP-dependent events; slow inactivation when calcium is not the charge carrier; steady-state inactivation only at positive holding potentials; lability of channel function in a cell-free environment (21, 54); and that the L-type VDCC has a single channel conductance of ~ 20 pS.

Whole-cell clamping and inside-out excised patch recording are techniques well suited to studying channel modulation. These techniques monitor channel function under conditions in which the molecular composition of the cytoplasmic and extracellular solutions can be controlled. The best-established mechanism of calcium channel modulation is that of the L-type calcium channels mediated by cAMP-dependent kinase. Both intracellular and extracellular stimulation can alter the function of these channels and modulate them (21, 54). Calcium current is activated by cAMP; protein kinase A in a preactivated form that requires no cAMP; by activation of endogenous protein kinase C by the tumor-promoting phorbol ester tetradecanoylphorbolacetate (TPA); and intracellular injection of the purified enzyme. In addition, the activation of protein kinase C (30); internal GTP binding proteins, specifically G_s and its subunits (59, 60); and internal inositol trisphosphate (55) have also been postulated to modulate DHP-sensitive calcium channels. This modulation may involve phosphorylation of the channel itself as the last step of the signaling cascade. Calcineurin is a calcium-sensitive protein phosphatase that removes the phosphate from the activated channels and results in channel inactivation (10).

Divalent ions, including Ni^{2+}, Cd^{2+}, Co^{2+}, Mn^{2+}, and La^{3+}, can block calcium channels (22). Because these ions move so slowly in the pore they interfere with more permeant ions, which then must wait their turn. Many pharmacological agents can modulate the calcium channel properties and block or activate the channels. Because they are not particularly specific to calcium channels, high concentrations can depress Na^+ and K^+ channel currents as well (22).

MODEL OF CALCIUM CHANNEL STRUCTURE/FUNCTION RELATIONSHIPS

It is thought that the calcium channel pore (see Fig. 4) is formed by four trans-membrane domains, each of which contributes one-fourth of the pore wall by contributing one H5 (or SS1) domain (18). It has been postulated that ion selectivity is due to the structural differences of the ion-conducting pores. Therefore, mutation or replacement of amino acids in the putative pore has been used as a way to study its structure. Tsien and colleagues demonstrated that four asymmetrically disposed glutamic acid residues located in the pore (H5) of the L-type channel are involved in determining the enormous Ca selectivity exhibited by this channel (58).

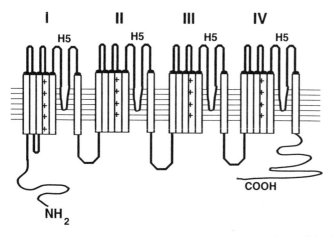

Figure 4 Model of proposed transmembrane topology of the VDCC. The twenty-four putative transmembrane segments of the α_1 subunit of the VDCC are shown with the H5 region that is thought to form the channel pore (see Fig. 3). The twenty-four transmembrane segments and four H5 regions are grouped in four repeating motifs (I–IV). Repeats I and III and II and IV are most homologous, suggesting that the channel structure evolved by gene duplication. The amino and carboxyl termini are intracellular. The four-transmembrane segment of each motif contains positively charged residues (denoted +) at every third position (arginines or lysines) and is believed to form the charge sensor of the channel.

Sensitivity and high affinity to DHP is a distinct characteristic that differentiates L-type calcium channels from other types of channels. The DHP-binding site has ben proposed to comprise a combination of the extracellular ends of the S6 helices of the third and fourth repeating domains as well as the loop linking S5 and S6 of the third domain, as determined using a photoaffinity labeling technique (37). Calcium channels can be viewed as a cylindrically symmetrical aggregate of multiple subunits (or of tandem-repeated homologous domains within a single polypeptide) with the ion conduction pore located on the axis of symmetry. The selectivity of calcium channels for calcium over more plentiful ions such as Na^+ or K^+ is determined by high-affinity binding of calcium within their pore. Four conserved glutamate residues in equivalent positions in the putative pore-lining regions of repeats I–IV in the calcium channel α_1 subunit have been identified as critical determinants of this selectivity (58). The model of calcium permeation based on these observations allows for binding of two calcium ions inside the pore in close proximity, within the sphere of influence of the four glutamates. The asymmetry of the four glutamates allows interactions with multiple calcium ions moving single-file within the pore.

The functional significance of each motif, and the putative cytoplasmic regions linking the repeats and the amino and carboxyl-terminal regions have also been studied. Repeat I of the DHPR is critical in determining calcium channel activation kinetics (51). The current produced with the chimeric constructs carrying the cardiac repeat I resembles the current produced by the native cardiac muscle DHPR. The current produced with the chimeric constructs carrying the skeletal repeat I resembles the current produced by the native skeletal muscle DHPR. The region of the skeletal muscle DHPR required for excitation–contraction coupling has been localized to the cytoplasmic loop between repeats II and III (49, 50). The chimeric construct containing skeletal II–III cytoplasmic loop expressed in dysgenic myotubes shows skeletal-type E-C coupling while the loop of I-II is more functionally interchangeable between the cardiac and skeletal muscle DHPR. Single amino-acid substitutions in the regions encompassing the short segment SS2 of the third and/or fourth repeats of sodium channel (such as replacing lysine at position 1422 in repeat III and/ or alanine at position 1714 in repeat IV of rat sodium channel II with the glutamic acid) can alter the ion-selectivity of the sodium channel to resemble those of calcium channels, suggesting that these residues constitute part of the selectivity filter of the channel (20).

Coexpression of the cardiac α_1 with the α_2 and β subunits in *Xenopus* oocytes accelerated the activation and inactivation of the channel and shifted the voltage dependence of inactivation to more negative membrane potentials (34). Coexpression of the cardiac α_1 subunit with the β_{1a} in *Xenopus* oocytes accelerated activation, increased peak current, and shifted the voltage dependence of activation to more negative membrane potentials (56). Using chimeras from channels with different inactivation rates. Tsien and colleagues showed that the amino acids responsible for kinetic differences are localized to membrane-spanning segment S6 of the first repeat of the α_1 subunit (IS6), and to putative extracellular and cytoplasmic domains flanking IS6 (61).

Further elucidation of the structure–function relationships will progress slowly until the three-dimensional structure at atomic resolution is achieved.

ACKNOWLEDGMENTS

This work was supported by the National Institutes of Health (RO1-NS29814). ARM is a Briston-Meyers/Squibb Established Investigator of the American Heart Association.

REFERENCES

1. Artman M. Development changes in myocardial contractile responses to inotropic agents. Cardiovasc Res 1992; 26:1–12.
2. Artman M, Graham T, Boucek R. Effects of postnatal maturation on myocardial contractile responses to calcium antagonists and changes in contraction frequency. J Cardiovasc Pharmacol 1985; 7:850–855.
3. Bers DM. Excitation–Contraction Coupling and Cardiac Contractile Force. Boston: Kluwer Academic Publishers, 1991.
4. Biel M, Ruth P, Bosse E, Hullin R, Stuhmer W, Flockerzi V, Hofman F. Primary structure and functional expression of a high voltage activated calcium channel from rabbit lung. FEBS 1990; 269:409–412.
5. Brillantes A-MB, Brezprozvannaya S, Marks A. Developmental and tissue-specific regulation of expression of the cardiac and skeletal muscle calcium channels involved in excitation-contraction coupling. Circ Res 1994; 75:503–510.
6. Brilliantes A, Allen P, Takahashi T, Izumo S, Marks A. Differences in cardiac calcium release channel (ryanodine receptor) expression in myocardium from patients with end-stage heart failure caused by ischemic versus dilated cardiomyopathy. Circ Res 1992; 71:18–26.
7. Catterall WA. Structure and function of voltage-sensitive ion channels. Science 1988; 242:50–61.
8. Catterall WA. Excitation-contraction coupling in vertebrate skeletal muscle: a tale of two calcium channels. Cell 1991; 64:871–874.
9. Catterall WA. Structure and function of voltage-gated ion channels. Annu Rev Biochem 1995; 64:493–531.
10. Chad JE, Eckert R. An enzymatic mechanism for calcium current inactivation in dialysed Helix neurones. J Physiol 1986; 378:31–51.
11. Chin T, Friedman W, Klitzner T. Developmental changes in cardiac myocyte calcium regulation. Circ Res 1990; 67:574–579.
12. De Jongh KS, Merrick DK, Catterall WA. Subunits of purified calcium channels:

a 212-kDa form of α1 and partial amino acid sequence of a phosphorylation site of an independent β subunit. Proc Natl Acad Sci 1389; 86:8585–8589.

13. DeJongh KS, Warner C, Catterall WA. Subunits of purified calcium channels. J Biol Chem 1990; 265:14738–14741.

14. Diebold R, Koch W, Ellinor P, Wang J, Muthuchamy M, Wieczorek D, Schwartz A. Mutually exclusive exon splicing of the cardiac calcium channel α₁ subunit gene generates developmentally regulated isoforms in the rat heart. Proc Natl Acad Sci 1992; 89:1497–1501.

15. Fabiato A, Fabiato F. Calcium and cardiac excitation-contraction coupling. Annu Rev Physiol. 1984; 41:743.

16. Go L, Moschella M, Fyfe B, Marks A. Differential regulation of calcium release channels in human heart failure. Clin Res 1994; 42(2):166A.

17. Grynkiewicz G, Poenie M, Tsien R. A new generation of calcium indicators with greatly improved fluorescence properties. J Biol Chem 1985; 260:3440–3450.

18. Guy HR, Seetharamulu P. Molecular model of the action potential sodium channel. Proc Natl Acad Sci 1986; 83:508–512.

19. Hamill OP, Marty A, Neher E, Sakmann B, Siqworth FJ. Improved patch-clamp techniques for high-resolution current recording from cells and cell-free membrane patches. Pflugers Arch 1981; 391:85–100.

20. Heinemann S, Terlau H, Stuhmer W, Imoto K, Numa S. Calcium channel characteristics conferred on the sodium channel by single mutations. Nature 1992; 356:441–443.

21. Hess P. Calcium channels in vertebrate cells. Annu Rev Neurosci 1990; 13:337–356.

22. Hille B. Ionic Channels of Excitable Membranes. Sunderland, MA: Sinauer Associates, 1992.

23. Hui A, Ellinor PT, Krizanova O, Wang J-J, Diebold RJ, Schwartz A. Molecular cloning of multiple subtypes of a novel rat brain isoform of the α₁ subunit of the voltage-dependent calcium channel. Neuron 1991; 7:35–44.

24. Huynh T, Chen F, Wetzel G, Friedman W, Klitzner T. Developmental changes in membrane Ca2+ and K+ currents in fetal, neonatal, and adult rabbit ventricular myocytes. Circ Res 1992; 508–515.

25. Jarmakani J, Nakanishi T, George B, Bers D. Effect of extracellular calcium on myocardial mechanical function in the neonatal rabbit. Dev Pharmacol Ther 1982; 5:1–13.

26. Jay SD, Ellis SB, McCue AF, Williams ME, Vedvick TS, Harpold MM, Campbell KP. Primary structure of the gamma subunit of the DHP-sensitive calcium channel from skeletal muscle. Science 1990; 248:490–492.

27. Klitzner T, Friedman W. Excitation-contraction coupling in developing mammalian myocardium: evidence from voltage clamp studies. Pediatr Res 1988; 23:428–432.

28. Koch WJ, Hiu A, Shull GE, Ellinor P, Schwartz A. Characterization of cDNA clones encoding two putative isoforms of the α₁ subunit of the dihydropyridine-sensitive voltage-dependent calcium channel isolated from rat brain and rat aorta. FEBS 1989; 250:386–388.

29. Koch WJ, Ellinor PT, Schwartz A. cDNA Cloning of a dihydropyridine-sensitive calcium channel from rat aorta. J Biol Chem 1990; 265:17786–17791.
30. Lacerda AE, Rampe D, Brown AM. Effects of protein kinase C activators on cardiac calcium channels. Nature 1988; 335:249–251.
31. Ma YS, Kobrinsky E, Marks A. Cloning and expression of a novel truncated calcium channel from non-excitable cells. J Biol Chem 1995; 270:483–493.
32. Mahony L, Jones L. Developmental changes in cardiac sarcoplasmic reticulum in sheep. J Biol Chem 1986; 261:15257–15265.
33. Mercardier J, Lompre A, Duc P, Boheler K, Fraysse J, Wisnewsky C, Allen P, Komajda M, Schwartz K. Altered sarcoplasmic reticulum Ca2+-ATPase gene expression in the human ventricle during end-stage heart failure. J Clin Invest 1990; 85:305–309.
34. Mikami A, Imoto K, Tanabe T, Niidome T, Mori Y, Takeshima H, Narumiya S, Numa S. Primary structure and functional expression of the cardiac dihydropyridine-sensitive calcium channel. Nature 1989; 340:230–233.
35. Minta A, Kao J, Tsien R. Fluorescent indicators for cytosolic calcium based on rhodamine and fluorescein chromophores. J Biol Chem. 1989; 264:8171–8178.
36. Morgan J, Erny R, Allen P, Grossman W, Gwathmey J. Abnormal intracellular calcium handling: a major cause of systolic and diastolic dysfunction in ventricular myocardium from patients with end-stage heart failure. Circulation 1990; 81(suppl III):III21–III32.
37. Nakayama H, Taki M, Striessnig J, Glossman H, Catterall W, Kanaoka Y. Identification of 1,4-dihydropyridine binding regions within the α_1 subunit of skeletal muscle Ca^{2+} channels by photoaffinity labeling with diazipine. Proc Natl Acad Sci 1991; 88:9203–9207.
38. Papazian DM, Timpe LC, Jan YN, Jan YJ. Alteration of voltage-dependence of Shaker potassium channel by mutations in the S4 sequence. Nature 1991; 349:305–310.
39. Perez-Reyes E, Kim H, Lacerda A, Horne W, Wei X, Rampe D, Campbell K, Brown A, Birnbaumer L. Induction of calcium currents by the expression of the alpha1-subunit of the dihydropyridine receptor from skeletal muscle. Nature 1989; 340:233–236.
40. Perez-Reyes E, Wei X, Castellano A, Birnbaumer L. Molecular Diversity of L-type calcium channels. J Biol Chem 1990; 265:20430–20436.
41. Ruth P, Rohrkasten A, Biel M, Bosse E, Regulla S, Meyer H, Flockerzi V, Hofman F. Primary structure of the B subunit of the DHP-sensitive calcium channel from skeletal muscle. Science 1989; 245:1115–1118.
42. Sakmann B, Neher E. Patch clamp techniques for studying ionic channels in excitable membranes. Annu Rev Physiol 1984; 46:455–472.
43. Seguchi M, Harding J, Jarmakani J. Developmental change in the function of sarcoplasmic reticulum. J Mol Cell Cardiol 1986; 18:189–195.
44. Seguchi M, Jarmakani J, George B, Harding J. Effect of Ca2+ antagonists on mechanical function in the neonatal heart. Pediatr Res 1986; 20:838–842.
45. Snutch TP, Leonard JP, Gilbert MM, Lester A, Davidson N. Rat brain expresses a heterogeneous family of calcium channels. Proc Natl Acad Sci Usa 1990; 87:3391–3395.

46. Snutch TP, Tomlinson WJ, Leonard JP, Gilbert MM. Distinct calcium channels are generated by alternative splicing and are differentially expressed in the mammalian CNS. Neuron 1991; 7:45-57.

47. Stuhmer W, Conti F, Suzuki H, Wang X, Noda M, Yahagi N, Kubo H, Numa S. Structural parts involved in activation and inactivation of the sodium channel. Nature 1989; 339:597-603.

48. Takahashi T, Allen PD, Lacro RV, Marks AR, Dennis AR, Schoen FJ, Grossman W, Marsh JD, Izumo S. Expression of dihydropyridine receptor (Ca2+ channel) and calsequestrin genes in the myocardium of patients with end-stage heart failure. J Clin Invest 1992; 90:927-935.

49. Tanabe T, Mikami A, Numa S, Beam KG. Cardiac-type excitation-contraction coupling in dysgenic skeletal muscle injected with cardiac dihydropyridine receptor cDNA. Nature 1990; 344:451-453.

50. Tanabe T, Beam KG, Adams BA, Niidome T, Numa S. Regions of the skeletal muscle dihydropyridine receptor critical for excitation-contraction coupling. Nature 1990; 346:567-569.

51. Tanabe T, Adams BA, Numa S, Beam KG. Repeat I of the dihydropyridine receptor is critical in determining calcium channel activation kinetics. Nature 1991; 352:800-803.

52. Tanabe T, Takeshima H, Mikami A, Flockerzi V, Takahashi H, Kangawa K, Kojima M, Matsuo H, Hirose T, Numa S. Primary structure of the receptor for calcium channel blockers from skeletal muscle. Nature 1987; 328:313-328.

53. Tanaka H, Shigenobu K. Effect of ryanodine on neonatal and adult rat heart: developmental increase in sarcoplasmic reticulum function. J Mol Cell Cardiol 1989; 21:1305-1313.

54. Tsien RW, Hess P, McCleskey E, Rosenberg R. Calcium channels: mechanisms of selectivity, permeation, and block. Annu Rev Biophys Chem 1987; 16:265-90.

55. Vilven J, Coronado R. Opening of dihydropyridine calcium channels in skeletal muscle membranes by inositol trisphosphate. Nature 1988; 336:587-589.

56. Wei X, Perez-Reyes E, Lacerda A, Schuster G, Brown A, Birnbaumer L. Heterologous regulation of the cardiac Ca2+ channel $\alpha 1$ subunit by skeletal muscle β and γ subunits. J Biol Chem 1991; 266:21943-21947.

57. Wetzel G, Chen F, Klitzer T. L- and T- type calcium channels in acutely isolated neonatal and adult cardiac myocytes. Pediatr Res 1991; 30:89-94.

58. Yang J, Ellinor PT, Sather WA, Zhang JF, and Tsien RW. Molecular determinants of Ca2+ selectivity and ion permeation in L-type Ca2+ channels. Nature 1993; 366:158-161.

59. Yatani A, Codina J, Imoto Y, Reeves J, Nirnbaumer L, Brown AM. A G protein directly regulates mammalian cardiac calcium channels. Science 1987; 238:1288-1292.

60. Yatani A, Imoto Y, Codina J, Hamilton SL, Brown AM, Birnbaumer L. The stimulatory G protein of adenylyl cyclase, Gs, also stimulates dihydroyridine sensitive Ca channels. J Biol Chem 1988; 263:9887-9895.

61. Zhang JF, Ellinor PT, Aldrich RW, Tsien RW. Molecular determinants of voltage-dependent inactivation in calcium channels. Nature 1994; 372:97-100.

12

Structure and Function of Calcium Release Channels

Andrew R. Marks
Mount Sinai School of Medicine
New York, New York

Intracellular calcium release channels form a unique family of ion channels that are differentiated from all others by their enormous size. These channels, located on the endoplasmic or sarcoplasmic reticuli of all types of cells, are among the largest proteins identified to date. The ryanodine receptor (RyR) is a tetramer with a molecular mass of ~ 2.3 million daltons and the inositol 1,4,5-trisphosphate receptor (IP3R, also a tetramer) has a molecular mass of ~ 1.2 million daltons. In contrast, the major subunit of the voltage-dependent calcium channels on the plasma membrane has a mass of $\sim 200,000$ daltons, and the entire five subunit structure is $\sim 400,000$ daltons. Elucidating the molecular structure of the calcium release channels (CRC) has provided substantial advances in our understanding of the mechanisms underlying excitation–contraction (EC) coupling in the heart.

Cloning studies have revealed that the calcium release channels of the sarcoplasmic and endoplasmic reticuli form a distinct gene family. This distinct gene family currently includes the two major channel types, RYR and IP3R. Each of these major channel types in turn is represented by three forms (Fig. 1).

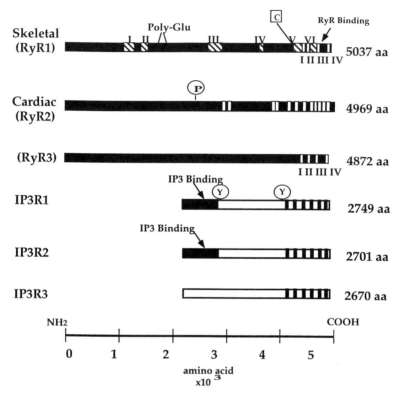

Figure 1   Calcium release channel structures. This representation of the topography of calcium release channels is based on the deduced amino acid sequence from cDNA cloning and protease sensitivity mapping of surface exposed regions. The skeletal RyR (8, 65, 97, 108), cardiac RyR (80, 83), and brain RyR (38) are approximately 66% identical at the amino acid level. Six regions of protease sensitivity have been identified in the skeletal RyR1 (cross-hatched boxes I–VI) (63). Four of these six regions are highly conserved between the skeletal and cardiac RyR1s, two of these regions (aa 1270-1431 and 4249-4626) are divergent and may represent sequences that are responsible for functional differences observed between the cardiac and skeletal muscle RyRs. The ryanodine binding site has been identified near the amino terminus (9). Three forms of IP3R have likewise been identified, type 1 (75), type 2 (95), and type 3 (5, 62). The IP3-binding site has been localized to the amino terminus in the types 1 (73) and 2 IP3R (95). Two putative tyrosine phosphorylation sites (Y) have been identified in the type 1 IP3R (40) and it has been shown that the channel is activated by tyrosine phosphorylation by nonreceptor protein tyrosine kinases in vitro and in vivo (50).

Additional structural complexity is achieved by the presence of alternative splicing. In the case of IP3R, alternative splicing generates specific neuronal and nonneuronal forms (18, 32).

The unifying characteristic of the CRCs is the fourfold symmetrical structure in each case of four subunits. Recent evidence suggests that, at least in the case of the IP3R, heterotetramers can be made from a mixture of two or three distinct IP3R subunits (74, 106). Another structural similarity is the clustering of the putative transmembrane segments near the carboxy terminus of each CRC (Fig. 1). Putative transmembrane segments are encoded by approximately 10% of the sequence, while the remainder of the sequence encodes large cytoplasmic structures that presumably participate in regulating channel function and interactions with other proteins. Functional expression of RyR has demonstrated that important modulatory binding sites are encoded by the 16 kb RyR mRNA and that a second protein, FKBP12, is required for optimal channel gating (8).

RYANODINE RECEPTORS

Intracellular calcium release channels are required for a wide variety of cellular signaling pathways including EC coupling, oocyte fertilization, hormone secretion, neurotransmitter release, and T-lymphocyte activation. Among these pathways EC coupling is one of the best characterized. Depolarization of the sarcolemma in striated muscle is coupled to the release of intracellular calcium from the SR. In cardiac muscle, the RyR is activated during EC coupling by calcium influx via the voltage-dependent calcium channel or dihydropyridine receptor (DHPR), a phenomenon referred to as calcium-induced calcium release (CICR) (21, 22, 25). The voltage dependence of an intramembrane charge movement postulated to be related to activation of skeletal muscle contraction was reported more than 20 years ago (89). A role for the voltage-dependent calcium channel or DHPR as a voltage sensor in skeletal muscle EC coupling was proposed (33, 86, 87). However, in the heart, the DHPR serves as a true calcium channel that is voltage activated, not simply as a voltage sensor. A physical relationship between the DHPR and RyR that could fit the model of direct interaction between the two types of calcium channels during EC coupling has been observed using electron microscopy (4). The DHPR and RyR are "coupled" across the intracellular junction between the transverse tubule and the terminal cisternae of the SR (triad junction). A region in the cytoplasmic loop of the DHPR located between domains II and III has been identified as that interacting with the RyR during EC coupling, resulting in activation of SR calcium release (61, 100). The space between these two membranes is joined by foot structures (30) that have been identified as the RyR and shown to be the calcium release channel of the SR (44, 47, 48, 57, 92).

STRUCTURE

RyRs have been purified from skeletal and cardiac muscle (47, 48, 57, 92) and single-channel measurements have determined the biophysical properties of the native calcium release channel (3, 16, 44, 45, 91). The essential role of the RyR in EC coupling has been well established (10, 29). The primary structures of RyRs from skeletal (65, 97, 108) and cardiac muscle (80, 83) and from brain (38) have been deduced from cDNA cloning (they have been designated RyR1, 2 and 3 respectively, Fig. 1). They are each tetramers comprised of four approximately 565,000 MW RyR subunits. The skeletal, cardiac, and brain forms share ~66% sequence homology. Significant divergence between the sequences of the cardiac and skeletal muscle forms, particularly in the region comprised of amino acids 1872–1923 corresponding to an area with high surface probability (63). A 2.4 kb transcript of the skeletal muscle RyR1 expressed in rabbit brain (98) is not detected in other closely related species.

The RyR is the major intracellular calcium release channel in striated muscle, it is also expressed at lower levels in a wide variety of cell types including brain (67), smooth muscle (42), and endothelial cells (58). The approximate 40% homology between the RyRs and IP3R1 in some of the putative transmembrane regions is sufficient to suggest that these two channels evolved from a common ancestral cation release channel. Recombinant RyR1 and RyR2 have been expressed in CHO cells and in *Xenopus* oocytes (80, 84). These studies have demonstrated that each of the these RyR cDNAs encodes the subunit of the calcium release channel in cardiac and skeletal muscle. More recently, single-channel recordings of the cloned skeletal RyR1 expressed in COS-1 cells have been reported; however, multiple conductances were observed from these cloned expressed channels including some channels with conductances >1 nS, which are not seen with native ryanodine receptors (13). Our group expressed the skeletal muscle RyR1 in *Xenopus* oocytes and in insect cells, showing that these recombinant channels behave like the native ryanodine receptor in terms of activation and inhibition by channel modulators, conductance, and cation selectivity (8, 55).

Important reagents have been characterized and used to probe calcium release channel function including antibodies (12, 28); ryanodine (14, 41, 68); and scorpion toxins (103). Divergences in the structure of the RyR1 and RyR2 are paralleled by subtle functional differences. The conductance for skeletal RyR1 (with 50 mM Ca as the charge carrier) is 120 ps, whereas that of cardiac RyR2 is 100 ps (20). Moreover, RyR2 is more sensitive to calcium than RyR1 (69). Using antibodies specific for regions near the carboxy terminus of the RyR1, MacLennan and colleagues have identified potential calcium-binding sites near the carboxy terminus (12) in regions that had previously been predicted to be surface exposed on the basis of proteolysis sensitivity. RyR3 has been reported to be most abundant in the muscles of the diaphragm (15) and its functional properties are distinct from those of RyR1 and RyR2 in that it exhibits approximately 10 times lower sensitivity to calcium compared to RyR-1 (99).

TOPOGRAPHY

Several models have been proposed for the surface topography of the RyR1 based on hydropathy analyses of the deduced amino acid sequences of the RyRs obtained by cDNA cloning. Numa originally identified four transmembrane segments located near the carboxy terminus (97), whereas MacLennan proposed that there may be as many as 10-12 transmembrane segments (108). Understanding the surface topography of the RyR1 provides the basis for designing strategies to dissect structure–function relationships. For example, one must know which regions are likely to be cytoplasmic and which are likely to be found within the SR in order to identify candidate modulator binding sites. The surface topography of the skeletal muscle RyR1 has been examined using protease sensitivity mapping (63) and the transmembrane topology has been studied with site-specific antibodies (37). The intact foot structure (a tetramer of four ryanodine receptor subunits) was digested with proteases and the resultant peptides were sequenced yielding thirty cleavage sites identified by microsequencing HPLC-purified peptides corresponding to six protease-sensitive regions that may represent surface-exposed regions of the molecule (Fig. 1). Several regions with high surface probability but protease resistance are candidates for sequences lining the calcium efflux pore(s) of the channel, and for regions of protein–protein interaction during formation of the foot structure. One of these regions, located between amino acids 1873 and 1890, contains 17 consecutive glutamic acid residues and is not found in the cardiac RyR2. The polyglutamic acid region could serve as a selectivity filter analogous to the ring of negative charges found in the mouth of the acetylcholine receptor (46).

Four site-directed antibodies that recognized epitopes near the carboxy terminus were used to analyze whether loops between putative transmembrane segments were luminal (inside the SR) or cytoplasmic (37).

Two recent studies have identified the high- and low-affinity ryanodine binding sites using different approaches. In collaboration with Dr. Susan Hamilton's group at Baylor we showed that the high- and low-affinity ryanodine binding sites were localized to a peptide fragment near the carboxy terminus of RyR1 that was recognized by a site-specific anti-RyR1 antibody directed against an epitope at amino acid 5029 (9, 49). A similar localization was achieved by Dr. Kevin Campbell's group by photoaffinity labeling RyR1 with an azido derivative of ryanodine (105).

FUNCTIONAL EXPRESSION OF RYANODINE RECEPTORS

In vitro transcribed RyR mRNA has been injected into *Xenopus* oocytes and RyR1 and RyR2 expression determined by recording the native Ca-activated Cl⁻ current of *Xenopus* oocytes using voltage clamp techniques (8, 80). This indicates that a caffeine-sensitive intracellular calcium release channel was expressed in oocytes injected with RyR mRNA. To obtain cloned RyR1 suitable for reconstitution in lipid bilayers, we infected insect cells with recombinant Baculovirus containing the RyR1 cDNA. We studied purified cloned expressed RyR to eliminate the effects of contaminating proteins that modify calcium release channel function (8). Recombinant RyR1 was purified from insect (Sf9) cells on a sucrose gradient using [^{3}H]ryanodine to monitor the degree of purification. After reconstitution into planar lipid bilayers, recombinant RyR1 formed a channel with properties similar to those of the native RyR (Fig. 2). This channel exhibited a conductance of 540 ± 49 ps (with Cs 250:50 mM as the charge carrier) and was modulated to the characteristic 1/2 conductance state by ryanodine (8). Recombinant RyR1 expressed in Sf9 cells formed a channel that was Ca-sensitive (activated by 100 mM Ca) and was activated by 1 mM ATP, and inhibited by 20 mM ruthenium red and by 1 mM $MgCl_2$ (8).

FKBP12 OPTIMIZES THE FUNCTION OF THE RYANODINE RECEPTOR/CALCIUM RELEASE CHANNEL

The Ca release channel/RyR1 consists of four 565 kDa protomers. A 12 kDa protein is tightly associated with highly purified RyR1 from rabbit skeletal muscle SR (49). A novel form of FKBP, FKBP12.6, is physically associated with the cardiac RyR2 (101), and modifies its function in a manner similar to the role of FKBP12 as a modifier of RyR1 function (52). The 12 kDa protein from skeletal muscle is the binding protein for the immunosupressant drug FK506 (FKBP12), an immumophillin originally identified by its ability to bind to the structurally related immunosuppressant drugs FK506 and rapamycin (90). FKBP12 is expressed at high levels in all types of muscle (49) and has the

---

Figure 2 Single-channel recordings from recombinant RyR1 expressed in insect cells. First tracing: Cloned expressed RyR1, isolated by sucrose gradient density purification, was incorporated into liposomes and fused to planar lipid bilayers. Second tracing: Channels with high cesium conductances were observed after activation with caffeine (5 mM). Third tracing: Expressed RyR1 was modulate by ryanodine (0.5 µM). Bottom graph: The slope conductance 540 ± 48 ps for the expressed channel. The reversal potential calculated for Cs was 32 mV ($P_{Cs}:P_{Cl} = 11.1$). In all cases dashed lines on the left of each tracing represent the closed state, channel openings are downward. (From Ref. 7.)

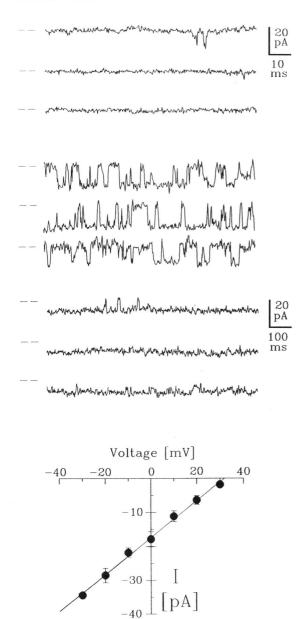

properties of a *cis-trans* peptidyl-prolyl isomerase. FK506 binds to FKBP12 and blocks calcium-dependent T-cell activation by inhibiting the phosphatase calcineurin and preventing translocation of the transcription factor NFAT to the nucleus (59). The molar ratio of FKBP to RyR1 is approximately 1:1 (102), indicating that one FKBP molecule is associated with each subunit of the calcium release channel/RyR.

FKBP12 optimizes RyR1 channel behavior (Fig. 3), an effect that can be reversed by adding FK506 or rapamycin, both of which inhibit the isomerase activity of FKBP12 (8). These results provided a cellular function for FKBP12, and established that the functional calcium release channel is a complex comprised of RyR and FKBP12. Since rapamycin and FK506, both of which inhibit the isomerase activity of FKBP12, reverse the channel optimizing effects of FKBP12 (Fig. 4), conserved prolines may be important in regulating channel function. Prolines were shown to be critical for voltage gating in gap junctions (94).

We have coined the term channel accessory protein (CAP) to explain the natural cellular function of FKBP12 (8). A hypothetical model depicting the role of FKBP12 in enhancing cooperativity between the four subunits of the ryanodine receptor is proposed (Fig. 5).

INOSITOL 1,4,5-TRISPHOSPHATE RECEPTORS

The major intracellular calcium release channel in most types of cells (with the exception of cardiac and skeletal muscle) is the IP3R located on the endoplasmic reticulum (ER). The second messenger inositol 1,4,5-trisphosphate (IP3) functions as a major regulator of intracellular calcium levels involved in diverse signaling pathways (2). The phosphoinositol pathway is activated by G-protein coupled or nonreceptor protein tyrosine kinase activation of cell surface receptors. For example angiotensin II (Ang II) mediates a rise in vascular smooth muscle intracellular calcium by activating the IP3R pathway. Upon binding to its cell surface receptor, Ang II activates the phosphoinositol pathway via phospholipase C, which converts phosphoinositides to diacylclycerol and IP3. DAG in turn activates protein kinase C pathways. IP3 binds to its receptor on the ER resulting in release of intracellular Ca. In T cells, activation of the T-cell receptor in turns activates members of the Src kinase family of nonreceptor protein tyrosine kinases including Fyn, which activates phospholipase γ_1, leading to the generation of IP3 and which activates the IP3R to release intracellular stores of calcium (40, 51). Recent data show that the IP3R is also directly tyrosine phosphorylated by Fyn during T-cell activation (50). Tyrosine phosphorylation of the IP3R increases the open probability of the channel. Thus, there is cross talk between the tyrosine kinase pathway and the IP3 pathway that results in modulation of cytoplasmic calcium concentrations (50).

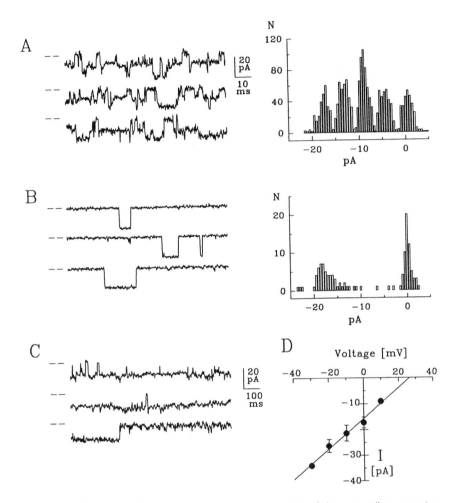

Figure 3 Effect of FKBP12 on subconductance states of the ryanodine receptor and FK506 reverses this stabilizing effect. A. Recombinant RyR1 expressed in insect cells and reconstituted in planar lipid bilayers exhibits multiple conductances including the fully open state (4 pA), and the subconductance states: 1/2 open (2 pA) and 1/4 open (1 pA). B. Recordings of the cloned expressed RyR plus FKBP12 are shown. The histogram on the right demonstrates two populations of channels closed (0 pA) and fully open (4 pA). This experiment demonstrates the stabilizing effect of FKBP12 on the RyR, which may be due to the prolyl isomerase activity of the enzyme. The channels shown in this figure were all recorded from a single experiment. The zero current is shown by the line on the left of each pair of tracings and channel openings are in the downward direction. The channels were recorded at 0 mV. The *trans* chamber contained 53 mM Ca, 250 mM Hepes, pH 7.35; the *cis* chamber contained 250 mM Hepes/Tris at pH 7.35. (From Ref. 8.)

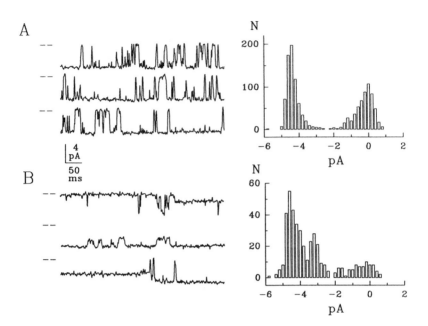

Figure 4 FK506 added to the RyR1-calcium release channel reverses the stabilizing effect of FKBP12. A. Recordings of the native RyR1 that copurifies with FKBP12 (with calcium as the charge carrier). The histogram on the right demonstrates two populations of channels closed (0 pA) and fully open (4 pA). B. Thirty minutes after addition of 12 μM FK506 (which inhibits the isomerase activity of FKBP12 and dissociates FKBP12 from the channel) multiple conductances are observed including the fully open state (4 pA), and the subconductance states: 1/2 open (2 pA) and 1/4 open (1 pA). The channels shown in this figure were all recorded from a single experiment. The zero current is shown by the line on the left of each pair of tracings and channel openings are in the downward direction. (From Ref. 8.)

Three forms of IP3R have been identified (Fig. 1). The type 1 IP3R has been isolated from brain (cerebellum), vas deferens, and aortic smooth muscle (11, 27, 77, 88). IP3R purified from bovine aortic smooth muscle has a MW of approximately 240 kDa, based on polyacrylamide gel electrophoresis (11) and a MW of 313 kDa based on cDNA cloning (31). The purified smooth muscle IP3R reconstituted in lipid vesicles displayed characteristics of the native intracellular Ca release channel on the ER (27, 66). IP3Rs have been identified as functional intracellular Ca release channels (3, 27, 66). IP3R1 has been cloned from rodent (31, 72), *Xenopus laevis* oocytes (56), and human T cells (40). A second IP3R cloned from rat cerebellum (IP3R type 2) shares 69% identity with the amino acid sequence of the type 1 IP3R (95, 107). A third

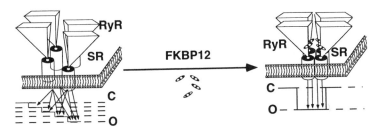

Figure 5   The Ca release channel may be formed by four pores through the membrane. Cooperativity between the four subunits, enhanced by FKBP12, would permit full conductance. Subconductance states would be generated when less than four channels are open.

(IP3R type 3) shares 64% identity with the amino acid sequence of the type 1 IP3R (5, 62).

A model for the transmembrane topography of the channel is based on primary sequence data obtained from the cloning of the cDNA encoding the IP3R from brain and smooth muscle (71). Most hydrophobic sequences are clustered in the carboxy terminal 25% of the linear sequence, reminiscent of the skeletal and cardiac muscle RyRs (Fig. 1). The remaining sequence encodes the large cytoplasmic portion of the receptor, analogous to the "foot structure" of the triad and dyad junctions in skeletal and cardiac muscle. The ligand binding region of the brain form of the receptor near the amino terminus has been identified using detelion mutants of the cloned expressed receptor (73).

Three domains have been identified for the IP3Rs: a ligand binding domain at the amino terminal end, a coupling domain linking IP3 binding to Ca release channel activation, and a carboxy-terminal channel region (72). Alternative splicing (73, 79) defining neuronal and non-neuronal forms of IP3R has been shown (18).

IP3R IN THE HEART

IP3 signaling pathway is the primary mechanism governing intracellular Ca release in most types of cells. In contrast, in the heart the major pathway for intracellular Ca release requires the RyR. Hormonal regulation of cardiac contractility may be mediated by IP3-induced intracellular Ca release. However, the significance of IP3-induced intracellular Ca release in the heart has been hotly debated. A role for IP3-mediated pathways in E-C coupling has been proposed based on studies suggesting IP3-induced Ca release and contraction in cardiac muscle (23-25). IP3-induced Ca release from cardiac SR has been observed in skinned ventricular fibers from rat (53) and cardiac SR vesicles (43). IP3 has also been shown to potentiate the effects of caffeine-induced Ca release in skinned guinea pig papillary muscle (81). IP3-induced intracellular Ca release has been reported with high concentrations of α-adrenergic agonists in rat left ventricular muscle (82, 85). In contrast, it has also been reported that IP3 has no effect on isolated cardiac SR or in permeabilized myocytes (78). The rate and degree of IP3-induced Ca release in the heart has been significantly lower than that observed for Ca-induced Ca release. Endothelin, a potent inducer of contraction in the heart, may activate IP32 cardiac myocytes (60).

The type 1 IP3R mRNA and protein are expressed in cardiac myocytes (76). On the basis of immunoreactivity with a sequence-specific anti-IP3R antibody and RNAse protection using a smooth muscle IP3R cRNA probe, the IP3R expressed in cardiac myocytes is structurally most similar to the type I IP3R expressed in vascular smooth muscle, the cerebellum, and in human T cells (31, 40, 64. 72). Northern blot and RNAse protection analyses of total heart RNA demonstrated a signal corresponding to IP3R mRNA (64, 79), and IP3 binding to a component of the canine cardiac SR has been reported (54). IP3R is expressed in cardiac myocytes and could be involved in physiological modulation of cardiac contractility in response to pharmacological agents and hormones. IP3R could mediate diastolic tone and/or hypertrophy signaling pathways in the heart, perhaps by regulating Ca-responsive genes. The levels of IP3R mRNA in the heart are lower ($\sim$ 50-fold) than that encoding the cardiac RyR, suggesting that the amount of IP3R in the heart is significantly less than that of the RyR (76). Increased expression in the Purkinje fibers has been reported (36).

REGULATION OF CALCIUM RELEASE CHANNEL EXPRESSION IN HUMAN HEART FAILURE

The molecular bases for systolic and diastolic dysfunction remain poorly understood. Both abnormal calcium handling and defects in the contractile apparatus may contribute to the myocardial dysfunction. Cardiac RyR2 mRNA and protein levels (assessed by [^{3}H]ryanodine binding) were significantly decreased in end-stage failing human hearts while the expression of a second form of intracellular calcium release channel, the IP3R (see below), was increased (6, 34). RyR2 mRNA levels in the left ventricle were decreased by 29% in patients with ischemic cardiomyopathy (ICM, $p < .05$) and were reduced by 32% in patients with idiopathic dilated cardiomyopathy (IDCM, $p < .05$) (34). Cardiac RyR2 mRNA levels were reduced in myopathic septum by 36–39% ($p < .05$), regardless of whether the tissue was obtained from ICM or IDCM patients (34). We had previously demonstrated that the heart contains at least two types of CRC: RyR2 and the type 1 IP3R (76). More recently we showed that the same two different types of calcium-release channels are expressed in the normal and failing human myocardium: RyR2 and the IP3R1; and that distinct and opposite regulation of each type of calcium-release channel mRNA levels occurs during end-stage heart failure (34). The same study also reported the upregulation of IP3R mRNA levels in the ventricles of patients with end-stage heart failure compared with normal patients, in contrast to other calcium channels, which are downregulated (Fig. 6). Levels of IP3R mRNA were markedly increased in the myopathic left ventricle: by 98% in ICM and by 143% in IDCM (p < .005 for both), and in the myopathic right ventricle by 80% in ICM and by 110% in IDCM (p < .005 for both), compared with normal tis-

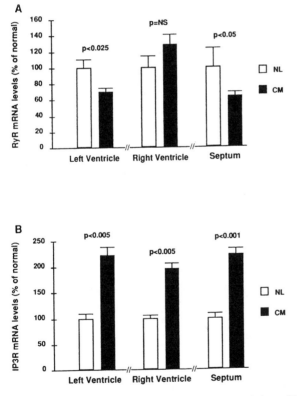

Figure 6   Downregulation of RyR2 and upregulation of IP3R1 during end stage human heart failure. mRNA levels for RyR2 and IP3R1 were determined using slot blot analyses of samples obtained from explanted human hearts of patients undergoing cardiac transplantation. (From Ref. 35.)

sue. IP3R levels were also significantly upregulated in the myopathic septum by 122–124% (p < .001), whether ICM or IDCM. IP3-binding sites increased 43% compared to ryanodine binding sites in the failing heart. Despite these descriptive studies of the regulation of CRC mRNA and protein, correlations between these observations and possible functional consequences in terms of cardiac contractility in the failing heart have not yet been established.

Previous studies on human heart failure had demonstrated downregulation of the mRNA encoding the excitation–contraction coupling calcium channels in myopathic left ventricular tissue. The mRNA level of SR calcium-ATPase has been shown to be reduced by 35–55% in end-stage heart failure (1, 26, 70, 96). Likewise, mRNA levels of the voltage-gated calcium channel DHPR were decreased in myopathic left ventricles by 47% (96). Our group and others have also shown that RyR2 mRNA levels in the left ventricle were decreased in patients with cardiomyopathy (6).

The simultaneously reduced RyR2 and elevated IP3R mRNA levels argue against a universal decrease or increase in either cardiac gene expression or number of myocytes as the explanation for the regulation of CRCs in the failing heart. Recent animal studies have reproduced this finding of decreased RyR2 calcium-release channel mRNA levels in heart failure using various animal models such as chronic doxorubicin cardiomyopathy in rabbits (19) and rapid ventricular pacing-induced or spontaneous heart failure in dogs (17, 104). Our preliminary studies using rats with acute doxorubicin-induced cardiomyopathy also showed downregulation of RyR2 mRNA levels, as well as upregulation of IP3R mRNA levels (39). That various processes leading to heart failure manifest similar changes in calcium-release channel regulation suggest that these changes may be fundamental to the pathophysiology of heart failure and not merely due to the effects of individual pharmacological agents or entities. In the context of the current study, this suggests that the regulation of RyR2 and IP3R mRNA levels cannot be attributed solely to drugs the patients were taking (e.g., angiotensin-converting enzyme inhibitors or positive inotropes), or as a result of end-stage cardiac decompensation. Further support for the concept that changes in calcium channel expression contribute to, as opposed to result from, heart failure comes from recent studies we have done using rats with hypertrophic cardiomyopathy induced by aortic banding. In these studies changes in CRC expression occurs early in the course of the development of hypertrophy before the onset of significant hemodynamic abnormalities (Go, Cross, and Marks, unpublished).

The IP3R could participate in regulating contractility in the failing heart by analogy to its role in controlling smooth muscle contraction via pharmacomechanical coupling (93). Heart failure is a disorder of the circulation characterized by increased neurohormonal activity. Due to the impaired systolic emptying that results from injury, the heart progressively becomes dependent upon the sympathetic nervous system to provide more efficient contractions. Studies using intracoronary infusions of adrenergic agonists in patients with heart failure have demonstrated both β-adrenergic receptor-mediated lusitropy and α-adrenergic receptor-mediated inotropy in such patients. Modulation of contractility by adrenergic agents could occur via IP3R-mediated intracellular calcium release, with upregulation of IP3R as a mechanism to increase sensitivity in the failing myocardium.

Armed with descriptive reports that now clearly show that calcium channel expression is regulated during heart failure, the challenge is to determine what role, if any, this regulation plays in the pathogenesis of heart failure. Ultimately, these studies of calcium channel modulation during heart failure could provide the basis for novel forms of therapy designed to target molecules that most directly regulate cardiac contractility: the intracellular calcium release channels.

ACKNOWLEDGMENTS

I am grateful to the members of my laboratory whose work forms the basis for much of this chapter, in particular Anne-Marie B. Brillantes, Karol Ondrias, Loewe O. Go, Andrew Scott, T. Jayaraman. Maria C. Moschella, Evgeny Kobrinsky, Elena Ondriasova, and David Harnick. I also wish to thank my colleagues Drs. Barbara Ehrlich, Sidney Fleischer, and Susan Hamilton for many helpful discussions over the years and for reviewing parts of the manuscript. This work was supported by grants to A.R.M. from the NIH (NS29814), the AHA, the NYHA Affiliate, and the MDA. A.R.M. is a Bristol-Meyers/Squibb Established Investigator of the American Heart Association. A-M.B.B. and D.H. were Howard Hughes Fellows, K.O. and E.O. are on leave from the Institute of Experimental Pharmacology, Bratislava, Slovakia.

REFERENCES

1. Arai M, Alpert NR, MacLennan DH, Barton P, Periasamy M. Alterations in sarcoplasmic reticulum gene expression in human heart failure. A possible mechanism for alterations in systolic nd diastolic properties of the failing myocardium. Circ Res 1993; 72:463–469.
2. Berridge MJ. Inositol trisphosphate and calcium signalling. Nature 1993; 361:314–325.
3. Bezprozvanny I, Watras J, Ehrlich B. Bell-shaped calcium response curves of Ins(1,4,5)P3- and calcium-gated channels from endoplasmic reticulum of cerebellum. Nature 1991; 351:751–754.

4. Block BA, Imagawa T, Campbell KP, Franzini-Armstrong C. Structural evidence for direct interaction between the molecular components of the transverse tubule/ sarcoplasmic reticulum junction in skeletal muscle. J Cell Biol 1988; 107:2587–2600.

5. Blondel O, Takeda J, Janssen H, Seino, Bell G. Sequence and functional characterization of a third inositol trisphosphate receptor subtype, IP3R-3, expressed in pancreatic islets, kidney, gastrointestinal tract, and other tissues. J Biol Chem 1993; 268:11356–11363.

6. Brillantes A, Allen P, Takahasi T, Izumo S, Marks A. Differences in cardiac calcium release channel (ryanodine receptor) expression in myocardium from patients with end-stage heart failure caused by ischemic versus dilated cardiomyopathy. Circ Res 1992; 71:18–26.

7. Ondrias K, Brillantes A-MB, Scott A, Ehrlich BE, Marks AR. Single channel properties and calcium conductance of the cloned expressed ryanodine receptor/ calcium release channel. Organellar Ion Channels and Transporters, Society of General Physiologists Series 1996; 51:29–45.

8. Brillantes A-MB, Ondrias K, Scott A, Kobrinsky E, Ondriasova E, Moschella MC, Jayaraman T, Landers M, Ehrlich BE, Marks AR. Stabilization of calcium release channel (ryanodine receptor) function by FK-506 binding protein. Cell 1994; 77:513–523.

9. Callaway C, Seryshev A, Wang J-P, Slavid K, Needleman D, Cantu C, Wu Y, Jayaraman T, Marks A, Hamilton S. Localization of the high and low affinity [3H]Ryanodine binding sites on the skeletal muscle Ca2+ release channel. J Biol Chem 1994; 269:15876–15884.

10. Caterall WA. Excitation-contraction coupling in vertebrate skeletal muscle: a tale of two calcium channels. Cell 1991; 64:871–874.

11. Chadwick CC, Saito A, Fleischer S. Isolation and characterization of the inositol trisphosphate receptor from smooth muscle. Proc Natl Acad Sci 1990; 87:2132–2136.

12. Chen SRW, Zhang L, MacLennan DH. Characterization of a Ca2+ binding and regulatory site in the Ca2+ release channel (ryanodine receptor) of rabbit skeletal muscle sarcoplasmic reticulum. J Biol Chem 1992; 267:23318–23326.

13. Chen SW, Vaughan DM, Airey JA, Coronado R, MacLennan DH. Functional expression of cDNA encoding the Ca2+ release channel (ryanodine receptor) of rabbit skeletal muscle sarcoplasmic reticulum in COS-1 cells. Biochemistry 1993; 32:3743–3753.

14. Chua A, Diaz-Munoz M, Hawkes M, Brush K, and Hamilton S. Ryanodine as a probe for the functional state of the skeletal muscle sarcoplasmic reticulum calcium release channel. Mol Pharmacol 1990; 37:735–741.

15. Conti A, Sorrentino V. Differential distribution of ryanodine receptor type 3 (RyR3) gene product n mammalian skeletal muscles. Biophys J 1996; 70:A124.

16. Coronado R, Kawano S, Lee C, Valdivia C, and Valdivia H. Planar bilayer recording of ryanodine receptors of sarcoplasmic reticulum. Methods Enzymol 1992; 207:699–707.

17. Cory R, McCutcheon L, O'Grady M, Pang A, Geiger J, O'Brien P. Compensatory downregulation of myocardial Ca channel in SR from dogs with heart failure. Am J Physiol 1993; 264:H926–H927.
18. Danoff S, Ferris C, Donath C, Fischer G, Munemitsu S, Ullrich A, Snyder S, Ross C. Inositol 1,4,5-trisphosphate receptors: distinct neuronal and nonneuronal forms derived by alternative splicing differ in phosphorylation. Proc Natl Acad Sci 1991; 88:2951–2955.
19. Dodd D, Atkinson J, Olson R, Buck S, Cusack B, Fleischer S, Boucek Jr R. Doxorubicin cardiomyopathy is associated with a decrease in calcium release channel of the sarcoplasmic reticulum in a chronic rabbit model. J Clin Invest 1993; 91:1697–1705.
20. Ehrlich B, Watras J. Inositol 1,4,5-trisphosphate activates a channel from smooth muscle sarcoplasmic reticulum. Nature 1988; 336:583–586.
21. Fabiato A. Calcium-induced release of calcium from the cardiac sarcoplasmic reticulum. Am J Physiol 1983; 245:C1–C14.
22. Fabiato A. Time and calcium dependence of activation and inactivation of calcium-induced release of calcium from the sarcoplasmic reticulum of a skinned canine cardiac purkinje cell. J Gen Physiol 1985; 85:247–289.
23. Fabiato A. Inositol (1,4,5)-trisphosphate induced release of Ca2+ from the sarcoplasmic reticulum of skinned cardiac cells. Biophys J 1986; 49:190a.
24. Fabiato A. Comparison and relation between inositol (1,4,5)-trisphosphate induced release and calcium induced release from the sarcoplasmic reticulum. In: Yamada K, Sibata S, eds. Recent Advances in Calcium Channels and Calcium Antagonists. Elmsford NY: Pergamon Press, 1990:35–39.
25. Fabiato A, Fabiato F. Calcium and cardiac excitation-contraction coupling. Annu Rev Physiol 1985; 41:743.
26. Feldman AM, Weinberg EO, Ray PE, Lorell BH. Selective changes in cardiac gene expression during compensated hypertrophy and the transition to cardiac decomposition in rats with chronic aortic banding. Circ Res 1993; 73:184–192.
27. Ferris CD, Huganir RL, Supattapone S, Snyder SH. Purified inositol 1,4,5-trisphosphate receptor mediates calcium flux in reconstituted lipid vesicles. Nature 1989; 342:87–89.
28. Fill M, Mejia-Alvarez R, Zorzato F, Volpe P, Stefani E. Antibodies as probes for ligand gating of single sarcoplasmic reticulum Ca2+-release channels. Biochem J 1991; 273:449–457.
29. Fleischer S, Inui M. Biochemistry and biophysics of excitation–contraction coupling. Annu Rev Biophys Biophys Chem 1989; 18:333–364.
30. Franzini-Armstrong C, Nunzi G. Junctional feet and membrane particles in the triad of a fast twitch muscle fiber. J Muscle Res Cell Motil 1983; 4:233–252.
31. Furuichi T, Yoshikawa S, Miyawaki A, Wada K, Maeda N, Mikoshiba K. Primary structure and functional expression of the inositol 1,4,5-trisphosphate-binding protein P400. Nature 1989; 342:32–38.
32. Futatsugi A, Kuwajima G, Mikoshiba K. Tissue-specific and developmentally regulated alternative splicing in mouse skeletal muscle ryanodine receptor mRNA. Biochem J 1995; 305:373–378.

33. Garcia J, McKinley K, Appel S, Stefani E. Ca2+ current and charge movement in adult single human skeletal muscle fibres. J Physiol 1992; 454:183–196.
34. Go LO, Moschella MC, Watras J, Handa KK, Fyfe BS, and Marks AR. Differential regulation of two types of intracellular calcium release channels during end-stage heart failure. J Clin Invest 1995; 95:888–894.
35. Go LO, Moschella MC, Watras J, Handa KK, Fyfe BS, Marks AR. Differential regulation of two types of intracellular calcium release channels during end-stage heart failure. J Clin Invest 1995; 95:888–894.
36. Gorza L, Schiaffino S, and Volpe P. Inositol 1,4,5-trisphosphate receptor in heart: evidence for its concentration in Purkinje myocytes of the conduction system. J Cell Biol 1993; 121:345–353.
37. Grunwald R, Meissner G. Lumenal sites and C terminus accessibility of the skeletal muscle calcium release channel (ryanodine receptor). J Biol Chem 1995; 270:11338–11347.
38. Hakamata Y, Nakai J, Takeshima H, Imoto K. Primary structure and distribution of a novel ryanodine receptor/calcium release channel from rabbit brain. FEBS 1992; 312:229–235.
39. Handa KK, Go LO, Marks AR. Regulation of calcium channel expression during heart failure. Circulation 1993; 88(suppl I):I-624.
40. Harnick DH, Jayaraman T, Go L, Ma Y, Mulieri P, Marks AR. The human type 1 inositol 1,4,5-trisphosphate receptor from T lymphocytes: structure, localization and phosphorylation. J Biol Chem 1995; 270:2833–2840.
41. Hawkes MJ, Nelson TE, Hamilton SL. [3H]Ryanodine as a probe of changes in the functional state of the Ca2+-release channel in malignant hyperthermia. J Biol Chem 1992; 267:6702–6709.
42. Herrmann-Frank A, Darling E, and Meissner G. Functional Characterization of the Ca^{2+}-gated Ca^{2+} release channel of vascular smooth muscle sarcoplasmic reticulum. Pflugers Arch 1991; 418:353–359.
43. Hirata M, Suematsu T, Hashimoto T, Hamachi T, Koga T. Release of Ca2+ from a non-mitochondrial store site in peritoneal macrophages treated with saponin by inositol (1,4,5)-trisphosphate. Biochem J 1984; 223:229–236.
44. Hymel L, Inui M, Fleischer S, Schindler HG. Purified ryanodine receptor of skeletal muscle forms Ca^{2+}-activated oligomeric Ca^{2+} channels in planar bilayers. Proc Natl Acad Sci USA 1988; 85:441–44.
45. Imagawa T, Smith J, Coronado R, Campbell K. Purified ryanodine receptor from skeletal muscle sarcoplasmic reticulum is the Ca2+-permeable pore of the calcium release channel. J Biol Chem 1987; 262:16636–16643.
46. Imoto K. Rings of negatively charged amino acids determine the acetylcholine receptor channel conductance. Nature 1988; 335:645–648.
47. Inui M, Saito A, Fleischer S. Isolation of the ryanodine receptor from cardiac sarcoplasmic reticulum and identity with the feet structures. J Biol Chem 1987; 262:15637–15642.
48. Inui M, Saito A, Fleischer S. Purification of the ryanodine receptor and identity with feet structures of junctional terminal cisternae of sarcoplasmic reticulum from fast skeletal muscle. J Biol Chem 1987; 262:1740–1747.

49. Jayaraman T, Brillantes A-MB, Timerman AP, Erdjument-Bromage H, Fleischer S, Tempst P, Marks AR. FK506 binding protein associated with the calcium release channel (ryanodine receptor). J Biol Chem 1992; 267:9474–9477.

50. Jayaraman T, Ondrias K, Ondriasova E, Marks AR. Regulation of the inositol 1,4,5-trisphosphate receptor by tyrosine phosphorylation. Science 1996; 272:1492–1494.

51. Jayaraman T, Ondriasova E, Ondrias K, Harnick D, Marks AR. The inositol 1,4,5-trisphosphate receptor is essential for T cell receptor signaling. Proc Natl Acad Sci USA 1995; 92:6007–6011.

52. Kaftan E, Marks AR, Ehrlich BE. Effects of rapamycin on ryanodine receptor/calcium release channels from cardiac muscle. Circ Res 1996; 78:990–997.

53. Kentish J, Barsotti R, Lea T, Mulligan I, Patel J, Ferenczi M. Calcium release from cardiac sarcoplasmic reticulum induced by photorelease of calcium or Ins(1,4,5)P3. Am J Physiol 1990; 258:H610–H615.

54. Kijima Y, and Fleischer S. Characterization of inositol 1,4,5-trisphosphate binding to canine cardiac sarcoplasmic reticulum. Biophys J 1992; 61:A423.

55. Kobrinsky E, Ondrias K, Marks AR. Expressed ryanodine receptor can substitute for the inositol 1,4,5-trisphosphate receptor during progesterone induced maturation in Xenopus oocytes. Dev Biol 1995; 172:531–540.

56. Kume S, Muto A, Aruga J, Nakagawa T, Michikawa T, Furuichi T, Nakade S, Okano H, Mikoshiba K. The Xenopus oocyte IP3 receptor: structure, function and localization in oocytes. Cell 1993; 73:555–570.

57. Lai FA, Erickson HP, Rousseau E, Liu QL, Meissner G. Purification and reconstitution of the calcium release channel from skeletal muscle. Nature (London) 1988; 331:315–319.

58. Lesh RE, Marks AR, Somlyo A, Fleischer S, Somylo A. Anti-ryanodine receptor antibody binding sites in aortic and endocardial endothelium. Circ Res 1993; 72:481–488.

59. Liu J, Farmer J, Lane W, Friedman J, Weissman I, Schreiber S. Calcineurin is a common target of cyclophilin-cyclosporin A and FKBP-FK506 complexes. Cell 1991; 66:807–815.

60. Lovenberg W, Miller RC. Endothelin: a review of its effects and possible mechanisms of action. Neurochem Res 1990; 15:407–417.

61. Lu X, Xu L, Meissner G. Activation of the skeletal muscle calcium release channel by a cytoplasmic loop of the dihydropyridine receptor. J Biol Chem 1994; 269:6511–6516.

62. Maranto A. Primary structure, ligand binding, and localization of the human type 3 inositol 1,4,5-trisphosphate receptor expressed in intestinal epithelium. J Biol Chem 1994; 269:1222–1230.

63. Marks AR, Fleischer S, Tempst P. Surface topography analysis of the ryanodine receptor/junctional channel complex based on proteolysis sensitivity mapping. J Biol Chem 1990; 265:13143–13149.

64. Marks AR, Tempst P, Chadwick CC, Riviere L, Fleischer S, Nadal-Ginard B. Smooth muscle and brain inositol 1,4,5-trisphosphate receptors are structurally and functionally similar. J Biol Chem 1990; 265:20719–20722.

65. Marks AR, Tempst P, Hwang KS, Taubman MB, Inui M, Chadwick C, Fleischer S, Nadal-Ginard B. Molecular cloning and characterization of the ryanodine receptor/junctional channel complex cDNA from skeletal muscle sarcoplasmic reticulum. Proc Natl Acad Sci USA 1989; 86:8683–8687.

66. MayrLeitner M, Chadwick C, Timmerman A, Fleischer S, Schindler S. Purified IP3-receptor from smooth muscle forms an IP3 gated and heparin sensitive channel in planar bilayers. Cell Calcium 1991; 12:505–514.

67. McPherson PS, Kim Y-K, Valdivia H, Knudson CM, Takekura H, Franzini-Armstrong C, Coronado R, Campbell K P. The brain ryanodine receptor: a caffeine-sensitive calcium release channel. Neuron 1991; 7:17–25.

68. Meissner G, and El-Hashem A. Ryanodine as a functional probe of the skeletal muscle sarcoplasmic reticulum Ca2+ release channel. Mol Cell Biochem 1992; 114:119–123.

69. Meissner G, Lai F, Anderson K, Xu L, Liu Q, Herrman-Frank A, Rousseau E, Jones R, Lee H. Purification and reconstitution of the ryanodine- and caffeine-sensitive Ca^{2+} release channel complex from muscle sarcoplasmic reticulum. Adv Exp Med Biol 1991; 304:241–256.

70. Mercardier J, Lompre A, Duc P, Boheler K, Fraysse J, Wisnewsky C, Allen P, Komajda M, Schwartz K. Altered sarcoplasmic reticulum Ca2+-ATPase gene expression in the human ventricle during end-stage heart failure. J Clin Invest 1990; 85:305–309.

71. Michikawa T, Hamanaka H, Otsu H, Yamamoto A, Miyawaki A Furuichi F, Tashiro Y, and Mikoshiba K. Transmembrane topology and sites of N-glycosylation of inositol 1,4,5-trisphosphate receptor. J Biol Chem 1994; 269:9184–9189.

72. Mignery GA, Newton CL, Archer BT, Sudhof TC. Structure and expression of the rat inositol-1,4,5-trisphosphate receptor. J Biol Chem 1990; 265:12679–12685.

73. Mignery GA, Sudhof TC. The ligand binding site and transduction mechanism in the inositol 1,4,5-trisphosphate receptor. EMBO J 1990; 9:3893–3898.

74. Monkawa T, Miyawaki A, Sugiyama T, Yoneshima H, Yamamoto-Hino M, Furuichi T, Saruta T, Hasegawa M, Mikoshiba K. Heterotetrameric complex formation of inositol 1,4,5-trisphosphate receptor subunits. J Biol Chem 1995; 270:14700–14704.

75. Mori Y, Friedrich T, Kim M-S, Mikami A, Nakai J, Ruth P, Bosse E, Hofmann F, Flockerzi V, Furuichi T, Mikoshiba K, Imoto K, Tanabe T, Numa S. Primary structure and functional expression from complementary DNA of a brain calcium channel. Nature 1991; 350:398–402.

76. Moschella MC, Marks AR. Inositol 1,4,5-trisphosphate receptor expression in cardiac myocytes. J Cell Biol 1993; 120:1137–1146.

77. Mourey RJ, Verma A, Supattapone S, Snyder SH. Purification and characterization of the inositol 1,4,5-trisphosphate receptor protein from rat vas deferens. Biochem J 1990; 272:383–389.

78. Movesian M, Thomas A, Selak M, Williamson J. Inositol trisphosphate does not

release Ca2+ from permeabilized cardiac myocytes and sarcoplasmic reticulum. FEBS Lett 1985; 185:328–332.

79. Nakagawa T, Okano H, Furuichi T, Aruga J, Mikoshiba K. The subtypes of the mouse inositol 1,4,5-trisphosphate receptor are expressed in a tissue-specific and developmentally specific manner. Proc Natl Acad Sci 1991; 88:6244–6248.

80. Nakai J, Imagawa T, Hakamata Y, Shigekawa M, Takeshima H, Numa S. Primary structure and functional expression from cDNA of the cardiac ryanodine receptor/calcium release channel. FEBS 1990; 271:169–177.

81. Nosek T, Williams M, Ziegler S, Godt R. Inositol trisphosphate enhances calcium release in skinned cardiac and skeletal muscle. Am J Physiol 1986; 250:C807–C811.

82. Otani H, Otani H, Das D. α1-Adrenoreceptor-mediate phosphoinositide breakdown and inotropic response in rat left ventricular papillary muscles. Circ Res 1988; 62:8–17.

83. Otsu K, Willard HF, Khanna VK, Zorzato F, Green NM, MacLennan DH. Molecular cloning of cDNA encoding the Ca2+ release channel (ryanodine receptor) of rabbit cardiac muscle sarcoplasmic reticulum. J Biol Chem 1990; 265:13472–13483.

84. Penner R, Neher E, Takeshima H, Nishimura S, Numa S. Functional expression of the calcium release channel from skeletal muscle ryanodine receptor cDNA. FEBS 1989; 259:217–221.

85. Poggioli J, Sulpice J, Vassort G. Inositol phosphate production following α1-adrenergic, muscarinic, or electrical stimulation in isolated rat heart. FEBS Lett 1986; 206:292–298.

86. Rios E, Brum G. Involvement of dihydropyridine receptors in excitation–contraction coupling in skeletal muscle. Nature 1987; 325:717–720.

87. Rios E, Pizarro G, Stefani E. Charge movement and the nature of signal transduction in skeletal muscle excitation-contraction coupling. Annu Rev Physiol 1992; 54:109–133.

88. Ross CA, Meldolesi J, Milner TA, Saloh T, Supattapone S, Snyder S H. Inositol 1,4,5-trisphosphate receptor localized to endoplasmic reticulum in cerebellar Purkinje neurons. Nature 1989; 339:468–470.

89. Schneider MF, Chandler WK. Voltage dependent charge movement in skeletal muscle: a possible step in excitation-contraction coupling. Nature 1973; 242:244–246.

90. Schreiber S. Chemistry and biology of the immunophilins and their immunosuppressive ligands. Science 1991; 251:283–287.

91. Smith JS, Coronado R, Meissner G. Single channel measurements of the calcium release channel from skeletal muscle sarcoplasmic reticulum. J Gen Physiol 1986; 88:573–588.

92. Smith JS, Imagawa T, Ma J, Fill M, Campbell KP, Coronado R. Purified ryanodine receptor from rabbit skeletal muscle is the calcium release channel of sarcoplasmic reticulum. J Gen Physiol 1988; 2:1–26.

93. Somlyo A. Excitation–contraction coupling and the ultrastructure of smooth muscle. Circ Res 1985; 57:497–507.

94. Suchyna TM, Xu LX, Gao F, Fourtner CR, Nicholson BJ. Identification of a proline residue as a transduction element involved in voltage gating of gap junctions. Nature 1993; 365:847–849.

95. Sudhof T, Newton C, Archer B, Ushkaryov Y, Mignery G. Structure of a novel InsP3 receptor. EMBO J 1991; 10:3199–3206.

96. Takahashi T, Allen PD, Lacro RV, Marks AR, Dennis AR, Schoen FJ, Grossman W, Marsh JD, Izumo S. Expression of dihydropyridine receptor (Ca2+ channel) and calsequestrin genes in the myocardium of patients with end-stage heart failure. J Clin Invest 1992; 90:927–935.

97. Takeshima H, Nishimura S, Matsumoto T, Ishida H, Kangawa K, Minamino N, Matsuo H, Ueda M, Hanaoka M, Hirose T, Numa S. Primary structure and expression from complementary DNA of skeletal muscle ryanodine receptor. Nature 1989; 339:439–445.

98. Takeshima H, Nishimura S, Nishi M, Ikeda M, Sugimoto T. A brain-specific transcript from the 3'-terminal region of the skeletal muscle ryanodine receptor gene. FEBS 1993; 322:105–110.

99. Takeshima H, Yamazawa T, Ikemoto T, Takekura H, Nishi M, Noda T, and Iino M. Ca(2+)-induced Ca2+ release in myocytes from despedic mice lacking the type-1 ryanodine receptor. EMBO J 1995; 14:2999–3006.

100. Tanabe T, Beam KG, Adams BA, Niidome T, Numa S. Regions of the skeletal muscle dihydropyridine receptor critical for excitation-contraction coupling. Nature 1990; 346:567–569.

101. Timerman AP, Jayaraman T, Wiederrecht G, Onoue H, Marks A, Fleischer S. The ryanodine receptor from canine heart sarcoplasmic reticulum is associated with a novel FK-506 binding protein. BBRC 1994; 198:701–706.

102. Timerman AP, Ogunbunmi E, Freund E, Wiederrecht G, Marks A, Fleischer S. The calcium release channel of sarcoplasmic reticulum is modulated by FK-506 binding protein. J Biol Chem 1993; 268:22992–22999.

103. Valdivia HH, Kirby MS, Lederer WJ, Coronado R. Scorpion toxins targeted against the sarcoplasmic reticulum Ca2+-release channel of skeletal and cardiac muscle. Proc Natl Acad Sci 1992; 89:12185–12189.

104. Vatner DE, Sato N, Kiuchi K, Shannon RP, Vatner SF. Decrease in myocardial ryanodine receptors and altered excitation-contraction coupling early in the development of heart failure. Circulation 1994; 90:1423–30.

105. Witcher DR, McPherson PS, Kahl SD, Lewis T, Bentley P, Mullinnix MJ, Windass JD, and Campbell KP. Photoaffinity labeling of the ryanodine receptor/Ca2+ release channel with an azido derivative of ryanodine. J Biol Chem 1994; 269:13076–13079.

106. Wojcikiewicz RJH, He Y. Type I, II, and III inositol 1,4,5-trisphosphate receptor co-immunoprecipitation as evidence for the existence of heterotetrameric receptor cojmplexes BBRC 1995; 213:334–341.

107. Yamamoto-Hino M, Sugiyama T, Hikichi K, Mattel M, Hasegawa K, Sekine S, Sakurada K, Miyakawa A, Furuichi T, Hasegawa M, Mikoshiba K. Cloning and characterization of human type 2 and type 3 inositol 1,4,5-Trisphosphate receptors. Recept Chan 1994; 2:9–22.

108. Zorzato F, Fujii J, Otso K, Phillips M, Green NM, Lai FA, Meissner G, MacLennan DH. Molecular cloning of cDNA encoding human and rabbit forms of the Ca2+ release channel (ryanodine receptor) of skeletal muscle sarcoplasmic reticulum. J Biol Chem 1990; 265:2244–2256.

13

Advances in the Molecular Characterization of the Na$^+$/Ca^{2+} Exchanger

Dan H. Schulze and W. J. Lederer
University of Maryland School of Medicine
Baltimore, Maryland

The Na$^+$/Ca^{2+} exchanger is an integral plasma membrane protein that extrudes Ca^{2+} from the cells under physiological conditions (1,2). While the exchanger has been demonstrated in many tissues including heart, brain, kidney, lung, large intestine, pancreas, and spleen (3-4), the most complete physiological characterization has been in cardiac muscle. In the heart the exchanger is the dominant transport system that extrudes Ca^{2+} from the cardiac myocyte to balance the calcium influx via I$_{Ca}$ (5-7).

The Na$^+$/Ca^{2+} exchanger under physiological conditions in all tissues appears to operate at a fixed stoichiometry, extruding one Ca^{2+} for three entering sodium ions (1,2). With this stoichiometry, the exchanger utilizes the energy stored in the electrochemical Na$^+$ gradient to pump Ca^{2+} out of the cell and produces a net movement of charge proportional to the turnover rate of the Na$^+$/Ca^{2+} exchanger. A secondary consequence is that the Na$^+$/Ca^{2+} exchanger is also voltage dependent (8,9). It should also be noted that the cardiac action potential makes it possible, in principle, for the Na$^+$/Ca^{2+} exchanger to reverse the direction of net Ca^{2+} transport as the electrochemical gradient changes. This has led to the intriguing, albeit controversial, proposal that the Na$^+$/Ca^{2+} exchanger may actually complement the I_{Ca}-dependent Ca^{2+}-influx (which triggers intracellular Ca^{2+} release in heart; 10,11) to activate the ryanodine receptor to release Ca^{2+} (12–14).

When examining Ca^{2+} homeostasis in diverse cells, it is clear that both the plasma membrane Ca^{2+} pump and the Na^+/Ca^{2+} exchangers play a role principally in extruding Ca^{2+}. This chapter will focus on the Na^+/Ca^{2+} exchanger specifically and more narrowly on molecular biological developments related to the Na^+/Ca^{2+} exchanger, beginning with the cloning of the exchanger and extending into an examination of the gene structure. Recent work focusing on transcription of the Na^+/Ca^{2+} exchanger, targeting of the protein via the signal sequences, and long-term research directions of physiological and molecular investigations will also be reviewed.

CLONING OF THE CANINE CARDIAC Na$^+$/Ca^{2+} EXCHANGER

The initial advance in the identification of the Na^+/Ca^{2+} exchanger protein was the production of polyclonal antisera that contained antibodies against the exchanger. Several laboratories, in preparing antibodies against the Na^+/Ca^{2+} exchanger, had demonstrated that several discrete sizes of protein fragments could be identified: 160, 120, and 70 Kd (15,16). The laboratory of Dr. Philipson screened a λgt11 expression library made from canine heart with polyclonal antisera against the Na^+/Ca^{2+} exchanger. Positive clones produced a protein product that was recognized by the antisera (17). After a full-length clone had been obtained and had characterized the cDNA, they demonstrated that cRNA injected into *Xenopus* oocytes resulted in an Na^+-dependent Ca^{2+} flux characteristic of the Na^+/Ca^{2+} exchanger function. The initial sequence of a canine Na^+/Ca^{2+} exchanger cDNA and the deduced amino acid sequence identified a potential Kozak consensus sequence (18) as the putative site of initiation of protein synthesis followed by an open reading frame of 970 amino acids. Hydrophobicity analysis of the predicted polypeptide sequence suggested that there were 6 N terminal and 6 C terminal potential transmembrane regions with a large hydrophilic stretch of amino acids thought to be located inside the cell (see Fig. 1). The N- terminal hydrophobic domain was shown to be a cleavable signal peptide, based on previous biochemical analysis of the mature bovine protein of the Na^+/Ca^{2+} exchanger (19). The signal peptide targets protein to the membrane. It was interesting that most polytopic membrane molecules characterized do not have cleavable signal sequences, because these proteins are thought to have transmembrane segments with the targeting information (20).

When the canine cardiac Na^+/Ca^{2+} exchanger sequence was compared to all published sequences, only a short putative transmembrane region of the exchanger displayed marginal homology in a 23 amino acid stretch with the Na^+, K^+-ATPase displaying significant levels of identity (21) (Fig. 1). The

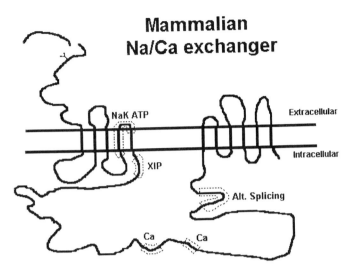

Figure 1   Representation of the Na$^+$/Ca^{2+} exchanger. The parallel horizontal lines represent the plasma membrane with intracellular region at the bottom and the exchanger passing through the membrane. Relevant sites are highlighted. The signal peptide is cleaved at the 5′ end. The position of glycosylation is represented (Ψ) (23). The region that displayed homology to Na$^+$K$^+$-ATPase (17), the position for hypothesized binding of calmodulin and the site of binding the inhibitory peptide (XIP) (22) and two regions for Ca^{2+} binding on the intracellular loop (51) are shown. The region in the intracellular loop that undergoes alternative splicing is noted (66,67). (Based on sequence analysis in Refs. 3 and 17.)

authors also described a cluster of basic amino acids in the protein (see XIP) at a region that is predicted to be the in the intracellular loop of the protein that they suggested could be a calmodulin-binding domain (17). More recent experiments have demonstrated that a peptide can bind to this region of the exchanger, inhibiting exchanger function (22). Other experiments demonstrated that the canine Na$^+$/Ca^{2+} exchanger polypeptide was glycosylated in a single N-terminal asparagine residue (25).

CLONING OF CARDIAC Na$^+$/Ca^{2+} EXCHANGER FROM HUMAN AND OTHER MAMMALIAN SPECIES

After the publication of the initial cloning of a canine Na$^+$/Ca^{2+} exchanger, using the deduced amino acid sequence we (3) and others (24) developed probes to be used in cloning the human cardiac Na$^+$/Ca^{2+} exchanger using homology-based strategies. Sequence analysis of a full-length clone demonstrated that the human Na$^+$/Ca^{2+} exchanger had a very similar overall structure of potential transmembrane regions and overall amino acid identity when compared to the canine exchanger (3). Sequence comparison demonstrated that there was only minor sequence divergence between the canine and human exchangers (98% at the deduced amino acid levels and 95% at the nucleic acid level) (3). About half of the amino acid differences resided in the putative leader peptide. The level of sequence divergence observed between the human and other mammalian Na^+/Ca^{2+} exchanger is comparable to the divergence demonstrated for other mammalian transporter molecules such as the Na^+ pump (21,25,26) and the β_1-subunit of the voltage-dependent calcium channel (27). After cloning of the human Na^+/Ca^{2+} exchanger, other mammalian cardiac Na^+/Ca^{2+} exchanger were published such as the rat (28), cow (29), guinea pig (30), and recently the mouse (31) and cat (32). All of these Na^+/Ca^{2+} exchanger clones display similar levels of sequence identity when compared to either the human or the canine cardiac exchangers (greater than 96% amino acid identity).

SIGNAL PEPTIDE COMPARISON OF MAMMALIAN Na^+/Ca^{2+}EXCHANGER SEQUENCES

Most of the diversity in the comparison between the mammalian Na^+/Ca^{2+} exchangers resides in the signal peptide, which was identified as being missing in the mature bovine protein (19). When all of the published mammalian sequences for putative signal peptides for the Na^+/Ca^{2+} exchanger are compared (Fig. 2), a pattern of conserved amino acids can be observed. The signal sequences have eight amino acids, which are identical in the same position relative to the initial methionine in all of the sequences compared. Twelve more of the positions in the signal sequence display conservative changes in amino acids (i.e., one hydrophobic or charged amino acid replaces another amino acid with similar biochemical characteristics). While the signal sequences are only between 59 and 75% identical depending on the comparison, the remaining part of the Na^+/Ca^{2+} exchanger proteins is greater than 97% identical when compared to the Na^+/Ca^{2+} exchanger proteins of other mammalian species. When compared to the Na^+/Ca^{2+} exchanger, most of the polytopic transport proteins do not contain a signal sequence but are still targeted properly to the plasma membrane (20,33–36). It is thought that the transmembrane-spanning segments of these proteins have targeting information. Such internal signal–anchor sequences have been identified in a number of eukaryotic transport proteins anion exchanger AE1 (35) and P-glycoprotein (37,38). Three groups recently have independently demonstrated that the signal sequence is not necessary to target the exchanger proteins to the plasma membrane (39–41). One possible role for the signal sequence is to enhance membrane insertion. This has been described in human B_2-adrenergic receptor (34) where it is demonstrated that when a cleavable signal peptide was fused to this protein, translocation of the receptor protein was doubled in the endoplasmic reticulum. Such an increase could

Na$^+$/Ca^{2+} Exchanger

Signal Sequences (AA)	Identity to human	Ref.
	↓	
Human	MRRLSLSPTFSMGFHLLVTVSLLFSHVDNVIA	–	3,24
Canine	MLQLRLLPTFSMGCHLLAVVALLFSHVDHVIA	23/32	15
Rat	MLRLSLPPNVSMGFRLVTLVALLFTHVDHITA	19/32	28
Bovine	MLQFSLSPTLSMGFHVIAMVALLFSHVDHISA	20/32	29
Rabbit	MPRFSLSSPFSMGFHLLAIVALFFFRVDHVSA	20/32	65
Guin.Pig	MLRLSLSPTYSLGFHLLAMMTLLISHVDHITA	21/32	20
Cat	MLRLSLSPTFSVGFHLLAFVPLLFSHVDLISA	24/32	32

```
Pos.of AA  | ||  |   | ||| || || |   ||| |
           *  CH  *   H*H*H HH HH *HH  ** H *
```

Figure 2 Comparison of signal sequences from mammalian Na$^+$/Ca^{2+} exchangers. Arrow at the top identifies the cleavage position of the signal peptide (19) and hydrophobic region with a bold line at the top. Underlined deduced amino acids are charged or polar residues and the highlighted residues are hydrophobic. An asterisk (*) at the bottom denotes the positions in the sequence where all are identical. C and H at the bottom represent the positions where all of the sequences being compared have only Charged or Hydrophobic residues, respectively. The cat sequence was obtained from Genbank accession number L35846.

enhance expression of the Na$^+$/Ca^{2+} exchanger in cell types that express low levels of the protein, as is the case in some tissues.

ALTERNATIVE ROLES OF THE SIGNAL PEPTIDE

Another possible role of the signal peptide is that cleavage of the signal may be required for the molecule to associate with itself or with other molecules. Most membrane transport proteins are oligomeric (42). The only information about the possible structure of the Na$^+$/Ca^{2+} exchanger resides in analysis of the molecular weight of identifiable protein (15,16). In some other transport proteins, it has not been demonstrated that oligomerization is always required for transport. For example, the Na$^+$/H$^+$ exchanger, which can form stable dimers, has been demonstrated to function in the monomeric form (43). The Na$^+$/Ca^{2+} exchanger could associate with other cellular proteins in order to be localized to particular subcellular regions. Philipson and his group have found that there is a biochemical association of the Na$^+$/Ca^{2+} exchanger with the cytoskeletal structural protein ankyrin (44). This raised the possibility that the Na$^+$/Ca^{2+} exchanger may be highly localized to a specific sarcolemmal domain. In our opinion, however, this has not been demonstrated in heart muscle. There is, nevertheless, some controversy about the immunolocalization of the Na$^+$/Ca^{2+} exchanger. Kieval et al. (45) found that, to a first approximation, in adult rat heart cells there was uniform distribution of the protein on the surface membrane including the transverse tubules. Frank et al. (46) argued, in contrast, that the Na$^+$/Ca^{2+} exchanger was preferentially localized to the t-tubules in heart. While immunolocalization in the kidney suggests that it may be enriched in the connecting tubules, there is some controversy in this finding as well (47,48). Specialized membrane-specific targeting of the protein does, however, seem likely if the focused transport function of the Na^+/Ca^{2+} exchanger is to be achieved. This is an important area for current and future investigations.

STRUCTURE/FUNCTION CHARACTERISTICS OF THE Na^+/Ca^{2+} EXCHANGER

Following the cloning of the Na^+/Ca^{2+} exchanger, progress has been made in identifying regions of the molecule that contribute to specific functional characteristics. For example, the large intracellular loop of the protein has been suggested to contain the Ca^{2+} regulatory domain since either deletion of the intracellular loop by cloning methods or putative deletion of the intracellular loop by proteolysis (chymotrypsin) removes the Ca^{2+} regulatory effect on the exchanger (50). Other experiments in which most of the intracellular loop was deleted (by engineering the construct that was used) show that the Na^+/Ca^{2+} exchanger still functions, indicating that this region of the protein is not essential for transport function. Also these constructs were not regulatable by free intracellular Ca^{2+}. To localize the Ca^{2+}-binding sites, portions of the exchanger intracellular loop were expressed as fusion proteins and examined in a gel-separation experiment using radioactive Ca^{2+} to overlay onto these proteins. The high-affinity sites could be identified by the co-localization of the radioactive Ca^{2+} and a specific fusion protein. The Ca^{2+} binding region identified by this experiment has two highly acidic sequences characterized by three aspartic acid residues. The Ca^{2+} affinity of this region of the protein is reduced when these residues are mutated, demonstrating the importance of these residues in Ca^{2+} binding (51).

The first direct demonstration that the Na^+/Ca^{2+} exchanger protein is phosphorylated was recently presented by Shigekawa and his colleagues (52). The protein had been immunoprecipitated in a phosphorylated state from smooth muscle cells. This group demonstrated that only serine residues are phosphorylated and they also suggest that the state of phosphorylation can affect the function of the exchanger. Other attempts to demonstrate direct phosphorylation of the Na^+/Ca^{2+} exchanger protein have not been as clear but these studies can demonstrate an ATP-dependent regulation of the exchanger (53,54). They show that ATP depletion inhibits both Ca^{2+}-dependent efflux and influx and may alter the competitive interactions of extracellular Na^+ and Ca^{2+}. When phorbol esters are administered to cells there appears to be a downregulation of Na^+/Ca^{2+} exchanger function (54). This study concludes that phorbol ester activation of protein kinase C downregulates the exchanger mRNA level, the Na$^+$/Ca^{2+} exchanger protein and the functional activity in renal epithelial cells.

Other studies are currently making site-directed mutations to particular regions of the exchanger to determine how they will alter function, One such study recently described site-specific mutations of particular amino acids within putative transmembrane regions and they have identified particular residues that appear to be important for the ion transport process (55).

TRANSCRIPTION OF THE Na$^+$/Ca^{2+} EXCHANGER

We and others have demonstrated that the Na$^+$/Ca^{2+} exchanger mRNA is present in many tissues, with heart tissue containing the highest levels. Brain and kidney also have high levels of transcript when compared to other tissues (3,4). In brain tissue the in situ hybridizations of Grayson and his colleagues, using a probe from the 3′ end of the coding sequence, demonstrate that exchanger transcripts are particularly prevalent in the hippocampus and the cortex with lower levels in the hypothalamus and midbrain (56).

Northern blot analysis from several laboratories demonstrated that multiple transcript sizes can be detected in a number of tissues (3,4, 17). A high-molecular-weight species(greater than 10 Kb) can be routinely observed in cardiac and brain total RNA (3). All tissues that have detectable levels of the transcript contain the 7.4 Kb transcript and many reveal a 1.7 Kb transcript. The 1.7 Kb transcript is not long enough to code for the full-length protein, however. We and others have had difficulty in cloning this short transcript. Another group suggested that this hybridization signal is an artifact due to large amounts of contaminating ribosomal RNA (17).

Since no drugs specifically block the exchanger, ameloride and its derivatives have been used as effective but nonspecific inhibitors (57,58) but have led to some confusing results concerning Na$^+$/Ca^{2+} exchanger function (59,60). Recently, an antisense strategy has been utilized by Niggli and his co-workers specifically to inhibit the function of the Na$^+$/Ca^{2+} function in cardiac cells (61). This approach utilized addition to the bathing solution of phosphothiolated antisense oligonucleotides that are complementary to the 3′ untranslated region of the Na$^+$/Ca^{2+} exchange transcript, suggesting that this method could represent a useful tool in describing cellular and molecular properties of the exchanger. Consistent with the antisense experiments, we have demonstrated that the 3′ untranslated region is highly conserved at the nucleic acid level and suggest that this region of the mRNA may play an important (albeit presently undefined) role in Na$^+$/Ca^{2+} exchanger processing or stability (62) (see below).

Na$^+$/Ca^{2+} exchanger transcription can vary from tissue to tissue but the absolute level of the 7.2 Kb transcript of the exchanger changes during development (63) and during the onset of specific cardiomyopathies (64). This alteration in Na^+/Ca^{2+} exchanger level is usually reflected in or in response to a concomitant change in the Ca^{2+}-ATPase levels. The fetal and newborn hearts in various species differ in contraction and relaxation processes when compared to adult heart. Since many developmental changes have been attributed to alterations in Ca^{2+} regulation, study of exchanger transcriptional activity in development has been undertaken. When the levels or exchanger transcript and plasma membrane Ca^{2+}-ATPase are compared using slot blot analysis and densitometry, the level of exchanger is high in the ventricular cells of the fetus while the Ca^{2+} pump is low (63). As the animal develops and the level of the Ca^{2+}-ATPase increases, there is a decrease in the amount of the exchanger.

In several studies that examine hearts during the onset of failure, reduced levels of mRNA and of protein for the plasma membrane Ca^{2+}-ATPase have been identified (64). While preliminary studies from pooled heart tissue did not demonstrate significant changes in the level of the Na^+/Ca^{2+} exchanger mRNA levels (24), in another study the mRNA for the exchanger increased in failing hearts (64). In a large series of defined failing human hearts, mRNA levels for the exchanger were elevated 55% in patients with dilated cardiomyopathy and a 41% increase was identified in patients with coronary artery disease. A concomitant decrease was observed for the plasma membrane Ca^{2+}-ATPase mRNA in these same patients when compared to nonfailing hearts. Western blot analysis of the amount of Na^+/Ca^{2+} exchanger and Ca^{2+} ATPase proteins, while not demonstrating as large a difference, as was shown for mRNA levels, agreed qualitatively with the results obtained for the mRNA. (65). While the results of these experiments show a compensatory relationship between the exchanger and plasma membrane Ca^{2+}-ATPase, more conclusive studies are needed to establish the direct links between heart failure and the Na^+/Ca^{2+} exchanger.

Na^+/Ca^{2+} EXCHANGER IN DIFFERENT TISSUES

When we saw the work of Reilly and co-workers, who published their study of the kidney Na^+/Ca^{2+} exchanger in rabbit (65), there were interesting differences between their sequence and other mammalian exchanger sequences published. While the N-terminal, C-terminal regions with the transmembrane regions and most of the intracellular loop of the kidney sequence were comparable to other previously published mammalian exchangers, there was a restricted region within the intracellular loop that was very different when compared to other mammalian sequences. For example, over a stretch of 34 amino acids only 11 were identical when compared to the equivalent region in the human Na^+/Ca^{2+} exchanger sequence (seen in Fig. 3 comparing human cardiac and rabbit kidney 1). There was also the deletion of 28 amino acids when the rabbit kidney sequence is compared to the human cardiac sequence (Fig. 3).

```
Human Cardiac  EFQNDEIVKTISVKVIDDEEYEKNKTFFLEIGKPRLVEMSEKKALLLNEL 610
Rabbit Cardiac -------------------------------E---------------- 610

Rabbit Kid.1   ---------I-TIRIF-R-----ECS-S-VLEE-KWICRRGM-------- 609
Rabbit Kid.2   ---------I-TIRIF-R-----ECS-S-VLEE-KWICRRGM-ββββββ 609


Human Cardiac  GGFTITGKYLFGQPVFRKVHAREHPILSTVITIADEYDDKQPLTSKEKEE 660
Rabbit Cardiac ----------Y----L------D--VP-------E-----------E-- 660

Rabbit Kid.1   ------ββββββββββββββββββββββββββββE-----------E-- 631
Rabbit Kid.2   ------βββββββββββββββββββββββββββββE-----------E-- 624


Human Cardiac  RRIAEMGRPILGEHTKLEVIIEE 683
Rabbit Cardiac ----------------------- 683

Rabbit Kid.1   ----------------------- 654
Rabbit Kid.2   ----------------------- 647
```

Figure 3 Deduced amino acid sequence comparison for human cardiac Na$^+$/Ca^{2+} exchanger clone 9-4 and PCR products from heart and kidney. Human sequence -, the deduced amino acid is identical the human heart. β, no amino acid in the equivalent position with the human heart sequence. (Human sequence from Ref. 3; rabbit cardiac and kidney forms from Ref. 66.)

To determine the nature of these differences and whether they were due to the species studied (e.g., rabbit vs. human or dog, or the tissue studied [kidney vs. cardiac]), PCR primers that flanked the region of diversity were used to amplify cDNA made from various rabbit tissues (66). When we sequenced the PCR products from the rabbit heart, we obtained a single sequence and that displayed expected amino acid identity to the human clone (Fig. 3: compare human and rabbit cardiac). The rabbit kidney had two detectable bands that are presented in Figure 3 when they were cloned and sequenced. The Na$^+$/Ca^{2+} exchanger isoform rabbit kidney 1 is identical to the sequence published by Reilly (65) in this region. A second kidney sequence, rabbit kidney 2, found in the majority of rabbit kidney clones, was identical to the rabbit kidney 1 sequence except for a 21 bp that resulted in a seven amino acid deletion shown in Figure 3. The large stretch of amino acid differences between the rabbit cardiac and kidney products suggested that either multiple genes existed or that alternative splicing had replaced one exon for another. If the latter hypothesis is correct the deletions could arise because exons had not been included in the mature transcripts of the kidney Na$^+$/Ca^{2+} exchanger. We demonstrated using RNase protection that the shorter form, rabbit kidney 2, is the predominant form of RNA present in the kidney (66). In analyzing the full set of sequences for the tissue and species-specific differences that have been identified, we proposed that alternative splicing of a single gene is the most likely mechanism.

ALTERNATIVELY SPLICED Na⁺/Ca²⁺ EXCHANGER TRANSCRIPTS

To test formally the possibility that alternative splicing is producing the differences in mRNA that have been found in different tissues, we needed to determine the germline configuration of the Na^+/Ca^{2+} exchanger sequence. A genomic phage clone that contained the region of the diversity was obtained by standard cloning and screening procedures. Analysis of a 15 Kb genomic phage clone (67) demonstrated that the region of divergence represented was by about 76 amino acids in the cardiac cDNA and is coded for by more than 10 Kb of the rabbit genome (Fig. 4). Sequence analysis of the intron/exon boundaries identified six distinct exons labeled A through F in order of their position in the genomic clone. These six exons could account for all of the sequences characterized in the three cloned PCR products shown in Figure 3. Further sequence analysis of the exons in this clone suggested that either exon A or B (but not both) must be used when these exons are assembled in order to maintain the appropriate reading from downstream. Exons A and B are thus "mutually exclusive" exons. The next four exons (C–F) that were identified are 7, 5, 6, and 23 amino acids long, respectively. Exons C through F are cassette-type exons: any combination of these exons could be assembled resulting in a protein that was in frame downstream from the sites of alternative splicing. A second group came to conclusions similiar to ours suggesting splicing generates the diversity, with their work based on Southern analysis and sequencing of PCR products (68).

REGULATION OF TRANSCRIPTION AND SPLICING OF THE Na⁺/Ca²⁺ EXCHANGER

More recently, alternative splicing has been described in the 5' untranslated region of the mammalian NCX1 gene (4,32). Analysis of the 5' untranslated region from several tissues identified three unique ends of different messages. This could occur by the use of three independent promoter regions and the subsequent splicing to the conserved region at –34 bp upstream of the start codon. Another explanation is that there is a single promotor and alternative

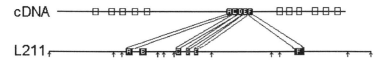

Figure 4   Rabbit cardiac cDNA for the Na^+/Ca^{2+} exchanger aligned with a genomic clone. cDNA containing exons A-C-D-E-F are shown with the genomic sequences from phage clone L211. (Based on data in Ref. 67.)

splicing of these different 5' ends onto the conserved sequences. We assume that these different 5' untranslated ends could reflect differential promotor activity and/or that splicing could be important for message stability or for the efficiency of translation in different tissues. Work on cat 5' splicing strongly suggests that the different 5' ends are due to the presence of tissue-selective promotors that are differentially expressed (32).

OTHER Na$^+$/Ca^{2+} EXCHANGER GENES

The Na$^+$/Ca^{2+} exchanger has recently been demonstrated to be a family of genes with very similar function but whose sequence can be remarkably different. Philpson's laboratory demonstrated that a second Na$^+$/Ca^{2+} exchanger gene, NCX2, exists and is expressed in rat brain. NCX2 was identified using their previously successful expression cloning strategy (69). The sequence has 66% amino acid identity when compared to the original Na$^+$/Ca^{2+} exchanger, NCX1. The NCX2-derived Na$^+$/Ca^{2+} exchanger appears to function in a similar manner to that derived from NCX1 except that it displays a decreased affinity for the binding of intracellular Ca^{2+} (69). The NCX2 gene has only been characterized in the rat.

Another Na$^+$/Ca^{2+} exchanger gene was originally described in the rods of the retina and is generally referred to as the Na$^+$/Ca^{2+}, K$^+$ exchanger. The rod exchanger has an activity quite similar to the classic Na$^+$/Ca^{2+} exchange activity. This exchanger produces an Na$^+$-dependent Ca^{2+} flux but differs in that high concentrations of K$^+$ inhibit and only 10 μM extracellular La^{3+} abolish the activity (71,72). The exchanger in the rods can transport Sr^{3+} but not Ba^{2+} or other divalent ions. Cloning of this exchanger has demonstrated that the rod Na$^+$/Ca^{2+}, K$^+$ exchanger has a similar overall structure to the heart form: there are the same number of putative transmembrane regions and an intracellular loop region and a potential leader peptide. There are only two regions in which there is reasonable amino acid identity between the bovine rod and the human or canine cardiac exchangers. The second and third transmembrane regions and the seventh and eighth transmembrane regions have about 40% amino acid identity in this restricted portion of these two proteins. Three proteins involved with Ca^{2+} movement including the Na$^+$/Ca^{2+} exchanger, the rod Na$^+$/Ca^{2+}, K exchanger (72), and the ryanodine receptor (73), have clustered stretches of acidic residues. The importance of these regions is not known.

PRESENT AND FUTURE WORK

Four questions are being investigated particularly vigorously today. First, what purpose is served by the multiple Na$^+$/Ca^{2+} exchanger genes and of the isoforms of NCX1? To date only modest functional differences have been identified and no clear physiological purpose has been determined. Nevertheless, it is an underlying assumption that the tissue-specific isoforms of NCX1 must be important. Do the different Na^+/Ca^{2+} exchanger proteins exist to facilitate subcellular localization? Are they important in protein–protein interactions with the Na^+/Ca^{2+} exchanger? Do they alter the biophysical properties of the Na^+/Ca^{2+} exchanger? The co-existence of NCX2 and NCX1 in the brain must also be important and all of these questions apply to the new gene products as well. Second, what is the nature of the physiological regulation of the Na^+/Ca^{2+} exchanger? It is certainly clear that intracellular and extracellular ion concentrations affect the turnover rate of the Na^+/Ca^{2+} exchanger. It is not at all clear *how* $[Ca^{2+}]_i$, $[Na^+]_i$ or $[H^+]_i$ acts as a regulator (rather than a transport factor) (see 76,77). Which phosphorylation sites on the Na^+/Ca^{2+} exchanger are important? What kinases actively modulate the function of the Na^+/Ca^{2+} exchanger? Are there additional modulatory proteins that affect the Na^+/Ca^{2+} exchanger? Third, what are the controls that regulate Na^+/Ca^{2+} exchanger gene expression? What are the regulatory domains of the gene(s)? What signals turn on gene expression? How are these signals recruited during development or disease? Finally, What are the biophysical properties of the Na^+/Ca^{2+} exchanger? Where do Ca^{2+} or Na^+ ions bind on the intracellular and on the extracellular face of the Na^+/Ca^{2+} exchanger protein? Is the binding site in the electrical field of the membrane? What is (are) the rate-limiting step(s) in transport? How does that change during physiological activation? Is the stoichiometry of transport always constant? How do cofactors change the biophysics?

The existence of multiple Na^+/Ca^{2+} exchanger genes and multiple isoforms of NCX1 will certainly facilitate the broad investigation of the structure and function of the Na^+/Ca^{2+} exchanger. Furthermore, the recently described *Drosophila* Na^+/Ca^{2+} exchanger (74,75) will undoubtedly aid in these investigations.

REFERENCES

1. Blaustein MP, Dipolo R, Reeves J. Sodium Calcium exchanger. Ann NY Acad Sci 1991; 639:1–667.
2. Allen, TJA, Nobel D, Reuter H, eds. Sodium-Calcium Exchange. Oxford, UK: Oxford University Press, 1989.
3. Kofuji P, Hadley RW, Keival RS, Lederer WJ, Schulze DH. Expression of the Na-Ca exchanger in diverse tissues: a study using the cloned human cardiac Na-Ca exchanger. Am J Physiol 1992; 263:C1241–C1249.
4. Lee S-L, Yu SL, Lytton J. Tissue specific expression of Na^+-Ca^{2+} isoforms. J Biol Chem 1994; 269:14849–14852.
5. Crespo LM, Grantham CJ, Cannell MB. Kinetics and stochiometry and role of Na-Ca exchange mechanism in isolated cardiac myocytes. Nature 1990; 345:618–621.
6. Bers DM, Bridge JHB. Relaxation of rabbit ventricular muscle by Na-Ca exchange and sarcoplasmic reticulum calcium pump. Circ Res 1989; 65:334–342.

7. Bers DM Lederer WJ Berlin JR. Intracellular Ca transients in rat cardiac myocytes: role of Na–Ca exchange in excitation–contraction coupling. Am J Physiol 1990; 258:C944–C954.

8. Reeves JP. The sarcolemmal sodium-calcium exchange system. Curr Top Membr Transport 1985; 25:77–125.

9. Eisner DA, Lederer WJ. Na-Ca exchange: stochiometry and electrogenicity. Am J Physiol 1985; 284:C189–C202.

10. Cheng H, Lederer WJ, Cannell MB. Calcium sparks: elementary events underlying excitation-contraction coupling in heart muscle. Science 1993;262:740–744.

11. Cannell MB, Cheng H, Lederer WJ. The control of calcium release in heart muscle. Science 1995; 268:1045–1050.

12. Leblanc N, Hume JR. Sodium-current-induced release of Ca from cardiac sarcoplasmic reticulum. Science 1990; 248:372–376.

13. Lipp P, Niggli E. Sodium-current induced calcium signals in isolated guinea-pig ventricular myocytes. J Physiol 1994; 474:439–446.

14. Sham JSK, Cleemann L, Morad M. Gating of the cardiac Ca^{2+} release channel: the role of Na$^+$ current and Na$^+$-Ca^{2+} exchange. Science 1992; 255:850–853.

15. Philipson KD, Longoni S, Ward R. Purification of the cardiac Na$^+$-Ca^{2+} exchange protein. Biochim Biophys Acta 1988; 945:298–306.

16. Ambesi A, Vanalstyne EL, Bagwell EE, Lindenmayer GE. Effect of polyclonal antibodies on the sodium-calcium exchanger. Ann NY Acad Sci 1991; 639:245–247.

17. Nicoll DA, Longoni S, Philipson KD. Molecular cloning and functional expression of the cardiac sarcolemmal Na$^+$-Ca^{2+} exchanger. Science 1990;250:562–565.

18. Kozak M. Structural features in eucaryotic mRNAs that modulate the initiation of translation. J Biol Chem 1991; 266:19867–19870.

19. Durkin JT, Ahrens DC, Pan Y-EC, Reeves JP. Purification and amino-terminal sequence of the bovine cardiac sodium-calcium exchanger: evidence for the presence of a signal sequence. Arch Biochem Biophys 1991; 290:369–375.

20. von Heijne G. Signal for protein targeting into and across membranes. Subcell Biochem 1994; 22:1–19.

21. Lebovitz RM, Takeyasu K, Fambrough DM. Molecular characterization and expression of the (Na$^+$ +K$^+$)-ATPase alpha subunit in *Drosophila melanogaster*. EMBO J 1989; 8:193–202.

22. Li Z, Nicoll DA, Collins A, Hilgemann DW, Filoteo AG, et al. Identification of a peptide inhibitor of the cardiac sarcolemmal Na$^+$-Ca^{2+} exchanger. J Biol Chem 1991; 266:1014–1020.

23. Hryshko LV, Nicoll DA, Weiss JN, Philipson KD. Biosynthesis and initial processing of the cardiac sarcolemmal Na$^+$-Ca^{2+} exchanger. Biochim Biophys Acta 1993; 1151:35–42.

24. Komuro I, Wenninger KE, Philipson DK, Izumo S. Molecular cloning and characterization of ther human cardiac Na$^+$/Ca^{2+} exchanger cDNA. Proc Natl Acad Sci 1992; 89:4769–4773.

25. Shull GE, Greeb J, Lingrel JB. Molecular cloning of three distinct forms of the Na$^+$, K$^+$-ATPase α-subunit from rat brain. Biochemistry 1986;25:8125–8132.

26. Takeyasu K, Tankum MM, Renaud KJ, Fambrough DM. Ouabain-sensitive (Na$^+$ + K$^+$)-ATPase activity expressed in mouse L cells by transfection with DNA encoding the α-subunit of an avian sodium pump. J Biol Chem 1988; 263:4347–4354.

27. Powers PA, Liu S, Hogan K, Gregg RG. Skeletal muscle and brain isoforms of a β-subunit of human voltage-dependent calcium channels are encoded by a single gene. J Biol Chem 1992; 267: 22967–22972.

28. Low W, Kasir J, Rahamimoff H. Cloning of the rat heart Na$^+$-Ca^{2+} exchanger and its functional expression in HeLa cells. FEBS Lett 1993; 316:63–67.

29. Aceto JF, Condresscu M, Kroupis C, Nelson H, Nicoll DA, et al. Cloning and expression of the bovine sodium-calcium exchanger. Arch Biochem Biophys 1992; 298:553–560.

30. Tsuruya Y, Bersohn MM, Li Z, Nicoll DA, Philipson KD. Molecular cloning and functional expression of the guinea pig cardiac Na$^+$-Ca^{2+} exchanger. Biochim Biophys Acta 1994; 1196:97–99.

31. Kim I, Lee CO. Cloning of mouse cardiac Na$^+$/Ca^{2+} exchanger and functional expression in *Xenopus* oocytes. Ann NY Acad Sci 1996; 779:126–128.

32. Barnes KV, Dawson MM, Menick DR. Initial characterization of the feline sodium-calcium exchanger. Ann NY Acad Sci 1996; 779.

33. von Heijne G. Patterns of amino acids near signal-sequence cleavage sites. Eur J Biochem 1983; 133:17–21.

34. Guan X-M, Kobilka TS, Kobilka BK. Enhancement of membrane insertion and function in type IIIb membrane protein following introduction of a cleavable signal peptide. J Biol Chem 1992; 267:21995–21998.

35. Tam LY, Loo TW, Clarke DM, Reithmeier RAF. Identification of an internal topographic signal sequence in human band 3, the erythrocyte anion exchanger. J Biol Chem 1994; 269:32542–32550.

36. Reithmeier RAF. Mammalian exchangers and cotransporters. Curr Opin Cell Biol 1994; 6:583–594.

37. Loo TW, Clarke DM. Prolonged association of temperature-sensitive mutants of human P-glycoprotein with calnexin during biogenesis. J Biol Chem 1994; 269:28683–28689.

38. Zhang J-T, Lee CH, Duthie M, Ling V. Topological determinants of internal transmembrane segments in P-glyocoprotein sequences. J Biol Chem 1995; 270:1742–1746.

39. Loo TW, Ho C, Clarke DM. Expression of a functionally active human renal sodium-calcium exchanger lacking a signal sequence. J Biol Chem 1995; 270:19345–19350.

40. Furman I, Cook O, Kasir J, et al. The putative amino-terminal signal peptide of the cloned rat brain Na$^+$-Ca^{2+} exchanger gene (RBE-1) is not mandatory for functional expression. J Biol Chem 1995; 270:19120–19127.

41. Sahin-Toth M, Nicoll DA, Franks JS, et al. The cleaved N-terminal signal sequence of the cardiac Na$^+$-Ca^{2+} exchanger is not required for functional membrane integration. Biochem Biophys Res Commun 1995; 212:968–974.

42. Klingenberg M. Membrane protein oligomeric structure and transport function. Nature 1981; 290:449–454.

43. Fafournoux P, Noel J, Pouyssegur J. Evidence that Na$^+$/H$^+$ exchanger isoforms NHE1 and NHE3 exist as stable dimers in membranes with a high degree of specificity for homodimers. J Biol Chem 1994; 269:2589–2596.

44. Li Z, Frank JS, Bennett V. et al. The cardiac Na$^+$-Ca^{2+} exchanger binds to the cytoskeletal protein ankyrin. J Biol Chem 1993; 268:11489–11491.

45. Kieval RS, Bloch RJ, Lindenmayer GE, et al. Immunofluorescence localization of the Na-Ca exchanger in heart cells. Am J Physiol 1992; 263:C545–C550.

46. Frank JS, Mottino G, Reid D, et al. Distribution of the Na$^+$-Ca^{2+} exchanger protein in mammalian cardiac myocytes: an immunofluorescence and immunocolloidal gold labeling study. J Cell Biol 1992; 117:337–345.

47. Reilly RF, Shugrue CA, Lattanzi D, Biemesderfer D. Immunolocalization of the Na$^+$/Ca^{2+} exchanger in rabbit kidney. Am J Physiol 1993; 265:F327–F332.

48. Bourdeau JE, Taylor AN, Iacopino AM. Immunocytochemical localization of the sodium-calcium exchanger in canine nephron. J Am Soc Nephrol 1993; 4:105–110.

49. Hilgemann DW, Nicoll DA, Philipson KD. Charge movement during Na$^+$ translocation by native and clone cardiac Na$^+$/Ca^{2+} exchanger. Nature 1991; 352:715–718.

50. Matsuoka S, Nicoll DA, Reilly RF, et al. Initial localization of regulatory regions of the cardiac sarcolemmal Na$^+$-Ca^{2+} exchanger. Proc Natl Acad Sci 1993; 90:3870–3874.

51. Levitsky DO, Nicoll DA, Philipson KD. Identification of the high affinity Ca^{2+}-binding domain of the cardiac Na$^+$-Ca^{2+} exchanger. J Biol Chem 1994; 269:22847–22852.

52. Iwamoto T, Wakabayashi S, Shigekawa M. Growth factor-induced phosphorylation and activation of aortic smooth muscle Na$^+$/Ca^{2+} exchanger. J Biol Chem 1995; 270:8996–9001.

53. Condrescu M, Gardner JP, Chernaya G, et al. ATP-dependent regualtion of sodium-calcium exchange in chinese hamster ovary cells transfected with bovine cardiac sodium-calcium exchanger. J Biol Chem 1995; 270:9137–9146.

54. Smith L, Prozig H, Lee H-W, et al. Phorbol esters downregulate expression of the sodium/calcium exchanger in renal epithelial cells. Am J Physiol 1995; 269:C457–C463.

55. Nicoll DA, Hryshko LV, Matsuoka S, et al. Mutagenesis studies of the cardiac Na$^+$-Ca^{2+} exchanger. Ann NY Acad Sci 1996; 779:86–92.

56. Marlier LNJ-L, Zheng T, Tang J et al. Regional distribution in the rat central nervous system of a mRNA encoding a portion of the cardiac sodium/calcium exchange isolated from cerebellar granule neurons. Mol Brain Res 1993; 20:21–39.

57. Moolenaar WH. Regulation of cytoplasmic pH by Na$^+$/H$^+$ exchange. Trends Biochem Sci 1986; 11:141–143.

58. Palmer RG. Voltage-dependent block by amiloride and other monovalent cations of apical Na channels in the toad urinary bladder. J Memb Biol 1984; 80:153–165.

59. Wacholtz MC, Cragoe EJ, Lipsky PE. Delineation of the role of the Na$^+$/Ca^{2+} exchanger in regulating intracellular Ca^{2+} in T cells. Cell Immunol 1993; 147:95–109.

60. Donnadieu E, Trautmann A. Is there a Na$^+$/Ca^{2+} exchanger in macrophages and in lymphocytes. Pflugers Arch 1993; 424:448–455.

61. Lipp P, Schwaller B, Niggli E. Specific inhibition of Na-Ca exchange function by antisense oligonucleotides. FEBS Lett 1995; 364:198–202.

62. Luo S, Lederer, WJ, Schulze, DH. Striking homology in the 3' untranslated region of NCX1 cDNAs. Biophys J 1996; 70:A202.

63. Boerth SR, Zimmer DB, Artman M. Steady-state mRNA levels of the sarcolemmal Na^+-Ca^{2+} exchanger peak near birth in developing rabbit and rat hearts. Circ Res 1994; 74:354–359.

64. Studer R, Reinecke H, Bilger J, et al. Gene expression of the cardiac Na^+-Ca^{2+} exchanger in end-stage human heart failure. Circ Res 1994; 75:443–453.

65. Reilly RF, Shugrue CA. cDNA cloning of a renal Na^+-Ca^{2+} exchanger. Am J Physiol 1992; 262:F1105–F1109.

66. Kofuji P, Lederer WJ, Schulze DH. Na/Ca exchanger isoforms expressed in the heart and kidney. Am J Physiol 1993;2 63:C1241–C1249.

67. Kofuji P, Lederer WJ, Schulze DH. Mutually exculsive and cassette exons underlie alternatively spliced isoforms of the Na/Ca exchanger. J Biol Chem 1994; 269:14849–14852.

68. Nakasaki Y, Iwamoto T, Hanada H, et al. Cloning of the rat aortic smooth muscle Na^+/Ca^{2+} exchanger and tissue-specific expression of isoforms. J Biochem 1993;144:528–534.

69. Li Z, Matsuoka S, Hryshko LV, et al. Cloning of the NCX2 isoform of the plasma membrane Na^+-Ca^{2+} exchanger. J Biol Chem 1994; 269:17434–17439.

70. Cervetto L, Lagnado L, Robinson DW, McNaughton PA. Extrusion of calcium from rod outer segments is driven by both sodium and potassium gradients. Nature 1989; 337:740–743.

71. Yau KW, Nakatani K. Electrogenic Na-Ca exchange in retinal rod outer segment. Nature 1984; 311:661–663.

72. Reilander HA, Achilles A, Friedel T, et al. The primary structure and functional expression of the Na/Ca, K exchanger from bovine rod photoreceptors. EMBO J 1992; 11:1689–1695.

73. Takeshima H, Nishimura S, Matsumoto T, et al. Primary structure and expression from complementary DNA to skeletal muscle ryanodine receptor. Nature 1989; 339:439–445.

74. Valdivia C, Kofuji P, Lederer WJ, Schulze DH. Characterization of the Na/Ca exchanger cDNA in *Drosophila*. Biophys J 1994; 68:A410.

75. Schulze DH, Valdivia C, Kofuji P, et al. Alternative splicing of the intracellular loop of the Na^+/Ca^{2+} exchanger. Ann NY Acad Sci 1996; 779:46–57.

76. Doering AE, Lederer WJ. The mechanism by which cytoplasmic protons inhibit the sodium-calcium exchanger in guinea pig heart cells. J Physiol 1993; 446:481–499.

77. Doering AE, Lederer WJ. The action of Na^+ as a cofactor in the inhibition by cytoplasmic protons of the cardiac Na^+/Ca^{+2} exchanger in the guinea pig. J Physiol 1994; 480:9–20.

14

Tyrosine Kinases in the Regulation of Vascular Smooth Muscle Function

Marshall A. Corson and Bradford C. Berk
University of Washington
Seattle, Washington

Vascular smooth muscle cells (VSMC) perform several functions in the blood vessel wall, according to their specific location and the presence or absence of disease. In normal vessels, VSMC exist in a nonproliferative, contractile phenotype and their level of activation by neurohumoral agonists is a major determinant of arterial and venous tone. With the development of vascular disease VSMC undergo a gradual shift to a less differentiated phenotype that is increasingly dedicated to reparative functions, such as migration, hypertrophy (increase in cell mass and ploidy), and hyperplasia (increase in cell number). These changes in VSMC biology are accompanied by fundamental alterations in protein and gene expression. A combination of biochemical and genetic approaches has yielded insights into the signal transduction mechanisms regulating these VSMC responses, which are stimulated in the pathological environment by autocrine-, paracrine- and locally derived mitogens, cytokines, and other trophic factors. Binding of these factors to their receptors triggers a pyramidal cascade of information transfer, mediated via several types of evolutionarily conserved signal processes: activation of protein kinases, direct protein–protein interactions, generation of soluble second messengers, and changes in metabolism of phosphoinositides and high-energy phosphates. These processes result in the transmission of signals positively "downstream" with consequent "upstream" negative feedback, constituting a system of checks and balances that requires sustained stimulation for cell growth. A critical role for regulation of cell function has been demonstrated for phosphorylation of signaling proteins on tyrosine residues by protein tyrosine kinases (PTK). Although phosphorylation on tyrosine constitutes only a fraction of the overall phosphorylation events in mammalian cells, it is of critical importance in signaling by myriad cell surface receptors.

This chapter will review the role of PTKs in VSMC function, with emphasis on the predominant role played by PTK cascades as a means of propagating growth signals to the cell interior. Initially we will review the major elements and principles of PTK signaling that have emerged from the study of relevant mammalian cells. Signaling components will be grouped according to their major function as receptors, adaptors, regulators, or effectors. We will compare and contrast the signal pathways activated by platelet-derived growth factor (PDGF) and angiotensin II, two important VSMC growth factors. We will then review how VSMC may adapt to changing circumstances through the utilization of PTK pathways that regulate contraction, migration, hypertrophy, and hyperplasia. Characterization of PTK pathways that mediate VSMC function should lead to the design and implementation of targeted molecular therapies to promote adaptive responses of VSMC to disease states.

RECEPTORS, ADAPTORS, REGULATORS, AND EFFECTORS OF PTK SIGNALING

Signal Initiation by Receptor PTKs

Growth factor receptors with tyrosine kinase activity possess structural features that transmit growth signals from the cell exterior to its interior. These conserved features include a large, glycosylated, extracellular ligand-binding domain, a single hydrophobic transmembrane region, and a cytoplasmic tail that contains a tyrosine kinase catalytic domain. Receptor PTKs exist in at least eight superfamilies, defined by similarities in their extracellular domains (e.g., cysteine-rich regions, immunoglobulin-like sequences), their existence as heterooligomers (hepatocyte growth factor [HGF] and insulin-like growth factor [IGF] receptor subclasses), or the presence of an insert region in their kinase domain (fibroblast growth factor [FGF] and PDGF receptor subclasses). Binding of growth factor activates the receptor by increasing phosphorylation of its intracellular domain on tyrosine residues. The precise activation mechanism is family-specific, but in all cases a conformational alteration of the receptor's extracellular domain facilitates receptor-receptor oligomerization (1). Concomitantly the tyrosine kinase activity of the oligomerized receptors is increased, resulting in transphosphorylation of neighboring intracellular domains. Receptor tyrosine phosphorylation establishes a conformation that is capable of recruiting, and forming high-affinity complexes with, cytoplasmic signaling molecules at the plasma membrane. The topography of signal molecule recruitment by the PDGF-R is shown in Figure 1. The activity of these bound molecules may be further regulated via phosphorylation by the receptor PTK, or their physical association with receptor may be sufficient to propagate mitogenic signals.

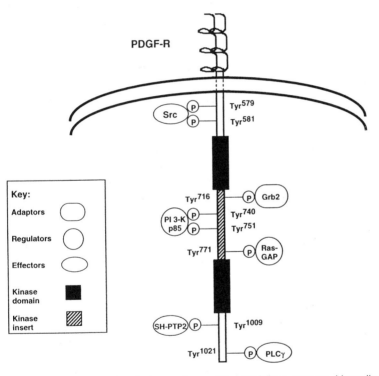

Figure 1 Signal molecule interactions of the PDGFβ receptors. Upon ligand binding, receptors oligomerize with resultant transphosphorylation of intracellular tails on multiple tyrosine residues. Only a single cytoplasmic PDGF-R domain is shown, which is notable for a long PTK domain, interrupted by a kinase insert region. The identity of tyrosines phosphorylated, as well as the signal molecules they bind, has been determined by deletion mutant analysis (9). The major adaptor recruited is Grb2, which couples PDGF-R to Ras via Sos. Regulators recruited include Ras-GAP and the p85 subunit of PI 3-K. Effectors shown to bind directly to the activated PDGF-R include Src, PLCγ, and Sh-phosphotyrosine phosphatases.

Signal Initiation by Receptors Lacking Intrinsic PTK Activity

Neurohumoral agonists that dynamically regulate vascular tone have been shown to initiate signal transduction via the seven transmembrane-spanning (heptahelical) G protein-coupled receptor superfamily. Physiologically important heptahelical receptors in VSMC include those for angiotensin II, thrombin, bradykinin, serotonin, endothelin, and the muscarinic and alpha- and beta-adrenergic agonists. These receptors share the properties that they bind to heterotrimeric G proteins and lack intrinsic PTK activity, in contrast to receptors for growth factors such as PDGF, FGF, and epidermal growth factor (EGF). The topography of heptahelical receptors is characterized by amino-terminal extracellular and carboxy-terminal intracellular "tails," connected by seven transmembrane segments with three intervening extracellular and three intracellular loops. Interactions among these domains impart specificity for agonist binding and initiate post-receptor signaling. Site-directed mutagenesis studies have shown that certain structural motifs are conserved within this superfamily of receptors and serve common functions, such as interaction with G proteins via the second transmembrane and third cytoplasmic loops (2). Additional specificity may be imparted by receptor-specific posttranslational modifications, such as palmitoylation, glycosylation, and phosphorylation. These heptahelical receptors have traditionally been viewed as evoking qualitatively similar contractile responses via Ca^{2+}-, phospholipid- and serine/threonine protein kinase-dependent pathways. More recently it has been appreciated that these receptors are also linked via PTKs to contraction in normal vessels (3), and to growth responses in pathological states (4). Although agonist-dependent tyrosine phosphorylation events have been well documented for many heptahelical receptors (see below), our understanding of the molecular bases for these interactions remains incomplete.

During inflammation and other forms of stress, VSMC are exposed to cytokines and interferons. Receptors for these ligands are composed of one to three polypeptides and are constitutively associated with members of the *Janus* *k*inase (JAK) PTK family. Although cytokine and interferon receptors are not PTKs per se, their activation mechanisms are so similar to the receptor PTKs that they should be considered in the same context. Ligand binding activities signal transduction by inducing receptor oligomerization and concomitant JAK activation, probably via a transmembrane signal resulting in the transphosphorylation of neighboring intracellular tails. As is the case for the receptor PTKs, this allows for binding of cytoplasmic signaling molecules, which may be substrates for JAK phosphorylation. The PTK substrates most often implicated in cytokine signaling are transcription factors designated Stat (*s*ignal *t*ransducers and *a*ctivators of *t*ranscription) proteins. These proteins bind specific phosphorylated tyrosines on the activated cytokine receptor, bringing them into a favored location for tyrosine phosphorylation by JAK. Upon phosphorylation they dimerize and are released for translocation to the nucleus (5). There they bind to specific promoter elements and induce gene expression. Activated and phosphorylated cytokine receptors also recruit adaptor proteins such as Shc, through which they couple to Ras, and the phosphatidylinositol 3-kinase (PI 3-K) pathways. Likewise, receptor PTKs can under some circumstances signal through JAK, although the physiological importance of this coupling has not been established (5).

Modular Domains in Intracellular Signaling

Specificity in the recruitment and activation of signaling molecules by receptor and nonreceptor PTKs is determined by sequences in both the kinases and the signaling molecules themselves. These protein–protein interactions are the consequence of highly specific interactions between tyrosine-phosphorylated proteins and modular domain-containing signaling adaptors,regulators, and effectors. Significant progress has been made recently in elucidating the bases for these interactions (6,7). For example, Src homology 2 (SH2) domains, found on many cytosolic signaling molecules, direct the interactions of these proteins with tyrosine phosphorylated receptor PTKs. Other domains, such as Src homology 3 (SH3), pleckstrin homology (PH), and the phosphotyrosine binding (PTB) domain, localize PTKs and their substrates to specific cell compartments and/or mediate specific interactions between signal and mediators.

Of these protein modules, the SH2 domain has been most extensively characterized. Consisting of approximately 100 amino acids, this globular region contains a pocket-like region that avidly binds phosphorylated tyrosines (6). Songyang and Cantley have utilized degenerate phosphopeptide libraries to identify sequence determinants of SH2 domain binding specificity. These investigators have proposed that the identity of the amino acids at the +1 and +3 positions on the carboxy-terminal side of the phosphorylated tyrosine, in combination with the identity of the residue at the 5th position of β-sheet D, is sufficient to define five functional subclasses of SH2 domains (7). For example, these sequences may dictate the preference of receptor PTKs for binding to targets such as the p85 regulatory subunit of PI 3-kinase or phospholipase C (PLC), whereas cytoplasmic PTKs such as Src may preferentially bind to other cytosolic targets.

SH3 domains are composed of approximately 60 amino acid residues and contain a proline-rich core of 10 amino acids (8). These sequences also mediate binding of molecules that are critical to PTK-based signal transduction. An example is the adaptor protein Grb2, which links activated receptor PTKs to the Ras regulator known as Sos. SH3 domains may also be important in directing the compartmentalization of cytosolic proteins, to locations such as the cytoskeleton or the plasma membrane (9). PH domains consist of two perpendicular antiparallel β-sheets followed by a C-terminal amphipathic α-helix. They are found in many types of proteins including PTKs, substrates for these kinases, effectors such as PLC and GTPases, and cytoskeletal proteins. In vitro studies suggest that PH domains function by tethering small signaling molecules to membranes, thus mediating protein–lipid interactions. However, the specific details of their function in intact systems remains to be determined. The most recently described modular domain has been designated the phosphotyrosine-binding (PTB) domain (10). First observed in Shc, a major substrate of several receptor PTKs, this domain has been found in several other important signaling proteins. In contrast to SH2 domains, PTB domains confer specificity through the amino acids located amino-terminal to phosphorylated tyrosine.

Adaptors

Various combinations of the signaling modules described above are utilized by adaptor proteins for amplification of receptor-dependent signals. For discussion purposes adaptors are defined as proteins without enzymatic activity that link activated receptors and downstream effectors through the formation of multimeric complexes. Adaptors function by providing recognition sequences that mediate binding and recruitment of effectors to specific cell locations, primarily at the cytoplasmic face of the cell membrane. In many, but not all cases, they are substrates for activated receptor PTKs, or may undergo other posttranslational modifications. Adaptors that have been particularly well studied include Grb2, Shc, and IRS-1. Grb2 is a bimodular protein that recognizes and binds to tyrosine-phosphorylated receptor PTKs via its SH2 domain, and to regulators or effectors via its SH3 domain. Much as the combination of SH2 and SH3 domains confer bifunctionality on Grb2, the combination of SH2 and PTB confers bifunctionality on Shc. In contrast to Grb2, Shc also appears to be regulated by tyrosine phosphorylation outside of its SH2 and PTB domains (11). IRS-1 is the major adaptor protein for receptor PTKs of the insulin/IGF-1 class, and has also been shown to bind to some cytokine receptors such as IL-4 (12). IRS-1 may be the most complex cytoplasmic adaptor molecular yet described: it contains a PH domain and at least eight tyrosine residues that are known to mediate interactions with SH2 domains of adaptors (e.g., Grb2), regulators (e.g., the 85 kD regulatory subunit of PI 3-K), and effectors (e.g., SH-phosphotyrosine phosphatase 2). A recent development is the identification of a novel IRS-1 analog, suggesting the possibility of further diversity in signaling through a multigene family (12).

The 14-3-3 family is a recently recognized class of adaptor proteins that mediates interactions between serine/threonine protein kinases and PTK signaling pathways. Because these proteins appear to function by recruiting Protein

Kinase C (PKC) and Raf-1 to the membrane and stabilizing their interaction with other effectors (e.g., Ras-Raf-1) or substrates, 14-3-3 proteins have been described as chaperones (13). 14-3-3 isoforms interact principally with the regulatory domain of Raf-1 at its zinc-finger domain, as well as less weakly interacting with its serine kinase domain (14). These proteins have been found to contain phosphoserine, -threonine and -tyrosine, but it is not known whether these modifications constitute regulatory events.

Regulators

Regulators are defined as adaptors that in addition to coupling receptor and effector also dynamically affect the latter's activity. This group includes the heterotrimeric G proteins, a novel class designated Regulators of G-protein Signaling (RGS), GTPase activators such as Ras-GTPase Activating Protein (Ras-GAP), and guanine nucleotide exchange factors such as Sos. The heterotrimeric G proteins have been well characterized in their ability to activate effectors such as phopholipases (A, C, and D), in VSMC as well as other mesodermal cells. Heterotrimeric G proteins consist of an α-subunit that contains the guanine-nucleotide-binding site and intrinsic GTPase activity, and a $\beta\gamma$-subunit complex (15). $G\beta\gamma$ increases the affinity of the $G\alpha$ subunit for receptors with which it interacts, and it regulates effectors, in combination with the $G\alpha$ subunit or as an isolated complex. There are currently 18 distinct $G\alpha$ subunits, organized into four subclasses on the basis of sequence and functional homology ($G\alpha s$, $G\alpha i$, $G\alpha o$, and $G\alpha q$). There are five known $G\beta$ subunits and seven $G\gamma$ subunits; $G\beta\gamma$ is cotranslationally expressed and always acts as a heterodimer. It now appears that $G\beta\gamma$ couples activated vasoconstrictor receptors to Ras-dependent responses (see below). RGS proteins comprise a multigene family that appears to regulate negatively the signals generated by heptahelical receptors through effects on $G\alpha$ subunits (16). The GTPase activators and guanine nucleotide exchange factors are negative and positive regulators, respectively, of the superfamily of effectors having in common a regulated GTPase cycle. These will be discussed in the following section.

Effectors

Ras, Raf

Like many other transducers of cell growth signals, *Ras* genes were first identified as the oncogenic principles of transforming retroviruses. Subsequently these oncogenes were found to represent the mutated alleles of cellular *Ras* genes. An important role for Ras in growth of normal cells was suggested by several findings. *Ras* genes are highly conserved throughout evolution. They encode proteins that bind guanine nucleotides, possess GTPase activity, and are associated with the plasma membrane. These properties, combined with their significant homology with heterotrimeric G proteins, suggested that Ras proteins participate in transmembrane signaling. A critical role for Ras in the transmission of signals from PTKs to cytoplasmic serine/threonine kinases was suggested by the observation that antibodies that neutralize Ras function could block transformation by PTK oncogenes but did not abrogate transformation by serine/threonine kinases (17).

Insights gained recently have markedly enhanced our understanding of the mechanisms utilized by Ras for transduction of growth signals. In particular three advances have made such a level of understanding possible: identification of the guanine nucleotide exchange factors of the Sos class, elucidation of the role of adaptor proteins such as Grb2 that link activated receptors to Sos, and the discovery that Raf kinase is a direct Ras effector. Early characterization of Ras proteins revealed that transforming mutations maintained the protein in a GTP-bound activated state, and these mutations were thought either to inhibit the intrinsic GTPase activity of Ras or to increase markedly the dissociation rate of GDP from (inactive) Ras. Either mechanism was consistent with the concept that Ras activity is dependent upon the nature of the guanosine-phosphorylated species bound, and upstream proteins that might affect the distribution of GTP- and GDP-bound Ras molecules within a given cell were then sought. The first such Ras exchange protein to be discovered was the CDC25 gene product in the yeast *Saccharomyces cerevisiae* (17). This protein and its subsequently described mammalian homologs accelerate the rate of GDP release, resulting in more rapid GTP binding and sustained Ras activation. Cycling of GTP-GDP occurs in a tightly regulated manner: the exchange protein binds to the GDP-bound form of Ras, reducing the affinity of Ras for GDP. GDP then dissociates from Ras and the resulting short-lived exchange factor–Ras complex is displaced by ambient GTP, again producing activated Ras.

Isolation of the *Drosophila* homolog of the CDC25 gene, named *SOS*, was followed by the cloning of two closely related mammalian counterparts, *Sos1* and *Sos2* (18). Biochemical studies revealed that recombinant Sos proteins are able to increase GDP/GTP exchange by Ras in vitro (17), confirming their identity as exchange factors. However the mechanism by which Sos activity could be increased after receptor activation was initially unknown. An additional adaptor protein was subsequently found utilizing a strategy in which the phosphorylated intracellular domain of the EGF-R was used as a probe to bind cytoplasmic molecules, one of which was isolated and characterized as Grb2 (19). Several groups were able to demonstrate that Grb2 and Sos are associated in a complex, and that the complex translocates to activated PTK receptors upon ligand binding and autophosphorylation. Thus the identity of the major pathway linking PTK receptors to Ras is now established, and assembly of the signal transfer complex upon PTK receptor phosphorylation is thought to be sufficient to stimulate guanine nucleotide cycling in Ras. While concurrent studies showed that RasGAP inhibits Ras by increasing the hydrolysis of GTP, Sos stimulates Ras by increasing the rate of release of GDP and reentry into the GTP-binding state. In contrast the links between heptahelical receptors and Ras are less clear.

Agonists for thrombin, lysophosphatidic acid, and m2 muscarinic heptahelical receptors have been shown to activate Ras (20,21). Several non-exclusive mechanisms have been proposed to explain this receptor coupling to ras: activation by G protein $\beta\gamma$ subunits, by adaptor(s) such as Grb2/Sos and/ or Shc, or a receptor-associated PTK. The G_i subclass of G proteins has recently been shown to mediate Ras activation through a multimeric signal complex involving the PH domain of its $G\beta\gamma$ subunit, Shc, Grb2, and Sos (22). Upon the interaction of $G\beta\gamma$ with Shc the latter becomes tyrosine phosphorylated by an unknown PTK, increasing its affinity for Grb2. Activation of Ras then proceeds through Gr2b/Sos, as is the case for activation by receptor PTKs (23). Linkage of other G proteins to Ras has not been directly demonstrated.

Ras is the principal member of a superfamily of over 50 low-molecular-weight GTPases, which can be further classified into five subfamilies according to structural and functional resemblance. Ras subfamily members play critical roles in cell growth and development. The Ras-related GTPase Rap1 has been found in VSMC and is upregulated by PDGF, but the physiological significance of these events remains to be proven (24). Rab/Arf subfamily members monitor and direct the movements of vesicles within cells. Ran is required for nuclear protein import, and Rho family members play dynamic roles in the regulation of the actin cytoskeleton (25). The activity of individual family members is similarly modulated, as is Ras, by guanine nucleotide exchange factors (positively) and by GTPase-activating proteins (negatively). A potentially important convergence point for pathways regulating growth and cytoskeletal rearrangement may be indicated by the recent observations that rho family members can associate directly with receptor PTKs (26) and may also regulate downstream mediators of the mitogen-activated protein kinase (MAPK) cascade through the intermediary kinase PAK (25).

Recent studies have established that activated Ras transmits a mitogenic signal downstream to the serine/threonine kinase Raf-1 and ultimately to downstream effector MAPKs as a consequence of direct Ras–Raf-1 intermolecular interactions. Raf-1 consists of three regions, CR1, CR2, and CR3, that are conserved through evolution and among the Raf-1 isoforms (27). CR1 consists of a Ras-binding domain, CR2 a serine/threonine-rich region with multiple phosphorylation sites, and CR3 is the carboxy-terminal catalytic domain. By covalently linking wild-type and mutant Ras proteins to an insoluble matrix, Wolfman and colleagues demonstrated that Raf-1 binding to Ras in stimulated cell lysates required the presence of GTP or a nonhydrolyzable GTP analogue to activate the MAPK cascade (28). Further evidence for direct interaction of activated Ras and Raf in signal transduction has come from studies using the yeast two-hybrid screening system to detect protein–protein interactions (29). These observations have been confirmed in several laboratories (30, 31). It is likely that additional modulators can further increase the activation of Raf-1 by Ras, such as the 14-3-3 proteins described above, which recruit Raf-1 to the cell membrane for interaction with Ras, and heat-shock proteins such as hsp50 and hsp90 (32).

The MAPK Superfamily

MAPKs are universal serine/threonine protein kinases activated in response to a variety of extracellular stimuli involved in cell growth, transformation, and differentiation (33). The MAPK superfamily is now recognized as comprising three major kinase subgroups, based on their activation motifs. The proximal activators of these subgroups are also distinct. The subgroup initially described, consisting of extracellular signal regulated kinase (ERK) 1 and ERK 2, are strongly activated by PTK receptors, as well as heptahelical receptors, through dual phosphorylation on threonine and tyrosine residues found within the motif Thr-Glu-Tyr (34). The kinases responsible for phosphorylation of ERK1/2 are designated MAP or ERK kinase (MEK). MEKs are unique because they can phosphorylate both tyrosine and threonine residues on ERK1/2 and are thus considered to be dual-specificity kinases (35). Overexpression of constitutively active MEK-1 protein in NIH 3T3 cells stimulates mitogenesis and transformation (36, 37), demonstrating the importance of ERK1/2 in the transduction of growth stimulatory signals. MEK-1 is thought to be regulated primarily via serine phosphorylation by the Raf-1 kinase; however, the possibility of MEK activation via non-Ras/Raf-dependent pathways has not been conclusively ruled out. A new member of this subclass, designated ERK5 or BMK-1, although possessing the Thr-Glu-Tyr motif, appears to be selectively responsive to certain forms of oxidative stress (38). It is specifically phosphorylated and activated by the recently cloned MEK-5 (39).

The MAPK subgroup containing the activation motif Thr-Pro-Tyr comprises the Jun N-terminal or stress-activated protein kinase (JNK/SAPK) family (40). These kinases are activated by a unique upstream SAPK kinase, known as MEK-4 or SEK, in response to cytokines and ultraviolet (UV) light. The third subfamily, possessing the activation motif Thr-Gly-Tyr, is currently known to consist of the 63 kD ERK3 (33) and the p38 MAPK (41). The latter kinase is activated by inflammatory stimuli such as interleukin-1, TNF and lipopolysaccharide (42) via phosphorylation by MEK-3 (43).

The in vivo substrates for ERK1/2 have not been conclusively identified; however, ERK1/2 can phosphorylate a wide variety of proteins in vitro, including the kinase that phosphorylates ribosomal S6 protein, pp90^{rsk} (44), cytosolic phospholipase A$_2$ (45), and the transcription factor p62^{TCF}, also called elk-1 or SAP-1). Phosphorylation of p62^{TCF} by ERK1/2 that has translocated to the nucleus may increase the expression of many growth-related genes via enhanced ternary complex formation among p62^{TCF}, serum response factor, and the serum response element in early immediate gene promoter regions (46). A cytoplasmic ERK1/2 substrate, involved in the initiation of the rate-limiting step in protein synthesis, is the mRNA cap-binding protein eukaryotic initiation factor 4E (eIF-4E) (47). This protein forms a complex with eIF-4A and p220 and binds mRNA to facilitate attachment of the ribosome (48). The eIF-4E protein is phosphorylated in response to mitogenic stimuli, resulting in partial enhancement of eIF-4E activity and initiation of translation. eIF-4E is also regulated by association with an inhibitory binding protein, 4E-BP1 (also known as PHAS-1). ERK1/2 was recently shown to phosphorylate 4E-BP1 and stimulate the release of eIF-4E, allowing it to interact with mRNA (49). This phosphorylation event provides a direct link between growth factor receptor binding and protein synthesis (independent of new gene expression) via the ERK1/2 pathway.

PI 3-K Pathway

Another important mitogenic pathway stimulated by receptor PTKs is initiated by the actions of phosphatidylinositol 3-K (PI 3-K). Analysis of PDGFβ-R deletion mutants by Williams and colleagues demonstrated that activation of PI 3-K is required for mitogenic signaling by PDGFβ-R. The 85 kD regulatory subunit of PI 3-K binds PDGFβ-R via its C-terminal SH2 domain (50). Subsequently the 110 kD PI 3-K effector subunit is recruited to a neighboring region of the 85 kD regulatory subunit and is activated. This kinase then phosphorylates membrane phosphatidylinositides (PtdIns) at the 3-position of the inositol ring, generating PtdIns3-P, PtdIns(3,4)P$_2$, and PtdIns(3,4,5) P$_3$. These phosphorylated species are thought to function as mitogenic second messengers, since no phospholipase has been found that can cleave inositol that is phosphorylated at the 3 position. However, until recently the targets of these phosphorylated lipid species were unclear.

Now there is growing evidence that targets include the serine/threonine kinase designated Akt/PKB, and some members of the PKC superfamily. Akt/PKB was discovered by virtue of its homology with PKC and PKA, and was found to be the cellular homolog of the transforming oncogene *v-Akt* (51). Akt/PKB consists of a carboxy-terminal catalytic domain and an amino-terminal PH domain, and is rapidly activated by a variety of mitogens. Three complementary lines of evidence have linked PDGFβ-R to Akt/PKB activation via PI 3-K: (a) PDGFβ-R mutants that fail to activate PI-3K also fail to activate Akt/PKB, (b) a dominant-negative mutant of PI 3-K inhibits PDGF-induced activation of Akt/PKB, and (c) activation of Akt/PKB by growth factors is inhibited by low concentrations of wortmannin, a specific inhibitor of PI 3-K (52). It has been suggested, but remains to be proven, that the lipid products of PI 3-K regulate the state of Akt/PKB dimerization and its consequent activation via intermolecular phosphorylation reactions (53). Such a phosphoinositide-protein regulatory mechanism has recently been demonstrated for the β-adrenergic-receptor kinase PH domain (54). Akt/PKB may further transmit mitogenic signals to the 70 kD S6 kinase, which is believed to be required for the transition of cells from G1 to S phase of the cell cycle (55). This S6 kinase has previously shown to be activated independently of the 90 kD ribosomal S6 kinase that is downstream of ERK1/2. Cotransfection of activated Akt/PKB mutants with 70 kD S6 kinase stimulate the latter's kinase activity (56), and wortmannin also inhibits its activation by PDGF (53). However, a dominant negative Akt/PKB experiment to test its role in 70 kD S6 kinase activation has not yet been reported.

Several additional considerations regarding the mitogenic signaling of PI 3-K are noteworthy. Isoform divesity of the 110 kD catalytic subunit has recently been reported. Of potential importance for VSMC signaling is the discovery of a γ form that does not interact with the 85 kD regulatory subunit but is activated by heterotrimeric G protein α_i and βγ subunits. Also, the α and β isoforms of the 110 kD PI 3-K catalytic subunit can under some circumstances be activated directly by Ras (52). Linkage of physiological VSMC receptors to PI 3-K targets via G proteins or via Ras is thus an attractive possibility that remains to be explored. It is also likely that other targets exist for the distinctive phospholipid products of activated PI 3-Ks.

Src Kinases

The 60 kD Src kinase is the best-characterized member of a family of nine cytoplasmic protein PTKs that participate in growth signal transduction. Tissue-specific expression of alternatively spliced gene products yields at least 14 different Src-related kinases (57). Three family members (Src, Fyn, and Yes) are expressed ubiquitously and studies utilizing transgenes suggest that their functions may be at least partially overlapping (58). Family members possess conserved functional domains that constitute a basis for common modes of regulation. These include an amino-terminal myristoylation sequence for membrane targeting, SH2 and SH3 domains, a kinase domain, and a carboxy-terminal noncatalytic domain. These regions participate in a complex tonic inhibition of Src kinases that can be overcome in cells exposed to mitogens.

Src kinase was initially identified as the cellular homolog of pp60^{v-Src}, the transforming gene of the Rous sarcoma virus. The oncogenic and cellular Src kinases resemble one another in overall domain structure. However, they differ significantly at the carboxy-terminus, where 19 amino acids of Src are replaced with 12 novel amino acids in v-Src, probably due to recombination events occurring during retroviral capture of the cellular *Src* gene. One of the residues that appears to be critical for regulation of Src is a Tyr at position 527, which is not present in v-Src. Phosphorylation of this tyrosine residue by C Src Kinase (Csk) family members inhibits Src kinase activity, whereas dephosphorylation of this residue appears to be an activating mechanism (59). Phosphorylation of Tyr^{416} in the catalytic domain may be an activating signal; the kinase(s) responsible have not been identified. Src activity is also inhibited via intramolecular interactions of the carboxy-terminal catalytic domains with both the SH2 and SH3 domains (60). In addition to these inhibitory functions of the SH2 and SH3 domains, they probably also stimulate Src activity through interactions with regulators and downstream kinase substrates.

The role of Src kinases in proliferation of somatic cells is under intense investigation. Following PDGF stimulation of quiescent fibroblasts, the Src, Yes, and Fyn kinases were shown to bind through their SH2 domains to the PDGFβ-R on phosphorylated Tyr^{579} and ^{581} (61). Mutant receptors lacking these tyrosines retain the ability to transduce PDGF-stimulated DNA synthesis as efficiently as wild-type, suggesting several possibilities: Src may not be required for PDGF-stimulated mitogenesis, it may be activated through another mechanism, or other intermediates may fulfill its signaling functions. In subsequent studies, microinjection of kinase-inactive forms of, or antibodies to, Src, Fyn, and Yes, markedly inhibited PDGF-stimulated mitogenesis, supporting a critical role for Src kinases (62). An alternative explanation for this series of findings is that a PDGF receptor-associated protein–tyrosine phosphatase (e.g., syp/SH-PTP) may dephosphorylate Src at Tyr^{527}, activating it in concert with the allosteric effects mediated by binding to receptor Tyr$^{579/581}$. A finding lending credence to this concept is that overexpression of receptor-like protein tyrosine phosphatase-α activates a signaling pathway that includes Src, activation and nuclear translocation of MAPK, with resultant phosphorylation and transactivation of c-Jun (63). Further evidence for an important role for Src kinases in mitogenesis was likewise suggested by a study in which coexpression of Src was necessary to obtain maximal kinase activity of Raf-1 by v-Raf using baculovirus expression vectors in insect cells (64).

FAK Family

Because changes in cytoskeletal architecture are intimately related to cell proliferation and differentiation, there has been intense interest in the role of PTKs in mediating these effects of growth factors. A heavily tyrosine-phosphorylated 125 kD protein, originally isolated from *v-Src*-transformed chicken embryo fibroblasts by Parsons and co-workers (65), was found to localize at specialized sites of cell adhesion known as focal adhesion complexes. Subsequent analysis revealed that this protein possesses PTK activity towards other proteins with which it colocalizes at these sites, such as paxillin (66). These findings indicated that this PTK, designated pp 125 focal adhesion kinase (FAK), may be a link between activated growth factor receptors and cytoskeletal rearrangements necessary for mitosis. This role is consistent with the observation in *v-src*-transformed fibroblasts that hyperphosphorylation of FAK occurs in concert with the loss of a requirement for cell attachment for cell growth (67).

Once cloned, FAK was found to lack previously characterized modular domains such as SH2 or SH3 and to resemble known PTKs only in its catalytic domain. Subsequently a carboxy-terminal sequence of 159 amino acids was determined to mediate its targeting to focal adhesion contacts (68). FAK is autophosphorylated at Tyr^{397} in resting, substrate-attached cells, and it possesses sites favored for phosphorylation by Src, such as $Tyr^{407, 576, and 577}$. Phosphorylation of these tyrosines markedly increases the PTK activity of FAK (69). Tyrosine phosphorylation of FAK in cultured VSMC increases upon attachment to substrate, and is mediated through integrin adhesion receptors (70). Stimulation of attached VSMC with soluble agonists for both PTK- and heptahelical receptors further stimulates FAK phosphorylation and activation. The precise sequence of signal events necessary for FAK activation is still unclear but Src and Csk appear to participate in integrin- and receptor PTK-dependent activation. A two-step mechanism has been proposed, with an initial event, possibly an attachment-dependent conformational change favoring the interaction of FAK with SH2 domains of Src (71). Activation by heptahelical receptors may be mediated by the rho family of GTPases, as suggested by studies using the rho inhibitor C3 botulinum exoenzyme (72). These stimulations have in common the formation of a multimeric complex within focal adhesion contacts that forms the nidus for assembly of other signal transducers, including adaptors such as paxillin and SH3-rich $p130^{Cas}$ (73), regulators of GTPases, and effectors such as PLCγ (71). The identity of additional downstream effectors is under active investigation.

Two laboratories have independently reported the cloning of a second FAK family member, denoted as Pyk2 (74) or cell adhesion kinase-β (75). In cells of neural origin, Pyk2 was found to be activated by heptahelical receptor agonists, PKC stimulation, or non-receptor-mediated interventions that increase cytoplasmic calcium levels, such as K^+ depolarization or calcium ionophore. This kinase has been postulated as a potential link between calcium-dependent signaling pathways and PTK pathways. As such it is a candidate to link heptahelical vasoconstrictor receptors with PTK-mediated contractile, migratory, and growth responses.

Modulation of PTK Signal Pathways: Protein Phosphatases, Cross-Talk, and Negative Feedback

The adaptors, regulators, and effectors discussed thus far function primarily in a positive forward fashion, with PTKs typically mediating signals that activate MAPK and cell growth. Because the network of signaling pathways may be stimulated by multiple agonists and must also be capable of terminating the signals produced, interactions both within and between the various pathways modulate signal outcome. Protein phosphatases appear to be the most important signal terminators. Like protein kinases, protein phosphatases can be grouped according to their affinity for phosphoserine/phosphothreonine, phosphotyrosine or, both. Early work suggested that phosphoserine/phosphothreonine phosphatases (PSPases) comprised a small family with constitutive activity towards phosphorylated substrates. It thus appeared that levels of protein serine/threonine phosphorylation were regulated exclusively by the state of kinase activation. Subsequently it has been recognized that PSPases are dynamically regulated by post-translational mechanisms, via Ca^{2+}/calmodulin dependence and phosphorylation, as well as by protein inhibitors (76). The diversity of the PSPase family is rapidly increasing as well, and studies from lower eukaryotic species indicate that the mammalian genome could encode as many as 500 PSPases and a like number of protein tyrosine phosphatases (PTPases) (77). PTPases appear to differ from PSPases in several ways. They are regulated through targeting to specific subcellular locations, as well as by serine/threonine or tyrosine phosphorylation. The consequences of PTPase phosphorylation are molecule-specific, as in some cases these events are stimulatory, while in other cases they are inhibitory. In contrast to PSPases, no PTPase regulatory subunits or protein inhibitors have yet been described. There appear to be major differences in the maximal activity of PTPases relative to PSPases, with the former being approximately threefold more active. This increased activity could be a major determinant of the relatively low levels of ambient tyrosine phosphorylation in cellular proteins and the transient nature of most phosphotyrosine responses (78). Thus the balance between PTK and PTPase activities must be highly shifted towards PTK activation for net phosphotyrosine signals to emerge.

Dual-specificity phosphatases have recently been isolated and characterized. The best known is the MAP kinase phosphatase (MKP-1), which is transcriptionally regulated, and upon induction is highly and specifically active towards threonine- and tyrosine-phosphorylated ERK1/2. Sun et al. demonstrated an important role for ERK1/2 and MKP-1 in regulating cell growth by showing that expression of MKP-1 quantitatively inhibited the ability of Ras to induce DNA synthesis in REF-52 cells (79). Mitogens such as FGF and PDGF stimulate a sustained increase in ERK1/2 activity (80). In contrast, nonmitogenic agents stimulate ERK1/2 only transiently (81), suggesting that dephosphorylation inhibits events required for cell proliferation. Our laboratory has recently shown that inhibition of MKP-1 expression with either actinomycin D or antisense oligonucleotides corresponding to MKP-1 sustains the activity of ERK1/2 (82), indicating that MKP-1 is the phosphatase responsible for inactivation of ERK1/2 in VSMC. Two recently isolated dual-specificity phosphatases designated MKP-2 (83) and MKP-3 (84) have been shown to possess partial sequence and functional homology to MKP-1, but it is not known at this time whether these phosphatases are important in VSMC biology.

Signaling cross-talk can be defined as interactions between pathways that modulate signal outcome. A primary example is the attenuation of growth factor-dependent stimulation of the MAPK pathway by activation of PKC or PKA. Pharmacological PKA activation or PLCγ overexpression has been shown to downregulate proximal PTK-dependent signal transduction at the level of receptor PTKs (85). Likewise, compounds that increase cAMP and activate PKA, such as forskolin and isoproterenol, have been found to inhibit PDGF-BB-induced activation of MEK and ERK1/2 in human VSMC (86). It has been suggested that cAMP inhibits the activity of Raf-1 kinase via PKA-mediated phosphorylation of critical negative regulatory residues in Raf-1 (87). In T lymphocytes PKA has been shown to inhibit selectively the SAPK/JNK pathway and not ERK1/2, reinforcing the concept that the precise "wiring" of these signal pathways is cell type-specific (88).

Through negative feedback, signal pathways "shut off" after a period of stimulation. This mechanism may resemble the end-product inhibition of proximal enzymatic mediators of metabolic pathways. Examples include the phosphorylations of the EGF-R (89), Sos (90), and MEK (91) by ERK1/2. These phosphorylations, although in some cases quantitatively impressive (e.g., EGF-R), appear to be only moderately inhibitory. The importance of these negative feedback phosphorylations in vivo is not substantiated.

SIGNALING BY RECEPTOR AND NONRECEPTOR PTKS IN VSMC

VSMC Signaling by Receptor PTKs

Thorough characterization of the physiological role of receptor PTKs expressed in normal and injured VSMC remains a high priority for vascular biologists. A detailed review of this subject can be found elsewhere in this volume. From the standpoint of signaling, however, it is probably instructive to comment on the current state of knowledge regarding the major receptor PTKs expressed in VSMC and differences in their signal initiation properties. Receptor PTKs that have historically been considered to be predominant include those for PDGF (α and β), FGF (92), EGF (EGF-R and the related heparin-binding EGF-like growth factor) (93), and IGF-1 (94). Recent studies have suggested the possibility that the function of a local HGF-HGFR system in the vascular wall may also be physiologically relevant (95).

There is a long history of investigation of the function of PDGF-R. A strict hierarchy of receptor tyrosine autophosphorylation reactions specifically couples its adaptors and regulators to effectors of cellular signal events. Early studies suggested that mitogenic signaling capacity of PDGF-R required an intact kinase insert domain, and the basis for this pathway was found to be obligatory binding of the 85 kD regulatory subunit of PI 3-K (50). PLCγ, which specifically binds to Tyr^{602} of PDGFβ-R, is activated by PDGF and in cultured VSMC mediates a moderate and relatively short-lived increase in intracellular calcium level (96). In intact rat aorta, PDGF stimulates a slow sustained contraction that is more potent on a molar basis than any known vasoconstrictor except endothelin, relative to which its potency is probably comparable (97). It is believed that sustained phosphatidylinositol turnover may be in part responsible for this contractile response, yet its attenuation by tyrosine kinase inhibitors would suggest a critical role for as yet undefined PTKs. Phosphatidylinositol turnover and calcium mobilization do not appear to be required for VSMC growth (98). Sustained Ras-dependent ERK1/2 activation, as a consequence of Grb2/Sos/Ras/Raf-1 stimulation, does, however, appear to be obligatory (99). PDGF is also a potent stimulus for VSMC migration and the determinants of PDGF-dependent migration vs. proliferation remain to be determined. It is likely that differences in VSMC PDGF responsiveness under different conditions are due to differences in quantitative PDGF-R expression as well as to phenotype-dependent differences in coupling to its various effectors.

Receptors of the EGF-R class appear to show two major differences in comparison with the PDGF-R. First, the adaptor protein Shc appears to play a more prominent role in mitogenic signaling (100). Second, the correspondence of specific phosphorylated tyrosines and adaptor/regulator/effector coupling displayed by the PDGF-R seems less strict for these receptors. These issues were explored by Soler and colleagues who assessed the capacity of wild-type and mutant EGF-R to associate with the SH2 domain-containing proteins PLCγ, Ras-GAP, PI 3-K p85 subunit, and Shc (101). Mutants included receptors with single site mutations at each of five autophosphorylation sites and receptors in which multiple sites were removed. In contrast to data obtained with PDGF-R single autophosphorylation site mutants, none of the EGF-R single site mutants was dramatically impaired in its capacity to associate with any of the SH2-containing proteins. However, association was completely abrogated when all five autophosphorylation sites were mutated or removed by deletion. These results indicate that individual autophosphorylation sites in the EGF-R are not stringently required for the recognition and association of different SH2-containing substrates. Thus, EGF-R autophosphorylation sites seem to be flexible and/or compensatory in their capacity to mediate association with these four SH2-containing substrates. The FGF-R family appear to resemble EGF-R in signaling via Shc, but they resemble PDGF-R in having fixed autophosphorylation site requirements (102).

IGF-1-R are another receptor PTK class likely to be important in VSMC physiology. This class differs from PDGF-R, EGF-R and FGF-R, in that the determinants for signal particle assembly reside in the recruited adaptor protein IRS-1 (12). The physiology of IGF-1 in VSMC is also distinctive; while being approximately 50% as effective on a molar basis as PDGF in stimulating migration of cultured human aortic VSMC, it is not coupled to activation of ERK1/2. This appears to represent a cell type-specific difference in IGF-1 signal transduction, as ERK1/2 activation is detectable in cells of adrenal or fibroblast origin (99). It is likely that the IGF-1 receptor is coupled to unique mitogenic pathway(s), since IGF-1 can synergize with other receptor PTK growth factors such as FGF or PDGF to enhance mitogenesis, acting as a progression factor according to the formalism of Stiles (103).

Heptahelical Receptors in VSMC

VSMC are exposed to many vasoconstrictors that signal through heptahelical receptors. Those best characterized for their ability to stimulate VSMC growth include angiotensin II, thrombin, endothelin, and serotonin. In general, these agents are capable of stimulating increases in cell size and protein content (hypertrophy) to a greater extent than they stimulate proliferation (104). Because few studies have compared the signaling events initiated by these agents under similar conditions or in human VSMC, only generalizations can be made. Interpretation of studies focused on single agents has been complicated by the fact that these agonists also stimulate autocrine and paracrine secretion of complementary growth factors (105). When VSMC are stimulated with these agonists, all have been shown to transduce activation of cellular PTKs, activate ERK1/2, induce early immediate gene expression, and to advance cells from the Go/G1 phase of the cell cycle (81, 106–108). Limited studies indicate that angiotensin II may be even more effective at advancing cells into S phase in vivo (109). This agonist will be discussed in greater detail because of its primary physiological importance and because its linkage to PTKs has been conclusively demonstrated.

Angiotensin II normally mediates vascular homeostasis through its effects on salt and water balance, blood pressure, and vascular tone. It is produced both systematically and locally in the vessel wall by the actions of renin, which converts antiotensinogen into angiotensin I, and angiotensin-converting enzyme, which cleaves angiotensin I to form angiotensin II. In addition to its vasoconstrictor activity, angiotensin II has been shown to stimulate VSMC growth, increase the expression of inflammatory mediators such as phospholipase A_2 and NAD(P)H oxidase, and activate transcription of protooncogenes. These data suggest that angiotensin II plays an important role in various cardiovascular diseases associated with VSMC growth and vessel wall inflammation such as hypertension, atherosclerosis and restenosis following angioplasty.

Signal Initiation by the AT_1 Receptor

The primary angiotensin II receptor expressed in VSMC is the high-affinity AT_1 receptor (AT_1R). Based on its cDNA sequence, the AT_1R is similar to other vasoconstrictor receptors in possessing seven transmembrane domains (110). The angiotensin II binding site appears to be the result of interactions among several of its transmembrane and extracellular domains. Recent modeling analysis suggests that an interaction between Asp^{74} and Tyr^{292} is critical for ligand binding and AT_1R activation (111, 112). Site-directed mutagenesis has established that conserved residues at the following positions are important in G-protein binding and activation: Asp^{74} within the second transmembrane domain, Tyr^{215} within the fifth transmembrane domain, Tyr^{292} within the sixth transmembrane domain, and the domain Asp^{125}–Arg^{126}–Tyr^{127} in the amino-terminal region of the third cytoplasmic loop (2). These same residues may also be important in angiotensin II-stimulated growth (111). Figure 2 schematically depicts the major PTK signal pathways activated by the AT_1R.

Receptor phosphorylation is a critical event mediating the internalization and downregulation of heptahelical receptors. Following activation by ligand binding these receptors are phosphorylated on serine and threonine residues by members of the G protein receptor kinase (GRK) family, of which the β-adrenergic receptor kinase is the prototypic member (113). It has recently been shown that the AT_1R is phosphorylated basally and in response to angiotensin II (114). The majority of receptor phosphorylation in vivo was found on serine and there was a small increase in total phosphoserine content following agonist exposure. AT_1R internalization is regulated by a motif in the cytoplasmic tail involving Thr^{332} . . . Ser^{335}-Thr^{336}-Leu^{337}-Ser^{338} that is similar to the phosphorylation motif present in the third loop of the adrenergic receptors (115). Based on this finding, it appears that the carboxyl tail of AT_1R may serve as the mediator of functions normally mediated by the third loop in other heptahelical receptors.

AT$_1$R

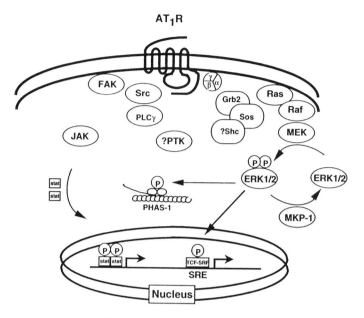

Figure 2 Major PTK pathways activated upon binding of angiotensin II to the AT$_1$R. Studies in cultured VSMC suggest that these pathways may be categorized as cytoplasmic PTKs (Src, FAK), PTKs with nuclear targets (JAK) and dual-specificity threonine/tyrosine kinases (MEK). Src is rapidly activated and is implicated as being "upstream" of both PLCγ and FAK. JAK phosphorylates the stat cytoplasmic transcription factors, causing them to translocate as a dimer to the nucleus, where they bind to gene promoters and induce mRNA expression (arrows). Activation of the ras/MEK/ERK pathway may occur through several regulatory pathways. Probable links of AT$_1$R to Ras include the βγ subunit of heterotrimeric G proteins and adaptors such as Shc/Grb2/Sos. In addition to Ras, PKC (not shown) and other undefined adaptors and/or regulators may also contribute to MEK activation. Activated MEK phosphorylates ERK1/2, increasing their serine/threonine kinase activity. Cytoplasmic targets include the PHAS-1 complex and the pp90[rsk] (not shown), resulting in increased protein synthesis. ERK1/2 also translocates to the nucleus, where it phosphorylates the complex of TCF and serum response factor at serum response elements, increasing early immediate gene expression. Undiscovered PTK(s) (?PTK) likely feed into these pathways, and may serve as further links between serine/threonine and tyrosine phosphorylation pathways. In contrast to the PDGF-R (shown in Fig. 1), the structural determinants of coupling of heptahelical receptors such as AT$_1$R to adaptors, regulators, and effectors are much less well defined.

Tyrosine phosphorylation of the AT$_1$R has also been observed. There is controversy regarding the extent to which tyrosine phosphorylation is regulated by agonist exposure. In our laboratories we found no net agonist-dependent increase in tyrosine phosphorylation up to 6 min after angiotensin II treatment followed by immunoprecipitation of the AT_1R and Western blot analysis using antiphosphotyrosine antibody (114). In contrast, when VSMC were metabolically labeled with [^{32}P]orthophosphate and the AT_1R was immunoprecipitated, phosphotyrosine could be demonstrated by amino acid analysis and there was a slow increase in the phosphotyrosine content following angiotensin II exposure (116). Because both of these techniques measure total phosphotyrosine content, increases and decreases in phosphorylation of individual tyrosine residues could be overlooked. There are several potential tyrosine phosphorylation sites within the AT_1R including amino acids 302, 312, 319, and 339 within the carboxyl tail. The tyrosine at position 319 is of special interest because it is part of the motif Tyr–Ile–Pro–Pro, which is analogous to an SH2 binding site within the PDGF receptor (Tyr-Ile-Ile-Pro), and within the EGF receptor (Tyr-Leu-Pro–Pro) (117). These receptor PTK motifs are target sequences for modular domain-containing signaling proteins when tyrosine is phosphorylated. We speculate that tyrosine phosphorylation of the AT_1 receptor may serve a similar function.

It has been appreciated for many years that angiotensin II stimulates a phosphoinositide-specific PLC to hydrolyze phosphatidylinositol 4,5-bisphosphate, thereby generating the second messengers inositol (1,4,5)-trisphosphate (IP_3) and diacylglycerol (DAG). The IP_3 released into the cytoplasm stimulates the mobilization of calcium from intracellular stores and DAG activates PKC. Several important observations regarding activation of PLC by angiotensin II in VSMC have recently been reported. PLC comprises a family of at least three related genes: PLC-β, PLC-γ, and PLC-δ (118). Many heptahelical receptors activate PLC-β via the α and $\beta\gamma$ subunits of G proteins (119,120). The PLC isoform mediating these VSMC responses in intact blood vessels is unknown. However, in cultured VSMC, the PLC-β isoforms are undetectable suggesting that another PLC isoform is responsible for signal transduction in these cells (121, 122). Because PLC-γ isoforms are activated by tyrosine phosphorylation following ligand binding to receptor PTKs, we sought evidence of angiotensin II-dependent tyrosine phosphorylation of PLC-γ in cultured VSMC. Within 1 min of angiotensin II stimulation an increase in PLC-γ tyrosine phosphorylation was detected, which returned to control levels within 6 min (122). The time course for tyrosine phosphorylation of PLC-γ is very similar to the time course for IP_3 formulation, suggesting that PLC-γ activation by tyrosine phosphorylation is responsible for IP_3 generation. These responses were completely abrogated by the AT_1R competitive inhibitor losartan, indicating that angiotensin II stimulates PLC-γ via the AT_1R.

Angiotensin II Activation of Cytoplasmic PTKs: Src and FAK

An increasing body of evidence suggests that Src plays an important role in angiotensin II signal transduction, which has been investigated in VSMC using several complementary strategies. After angiotensin II stimulation of VSMC the activity of immunoprecipitated Src was measured by both its autophosphorylation and its phosphotransferase activity towards enolase. Both assays demonstrated an approximate threefold increase in Src activity that was maximal within 1 min of angiotensin II stimulation (123). A search for a signaling complex involving cytoplasmic domain(s) of the AT_1R and Src, by AT_1R immunoprecipitation and anti-Src Western blot, did not show evidence for direct binding of these molecules. However the early and transient activation of Src that was detected implicated it as a potential PLCγ tyrosine kinase, which was tested using electroporation of a monoclonal anti-Src antibody into VSMC. Under these conditions both angiotensin II-stimulated PLC-γ phosphorylation and IP_3 formation were significantly inhibited relative to cells electroporated with purified IgG (124). In contrast, PDGF-dependent PLC-γ phosphorylation was unaffected, consistent with its direct activation by tyrosine phosphorylated PDGF-R. These findings demonstrate that Src activation is one of the earliest signal events stimulated by angiotensin II and strongly suggest that Src is the kinase responsible for tyrosine phosphorylation of PLC-γ. However, the lack of direct association of Src with the AT_1R suggests that other adaptor-type molecules are required to link the AT_1R to Src activation.

The AT_1R also exhibits similarities to integrin receptors based on several recent studies. Integrin-mediated signal transduction requires activation of the integrin receptor (e.g., $\alpha_2\beta_1$) by interactions with extracellular matrix ligands (e.g., fibronectin) and recruitment of intracellular kinases (125). Integrin activation leads to tyrosine phosphorylation of the PTK FAK, which appears to be due to autophosphorylation and activation by unclear mechanisms. Autophosphorylation of FAK on tyrosine generates a site for binding of SH2-domain-containing proteins and leads to recruitment and activation of Src-like protein kinases including Src itself, Fyn, and Csk (126). The signal transduction complex consisting of FAK and a Src-like kinase then phosphorylates another focal adhesion protein, paxillin (66). It has become clear that phosphorylation of FAK and paxillin in response to angiotensin II is one of the earliest and most prominent tyrosine phosphorylation events in VSMC (70, 127). The functional significance of this activation and the possible participation of integrins in this signal pathway remain to be determined.

Angiotensin II Activation of Ras, MEK, and ERK Pathways

One of the first molecules to be identified as being phosphorylated on tyrosine in response to angiotensin II was ERK1/2 (81, 128). Angiotensin II rapidly and transiently stimulates the activity of the p42 and p44 isoforms of MAPK in VSMC, as determined by phosphorylation of myelin basic protein. The activation of ERK1/2 by angiotensin II is partially dependent on PKC, as determined by prolonged exposure to phorbol ester (128). However, a significant amount of ERK1/2 activation by angiotensin II is PKC-independent (129). These data suggest that while separate pathways for ERK1/2 and PKC may exist in VSMC, there is considerable cross-talk between the two pathways, allowing for greater regulation of downstream events.

The pathways linking AT_1R to ERK1/2 are only beginning to be defined. By homology with receptor PTKs, it is likely that this pathway includes Ras. As discussed above, the regulation of Ras activity is complex, involving several adaptor proteins and guanine–nucleotide exchange factors. Tyrosine phosphorylation of the adaptor protein Shc may be utilized by angiotensin II in VSMC (130), as in in cardiac fibroblasts (131). We have also found that the tyrosine kinase inhibitor genistein inhibits PLC-γ phosphorylation and ERK1/2 activation in response to angiotensin II, suggesting that a receptor-associated PTK may link angiotensin II signaling through the AT_1 receptor to the Ras/ERK pathway (132).

We have explored the linkage of AT_1R to Raf-1 activation in cultured rat aortic VSMC, and found that angiotensin II causes translocation of Raf-1 to the membrane fraction. Translocation resulted in association with Ras as shown by Raf-1 coprecipitation with anti-Ras antibodies, and occurred earlier than ERK1/2 activation, suggesting that Ras–Raf complex formation precedes ERK1/2 activation (129). The complex of Ras, Raf, and other coimmunoprecipitates so formed was catalytically active, as demonstrated by an in vitro kinase reaction of the immunoprecipitated complex, a GST-MEK1 fusion protein and catalytically inactive ERK2. This activation of ERK2 was stimulated threefold by angiotensin II with maximal activation at 5 min. Inhibition of PKC activity by preincubation with phorbol ester blocked angiotensin II-stimulated Ras–Raf interaction, but a Ras–Raf-independent ERK2 activation was still detected, suggesting the existence of alternative pathways that remain to be defined.

One of the most important actions of angiotensin II is the stimulation of VSMC growth (133, 134). Substrates for ERK1/2 include both nuclear and cytosolic proteins involved in the regulation of DNA and protein synthesis. The serine/threonine kinase pp90[rsk], which phosphorylates the S6 ribosomal protein and stimulates protein synthesis, has been demonstrated to be a substrate for ERK1/2 (135). Angiotensin II has been shown to stimulate the phosphorylation of ribosomal S6 protein in VSMC within 30 min (136). This early event may explain the rapid increase in protein synthesis stimulated by angiotensin II that precedes VSMC hypertrophy (133). Other potential ERK1/2 substrates are proteins involved in the initiation of protein synthesis, such as the mRNA cap-binding protein eIF-4E (47). The role of this pathway in angiotensin II stimulation of VSMC hypertrophy is not known; however, it was recently shown that angiotensin II stimulates the serine phosphorylation of eIF-4E in VSMC (137).

Angiotensin II Signaling to the Nucleus via JAKs

A substantial body of evidence indicates that heptahelical receptors such as the AT_1R mediate signal events through activation of PTKs. In the case of the receptors for cytokines such as the interferons and interleukins, tyrosine phosphorylation is mediated by several cytosolic PTKs that associate with the receptor, including JAKs and the Src-related kinases Lck and Fyn (5). A variety of recent studies indicate that the AT_1R is likely to share properties with cytokine receptors. In parallel with the interleukin-2, interferon-γ, and interferon-α receptors, the AT_1R stimulates tyrosine phosphorylation, activates the ERK1/2 pathway, and induces c-*fos* mRNA expression (81, 107, 128, 138). A *sis*-inducing factor is present in the c-*fos* promoter and interacts with members of the STAT family of transcription factors (including Stat91 and Stat113) in a tissue and hormone-specific manner (139, 140). The recent demonstrations that angiotensin II activates Stat91 in cultured neonatal cardiac fibroblasts (141) and that thrombin activates JAK2 in platelets (142) suggested that AT_1R might activate these pathways in VSMC. Recently this hypothesis was confirmed by Marrero and co-workers, who reported that the tyrosine phosphorylation of JAK2, the related kinase TYK2, and Stat113 is significantly increased within 5 min of angiotensin II treatment (143). These observations suggest that seven transmembrane receptors may signal using some of the same mechanisms observed with cytokine and PTK receptors.

VSMC PTKS IN HEALTH AND DISEASE

PTK in Smooth Muscle Contraction in Normal Vessels

Due to the technical difficulties in analyzing signal transduction at a biochemical level in normal intact nonhuman or human vessels, we do not yet fully understand the hierarchy of signal pathways that regulate contraction of VSMC. For example, vasoconstrictor-dependent myosin light chain phosphorylation by calcium/calmodulin-dependent myosin light chain kinase has historically been accorded the role of primary mediator of active VSMC contraction (144). Subsequent attention was focused on identifying the mediators of the sustained phase of VSMC, a condition in which calcium levels have returned towards baseline and phosphorylation of myosin light chain has declined. Work over the past 5 years has suggested the existence of PKC-dependent and PTK-dependent aspects of this phase of contraction (3). The PTK-dependent component may be mediated by both MEK/ERK1/2-dependent and MEK/ERK1/2-independent pathways. The MEK/ERK1/2-dependent pathway may be due to phosphorylation by ERK1/2 of the thin filament-associated protein caldesmon to form latch bridges, with low ATP cycling and oxygen consumption requirements (145). The existence of an MEK/ERK1/2-independent pathway is suggested by the

following. Contractions stimulated by PTK (e.g., EGF, PDGF) or certain heptahelical receptor agonists (angiotensin II and thrombin but not carbachol or
bradykinin) can be inhibited by the PTK inhibitors genistein or tyrphostin (3).
Because Src has long been known to be present in VSMC, it was hypothesized
to be the mediator of this response. However, the K_i values for these inhibitors differed significantly among various smooth muscles, and, more importantly, bore no relationship to the published K_i values for inhibition of the respective receptor PTK, Src (3), or ERK1/2 (146). Many vasoconstrictors also
require the presence of intracellular and/or extracellular calcium for contraction (144). Taken together these findings suggest that these agonists stimulate
contraction via a yet to be defined non-Src, calcium-sensitive PTK.

PTKs in Reparative Functions of VSMC: Hypertrophy,
Hyperplasia, and Migration

VSMC are subject to both quantitative and qualitative changes in agonist stimulation during the development of pathologic states. Through phenotypic modulation, VSMC acquire the capacity to migrate and/or to proliferate in response
to these stimuli. A relatively underexplored area is the extent to which PTK
signaling is convergent or divergent for these outcomes. According to Schwartz,
the waves of migration and proliferation involve distinctly differing populations
of VSMC, based on spatial and temporal differences in cell stimulation (147).
Because these responses are so intimately linked, it is likely that similar signal mechanisms are utilized, but the specific alterations in signal pathways that
determine their nature are relatively unknown. Current studies suggest that these
alterations include phenotype-dependent changes in receptors, adaptors, regulators, and effectors. For example, when cells migrate in response to physical
or metabolic injury they must reassemble directionally, in a complex process
requiring cytoskeletal rearrangements to remodel sites of attachment. Given the
primary participation of FAK in focal adhesion contact signal events, it is likely
that FAK or a related kinase is an important mediator. Migration also requires
increased secretion of proteases and elastolytic enzymes that allow VSMC to
disattach from neighboring cells and directionally reassemble. In this context,
a recent report that PTK regulate the induction of these enzymes is provacative
(148).

SUMMARY

For several years our laboratories have intensively investigated the paradigm
that under the appropriate conditions vasoconstrictor agonists can stimulate
VSMC growth via heptahelical receptors while growth factors may stimulate

VSMC contraction via receptor PTKs. The basis for this paradigm is the utilization of common signal pathways by both receptor classes. We have reviewed the major receptors, adaptors, regulators, and effectors mediating these events, with particular emphasis on the PTK pathways that are activated following VSMC stimulation. Many areas of important future research remain to be explored. Only a fraction of the PTKs and PTPases that are likely to be physiologically relevant have been characterized. As the factors that regulate modulation of VSMC phenotype are more precisely defined, increased insight should be gained into signaling pathway modulations that determine the physiological outcome (i.e., contractile, migratory, hypertrophic, or hyperplastic) of a given neurohumoral stimulus. Transgenic animals lacking one or more signaling components should yield more substantive insights into the hierarchies of these pathways in vivo. Finally, mechanistic insights gained from basic cellular and molecular investigations should lead to the development of therapies targeted to specific signal pathway abnormalities that will be applicable to the treatment of human cardiovascular diseases.

REFERENCES

1. Heldin CH. Dimerization of cell surface receptors in signal transduction. Cell 1995; 80:213–223.
2. Ohyama K, Yamano Y, Chaki S, Kondo T, Inagami T. Domains for G-protein coupling in angiotensin II receptor type I: studies by site-directed mutagenesis. Biochem Biophys Res Commun 1992; 189:677–683.
3. Hollenberg MD. Tyrosine kinase pathways and the regulation of smooth muscle contractility. Trends Pharmacol Sci 1994; 15:108–114.
4. Ito A, Shimokawa H, Kadokami T, Fukumoto Y, Owada MK, et al. Tyrosine kinase inhibitor suppresses coronary arteriosclerotic changes and vasospastic responses induced by chronic treatment with interleukin-1 beta in pigs in vivo. J Clin Invest 1995; 96:1288–1294.
5. Ihle JN. Cytokine receptor signalling. Nature 1995; 377:591–594.
6. Pawson T. Protein modules and signalling networks. Nature 1995; 373:573–580.
7. Songyan Z, Cantley LC. Recognition and specificity in protein tyrosine kinase-mediated signalling. TIBS 1995; 20:470–475.
8. Cohen GB, Ren R, Baltimore D. Modular binding domains in signal transduction proteins. Cell 1995; 80:237–248.
9. Malarkey K, Belham CM, Paul A, Graham A, McLees A, et al. The regulation of tyrosine kinase signalling pathways by growth factor and G-protein-coupled receptors. Biochem J 1995; 309:361–375.
10. Kavanaugh WM, Turck CW, Williams LT. PTB domain binding to signalling proteins through a sequence motif containing phosphotyrosine. Science 1995; 268:1177–1179.
11. van der Geer P, Hunter T, Lindberg RA. Receptor protein-tyrosine kinases and their signal transduction pathways. Annu Rev Cell Biol 1994; 10:251–337.

12. White MF. The IRS-1 signalling system. Curr Opin Genet Dev 1994; 4:47–54.
13. Freed E, Symons M, Macdonald SG, McCormick F, Ruggieri R. Binding of 14-3-3 proteins to the protein kinase Raf and effects on its activation. Science 1994; 265:1713–1716.
14. Aitken A. 14-3-3 proteins on the map. Trends Biochem Sci 1995; 20:95–97.
15. Rens D-S, Hamm HE. Structural and functional relationships of heterotrimeric G-proteins. Faseb J 1995; 9:1059–1066.
16. Druey KM, Blumer KJ, Kang VH, Kehrl JH. Inhibition of G-protein-mediated MAP kinase activation by a new mammalian gene family. Nature 1996; 379:742–746.
17. McCormick F. Activators and effectors of ras p21 proteins. Curr Opin Genet Dev 1994; 4:71–76.
18. Bowtell D, Fu P, Simon M, Senior P. Identification of murine homologues of the Drosophila son of sevenless gene: potential activators of ras. Proc Natl Acad Sci USA 1992; 89:6511–6515.
19. Lowenstein EJ, Daly RJ, Batzer AG, Li W, Margolis B, et al. The SH2 and SH3 domain-containing protein GRB2 links receptor tyrosine kinases to ras signalling. Cell 1992; 70:431–442.
20. van Corven EJ, Hordijk PL, Medema RH, Bos JL, Moolenaar WH. Pertussis toxin-sensitive activation of p21 ras by G protein-coupled receptor agonists in fibroblasts. Proc Natl Acad Sci USA 1993; 90:1257–1261.
21. Winitz S, Russell M, Qian N-X, Gardner A, Dwyer L, et al. Involvement of ras and raf in the G_i-coupled acetylcholine muscarininc m2 receptor activation of mitogen-activated protein (MAP) kinase kinase and MAP kinase. J Biol Chem 1993; 268:19196–19199.
22. Inglese J, Koch WJ, Touhara K, Lefkowitz RJ. G beta gamma interactions with PH domains and Ras-MAPK signalling pathways. Trends Biochem Sci 1995; 20:151–156.
23. van Biesen T, Hawes BE, Luttrell DK, Krueger KM, Touhara K, et al. Receptor-tyrosine-kinase- and G beta gamma-mediated MAP kinase activation by a common signalling pathway. Nature 1995; 376:781–784.
24. Quarck R, Bryckaert M, Magnier C, Corvazier E, Bredoux R, et al. Evidence for Rap1 in vascular smooth muscle cells. Regulation of their expression by platelet-derived growth factor BB. FEBS Lett 1994; 342:159–164.
25. Vojtek AB, Cooper JA. Rho family members: activators of MAP kinase cascades. Cell 1995; 82:527–529.
26. Zubiaur M, Sancho J, Terhorst C, Faller DV. A small GTP-binding protein, Rho, associates with the platelet-derived growth factor type-beta receptor upon ligand binding. J Biol Chem 1995; 270:17221–17228.
27. Daum G, Eisenmann-Tappe I, Fries HW, Troppmair J, Rapp UR. The ins and outs of Raf kinases. Trends Biochem Sci 1994; 19:474–480.
28. Moodie SA, Willumsen BM, Weber MJ, Wolfman A. Complexes of Ras·GTP with Raf-1 and mitogen-activated protein kinase kinase. Science 1993; 260:1658–1661.
29. Fields S, Song O. A novel genetic system to detect protein-protein interactions. Nature 1989; 340:245–246.

30. Vojtek AB, Hollenberg SM, Cooper JA. Mammalian Ras interacts directly with the serine/threonine kinase. Raf Cell 1993; 74:205–214.

31. Warne PH, Viciana PR, Downward J. Direct interaction of Ras and the amino-terminal region of Raf-1 in vitro. Nature 1993; 364:352–355.

32. Wartmann M, Davis RJ. The native structure of the activated Raf protein kinase is a membrane-bound multi-subunit complex. J Biol Chem 1994; 269:6695–6701.

33. Boulton TG, Nye SH, Robbins DJ, Ip NY, Radziejewska E, et al. ERKs: a family of protein-serine/threonine kinases that are activated and tyrosine phosphorylated in response to insulin and NGF. Cell 1991; 65:663–675.

34. Payne DM, Rossomando AJ, Martino P, Erikson AK, Her J-H, et al. Identification of the regulatory phosphorylation sites in pp42/mitogen-activated protein kinase (MAP kinase). EMBO J 1991; 10:885–892.

35. Crews CM, Erikson RL. Purification of a murine protien-tyrosine/threonine kinase that phosphorylates and activates the Erk-1 gene product: relationship to the fission yeast byr1 gene product. Proc Natl Acad Sci USA 1992; 89:8205–8209.

36. Mansour SJ, Matten WT, Hermann AS, Candia JM, Rong S, et al. Transformation of mammalian cells by constitutively active MAP kinase kinase. Science 1994; 265:966–970.

37. Cowley S, Paterson H, Kemp P, Marshall CJ. Activation of MAP kinase kinase is necessary and sufficient for PC12 differentiation and for transformation of NIH 3T3 cells. Cell 1994; 77:841–852.

38. Abe J, Kusuhara M, Ulevitch RJ, Berk BC, Lee JD. Big MAP kinase 1 (BMK1) is a redox sensitive kinase. J Biol Chem 1996; 271:16586–16590.

39. Zhou G, Bao ZQ, Dixon JE. Components of a new human protein kinase signal transduction pathway. J Biol Chem 1995; 270:12665–12669.

40. Kyriakis JM, Banerjee P, Nikolakaki E, Dai T, Rubie EA, et al. The stress-activated protein kinase subfamily of c-Jun kinases. Nature 1994; 369:156–160.

41. Lee JC, Laydon JT, McDonnell PC, Gallagher TF, Kumar S, et al. A protein kinase involved in the regulation of inflammatory cytokine biosynthesis. Nature 1994; 372:739–746.

42. Raingeaud J, Gupta S, Rogers JS, Dickens M, Han J, et al. Pro-inflammatory cytokines and environmental stress cause p38 mitogen-activated protein kinase activation by dual phosphorylation on tyrosine and threonine. J Biol Chem 1995; 270:7420–7426.

43. D'Erijard B, Raingeaud J, Barrett T, Wu IH, Han J, et al. Independent human MAP-kinase signal transduction pathways defined by MEk and MKK isoforms. Science 1995; 267:682–685.

44. Sturgill TW, Ray BL, Erikson E, Maller JL. Insulin-stimulated MAP-2 kinase phosphorylates protein S6 kinase II. Nature 1988; 334:715–718.

45. Lin LL, Wartmann M, Lin AY, Knopf JL, Seth A, et al. cPLA2 is phosphorylated and activated by MAP kinase. Cell 1993; 72:269–278.

46. Gille H, Kortenjann M, Thomae O, Moomaw C, Slaughter C, et al. ERK phosphorylation potentiates Elk-1 mediated ternary complex formation and transactivation. Embo J 1995; 14:951–962.

47. Joshi B-S, Rychlik W, Rhoads RE. Alteration of the major phosphorylation site

of eukaryotic protein synthesis initiation factor 4E prevents its association with the 48 S initiation complex. J Biol Chem 1990; 265:2979-2783.

48. Pause A, Belsham GJ, Gingras AC, Donz'e O, Lin TA, et al. Insulin-dependent stimulation of protein synthesis by phosphorylation of a regulator of 5'-cap function. Nature 1994; 371:762-767.

49. Lin T-A, Kong X, Haystead TAJ, Pause A, Belsham G, et al. PHAS-1 as a link between mitogen-activated protein kinase and translation initiation. Science 1994; 266:653-656.

50. Klippel A, Escobedo JA, Fantl WJ, Williams LT. The C-terminal SH2 domain of p85 accounts for the high affinity and specificity of the binding of phosphatidylinositol 3-kinase to phosphorylated platelet-derived growth factor beta receptor. Mol Cell Biol 1992; 12:1451-1459.

51. Bellacosa A, Testa JR, Staal SP, Tsichlis PN. A retroviral oncogene, akt, encoding a serine-threonine kinase containing an SH2-like region. Science 1991; 254:274-277.

52. Bos JL. A target for phosphoinositide 3-kinase: Akt/PKB. TIBS 1995; 20:441-442.

53. Downward J. Signal transduction. A target for PI(3) kinase. Nature 1995; 376:553-554.

54. Pitcher J, Touhara K, Payne E, Lefkowitz R. Pleckstrin homology domain-mediated membrane association and activation of the β-adrenergic receptor kinase requires cocordinate interaction with Gβγ subunits and lipid. J Biol Chem 1995; 270:11707-11710.

55. Lane HA, Fernandez A, Lamb NJ, Thomas G. p70S6 kinase function is essential for G1 progression. Nature 1993; 363:170-172.

56. Burgering BM, Coffer PJ. Protein kinase B (c-Akt) in phosphatidylinositol-3-OH kinase signal transduction. Nature 1995; 376:599-602.

57. Bolen JB, Rowley RB, Spana C, Tsygankov AY. The Src family of tyrosine protein kinases in hemopoietic signal transduction. Faseb J 1992; 6:3403-3409.

58. Lowell CA, Soriano P, Varmus HE. Functional overlap in the src gene family: inactivation of hck and fgr impairs natural immunity. Genes Dev 1994; 8:387-398.

59. Klages S, Adam D, Class K, Fargnoli J, Bolen JB, et al. Ctk: a protein-tyrosine kinase related to Csk that defines an enzyme family. Proc Natl Acad Sci USA 1994; 92:2597-2601.

60. Cooper JA, Howell B. The when and how of Src regulation. Cell 1993; 73:1051-1054.

61. Mori S, Ronnstrand L, Yokote K, Engstrom A, Courtneidge SA, et al. Identification of two juxtamembrane autophosphorylation sites in the PDGF beta-receptor; involvement in the interaction with Src family tyrosine kinases. Embo J 1993; 12:2257-2264.

62. Twamley S-GM, Pepperkok R, Ansorge W, Courtneidge SA. The Src family tyrosine kinases are required for platelet-derived growth factor-mediated signal transduction in NIH 3T3 cells. Proc Natl Acad Sci USA 1993; 90:7696-7700.

63. Zheng XM, Pallen CJ. Expression of receptor-like protein tyrosine phosphatase

alpha in rat embryo fibroblasts activates mitogen-activated protein kinase and c-Jun. J Biol Chem 1994; 269:23302–23309.

64. Williams NG, Roberts TM, Li P. Both p21ras and pp60v-src are required, but neither alone is sufficient, to activate the Raf-1 kinase. Proc Natl Acad Sci USA 1992; 89:2922–2926.

65. Kanner SB, Reynolds AB, Vines RR, Parsons JT. Monoclonal antibodies to individual tyrosine-phosphorylated protein substrates of oncogene-encoded tyrosine kinases. Proc Natl Acad Sci USA 1990; 87:3328–3332.

66. Burridge K, Turner CE, Romer LH. Tyrosine phosphorylation of paxillin and pp125[FAK] accompanies cell adhesion to extracellular matrix: a role in cytoskeletal assembly. J Cell Biol 1992; 119:893–903.

67. Guan JL, Shalloway D. Regulation of focal adhesion-associated protein tyrosine kinase by both cellular adhesion and oncogenic transformation. Nature 1992; 358:690–692.

68. Hildebrand JD, Schaller MD, Parsons JT. Identification of sequences required for the efficient localization of the focal adhesion kinase, pp125FAK, to cellular focal adhesions. J Cell Biol 1993; 123:993–1005.

69. Calalb MB, Polte TR, Hanks SK. Tyrosine phosphorylation of focal adhesion kinase at sites in the catalytic domain regulates kinase activity: a role for Src family kinases. Mol Cell Biol 1995; 15:954–963.

70. Polte TR, Naftilan AJ, Hanks SK. Focal adhesion kinase is abundant in developing blood vessels and elevation of its phosphotyrosine content in vascular smooth muscle cells is a rapid response to angiotensin II. J Cell Biochem 1994; 55:106–119.

71. Richardson A, Parsons JT. Signal transduction through integrins: a central role for focal adhesion kinase? Bioessays 1995; 17:229–236.

72. Rozengurt E. Convergent signalling in the action of integrins, neuropeptides, growth factors and oncogenes. Cancer Surv 1995; 24:81–96.

73. Nojima Y, Morino N, Mimura T, Hamasaki K, Furuya H, et al. Integrin-mediated cell adhesion promotes tyrosine phosphorylation of p130Cas, a Src homology 3-containing molecule having multiple Src homology 2-binding motifs. J Biol Chem 1995; 270:15398–15402.

74. Lev S, Moreno H, Martinez R, Canoll P, Peles E, et al. Protein tyrosine kinase PYK2 involved in Ca^{2+}-induced regulation of ion channel and MAP kinase functions. Nature 1995; 376:737–745.

75. Sasaki H, Nagura K, Ishino M, Tobioka H, Kotani K, et al. Cloning and characterization of cell adhesion kinase beta, a novel protein-tyrosine kinase of the focal adhesion kinase subfamily. J Biol Chem 1995; 270:21206–21219.

76. Cohen P. Signal integration at the level of protein kinases, protein phosphatases and their substrates. Trends Biochem Sci 1992; 17:408–413.

77. Hunter T. 1001 protein kinases redux—towards 2000. Semin Cell Biol 1994; 5:367–376.

78. Hunter T. Protein kinases and phosphatases: the yin and yang of protein phosphorylation and signaling. Cell 1995; 80:225–236.

79. Sun H, Tonks NK, Bar-Sagi D. Inhibition of ras-induced DNA synthesis by expression of the phosphatase MKP-1. Science 1994; 266:285–288.

80. Meloche S, Seuwen K, Pages G, Pouyssegur J. Biphasic and synergistic activation of pp44^{mapk} (ERK1) by growth factors: correlation between late phase activation and mitogenicity. Mol Endocrinol 1992; 6:845–854.

81. Duff JL, Berk BC, Corson MA. Angiotensin II stimulates the pp44 and pp42 mitogen-activated protein kinases in cultured rat aortic smooth muscle cells. Biochem Biophys Res Commun 1992; 188:257–264.

82. Duff JD, Monia BP, Berk BC. Mitogen-activated protein (MAP) kinase is regulated by the MAP kinase phosphatase (MKP-1) in vascular smooth muscle cells. J Biol Chem 1995; 270:7161–7166.

83. Misra P-A, Rim CS, Yao H, Roberson MS, Stork PJ. A novel mitogen-activated protein kinase phosphatase. Structure, expression, and regulation. J Biol Chem 1995; 270:14587–14596.

84. Muda M, Boschert U, Dickinson R, Martinou J-C, Martinou I, et al. MKP-3, a novel cytosolic protein-tyrosine phosphatase that exemplifies a new class of mitogen-activated protein kinase phosphatase. J Biol Chem 1996; 271:4319–4326.

85. Seedorf K, Sherman M, Ullrich A. Protein kinase C mediates short- and long-term effects on receptor tyrosine kinases. Regulation of tyrosine phosphorylation and degradation. Ann NY Acad Sci 1995; 766:459–462.

86. Graves LM, Bornfeldt KE, Raines EW, Potts BC, Macdonald SG, et al. Protein kinase A antagonizes platelet-derived growth factor-induced signaling by mitogen-activated protein kinase in human arterial smooth muscle cells. Proc Natl Acad Sci USA 1993; 90:10300–10304.

87. Cook SJ, McCormick F. Inhibition by cAMP of Ras-dependent activation of Raf. Science 1993; 262:1069–1072.

88. Hsueh YP, Lai MZ. c-Jun N-terminal kinase but not mitogen-activated protein kinase is sensitive to cAMP inhibition in T lymphocytes. J Biol Chem 1995; 270:18094–18098.

89. Northwood IC, Gonzalez FA, Wartmann M, Raden DL, Davis RJ. Isolation and characterization of two growth factor-stimulated protein kinases that phosphorylate the epidermal growth factor receptor at threonine 669. J Biol Chem 1991; 266:15266–15276.

90. Cherniack AD, Klarlund JK, Czech MP. Phosphorylation of the Ras nucleotide exchange factor son of sevenless by mitogen-activated protein kinase. J Biol Chem 1994; 269:4717–4720.

91. Campbell JS, Seger R, Graves JD, Graves LM, Jensen AM, et al. The MAP kinase cascade. Recent Prog Horm Res 1995; 50:131–159.

92. Xin X, Johnson AD, Scott B-T, Engler D, Casscells W. The predominant form of fibroblast growth factor receptor expressed by proliferating human arterial smooth muscle cells in culture is type I. Biochem Biophys Res Commun 1994; 204:557–564.

93. Peoples GE, Blotnick S, Takahashi K, Freeman MR, Klagsbrun M, et al. T lymphocytes that infiltrate tumors and atherosclerotic plaques produce heparin-

binding epidermal growth factor-like growth factor and basic fibroblast growth factor: a potential pathologic role. Proc Natl Acad Sci USA 1995; 92:6547–6551.

94. Delafontaine P, Anwar A, Lou H, Ku L. G-protein coupled and tyrosine kinase receptors: evidence that activation of the insulin-like growth factor I receptor is required for thrombin-induced mitogenesis of rat aortic smooth muscle cells. J Clin Invest 1996; 97:139–145.

95. Nakamura Y, Morishita R, Higaki J, Kida I, Aoki M, et al. Expression of local hepatocyte growth factor system in vascular tissues. Biochem Biophys Res Commun 1995; 215:483–488.

96. Berk BC, Alexander RW, Brock TA, Gimbrone MA Jr., Webb RC. Vasoconstriction: a new activity for platelet-derived growth factor. Science 1986; 232:87–90.

97. Masaki T. Endothelin in vascular biology. Ann NY Acad Sci 1994; 714:101–108.

98. Kobayashi S, Nishimura J, Kanaide H. Cytosolic Ca^{2+} transients are not required for platelet-derived growth factor to induce cell cycle progression of vascular smooth muscle cells in primary culture. Actions of tyrosine kinase. J Biol Chem 1994; 269:9011–9018.

99. Bornfeldt KE, Raines EW, Graves LM, Skinner MP, Krebs EG, et al. Platelet-derived growth factor. Distinct signal transduction pathways associated with migration versus proliferation. Ann NY Acad Sci 1995; 766:416–430.

100. Klint P, Kanda S, Claesson W-L. Shc and a novel 89-kDa component couple to the Grb2-Sos complex in fibroblast growth factor-2-stimulated cells. J Biol Chem 1995; 270:23337–23344.

101. Soler C, Beguinot L, Carpenter G. Individual epidermal growth factor receptor autophosphorylation sites do not stringently define association motifs for several SH2-containing proteins. J Biol Chem 1994; 269:12320–12324.

102. Huang J, Mohammadi M, Rodrigues GA, Schlessinger J. Reduced activation of RAF-1 and MAP kinase by a fibroblast growth factor receptor mutant deficient in stimulation of phosphatidylinositol hydrolysis. J Biol Chem 1995; 270:5065–5072.

103. Stiles CD, Capone GT, Scher CD, Antoniades HN, Van W-JJ, et al. Dual control of cell growth by somatomedins and platelet-derived growth factor. Proc Natl Acad Sci USA 1979; 76:1279–1283.

104. Bell L, Madri JA. Effect of platelet factors on migration of cultured bovine aortic endothelial and smooth muscle cells. Circ Res 1989; 65:1057–1065.

105. Berk BC, Corson MA. Autocrine and paracrine growth mechanisms in vascular smooth muscle. Curr Opin Cardiol 1992; 7:739–744.

106. Force T, Kyriakis JM, Avruch J, Bonventre JV. Endothelin, vasopressin, and angiotensin II enhance tyrosine phosphorylation by protein kinase C-dependent and -independent pathways in glomerular mesangial cells. J Biol Chem 1991; 266:6650–6656.

107. Molloy CJ, Taylor DS, Weber H. Angiotensin II stimulation of rapid protein tyrosine phosphorylation and protein kinase activation in rat aortic smooth muscle cells. J Biol Chem 1993; 268:7338–7345.

108. Corson MA, Alexander RW, Berk BC. 5-HT2 receptor mRNA is overexpresssed

in cultured rat aortic smooth muscle cells relative to normal aorta. Am J Physiol 1992; 262:C309–315.

109. Daemen MJAP, Lombardi DM, Bosman FT, Schwartz SM. Angiotensin II induces smooth muscle cell proliferation in the normal and injured rat arterial wall. Circ Res 1991; 68:450–456.

110. Murphy TJ, Alexander RW, Griendling KK, Runge MS, Bernstein KE. Isolation of a cDNA encoding the vascular type-1 angiotensin II receptor. Nature 1991; 351:233–235.

111. Bihoreau C, Monnot C, Davies E, Teutsch B, Bernstein KE, et al. Mutation of Asp74 of the rat angiotensin II receptor confers changes in angiotensin affinities and abolishes G-protein coupling. Proc Natl Acad Sci USA 1993; 90:5133–5137.

112. Marie J, Maigret B, Joseph MP, Larguier R, Nouet S, et al. Tyr292 in the seventh transmembrane domain of the AT1A angiotensin II receptor is essential for its coupling to phospholipase C. J Biol Chem 1994; 269:20815–20818.

113. Lefkowitz RJ, Inglese J, Koch WJ, Pitcher J, Attramadal H, et al. G-protein-coupled receptors: regulatory role of receptor kinases and arrestin proteins. Cold Spring Harb Symp Quant Biol 1992; 57:127–133.

114. Paxton WG, Marrero MB, Klein JD, Delafontaine P, Berk BC, et al. The angiotensin II AT$_1$ receptor is tyrosine and serine phosphorylated can serve as a substrate for the SRC family of tyrosine kinases. Biochem Biophys Res Commun 1994; 200:260–267.

115. Hunyady L, Baukal AJ, Balla T, Catt KJ. Independence of type I angiotensin II receptor endocytosis from G protein coupling and signal transduction. J Biol Chem 1994; 269:24798–24804.

116. Kai H, Griendling KK, Lassegue B, Ollerenshaw JD, Runge MS, et al. Agonist-induced phosphorylation of the vascular type I angiotensin receptor. Hypertension 1994; 24:523–527.

117. Fantl WJ, Johnson DE, Williams LT. Signalling by receptor tyrosine kinases. Annu Rev Biochem 1993; 62:453–481.

118. Rhee SG, Choi KD. Regulation of inositol phospholipid-specific phospholipase C isozymes. J Biol Chem 1992; 267:12393–12396.

119. Smrcka AV, Hepler JR, Brown KO, Sternweis PC. Regulation of polyphosphoinositide-specific phospholipase C activity by purified Gq. Science 1991; 251:804–807.

120. Taylor SJ, Chae HZ, Rhee SG, Exton JH. Activation of the beta 1 isozyme of phospholipase C by alpha subunits of the Gq class of G proteins. Nature 1991; 350:516–518.

121. Homma Y, Sakamoto H, Tsunoda M, Aoki M, Takenawa T, et al. Evidence for involvement of phospholipase C-gamma 2 in signal transduction of platelet-derived growth factor in vascular smooth muscle cells. Biochem J 1993; 290:649–653.

122. Marrero MB, Paxton W, Duff JD, Berk BC, Bernstein KC. Angiotensin II stimulates tyrosine phosphorylation of phosplipase C-γ1 in vascular smooth muscle cells. J Biol Chem 1994; 269:10935–10939.

123. Ishida M, Marrero MB, Schieffer B, Ishida T, Bernstein KE, et al. Angiotensin

II activates pp60[c-src] in vascular smooth muscle cells. Circ Res 1995; 77:1053–1059.

124. Marrero MB, Schieffer B, Bernstein KE. Electroporation of pp60[c-src] antibodies inhibits the angiotensin II activation of phospholipase C-γ1 in rat aortic smooth muscle cells. J Biol Chem 1995; 270:15734–15738.

125. Luscinskas FW, Lawler J. Integrins as dynamic regulators of vascular function. FASEB J 1994; 8:929–938.

126. Schaller MD, Parsons JT. Focal adhesion kinase and associated proteins. Curr Opin Cell Biol 1994; 6:705–710.

127. Leduc I, Meloche S. Angiotensin II stimulates tyrosine phosphorylation of the focal adhesion-associated protein paxillin in aortic smooth muscle cells. J Biol Chem 1995; 270:4401–4404.

128. Tsuda T, Kawahara Y, Ishida y, Koide M, Shii K, et al. Angiotensin II stimulates two myelin basic protein/microtubule-associated protein 2 kinases in cultured vascular smooth muscle cells. Circ Res 1992; 71:620–630.

129. Liao D-F, Duff JL, Daum G, Pelech ST, Berk BC. Angiotensin II stimulates MAP kinase kinase kinase activity in vascular smooth muscle cells: role of raf. Circ Res 1996; in press.

130. Linseman DA, Benjamin CW, Jones DA. Convergence of angiotensin II and platelet-derived growth factor receptor signaling cascades in vascular smooth muscle cells. J Biol Chem 1995; 270:12563–12568.

131. Schorb W, Peeler TC, Madigan NN, Conrad KM, Baker KM. Angiotensin II-induced protein tyrosine phosphorylation in neonatal rat cardiac fibroblasts. J Biol Chem 1994; 269:19626–19632.

132. Duff JL, Marrero MB, Berk BC. Unpublished observations.

133. Berk BC, Vekshtein V, Gordon HM, Tsuda T. Angiotensin II-stimulated protein synthesis in cultured vascular smooth muscle cells. Hypertension 1989; 13:305–314.

134. Geisterfer AAT, Peach MJ, Owens GK. Angiotensin II induces hypertrophy, not hyperplasia, of cultured rat aortic smooth muscle cells. Circ Res 1988; 62:749–756.

135. Sturgill TW, Wu J. Recent progress in characterization of protein kinase cascades for phosphorylation of ribosomal protein S6. Biochem Biophys Acta 1991; 1092:350–357.

136. Scott-Burden T, Resink TJ, Baur U, Burgin M, Buhler FR. Activation of S6 kinase in cultured vascular smooth muscle cells by submitogenic levels of thrombospondin. Biochem Biophys Res Commun 1988; 150:278–286.

137. Rao GN, Griendling KK, Frederickson RM, Sonenberg N, Alexander RW. Angiotensin II induces phosphorylation of eukaryotic protein synthesis initiation factor 4E in vascular smooth muscle cells. J Biol Chem 1994; 269:7180–7184.

138. Taubman MB, Berk BC, Izumo S, Tsuda T, Alexander RW, et al. Angiotensin II induces c-fos mRNA in aortic smooth muscle. Role of Ca^{2+} mobilization and protein kinase C activation. J Biol Chem 1989; 264:526–530.

139. Darnell JEJ, Kerr IM, Stark GR. Jak-STAT pathways and transcriptional activation in response to IFNs and other extracellular signaling proteins. Science 1994; 264:1415–1421.

140. Wagner BJ, Hayes TE, Hoban CJ, Cochran BH. The SIF binding element confers sis/PDGF induciblity onto the c-fos promoter. Embo J 1990; 9:4477–4484.
141. Bhat GJ, Thekkumkara TJ, Thomas WG, Conrad KM, Baker KM. Angiotensin II stimulates sis-inducing factor-like DNA binding activity. J Biol Chem 1994; 269:31443–31449.
142. Chen YH, Pouyssegur J, Courtneidge SA, Van Obberghen-Schilling E. Activation of Src family kinase activity by the G protein-coupled thrombin receptor in growth-responsive fibroblasts. J Biol Chem 1994; 269:27372–27377.
143. Marrero MB, Schieffer B, Paxton WG, Heerdt L, Berk BC, et al. Direct stimulation of Jak/STAT pathway by the angiotensin II AT1 receptor. Nature 1995; 375:247–250.
144. Rembold CM. Regulation of contraction and relaxation in arterial smooth muscle. Hypertension 1992; 20:129–137.
145. Adam LP, Franklin MT, Raff GJ, Hathaway DR. Activation of mitogen-activated protein kinase in porcine carotid arteries. Circ Res 1995; 76:183–190
146. Adam L, Kalinowski E, Hathaway D. Mitogen-activated protein kinase and contractility in carotid arteries: effects of the tyrosine kinase inhibitor genistein. Circulation 1994; 90:I-356a.
147. Schwartz SM, deBlois D, O'Brien ER. The intima. Soil for atherosclerosis and restenosis. Circ Res 1995; 77:445–465.
148. Kobayashi J, Wigle D, Childs T, Zhu L, Keeley FW, et al. Serum-induced vascular smooth muscle cell elastolytic activity through tyrosine kinase intracellular signalling. J Cell Physiol 1994; 160:121–131.

15

Myocardial Growth Factors

**W. Robb MacLellan, James Hawker,
and Michael D. Schneider**
Baylor College of Medicine
Houston, Texas

Heart failure in the setting of an increased hemodynamic burden (the so-called cardiomyopathy of overload) has been described in terms of a progressive paradigm shift within cardiovascular reasoning whose stages comprise, first, an emphasis on moment-to-moment mechanical adaptation, via sarcomere length and Starling's law; second, later biochemical inquiries into excitation–contraction coupling and short-term adaptation by protein phosphorylation; and, third, insights into long-term structural and functional adaptation via altered cardiac gene expression (1). One key component of the "hypertrophic phenotype" now is recognized to be the induction of an array of polypeptide growth factors, which are secreted proteins that play a vital role as regulators of growth and differentiation in various cells and tissues (2–5). Altered expression of peptide growth factors has been identified not only during hypertrophy of myocardium but also in other clinical contexts, including ischemia, myocarditis, and allograft rejection. The concept that growth factors might act in autocrine or paracrine circuits that mediate critical steps in normal cardiac development, as well as adaptation to abnormal stress, has been inferred on the basis of several lines of evidence (2–4), enumerated here and amplified below. (a) Peptide growth factors are expressed in a tightly regulated spatial and temporal pattern during cardiac development. (b) Growth factors that are upregulated in myocardium in vivo in the settings cited earlier can be induced, in cultured cardiac cells, by many conventional cardiac agonists. (c) Certain peptide growth factors promote cardiac muscle formation in vitro, using explants of cardiac progenitor cells or pluripotent cell lines. (d) Cardiac myocytes themselves are responsive to multiple growth factors, at least in vitro, and can be induced to reexpress a series of embryonic genes, duplicating many of the characteristic changes elicited by load (6, 7).

Hence, the myocardium is both a local source for numerous growth factors and an end-organ that possesses an unusually complex array of growth factor responses. The slate of trophic peptides implicated in these events is extensive, encompassing members of the type beta transforming growth factor (TGFβ), fibroblast growth factor (FGF), and insulin-like growth factor (IGF) superfamilies, among others. The present chapter will outline available evidence regarding the expression of cardiac growth factors, mechanisms of growth factor signal transduction in the context of other cardiac signaling cascades, and the involvement of peptide growth factors in the origin, development, and pathology of myocardium. Related issues (control of vascular smooth muscle proliferation by many of the same proteins, and the role played by angiotensin II produced within the myocardium itself) are reviewed elsewhere in this volume.

GROWTH FACTORS AND THEIR RECEPTORS

Transforming Growth Factor β

The type-beta transforming growth factors comprise a large superfamily of closely related multifunctional peptides. The prototypical member, TGFβ, is expressed as three isoforms in mammalian systems: TGFβ-1, TGFβ-2, and TGFβ-3 (see [4] for a recent review). More distant members, with diverse effects on morphogenesis, growth, and differentiation, include activins, bone morphogenetic proteins, Müllerian inhibitory substance, the *Drosophila* protein decapentaplegic, and the vegetal pole protein of *Xenopus laevis*, Vg-1. The biologically active mature peptides form the carboxy-terminus of each precursor protein, share 70% sequence homology at the amino acid level, and are highly conserved among species. Production of active TGFβ requires a complex series of processing events. First, intracellular cleavage of the TGFβ precursor releases a homodimer of the C-terminal protein plus the N-terminal remnant, called latency-associated peptide for reasons explained below. Once secreted, the mature TGFβ dimer associates noncovalently with latency-associated peptide, which in turn is linked through disulfide bonds to a 125–160 kDa TGFβ-binding protein. Latent TGFβ is not accessible to the TGFβ receptor, but can subsequently be activated by exposure to heat or acid, or by proteases such as plasmin. Multiple levels of posttranslational control thus influence the abundance of biologically active TGFβ, allowing precise regulation of TGFβ-mediated events.

In situ hybridization studies to define the distribution of TGFβ mRNA have demonstrated that TGFβ1 mRNA is first detected in the murine heart at day 7 postcoitum (p.c.) and is localized to endocardial cells but not myocardium (8). The TGFβ1 gene continues to be expressed at high levels until the perinatal period, when the mRNA is no longer detectable by in situ hybridization. By immunocytochemistry, extracellular TGFβ1 was detected predominantly in the endocardium and cardiac jelly, yet immunoreactive TGFβ1 also was highly abundant within murine ventricular muscle cells at 9–10.5 days p.c. (9). Indeed, myocardium was the most intensely stained region of the embryo. The apparent discrepancy in TGFβ1 RNA and protein expression is currently believed to intimate that TGFβ1 synthesized in epithelial cells may act in a paracrine fashion, upon the adjacent ventricular muscle cells. TGFβ1 is also proposed to act as a paracrine factor during cardiac morphogenesis in the chick, to mediate the conversion of endocardial epithelium into valve-forming mesenchymal cells (10, 11).

The distributions of TGFβ2 mRNA and protein likewise show disparities from one another. In the murine heart at 8.5 to 9.5 days of gestation, TGFβ2 mRNA is expressed at high levels in cardiac progenitor cells and the adjacent foregut endoderm (12). Subsequently, TGFβ2 mRNA is downregulated in myocardial cells, reciprocal with an accumulation of TGFβ2 protein (12). By days 9.5–10.5 p.c., TGFβ2 transcripts were restricted to prevalvular mesenchyme, the atrioventricular cushion, and ventricular outflow tract (13), yet the peptide was seen throughout all regions of myocardium (9). Neonatal rat cardiac myocytes in culture secrete large amounts of TGFβ2 (14), and expression of TGFβ2 protein continues even in adult ventricular muscle of the mouse (12). In the case of TGFβ3, neither transcripts nor peptide was detected in embryonic mouse myocardial cells: TGF-β3 mRNA was restricted to valvular mesenchyme (13), while the protein was most abundant in pericardium (9). Rather than reflecting methodological differences between the RNA and protein studies (such as the stringent specificity of reagents for one TGFβ isoform among several, and the comparative threshold for detection by each technique, respectively), these differences have been rationalized in conjunction with paracrine models for the specialization of valve mesenchyme (15) and cardiac myogenesis itself (12).

TGFβ Receptors

Three major TGFβ-binding cell surface proteins predominate in cardiac myocytes and most other mammalian cells, which are denoted receptors I, II, and III, in increasing order of size (TβR-1, TβR-II, TβR-III) (16, 17). Expression cloning of the type II receptor, identification of the similar but distinctive type I receptor, proof that each is a transmembrane serine-threonine kinase, and emergence of a superfamily of receptors for other TGFβ-related proteins have together led to rapid progress in elucidating mechanisms of TGFβ-dependent signal transduction (18–21) (Fig. 1).

The type III receptor (TβR-III), betaglycan, is a large (M_r 200–400 kDa) membrane-spanning proteoglycan, with an extensive extracellular domain capable of binding TGFβ, but a minimal intracellular tail with no known signaling function. Since cell lines devoid of TβR-III retain their responsiveness to TGFβ, betaglycan is dispensable for the biological actions of TGFβ, but participates in presentation of TGFβ to the signaling receptors, TβR-I and -II: overexpression of betaglycan in L6E9 cells deficient in TβR-II augmented the cells' response to ligand, especially TGFβ2, chiefly through an increase in receptor affinity (22).

Functional distinctions between TβR-I and TβR-II have been discerned largely through the use of a mink lung epithelial cell line, Mv1Lu, subjected to a chemical mutagen and selection of derivative clones that had lost their growth-inhibitory response to TGFβ (23). Evidence acquired from these TGFβ-resistant mutants suggested the tenets that TβR-I and TβR-II were both neces-

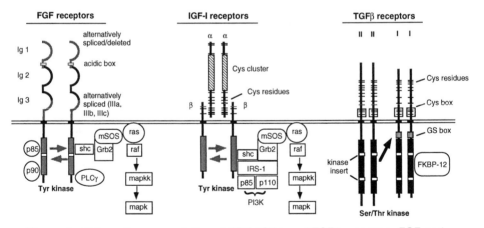

Figure 1 Schematic representation of FGF, IGF-I, and TGFβ receptors. FGF and IGF-I receptors share related protein tyrosine kinase signaling domains (shaded), which mediate receptor autophosphorylation in trans after ligand-induced dimerization. TGFβ signal transduction involves type I and type II serine/threonine kinases (solid) in a heterotetrameric complex, resulting in phosphorylation of the type I receptor GS box by the type II receptor kinase. Receptor-associated proteins and putative downstream targets are indicated for each growth factor family, respectively. See text for details.

sary and sufficient for TGFβ-signaling, that TβR-II is necessary for binding of TGFβ to TβR-I, and that TβR-I is required for signal transduction (19, 24). Each of these conclusions was subsequently confirmed by expression cloning of TβR-II, a transmembrane protein featuring a short, cysteine-rich extracellular ligand-binding domain, single transmembrane segment, and characteristic cytoplasmic Ser/Thr kinase domain, the hallmark of this receptor superfamily (25). Based on regions conserved among the Ser/Thr kinase domains of this family, and using degenerate primers for the polymerase chain reaction, a further subset of transmembrane Ser/Thr kinases has been cloned, comprising the type I receptors that had been visualized by affinity-labeling. The type I receptors share high homology to one another within their kinase domains (60–90%, at the amino acid level), and show lesser homology to TβR-II (37–42%) or other members of the type II receptor class. In addition, type I receptors share other features that differentiate them from type II receptors, which include the positioning of cysteine residues in the extracellular region, the presence of a serine/glycine-rich segment (GS box) at the amino-terminal portion of the intracellular domain, and an abbreviated carboxy-terminal tail.

Affinity labeling with radioiodinated TGFβ has directly demonstrated the presence of all three TGFβ-receptor types in cultured cardiac cells (14). As shown by coimmunoprecipitation, the type I and type II receptors detected in cardiac myocytes, as in other cell types, form a heteromeric complex with one another in the presence of TGFβ (26). TβR-II transcripts are expressed at low levels in embryonic and adult mouse cardiac tissue (21, 27). TβR-I mRNA is likewise expressed in both embryonic mouse and adult human heart (21, 28).

The availability of cloned receptors for TGFβ has clarified molecular mechanisms underlying the intricate interdependence of TβR-I and TβR-II: TβR-I fails to bind TGFβ in the absence of TβR-II, and, conversely, TβR-II is insufficient to propagate signal without TβR-I (19, 29). Although TβR-II can interact physically with all members of the type I receptor family when each is overexpressed in COS cells, only the complex of TβR-II with TβR-I had the capacity to bind TGFβ efficiently, transduce ligand-dependent signals, and restore TGFβ responses to MvlLu cells lacking endogenous TβR-I (30, 31). Recent data suggest that the TβR-II kinase exists as a spontaneous homodimer in the absence of ligand (32), and that the TβR-II kinase is constitutively active (29). Binding of TGFβ recruits TβR-I into a heterotetrameric protein kinase complex (33), leading to phosphorylation of the TβR-I GS box by TβR-II (29). The kinase activity of TβR-II thus is imperative for directional phosphorylation of TβR-I, and the kinase activity of TβR-I is necessary for downstream signal generation. These results, and the corresponding model of two interdependent protein kinases, predict that the operation of both receptors in tandem is required for all actions of TGFβ including gene induction, gene repression, and control of the cell cycle (often, as an antimitogen). Contrasting results include an apparently preferential loss of TβR-II in certain cancer cells that escape from growth inhibition by TGFβ (34, 35), and have raised the possibility, instead, that TβR-II and TβR-I might mediate distinguishable subsets of responses (growth inhibition and gene induction, respectively); see (36).

Fibroblast Growth Factor

Remarkable complexity also is seen in the fibroblast growth factor superfamily, which comprises at least nine members: the prototypes acidic and basic FGF (aFGF, FGF-1; bFGF, FGF-2), int-2 (FGF-3), hst-1/k-FGF (FGF-4), FGF-5, FGF-6, keratinocyte growth factor (FGF-7), androgen-induced growth factor (FGF-8), and glia-activating factor (FGF-9) (37–39). These range in size from 16 to 32 kDa, with 30–55% homology between different family members. FGF-1 and -2 first were purified as fibroblast mitogens from brain extracts, and subsequently were recognized in a variety of tissues. FGFs commonly accumulate in the extracellular matrix, including that of cardiac myocytes, where they are bound to heparan sulfate proteoglycans (HSPG) (40–42). The characteristic high affinity of FGFs for heparin and HSPGs has greatly facilitated their purification. Moreover, heparin protects FGFs from heat, acid, and proteolytic degradation. The role of heparin or HSPGs in the presentation of FGF to its signaling receptor will be discussed subsequently.

FGF-1 and -2 have been purified from the heart in numerous species (43–46), and have been localized to ventricular myocytes, among other cell types, by immunocytochemistry (43, 46, 47). Although historically FGF-1 and -2 were the initial members of this family to be discovered and remain the most thoroughly studied, FGF-1 and -2 in fact are rather atypical: they each lack a signal peptide sequence for secretion from cells, and their mechanism of export is unclear. Some have postulated that these FGFs might be chiefly released from injured or "wounded" cells. By contrast, most other FGFs contain this motif for protein secretion; FGF-9 also is efficiently secreted, despite the lack of this signal, by an unknown mechanism.

FGF-2 also is noteworthy for the existence of higher-molecular-weight isoforms, produced by initiating protein translation at alternative, upstream CUG codons, resulting in 21, 22, and 24 kDa forms, distinct from 18 kDa, AUG-initiated FGF-2 species (48). In cardiac myocytes, preferential expression of the larger FGF-2 isoforms is associated with proliferative neonatal cells, whereas postmitotic adult ventricular myocytes express predominantly 18 kDa FGF-2 (49). Transfection of cardiac myocytes has confirmed the expectation that 22 kDa FGF-2 preferentially translocates to the nucleus (50). Nuclear targeting of FGFs translated from alternative CUG initiation sites also has been described for int-2 (51) and FGF-3 (52) FGF-2 itself harbors an amino-terminal motif for nuclear translocation, whose effect may be limited, however, to determining the distribution of exogenously supplied FGF-1 (53). The presumptive nuclear targeting sequence found at the amino-terminus of FGF-1 appears crucial for transcriptional and mitogenic actions of the growth factor in endothelial cells, fibroblasts (54), and cardiac myocytes (55). Characteristically, exogenous FGF-1 and FGF-2 preferentially accumulate in the nucleus during G1, and peak before initiation of DNA synthesis (56, 57). However, the functional significance of nuclear targeting remains controversial both for FGF-1 and for other FGF isoforms.

Like their pattern of distribution, the spectrum of action for FGFs is much broader than was first surmised, and encompasses control of the cell cycle, tissue-specific transcription, and organogenesis. FGFs serve as mitogens for wide variety of mesoderm- and neuroectoderm-derived cells, including endothelium, vascular smooth muscle, glia, and neurons (37, 38), in addition to embryonic and neonatal ventricular myocytes (7, 44). FGF-1 and -2 are angiogenic factors, which induce vessel formation both in vitro and in vivo (58). As detailed in subsequent sections of this chapter, FGF-1 and -2 each upregulate the fetal program of gene expression in cardiac myocytes (6, 7, 55). FGF-1 (7) and possibly FGF-2 (59) also act as mitogens for ventricular myocytes from the neonatal rat and embryonic chick heart, respectively.

In avian embryos, FGF-2 was detected as punctate cytoplasmic aggregates in cells of the developing myocardium at the time of heart tube fusion (stage 9+), and the presence of 19 kDa FGF-2 was corroborated by immunoblotting (60). While FGF-2 was readily detected only in developing myocardium at this stage, FGF receptor was widely distributed in the embryo, although more abundant in ventricular myocytes and endothelial cells. By day 2–6 in ovo, FGF staining also is conspicuous in striated muscle and limb bud, in addition to myocardium (61). Both FGF-1 and -2 were widely distributed in developing rat embryo (11-20 d), with similar distributions in tissues of neurectodermal and mesodermal origin (62). FGF immunoreactivity in myocardium was found within cardiac myocytes, valve mesenchyme, and the ventricular outflow tracts.

Although no specific role for FGF-7 in the cardiovascular system has been suggested, FGF-7 transcripts are transiently detected in developing mouse myocardium, and are differentially regulated between the atrium and ventricle (63). Atrial expression of FGF-7 was first seen at 8.5 days p.c., and was maximal at 11 days p.c.; ventricular expression spanned 9.5–10.5 days p.c. FGF-7 also was seen in the somites of developing skeletal muscle, coincident with FGF-4 and -5, which were not expressed in the heart (63). By in situ hybridization of murine embryos, FGF-6 was shown to be exclusive to developing skeletal muscle (64), although RNA blots reveal faint expression of FGF-6 in the adult mouse heart (65).

FGF Receptors

The structural diversity, expression, and signaling mechanisms of FGF receptors have been recently reviewed (66–68). The cytoplasmic tyrosine kinase overall is similar in structure to that of other receptor tyrosine kinases (e.g., >50% amino acid identity with the receptor for PDGF), however a number of identifying features mark each of these tyrosine kinase families (Fig. 1). The FGF receptors share extracellular domains that are characterized by immunoglobulin-like (Ig) loops, formed by intrachain disulfide bonds. Other structural hallmarks of FGF receptors include a cluster of 6-9 acidic residues between loops I and II, a single membrane-spanning domain, a long juxtamembrane region of ~79 amino acids, a tyrosine kinase domain interrupted by one kinase insert of ~14–20 residues, and a C-terminal tail.

Four FGFR genes exist, which encode the receptors designated FGFR1-4. Overall homology among these ranges from 56 to 92%. Diversity of FGF receptors also arises from alternative mRNA splicing: FGFR1, -2, and -3 each have been shown to be expressed as alternative splice variants (69–72). One feature determined by splicing is the presence of 2 vs. 3 Ig loops in the extracellular ligand-binding domain. Thus far, Ig loop 1 (the most N-terminal loop) appears dispensable for ligand binding, and its function is unknown, whereas both loops II and III are required for binding. Different exons encode the different loops. For example, three alternative exons encode the C-terminal half of Ig loop III (IIIa, IIIb, and IIIc). Among these, IIIa is seen only in a naturally occurring, secreted form of receptor, truncated N-terminal to the transmembrane domain (73). IIIb and IIIc are found in alternative spliced forms of FGFR1, 2, and 3 (71), and influence the relative affinity of each receptor for particular FGF proteins. Thus, the binding affinities shown by FGFR1 isoforms are: IIIa, FGF-2 > FGF-1; IIIb: FGF-1 > FGF-2; IIIc FGF-1 = FGF-2. The corresponding affinities for the IIIb form of FGFR2 are: FGF-1 = FGF-7 > FGF-2; by contrast, IIIc binds FGF-1 and -2 equivalently, with no binding to FGF-7. The IIIb form of FGFR3 binds only FGF-1. Alternative exons also contribute to diversity in the carboxy-terminal tail (74).

Apart from the four high-affinity receptor tyrosine kinases, other cell surface molecules, whose significance is unproven, also binds FGFs. These include a cysteine-rich transmembrane receptor of unknown function, with a short cytoplasmic tail (75), and various HSPGs (76).

Early studies of FGF receptor expression by [^{125}I]-FGF-1 affinity-labeling established that receptor content in avian embryos is relatively constant from day 2 to 7 in ovo, but declines fivefold by day 13 (77). By day 19, little or no receptor was detected in cardiac or skeletal muscle (77). In ovo, the chicken fibroblast growth factor receptor CEK-1 is expressed in most tissues, whereas CEK-2 and -3 are more restricted (78). Highest expression of FGF receptor was seen in bone, skeletal muscle, cardiac muscle, vascular smooth muscle, and brain, with CEK-1 the predominant form in myocardium. Downregulation of FGF receptor immunostaining was seen in avian ventricular myocytes by stage 15 (60).

In the mouse, cardiac expression of the FGFR1 gene likewise declines more than eightfold between the embryo and the adult (79). The murine heart contains transcripts for predicted short (86 kDa, 2 loop) and long (102 kDa, 3 loop) forms of FGFR1 (79). The long form predominates in embryos, and the shorter form in adult heart, although the majority at both stages contain exon IIIc, an isoform associated with high-affinity binding of FGF-2.

Despite the obvious distinction that the signaling domains of FGF receptors harbor a canonical tyrosine kinase, rather than a serine/threonine kinase as seen for TGFβ, certain functional homologies are worth noting in the respective mechanisms of receptor activation. FGF binding to the FGFR induces receptor dimerization, intermolecular and phosphorylation of receptor dimers on tyrosine residues, activation of receptor tyrosine kinase activity, recruitment and tyrosine phosphorylation of intracellular substrates, and receptor internalization. However, FGF, unlike TGFβ, is a monomeric ligand. Recent data indicate that heparin causes oligomerization of FGF-1, enabling its binding to provoke dimer formation and subsequent activation of FGF receptor (80). Whether this mechanism applies to other FGFs is uncertain. Mutagenesis of FGF-2 suggests the existence of two distinct receptor-binding sites on each molecule, distinct from the heparin-binding domain, which act in concert. Hence, even a monomer of FGF-2 can promote FGFR dimerization, provided that both binding surfaces are available (81).

Others have indicated that heparin or HSPG may even be obligatory for FGF-1 and FGF-2 to bind the high-affinity, signaling receptors (82–84), a role far beyond the modulatory effect of betaglycan in presenting TGFβ to TGFβ receptors. This model is supported by the identification of the minimal oligosaccharide sequences within heparin that are necessary to enable FGF binding and signal transduction (85, 86), and by the formation of a ternary complex among FGF, heparin or HSPG, and FGFR, via a distinct K18K heparin-binding sequence in the FGFR extracellular domain (87); cf. (88).

The first identified substrate for tyrosine phosphorylation by the ligand-activated FGFR was phospholipase Cγ1; however, a mutation of FGFR1 that abolishes FGF-induced calcium release and PI hydrolysis (Y766F) did not impair mitogenic activity, suggesting that these biochemical responses are not needed for proliferation to occur (89, 90). Activation of PLCγ likewise was dispensable for mesoderm induction by FGF receptor in *Xenopus* animal caps (91). Other substrates that are phosphorylated or activated by FGF binding to FGFR are the SH2 adaptor protein Shc (92), the Src tyrosine kinase (93), and cortacin, a putative substrate for Src (93). Downstream, signaling proteins activated by FGFR are Raf-1 and mitogen-activated protein kinase (92). A role for Raf-1 in mesoderm induction by FGF has been confirmed using a kinase-defective, dominant-negative form of this serine/threonine kinase (94).

Distinctions have been noted, between FGFR classes, in their activation of signaling intermediaries (95). For example, by comparison to FGFR1, FGFR4 leads to much weaker tyrosine phosphorylation of PLCγ1, Raf-1, and MAP kinase, and no phosphorylation of Shc, yet both receptors could activate DNA synthesis in response to FGF (92). Certain proteins that have been implicated as direct or indirect substrates for other receptor tyrosine kinases (EGF or PDGF receptors) appears not to mediate signaling by FGFR. These include the receptor-binding protein Grb2, the protein tyrosine phosphatase p64 Syp/PTP1D, and two proteins that bind the Ras effector domain: GTPase-activating protein and the p85 regulatory subunit of PI-3 kinase (92).

Insulin-Like Growth Factors

The insulin-like growth factors, IGF-I and -II, are single-chain polypeptides containing ~70 amino acids (7.5 kDa). IGF-I is homologous with insulin itself (49%) and with IGF-II (61%) (96). IGF-I and -II both are synthesized in most tissues of the body and are abundant in the circulation, usually complexed with IGF-binding proteins (IGFBP). Apart from local autocrine or paracrine circuits, there also is likely importance to systemic IGF-I and -II. Conversely, the liver is the principal source of circulating IGFs, whereas local production by diverse cells and tissues can be regulated independently. The spatial and temporal distributions of IGF-I and -II differ. In embryonic day 14–15 rat embryos, IGF-I transcripts were particularly abundant in undifferentiated mesenchyme and sites of active remodeling such as the ventricular outflow tract; IGF-II mRNA was associated with developing muscle, cartilage, and vasculature (97). IGF-II is more prevalent in fetal tissues whereas IGF-I is more prevalent after birth (97). Lateral plate mesoderm, containing the progenitors of myocardium, is among the earliest sites expressing IGF-II RNA and protein in early mouse embryos (98).

Both IGF-I and -II circulate largely as part of a heterotrimeric, 125–150 kDa complex comprising IGFs, the IGF binding protein-3, and an acid-labile subunit (99). At least six IGFBPs have been identified, comprising 200–300 amino acids, with a 20–40 amino acid signal peptide sequence. Conserved residues include 18 cysteine residues in the amino- and carboxy-termini of IGFBPs 1–6, which may have importance for IGF binding. While growth hormone regulates local production and circulating levels of IGF-1, IGFBP-3 and -4 (at least) are regulated by the IGFs themselves and other growth factors including TGFβ.

The importance of IGFBPs lies in their ability to inhibit or potentiate the diverse metabolic and mitogenic effects of IGFs. IGFBP-1, -2, -3, and -4 decrease biological activity by inhibiting IGF binding to cells, sequestering the peptides, and preventing interaction with receptor (100, 101). IGFBP-3 in particular is more effective than IGFBP-1 or -2 in blocking cell surface binding. In paradoxical fashion, pretreating fibroblasts with IGFBP-3 increases IGF-I bioactivity, while coincubation decreases activity (102). Potentiation is ascribed to an increase in IGF-I binding via cell-associated IGFBP-3. Potentiation is also reported for IGFBP-1 and -2, when associated with the cell surface (103). Proteolysis of IGFBP-3 may represent a physiological posttranslational mechanism to regulate IGF bioavailability by decreasing its affinity for IGF and hence promoting the release of bound IGF (101).

IGF Receptors

The IGF-I receptor (IGF1R) is widespread in distribution and is chiefly responsible for the biological actions of both IGF-I and -II (104, 105). Its dissociation constants for binding different members of the insulin family are IGF-I, 1 nM; IGF-II, 2–10 nM; and insulin, 100–500 nM. Thus, the order of relative affinities for IGF1R is IGF-I > IGF-II >> insulin. IGF1R is a tetrameric transmembrane glycoprotein with the subunit structure, $\alpha_2\beta_2$. Its overall structure resembles that of the insulin receptor (IR). Each contains a tyrosine kinase signaling domain in the cytoplasmic segment of its β subunit, linked by disulfide bonds to the α subunit; the α-subunit, in turn, contains cysteine-rich regions that comprise the primary ligand-binding domain (Fig. 1). Certain differences are worth noting. Insulin and IGF-I bind distinguishable regions of their respective α subunits (106). Investigations of chimeric insulin/IGF1 receptor indicate that both tyrosine kinase domains can mediate short-term metabolic effects such as glucose transport, yet the IGF1R protein kinase is 10-fold more effective at inducing DNA synthesis (107). Naturally occurring hybrid receptors exist that comprise one insulin receptor α/β subunit pair with one IGF1R α/β subunit pair, a configuration resulting in increased affinity for, and activation by, IGF-I (108).

By mutation of the invariant lysine in the cytoplasmic domain ATP-binding site, tyrosine kinase activity was shown to be necessary for receptor autophosphorylation, activation of PI-3-kinase and 2-deoxyglucose uptake, induction of ornithine decarboxylase gene expression, and stimulation of DNA synthesis (109). Other regions critical for function include tyrosine residues 1131, 1135, 1136 of the kinase domain (110), and a NPXY sequence C-terminal to the transmembrane domain, needed both for signaling and for internalization (111). Ligand-induced autophosphorylation, for both IGF1R and IR, occurs as an intermolecular phosphorylation, in *trans* (112). A major substrate for tyrosine phosphorylation by both IR and IGF1R is a 185 kDa phosphoprotein, insulin receptor substrate-1 (IRS-1) (113). The phosphotyrosine residues of IRS-1 mediate association with cellular effector proteins such as PI3-kinase, through SH2 domains. IRS-1contains >10 potential tyrosine phosphorylation sites, of which six are found within a Y-M-X-M motif. A more general form of this, Y-X-X-M, is present in all proteins known to associate with PI-3 kinase.

The majority of metabolic and mitogenic responses to IGF-II also are mediated by the two receptor tyrosine kinases, IGF1R and IR. The so-called IGF2R, synonymous with the cation-independent mannose 6-phosphate (M6P) receptor, is a single-chain peptide characterized by a large extracellular domain, separable binding sites for IGF-II and M6P, a single transmembrane domain, and a short cytoplasmic tail which contains no kinase domain and has no known signaling activity. The functional importance of this receptor appears to lie, largely, in providing a degradative pathway for IGF-II, via receptor internalization (114). However, this view may be simplistic: in skeletal muscle cells, myogenin gene expression and the program of myogenic differentiation could be stimulated by L27 IGF-II, a substitution with normal affinity for IGF2R but markedly impaired affinity for IGF1R and IR (115). Moreover, a signaling pathway via Gi2 also has been ascribed to IGF2R (116).

Ligand binding stimulates autophosphorylation of IGF1R on the β subunit and activates tyrosine phosphorylation of cytoplasmic signaling molecules including IRS-1 (104, 117). Tyrosine phosphorylation of Shc also is induced by IGF-I, and was proven to be part of mitogenic cascade for IGF-I, insulin, and EGF action by microinjection of neutralizing antibodies directed against Shc (118, 119). Mice homozygous for a null mutation of IRS-1 are insulin resistant and exhibit growth retardation, but with normal histology (120); together with biochemical evidence for Shc phosphorylation and PI3K activation in the receptor-deficient animals, this suggests that IRS-1-dependent and IRS-1-independent pathways both exist. Tyrosine phosphorylation of nuclear proteins is induced within minutes of IGF-I treatment of cells (121).

IGF-I is a so-called progression factor for cell cycle control in fibroblasts, which is needed in synergy with competence factors (PDGF, EGF, and FGF). In BALB/c 3T3 fibroblasts, IGF-I is the only growth factor required late in G1, 6–2.5 h before the start of S phase, for the onset of DNA synthesis. In agreement with this model of discrete competence and progression factors, mouse embryo fibroblasts that lack endogenous IGF1R require functional IGF1R for mitosis and transformation in response to EGF (122). Although IGF-I can stimulate differentiation of skeletal myoblasts, by inducing myogenin expression (123), forced expression of IGF1R, like higher concentrations of IGF-I, induces proliferation instead (124).

Expression of IGF1R mRNA is widespread during early organogenesis, and is most prominent in neural and muscle tissue including myocardium (125, 126). As in most tissues, expression of IGF1R mRNA declines after birth. In the rat heart, IGF1R mRNA expression is maximal on the first day after birth, and decreases dramatically, to 17% of the peak abundance by 50 days of age (125). IGF2R is most abundant in the heart and vasculature, and, like IGF1R, declines rapidly after birth (114, 127, 128).

GROWTH FACTOR SIGNALING CASCADES IN MYOCARDIUM

p21 Ras

One area of particularly active research in cardiovascular medicine has been the attempt to explicate the linkage between ligand-induced trophic signals and subsequent regulation of the cardiac phenotype. An intricate web of effector molecules has been implicated in the transduction of growth factor-initiated signals in other systems, whose applicability is uncertain in the context of cardiac muscle (Fig. 1). Ras proteins are membrane-associated guanine nucleotide-binding proteins, distantly related to α subunits of the heterotrimeric G-proteins that mediate signaling by adrenergic, muscarinic, and other "heptahelical" receptors. Classically, Ras plays a pivotal role in transduction of receptor tyrosine kinases, such as the receptors for FGF, IGFs, and platelet-derived growth factor (129), but the importance of Ras in propagating signals induced by TGFβ and conventional cardiac agonists remains less well defined. Both passive mechanical stretch (130) and angiotensin II (131) increase the proportion of Ras that is GTP-bound, the active state. It has been suggested that mutationally activated Ras proteins can serve as surrogates for ligands that provoke the hypertrophic "program," and that, conversely, dominant-inhibitory forms of Ras selectively inhibit gene induction associated with hypertrophy (132); comparable findings have been reported for the Ras-dependent protein kinases, Raf and mitogen-activated protein kinase (133, 134).

However, gain-of-function mutations in growth factor signaling proteins are subject to the criticism that they do not address the physiological role of the wild-type protein at wild-type levels of expression (mediator vs. phenocopy?), and might merely induce or activate a secondary autocrine or paracrine peptide (135, 136). Indeed, Ras has even been reported to favor selectively the translation of certain growth factor mRNAs (137); increased formation of activin, rather than a specific role for Ras in activin signal transduction, thus is thought to explain the seeming involvement of Ras in signaling by this TGFβ-related peptide (138). Conversely, loss-of-function mutations often are confounded by issues of experimental design that impair the ability to discriminate between specific and global effects, including bias of ascertainment (negligible expression of the test gene in the absence of agonist), inadequate duration to permit downregulation of "constitutive" control genes, and unequal stability of proteins commonly used to compare the transcriptional activity of two co-transfected promoters.

Work from our laboratory suggests, instead, a revisionist interpretation, that Ras activity is required for efficient expression of an unexpectedly inclusive or generalized set of genes, both in cardiac muscle and in noncardiac cells (139) (Fig. 2). Although TGFβ-dependent transcription of the skeletal α-actin promoter can be inhibited by the N17 mutation of c-H-ras, basal transcription of the promoter is equally affected, even in defined medium lacking all exogenous growth factors. Indeed, all promoters examined were repressed with very similar dose-response relations, including β-myosin heavy chain (βMHC), which, like skeletal α-actin, is highly induced by TGFβ, FGFs, and other trophic factors; cardiac α-actin, which shows little or no induction; and nominally constitutive viral elements. Parallel effects were observed in mink lung epithelial cells using the TGFβ-inducible promoter for plasminogen activator inhibitor-1, herpes simplex virus thymidine kinase promoter, and a TATA-less promoter derived from the adenoassociated virus initiator element. The finding that dominant-negative Ras is an inhibitor of basal transcription has since been corroborated in two ways (unpublished results): using the catalytic domains of Ras GTPase-activating proteins, converting exogenous Ras to the inactive (GDP-bound) form, and using a recombinant adenovirus expressing N17 Ras, which markedly inhibited total run-off transcription in isolated nuclei. The linkage of dominant-negative Ras to impaired basal transcription is consistent with recent reports that an inhibitory Ras gene elicits programmed cell death (140).

FKBP-12

A TGFβ signaling pathway distinct from those defined for other classes of growth factors (Fig. 1) has been suggested by evidence that the immunophilin FKBP-12, an immunosuppressant-binding protein, physically interacts with the cytoplasmic domain of TβR-I, as revealed by interaction cloning, using a rat cardiac library (141). This implication of FKBP-12 in TGFβ signal transduction is intriguing, given the profound immunosuppressant effects of TGFβ (142), and the antiproliferative effects of rapamycin and FK506, the ligands for FKBP-12 (143). One plausible mechanism could entail intracellular calcium levels, since FKBP-12 specifically associated with the sarcoplasmic reticulum calcium release channel (ryanodine receptor) and modulates gating by the channel (144). However, the ability of FKBP-12 to mediate either the antimitogenic or transcriptional effects of TGFβ is unproven thus far. Indeed, mutation of the invariant proline adjacent to the TβR-I GS box indicates that FKBP-12 recognition is dispensable for TGFβ signal generation (144a).

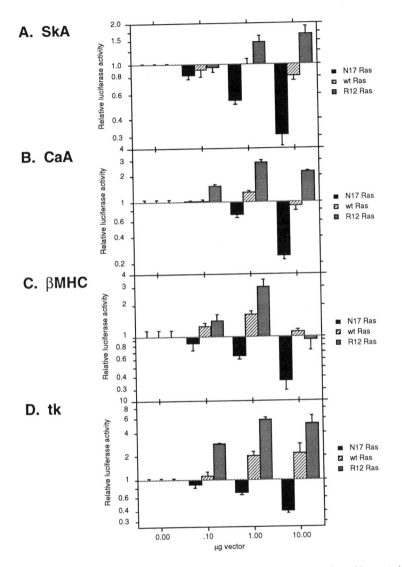

Figure 2 p21 Ras as a governor of global gene expression. Neonatal cardiac myocytes were transfected with the luciferase expression vectors shown in the presence of dominant-negative, wild-type, or activated Ras vectors. Results are expressed relative to the activity of each promoter in vector-transfected cells. All constructs were inhibited by N17 Ras with similar dose–response relations; comparable results were obtained for growth-factor-dependent and nominally constitutive promoters in Mv1Lu cells. (From Ref. 139.)

"Immediate-Early" Genes

Given that receptors for TGFβ differ fundamentally from receptor tyrosine kinases, such as those for FGFs, and from the G-protein-coupled receptors for endothelin and norepinephrine, one perplexity is that all four classes of agonist share the ability to activate a similar array of promoters for hypertrophy-associated genes (145–150). Viewed from the perspective of efforts to explicate signal transduction mediating hypertrophy, the paradox pertains both to convergence (How do disparage agonists evoke such similar responses?) and divergence (How does even one of these ligands regulate so extensive an array of cardiac genes?). Downstream from the multitude of cytoplasmic "second" messengers, immediate-early genes including c-fos, c-jun, and c-myc have been postulated to act as the "third" messengers for diverse ligand-dependent signals (151–153). These nuclear oncogenes encode sequence-specific DNA-binding proteins that are upregulated within minutes by various agonists and have been implicated in regulating both the cell cycle and gene transcription. In cultured cardiac myocytes, immediate-early transcription factors can be acutely induced, for example, by serum (145, 146), adrenergic agonists (154, 155), endothelin (148), FGFs (156), angiotensin II (157), or passive mechanical stretch (158, 159). In the intact myocardium, immediate-early genes are rapidly induced by aortic banding (160–164), adrenergic agonists (165), or ischemia (166); in the isolated rat heart, induction of Fos and Jun in ventricular myocytes was specifically associated with systolic wall stress, rather than diastolic stretch (167). The sequential temporal relationship between induction of these transcription factors and later changes in cardiac phenotype, taken together with regulatory properties defined for Myc, Fos, and Jun in skeletal muscles and other lineages (168–171), supports this hypothesis that such genes might mediate the hypertrophic program, at least in part.

    Relatively few experiments with cardiac cells have directly addressed the transcriptional equivalent of Koch's postulates: namely, whether Myc, Fos, and Jun can be shown to be sufficient and necessary for hypertrophic growth, fetal gene induction, or both. Forced expression of Fos and Jun in cultured cardiac myocytes can induce skeletal α-actin (172), ANF (173), and βMHC (T. Parker, personal communication), genes that are upregulated in this hypertrophic ventricle; however, dichotomous results, repression of hypertrophy-associated genes by these transcription factors, also have been reported (174, 175). An obvious concern is that induction of endogenous Fos/Jun by agonists or load is relatively transient, not sustained as with transfection. It is interesting that both TGFβ (176) and endothelin (177) are upregulated by Jun, suggesting that positive feedback via these autocrine factors might perpetuate the signals initiated by load. In transgenic mice, targeted expression of c-myc in myocardium causes ventricular enlargement, via an increase in cell number

(178); transcriptional effects of Myc in ventricular myocytes, if any, remain to be shown.

Loss-of-function mutations to abrogate the function of Fos/Jun, comparable to those discussed for Ras, have not yet been applied to these postulated nuclear mediators of hypertrophic signals. Although "knock-out" mutations of Fos and Jun have been generated in mice without evidence of a cardiac defect (179, 180), the existence of multiple *fos* and *jun* genes (with the likelihood of at least partial functional redundancy) suggests caution in interpreting this lack of an obvious cardiac phenotype. Cardiac abnormalities have, however, been seen with an embryonic-lethal null mutation of *c-myc* (181). Even more conspicuously, hypoplasia of the compact subepicardial layer of myocardium is the likely basis for early lethality in a compound heterozygote of the related N-*myc* gene, expressing N-*myc* at ~15% of normal levels (182). It also is important to recognize a point better appreciated, perhaps, for cardiac physiology and pharmacology: that genetic manipulations affecting embryonic hearts need not predict the requirement for or role of a protein in adult myocardium. Gene transfer to the adult ventricular muscle cell via recombinant adenovirus (183) therefore holds particular promise as a means of dissect signal transduction cascades in cells that have been otherwise refractory to mechanistic studies.

SRF and TEF-1

A prerequisite for any model proposing autocrine or paracrine control of cardiac myocyte growth and differentiated gene expression by peptide growth factors is to demonstrate that cardiac myocytes are in fact targets for the actions of the presumptive agonists. The authors' laboratory has shown that both TGFβ and FGF induce a panel of genes normally associated with the embryonic ventricle, including skeletal and smooth muscle α-actin, β-MHC, and atrial natriuretic factor, in concert with downregulation of α-MHC and SRCA2, the calcium-sequestering ATPase of sarcoplasmic reticulum (6, 7); this continuum of positive and negative responses shows noteworthy fidelity to the program activated by mechanical stress in vitro and in vivo. The skeletal α-actin promoter was selected for subsequent emphasis, as a representative cardiac-restricted gene that is inducible by peptide growth factors as well as other trophic signals. Two generic models for growth factor responsiveness exist, in connection with a gene's transcription in differentiated tissues. First, regulation might occur via discrete growth factor response elements, such as AP-1 (176) or NF-1 (184) in the case of TGFβ. Alternatively, growth factors might influence expression of a gene by altering the abundance or activity of tissue-specific transcription factors, as shown for the myogenic helix–loop–helix proteins in skeletal muscle (185, 186). A necessary step to discriminate between these models is to map minimal regions that mediate responsiveness of the promoter. Initial analysis of the SkA promoter revealed that the proximal 200 base pairs were sufficient for high-level tissue-restricted transcription in cardiac myocytes, and for responsiveness both to TGFβ and to FGFs (6). Mutational analysis of the promoter and identification of the corresponding transcription factors bound to the promoter revealed that tissue-restricted expression in cardiac myocytes relied on the collaborative function of three positive-acting factors present in ventricular myocyte extracts (serum response factor [SRF]. TEF-1, and Sp1) and was antagonized by a negative-acting zinc finger protein, YY1, whose binding site overlaps the proximal site for SRF (187) (Fig. 3). Functional binding sites for SRF were sufficient to enable a neutral, minimal promoter to respond to both TGFβ and basic FGF; at least the case of TGFβ, the TEF-1 site likewise can confer responsiveness. Thus, SRF and TEF-1 act as TGFβ response factors in cardiac muscle. SRF also mediates induction of the skeletal

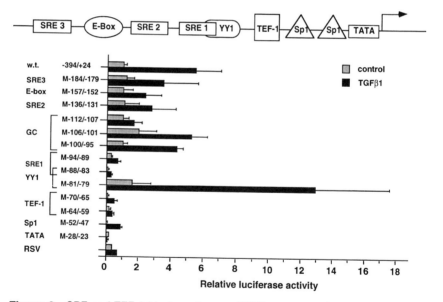

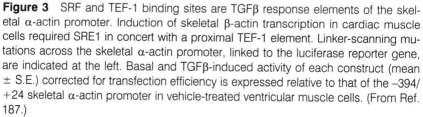

Figure 3 SRF and TEF-1 binding sites are TGFβ response elements of the skeletal α-actin promoter. Induction of skeletal β-actin transcription in cardiac muscle cells required SRE1 in concert with a proximal TEF-1 element. Linker-scanning mutations across the skeletal α-actin promoter, linked to the luciferase reporter gene, are indicated at the left. Basal and TGFβ-induced activity of each construct (mean ± S.E.) corrected for transfection efficiency is expressed relative to that of the −394/+24 skeletal α-actin promoter in vehicle-treated ventricular muscle cells. (From Ref. 187.)

α-actin promoter by FGF-2 (55); however, the proximal serum response element by itself is not sufficient for inhibition of the promoter by FGF-1.

Both SRF and TEF-1 already are known to play additional roles, in connection with myocardial hypertrophy and cardiac gene expression. SRF was first described as a protein mediating serum induction of the *c-fos* oncogene (188), and induction of *c-fos* in ventricular muscle cells by stretch or angiotensin II maps to the SRF binding site (130, 189). SRF is enriched in both skeletal (190) and cardiac muscle (187), but it is unknown whether differences in abundance or a tissue-restricted coactivator enable SRF binding sites to mediate preferential transcription in striated muscle (55, 191, 192). Since transcription factors related to SRF in yeast and plants can depend on associated homeobox proteins, the cardiac-specific homeobox protein Csx/Nkx-2.5 (193) is an exceptionally promising candidate to be a coactivator for SRF, TEF-1 participates not only in TGFβ induction of the skeletal α-actin promoter, but also in α_1-adrenergic and protein kinase C-dependent induction of β-MHC (194). Although muscle-enriched isoforms of TEF-1 exist (195), which forms mediate which trophic signals is conjectural at present.

ROLE OF PEPTIDE GROWTH FACTORS IN CARDIAC FUNCTION AND DISEASE

Cardiac Morphogenesis

Formation of cardiac muscle in early embryos requires the recruitment of pluripotent cells within the heart-forming region of lateral plate mesoderm, to establish the cardiac lineage. Seminal experiments pointing to the importance of diffusible signals in embryogenesis (arising from the ability of vegetal pole cells to convert animal pole explants of *Xenopus* embryos [presumptive ectoderm] into dorsal mesoderm) have led in recent years to identifying members of the TGFβ, FGF, and Wnt gene families that can act as mesoderm inducers (196). Whereas details of the spatial and temporal expression of TGFβ (4) have been taken to suggest a paracrine mechanism underlying the induction of cardiac myocytes and the cardiac valves as well, there is a clear need for more conclusive forms of proof. In addition to a role for the TGFβ superfamily in the induction of dorsal mesoderm, TGFβ is reported to provoke cardiac muscle formation in progenitor regions of the axolotl (197), the cardiogenic quail cell line QCE-6 (198), and *Xenopus laevis* (199). Notwithstanding the effect of activin on *Xenopus* dorsal mesoderm and the skeletal muscle lineage, both positive (200) and negative (199) results are reported for induction of a cardiac phenotype. Corresponding evidence for mammals has been quite limited, until recently, by the lack of practicable model systems that recapitulate cardiac myogenesis. One approach taken to delineate genes crucial for normal development, insertional mutagenesis, involves the use of retroviral vectors that integrate randomly into the mouse genome. A recessive, embryonic-lethal mutation was identified that prevents mesoderm formation in vivo, which has been traced to disruption of *nodal*, a TGFβ-related gene expressed specifically in the node of the anterior primitive streak, the mammalian equivalent of the Spemann organizer in *Xenopus* (201). A second strategy is the use of teratocarcinoma and embryonic stem cells, which provide access to the onset of cardiac gene transcription (202, 203), and in which TGFβ itself has been shown to provoke heart muscle formation (204, 205). To overcome the limitation that the impact of exogenous growth factors need not predict the function of the corresponding endogenous protein, a complementary line of evidence relies on inhibitors of growth factor expression or activity, such as antibodies or antisense oligonucleotides against TGFβ, which interfere with the conversion of endocardium into mesenchymal cells that make up the atrioventricular valves (10, 11). Antisense oligonucleotides that downregulate basic FGF have, analogously, been successfully employed to confirm that basic FGF is a mitogen for primitive cardiac myoblasts from anterior lateral plate mesoderm (Hamburger-Hamilton stage 6) (206).

Genetic ablation of growth factors or their receptors in vivo can provide insights that are potentially free of the ambiguities associated with model systems, overexpression, or antisense artifacts. By homologous recombination, two groups of investigators have engineered FGFR1 knockout mice, to ascertain the roles of FGF in development. FGFR1-deficient embryos, blastocyst culture, and embryonic stem (ES) cells indicate that FGFR1 is required for ES cell proliferation and axial organization (despite the existence of other, intact FGFR genes) but is dispensable for mesoderm induction (207). All embryos lacking FGFR1 display severe growth defects and die before or during gastrulation, with aberrant patterning of mesoderm and the absence of somites: the complex phenotype resulting from this mutation is viewed as implying a crucial role not only for cell proliferation in the early embryo but also in specifying mesodermal cell fates and pattern formation during gastrulation (207, 208).

By comparison, null mutations of IFG1R are lethal at birth, due to respiratory failure, in the setting of generalized organ hypoplasia (45% of normal weight); IGF-I knockouts have a more mild phenotype (60% of normal weight at birth), can survive to adulthood depending on the genetic background, and show no additive effect with the null mutation of IGF1R (209, 210) (Fig. 4). This generalized retardation of growth was exacerbated in double mutations of IGF-II plus IGF-I, or IGF-II plus IGF1R (209). The gene for IGF2R is one of several genes whose expression during embryogenesis depends on its parental origin, and is not expressed from the paternal allele (paternally imprinted) (211). Disruption of the IGF2R/M6PR gene hence has no effect, when inherited through the paternal germ line (a m^+/p^- phenotype). By contrast, inheriting the

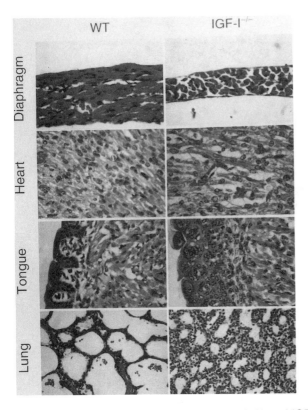

Figure 4 Histological analysis of wild-type (left) and IGF-I deficient (-/-) neonatal mice (right). The IGF-I-null mice are characterized by disorganization and vacuolization of muscle tissue (diaphragm, heart, and tongue), and by pulmonary atelectasis with alveolar hypercellularity. (From Ref. 210.)

mutated allele from the mother (m^-/p^+) results in threefold elevation of circulating IGF-II, a 30% generalized increase in organ growth, a disproportionate threefold increase in heart size, ventricular hyperplasia, and valvular and septal defects (212) (Fig. 5). The one m^-/p^+ heterozygote surviving to adulthood showed pathological features consistent with heart failure. That the perinatal lethality of IGF2R knockouts is contingent on overabundance of IGF-II is shown by crossing IGF2R-deficient T^{hp} mice with mice that lack IGF-II, resulting in a partial improvement in viability (213). As the improvement was incomplete, other explanations have been proposed, including the possibility that IGF2R binds the TGFβ1 precursor (a mannose-6-phosphate-containing protein), and facilitates the processing of TGFβ1 to its active, antimitogenic form (212).

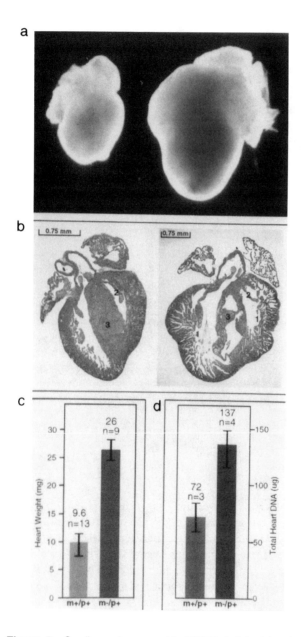

Figure 5   Cardiac enlargement in IGF2R deficient (m–/p+) mice. (a) Exterior and
(b) cross-sectional view. (c) Heart weight. (d) Cardiac DNA content. (From Ref. 212.)

A widespread requirement for any molecule in cell proliferation, such as FGFR1 or IGF1R, could potentially confound interpretation of the null phenotype in particular organ systems, given the risk of humoral, metabolic, or mechanical interference with normal events. Dominant-acting inhibitory mutations of the receptors for peptide growth factors provide an especially powerful means to ablate growth factor signaling pathways (138, 147, 214–216), which by contrast to knocked-out mutations, can be selectively targeted to particular cell types, or, potentially, developmental windows. Enzymatically effective mutations of receptor tyrosine kinases presumably act, in large part, by sequestering wild-type receptor monomers, resulting in a block to the autophosphorylation in *trans* that occurs after ligand-induced receptor dimerization. For the conspicuously different class of receptors for the TGFβ superfamily, kinase-defective mutations of the type II receptor would prevent activation of the type I receptor, and kinase-defective mutations of type I receptor would be unable to trigger downstream events. In essence, homologous partners are sequestered in the case of receptor tyrosine kinases, and heterologous partners in the case of receptors with serine/threonine kinase domains. An analogous kinase-defective truncation of the activin receptor blocks mesoderm induction and promotes neurulation in *Xenopus* embryos (138, 217). Despite evidence for TGFβ and activin as cardiogenic factors in model systems, it has not been proven that the endogenous growth factors play this role.

Recently, kinase-defective FGFR1 has been introduced into embryonic avian myocardium by means of a recombinant retrovirus, causing a relative decrease in clonal expansion by comparison to a control virus, and demonstrating that endogenous FGF is indeed a mitogen or survival factor for ventricular muscle cells between day 3 and 7 in ovo (218) (Fig. 6). No inhibition of subsequent growth resulted when hearts were infected on day 7, consistent with the known decline of endogenous FGF receptor during embryogenesis. This truncated FGF receptor forms heterodimers with all known FGFR classes and had been shown to block FGF signaling in *Xenopus* oocytes, early *Xenopus* embryos, L6 myoblasts, and transgenic mice (215, 219, 220). Forced expression of full-length FGFR1 had no effect on clonal growth, suggesting that endogenous FGF is limiting in the embryonic heart (218). Kinase-defective FGFR1 has also been used to implicate FGFs in the origin of smooth muscle during regional specification of *Xenopus laevis* mesoderm (221).

Given the known requirement that the type I and type II receptors for TGFβ form a heteromeric complex to initiate signaling events, we hypothesized that a kinase-deficient truncation of the TβR-II would act as a dominant negative inhibitor of TGFβ-induced signals, the approach used to explore the functional role of FGF (216, 219) and type II activin receptor (138, 217) in mesoderm formation. To construct the truncated TβR-II (ΔkTβR-II), a fragment consisting of the extracellular domain and membrane-spanning segments was ampli-

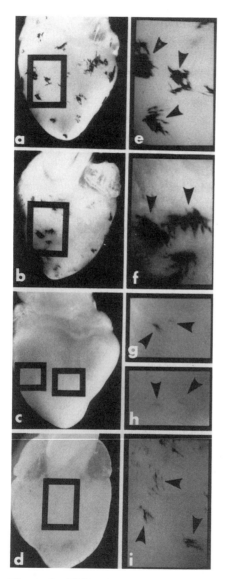

Figure 6 FGF receptor mediates cardiac myocyte proliferation in early avian cardiac development. Chicken hearts were inoculated on day 3 in ovo with replication-defective, helper virus-free retroviruses (~10 nl) and were stained for β-galactosidase activity on embryonic day 14. (a, e) *E. coli* lacZ; (b, f) full-length FGFR1 + lacZ; (c, g, h) kinase-defective truncation of FGFR1 + lacZ; (d, i) truncated FGFR1 in the antisense orientation + lacZ; (e–i) 3 X magnification of the boxed areas in a–d. (From Ref. 218.)

fied by PCR and cloned into a eukaryotic expression vector (Fig. 7). To determine whether ΔTβR-II could inhibit TGFβ signaling events, ΔTβR-II was overexpressed in neonatal cardiac myocytes. This construct blocked TGFβ-induced upregulation of skeletal α-actin by all three isoforms of TGFβ (147) (Fig. 7). Inhibition could be rescued by overexpression of the wild-type receptor, showing the specificity of the interaction, and was not seen with a comparable truncation of the type II activin receptor. Subsequent experiments by the authors have shown that a kinase-deficient truncations of the type I receptor, as well as point mutations in essential residues of the TβR-II kinase domain, likewise are dominant-acting inhibitors of signal transduction by the TGFβ receptor complex (26) (Figs. 8–10). All mutations that were inactive at rescuing receptor-deficient cells were, uniformly, dominant inhibitors in a wild-type background. Many of the residues selected for substitution by alanine (including K277, R378/D379, K381, D397, and R528) are invariant or highly conserved, charged amino acids known to be essential for activity of cyclic AMP-dependent protein kinase, the best-characterized serine/threonine kinase so far (38). These dominant-negative receptors thus provide a means to explore the role of TGFβ in vivo, which circumvents problems identified with "knock out" mutations including redundancy (222), embryonic or perinatal lethality (if used in conjunction with an inducible promoter [223]), and global phenotypes (224).

In *Drosphila*, dominant-negative mutations that disrupt morphogenetic signals by the TGFβ homologue, *decapentaplegic*, include substitutions in the kinase domain of *saxophone* and *thick veins*, the corresponding type I receptor genes (56, 57), Thus, dominant-negative receptors for the TGFβ superfamily exist in nature, but have not yet been identified for TGFβ itself. One a priori limitation of dominant-negative receptors is their inability, by themselves, to establish exactly which ligand is needed, if they have the property of binding multiple isoforms or relatives. The outcome of experiments with dominant-negative activin receptor, for example, is believed to reflect a block to signaling by the related peptide, Vg-1 (225). A second is the potential interplay among peptide growth factors acting in series: dominant-negative FGF receptor impairs activin signal transduction, in this manner, preventing mesoderm formation including the induction of muscle actin and the *Xenopus* brachyury gene (226, 227).

Hypertrophy

The fact that genes encoding peptide growth factors are induced in the ventricle after interventions that produce hypertrophy, taken in tandem with proof of cardiac myocytes' responsiveness to these factors, has provided cogent support for the concept that peptide growth factors might serve as autocrine or paracrine mediators of load. Upregulation of TGFβ is evoked in ventricular myocardium

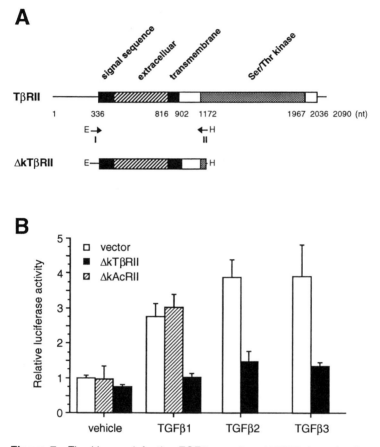

Figure 7 The kinase-defective TGFβ receptor, ΔkTβRII, is a dominant-negative suppressor of TGFβ signal transduction in cardiac muscle cells. (A) Schematic representation of the wild-type and truncated TβRII. Arrowheads indicate the positions of PCR amplification primers. (B) βkTβRII blocks induction of the skeletal α-actin promoter by all three mammalian isoforms of TGFβ. Neonatal rat ventricular muscle cells, transfected with skeletal α-actin-luciferase and constitutive β-galactosidase reporter genes, were cultured in absence or presence of TGFβs for 36 h. Activity of the skeletal α-actin promoter, corrected for transfection efficiency, is shown relative to that in vehicle-treated, vector-transfected cells. Error bars indicate standard error of the mean. Open bar: Control vector, lacking insert. Solid bar; ΔkTβRII, kinase-defective TβRII. Hatched bar: ΔkAcRII, an analogous truncation of the type II activin receptor. (From Ref. 147.)

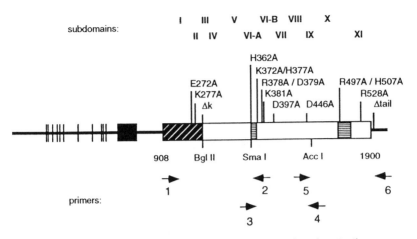

Figure 8 Structure of the TβRII mutations. Subdomains denote the consensus subdomains conserved within the serine/threonine and tyrosine kinase superfamilies (287). The schematic representation indicates the extracellular cysteines as vertical lines at the left of the figure and the transmembrane domain as a solid bar (■). Open bar (□), subdomains II–XI of the cytoplasmic serine/threonine kinase domain; Diagonally hatched bar, the amino-terminal remnant of the kinase domain retained in ΔkTβRII; Horizontally hatched bar, kinase insert-1 and -2. PCR amplification primers used in conjunction with the mutagenic oligonucleotides are illustrated below. (From Ref. 26.)

by pressure overload or norepinephrine infusion, and has been localized to the ventricular muscle cells themselves (228–230); induction also is seen in the cardiomyopathic hamster (231) Conversely, the angiotensin type I receptor antagonist DuP 753 prevented both hypertrophic growth and TGFβ induction after aortic banding (232). FGF-2 and IGF-I are likewise induced by aortic banding (233, 234); IGF-II may remain unchanged, despite induction of IGF-I (235). The association of IGF-I with ventricular hypertrophy also is noted in other models of systolic hypertension: uninephrectomized spontaneously hypertensive rats (by comparison to uninephrectomized Wistar-Kyoto controls) and uninephrectomized, deoxycorticosterone-treated, saline-fed rats (234), and is found in the right ventricle in hypertrophy produced by chronic hypoxia (236) or volume overload from an aortocaval shunt (237). IGF-I gene induction is accompanied by accumulation of IGF-I protein in ventricular myocytes (234) and returns toward normal as the increase in ventricular mass alleviates the increase in wall stress (234). Highlighted earlier in the review of transcriptional regulation, TGFβ and FGFs suffice to activate the "fetal" program in isolated cardiac myocytes (6, 7); see also (238). Comparable results have been reported for IGF-I (239) and IGF-II (237).

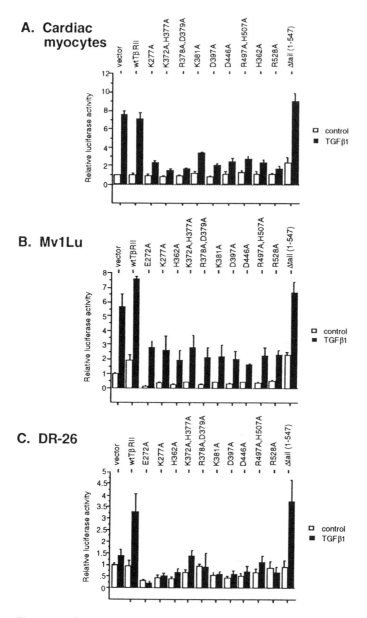

Figure 9 Dominant-negative activity of point mutations of the kinase domain of TβRII. (A) Cardiac myocytes, (B) Mv1Lu cells, and (C) TβRII-deficient DR-26 cells were transfected with vector or the mutations indicated. Cell lysates were analyzed for the activity of skeletal α-actin- (A) or p3TP-luciferase (B, C) and CMV-β-galatosidase reporter genes in the absence (□) and presence (■) of 1 ng/ml TGFβ1. Activity of each promoter is expressed relative to that in vehicle-treated, vector-transfected cells. (From Ref. 26.)

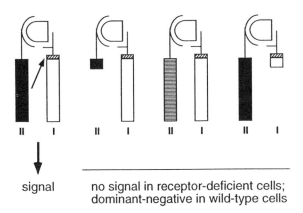

signal   no signal in receptor-deficient cells;
                dominant-negative in wild-type cells

Figure 10   Three classes of dominant-negative receptor inhibit TGFβ-dependent transcription. (Far left) TGFβ induces signal generation via association of TβRII and TβRI, and directional phosphorylation of the TβRI GS box by the TβRII kinase. Homodimerization of TβRII and activity of the TβRII serine/threonine kinase are ligand independent. (Left to right) Kinase-defective truncations of TβRII, missense mutations of TβRII that prevent the rescue of receptor-deficient cells, and kinase-defective truncations of TβRI each can disrupt TGFβ-dependent gene expression in cardiac myocytes or wild-type Mv1Lu mink lung epithelial cells. (From Ref. 26.)

As one approach to defining candidate intracellular signals that might couple wall stress to transcription, in vitro models using cardiac myocytes grown on silastic membranes have proven to be especially informative. Passive, linear stretch activates a host of signaling molecules including protein kinase C, Ras, and MAP kinase (130), upregulates immediate-early transcription factors (Myc, Fos, Jun, and Egr-1) and activates, at later intervals, the panel of genes associated with embryonic and hypertrophic ventricular muscle (SkA, βMHC, and ANF) (159, 240). Further credence for the hypothesis that growth factors are involved in a feedback loop sustaining the effects of mechanical load comes from observations that one factor released acutely after hemodynamic load, angiotensin II (241), can induce TGFβ in cardiac myocytes (157). Stretch-activated ion channels that have been postulated to serve as a mechanical sensor for load-induced hypertrophy are themselves upregulated by FGF-2 (242).

Although information regarding potential changes in growth factor receptor expression in hypertrophy or failure by contrast is scant, upregulation of IGF receptor has been reported in ventricular myocytes from patients with hypertrophic or dilated cardiomyopathy (243). A similar response is seen experimentally during compensatory hypertrophy of myocytes surviving infarction (244). In vitro, adult rat ventricular myocytes subjected to cell culture in the presence of growth factors respond with structural reorganization, re-expression of fetal genes including ANF and smooth muscle α-actin, and the induction of receptors for both FGFs (245) as well as IGFs (246). Prior to this adaptation in cell culture, adult rat ventricular myocytes were shown to increase protein synthesis when stimulated with insulin or IGF-I, but not FGF, PDGF, or EGF (247).

Myocarditis and Transplantation

Until recently, few investigations have addressed potential growth factor involvement in immunologically mediated cardiac disease, despite the presence of myocardial inflammation in many forms of cardiovascular pathology (248). TGFβ in particular has undergone scrutiny, due to its properties as a immuno-modulator (142, 249). Mice homozygous for a null mutation of TGFβ1 develop normally and survive until 3–4 weeks of age, but develop a multifocal inflammatory disease involving multiple organs including the heart (250, 251). Homozygous–null mice are indistinguishable from litter mates at birth, but at 7 days of life begin to display histological abnormalities consisting of mononuclear cell adherence to vascular endothelium (224). Aberrant overexpression of both class I and II antigens of the major histocompatibility complexes is noted prior to the initiation of a progressive inflammatory cardiomyopathy (252). Although multiple explanations exist to explain the unexpected normal phenotype of TGFβ null mice at birth given the postulated vital role of TGFβ in development, demonstration of significant amounts of immunoreactive TGFβ in null newborn mice led to the discovery that transplacental delivery of maternal TGFβ was responsible for the rescue of the null mutation (224). TGFβ null mice born to a homozygous null mother, kept viable by immunosuppression, displayed both thickening of the ventricle and valvular abnormalities (224). However, these cardiac abnormalities were not seen when the TGFβ null mutation was bred into immunodeficient strains (T. Doetschmann, personal communication).

Aberrant expression of class I and class II mixed histocompatibility antigens in TGFβ1-deficient animals suggests that one function of TGFβ1 is to restrain expression of these cell surface proteins. Conversely, since enhanced expression of mixed histocompatibility antigens was found both in autoimmune diseases (253, 254) and in allograft rejection (255), such results suggest a potential role for TGFβ in the management of these disorders. TGFβ is upregulated in models of allograft rejection (256) and correlates with the histological grade of rejection in humans (257). Exogenous TGFβ has been shown to prolong cardiac allograft survival (258, 259) and was efficacious even for xenografts of islet cells (260). Survival of cardiac allografts was also extended by direct injection of TGFβ expression vectors (261), suggesting the feasibility of gene therapy in this clinical setting. Mechanisms for immunosuppression by TGFβ include reduced neutrophil adherence (262), through control of cell adhesion molecules including integrins and selectins (263, 264), suppression of

MHC antigens cited earlier, or both. Less is known of other growth factors in cardiac allografts; however, increased expression of FGF-2 (265), FGF-1 (266), and their receptor, FGFR1 (267) has been observed, which might augment smooth cell hyperplasia and graft arteriopathy.

Myocardial inflammation, whether the primary insult is myocarditis or rejection, is accompanied by the production of proinflammatory cytokines (IL-1, TNF) known to contribute to cardiac dysfunction either directly (14, 268, 269) or indirectly, through attenuation of catecholamine responsiveness (270). TGFβ antagonizes the negative inotropic effects of IL-1 through attenuation of nitric oxide synthesis (269, 271). FGF at least in some cell types, also can inhibit induction of nitric oxide (272). A potential application for these factors thus may be in the management of reversible cardiac dysfunction seen in inflammatory cardiac disease.

Ischemia

Growth factors play a key role in response to tissue injury and wound healing in many biological systems. Therefore, it is not surprising that they have been implicated as cardioprotective agents. Intravenous TGFβ has been shown to reduce infarct size possibly by decreasing neutrophil adherence and subsequent migration into the periinfarct zone (262, 273). In models of acute myocardial ischemia, TGFβ message is upregulated more than sixfold (274, 275). The observation that TGFβ expression is highest at the margins of the infarct zone (274) and persisted for weeks after the initial insult, taken with its ability to regulate components of the extracellular matrix (276), suggest a role for this factor in mediating myocardial fibrosis and healing. FGF is upregulated in isolated cardiac myocytes in response to hypoxia (277) and has been shown to reduce infarct size (278, 279). Although FGFs are well known to induce angiogenesis (58), it is presently unknown if this or improved endothelium-dependent relaxation (280) is the mechanisms underlying the observed increase in collateral flow after FGF administration (281). Hypoxia also suffices to induce VEGF in cardiac myocytes (282), Induction of IGF-I and IGF receptor is reported to occur in myocardium surviving infarction (244).

Although it is beyond the scope of this discussion to review the wealth of data implicating growth factors in regulating both normal vascular biology and atherosclerosis, recent data have implicated TGFβ and the renin–angiotensin systems (283) as nonclassic risk factors in the premature development of coronary artery disease. Grainger and colleagues noted that a defect in the conversion of latent to active TGFβ in transgenic mice overexpressing apolipoprotein (a) resulted in development of preatherosclerotic lesions (284). The ability of active TGFβ to inhibit vascular smooth muscle cell growth (285) may explain why patients with decreased levels of TGFβ circulating in the active form have more advanced coronary artery disease (286).

CONCLUSIONS

Although encouraging progress has been made in recent years toward explaining the functional contribution of peptide growth factors in normal and abnormal cardiac biology, and the molecular basis for their effects, much remains to be elucidated. The majority of results available at this date remain descriptive, whereas mechanistic studies are more limited in number, and unanswered questions abound. With the potential for multiple growth factors to act in parallel as well as in series, precisely which factors are most critical in vivo, in governing recruitment of cells to the cardiac "fate," or in other aspects of cardiac organogenesis? Which govern the cell cycle in ventricular myocytes, and does downregulation of the mitogenic factors, downregulation of their receptors, or a postreceptor mechanism lock ventricular myocytes into their postmitotic state? What is the comparative importance of local circuits vs. systemic, circulating growth factors, and what mechanisms ulitmately determine growth factor availability and access to receptor in development or disease? Given the diversity of receptor forms and isoforms that bind many of the peptides reviewed here, what is the exact complement of growth factor receptors expressed in myocardium, and how are manifold responses allocated among these? What intracellular molecules couple receptor activation to hypertrophic growth and the plasticity of the cardiac genome? What components of the signal transduction machinery are invariant, among cardiac agonists with overlapping but distinguishable effects? As we begin to comprehend more regarding the biology of myocardial growth factors, we must consider how to manipulate growth factor levels and growth factor signaling cascades, to reengineer ventricular mass and function in the context of human disease.

ACKNOWLEDGMENTS

This work was supported by grants to M. D. S. from the National Institute of Health (R01 HL39141, R01 HL47567, P01 HL49953, T32 Hl07706) and the American Heart Association (91-009790) and by a National Research Service Award to J. H. (F32 HL09222). W. R. M. was a Fellow of the Medical Research Council of Canada and the American Heart Association-Bugher Foundation Center for Molecular Biology of the Cardiovascular System. W. R. M. and J. H. contributed equally to preparation of this work. The authors are grateful to Takashi Mikawa for discussion of results prior to publication, and to the current and former members of our laboratory whose work is cited here.

REFERENCES

1. Katz AM. Cardiomyopathy of overload: a major determinant of prognosis in congestive heart failure. N Engl J Med 1990; 322:100–110.

2. Parker TG, Schneider MD. Growth factors, proto-oncogenes, and plasticity of the cardiac phenotype. Annu Rev Physiol 1991; 53:179–200.

3. Schneider MD, Parker TG. Cardiac growth factors. Progr Growth Factor Res 1991; 3:1–26.

4. MacLellan WR, Brand T, Schneider MD. Transforming growth factor-beta in cardiac ontogeny and adaptation. Circ Res 1993; 73:783–791.

5. Komuro I, Yazaki Y. Control of cardiac gene expression by mechanical stress. Annu Rev Physiol 1993; 55:55–75.

6. Parker TG, Chow K-L, Schwartz RJ, Schneider MD. Differential regulation of skeletal α-actin transcription in cardiac muscle by two fibroblast growth factors. Proc Natl Acad Sci USA 1990; 87:7066–7070.

7. Parker TG, Packer SE, Schneider MD. Peptide growth factors can provoke "fetal" contractile protein gene expression in rat cardiac myocytes. J Clin Invest 1990; 85:507–514.

8. Akhurst RJ, Lehnert SA, Faissner A, Duffie E. TGF beta in murien morphogenetic processes: the early embryo and cardiogenesis. Development 1990; 108:645–656.

9. Mahmood R, Flanders KC, Morisskay GM. Interactions between retinoids and TGF betas in mouse morphogenesis. Development 1992; 115:67–74.

10. Potts JD, Runyan RB. Epithelial–mesenchymal cell transformation in the heart can be mediated, in part, by transforming growth factor β. Dev Biol 1989; 134:392–401.

11. Potts JD, Dagle JM, Walder JA, Weeks DL, Runyan RB. Epithelial-mesenchymal transformation of cardiac endothelial cells is inhibited by a modified antisense oligodesoxynucleotide to TGFβ3. Proc Natl Acad Sci USA 1991; 88:1516–1520.

12. Dickson MC, Slager HG, Duffie E, Mummery CL, Akhurst RJ. RNA and protein localisations of TGF-beta-2 in the early mouse embryo suggest an involvement in cardiac development. Development 1993; 117:625–639.

13. Millan FA, Denhez F, Kondaiah P, Akhurst RJ. Embryonic gene expression patterns of TGFβ1, β2 and β3 suggest different developmental functions in vivo. Development 1991; 111:131–144.

14. Roberts AB, Roche NS, Winokur TS, Burmester JK, Sporn MB. Role of transforming growth factor-beta in maintenance of function of cultured neonatal cardiac myocytes: autocrine action and reversal of damaging effects of interleukin-1. J Clin Invest 1992; 90:2056–2062.

15. Potts JD, Vincent EB, Runyan RB, Weeks DL. Sense and antisense TGFbeta3 messenger RNA levels correlate with cardiac valve induction. Dev Dynam 1992; 193:340–345.

16. Attisano L, Wrana JL, Lopez-Casillas F, Massagué J. TGF-beta receptors and actions. Biochim Biophys Acta 1994; 1222:71–80.

17. Lin HY, Moustakas A. TGF-beta receptors: structure and function. Cell Mol Biol 1994; 40:337–349.

18. Lin HY, Wang X-F, Ng-Eaton E, Weinberg RA, Lodish HF. Expression cloning of the TGF-beta type II receptor, a functional transmembrane serine/threonine kinase. Cell 1992; 68:775–785. Erratum: Cell 70(6).

19. Wrana JL, Attisano L, Carcamo J, Zentella A, Doody J, Laiho M. Wang XF,

Massague J. TGFβ signals through a heteromeric protein kinase receptor complex. Cell 1992; 71:1003–1014.

20. Barnett JV, Moustakas A, Lin W, Wang XF, Lin HY, Galper JB, Maas RL. Cloning and developmental expression of the chick type II and type III TGF beta receptors. Dev Dynam 1994; 199:12–27.

21. Lawler S, Candia AF, Ebner R, Shum L, Lopez AR, Moses HL, Wright CVE, Derynck R. The murine type II TGF-β receptor has a coincident embryonic expression and binding preference for TGF-β1. Development 1994; 120:165–175.

22. Lopez-Casillas F, Wrana JL, Massagué J. Betaglycan presents ligand to the TGF beta signaling receptor. Cell 1993; 73:1435–1444.

23. Laiho M, Weis MB, Masagué J. Concomitant loss of transforming growth factor (TGF)-beta receptor types I and II in TGF-beta-resistant cell mutants implicates both receptor types in signal transduction. J Biol Chem 1990; 265:18518–18524.

24. Laiho M, Weis FM, Boyd FT, Ignotz RA, Massagué J. Responsiveness to transforming growth factor-beta (TGF-beta) restored by genetic complementation between cells defective in TGF-beta receptors I and II. J Biol Chem 1991; 266:9108–9112.

25. Kingsley DM. The TGF-β superfamily: new membranes, new receptors, and new genetic tests of function in different organisms. Genes Dev 1994; 8:133–146.

26. Brand T, Schneider MD. Inactive type I and type II receptors for TGFβ are dominant inhibitors of TGFβ-dependent transcription. J Biol Chem 1995.

27. Matzuaki K, Xu J, Wang F, McKeehan WL, Krummen L, Kan M. A widely expressed transmembrane serine/threonine kinase that does not bind activin, inhibin, transforming growth factor β, or bone morphogenic protein. J Biol Chem 1993; 268:12719–12723.

28. Franzén P, Tendijke P, Ichijo H, Yamashita H, Schulz P, Heldin CH, Miyazono K. Cloning of a TGF beta type-I receptor that forms a heteromeric complex with the TGF beta type-II receptor. Cell 1993; 75:681–692.

29. Wrana JL, Attisano L, Wieser R, Ventura F, Massague J. Mechanism of activation of the TGF-beta receptor. Nature 1994; 370:341–347.

30. ten Dijke P, Yamashita H, Ichijo H, Franzen P, Laiho M, Miyazono K, Heldin CH. Characterization of type-I receptors for transforming growth factor-beta and activin. Science 1994; 264:101–104.

31. Bassing CH, Yingling JM, Howe DJ, Wang TW, He WW, Gustafson ML, Shah P, Donahoe PK, Wang XF. A transforming growth factor-beta type-I receptor that signals to active gene expression. Science 1994; 263:87–89.

32. Henis YI, Moustakas A, Lin HY, Lodish HF. The types II and III transforming growth factor-beta receptors form homo-oligomers. J Cell Biol 1994; 126:139–154.

33. Yamashita H, ten Dijke P, Franzen P, Miyazono K, Heldin CH. Formation of hetero-oligomeric complex of type I and type II receptors for transforming growth factor-beta. J Biol Chem 1994; 269:20172–20178.

34. Geiser AG, Burmester JK, Webbink R, Roberts AB, Sporn MB. Inhibition of growth by transforming growth factor-beta following fusion of two nonrespon-

sive human carcinoma cell lines: implication of the type II receptor in growth inhibitory responses. J Biol Chem 1992; 267:2588-2593.

35. Filmus J, Zhao J, Buick RN. Overexpression of H-ras oncogenes induces resistance to the growth-inhibitory action of transforming growth factor beta-1 (TGF-beta-1) and alters the number and type of TGF-beta 1 receptors in rat intestinal epithelial cell clones. Oncogene 1992; 7:521-6.

36. Chen RH, Ebner R, Derynck R. Inactivation of the type-II receptor reveals two receptor pathways for the diverse TGF-beta activities. Science 1993; 260:1335-1338.

37. Burgess WH, Maciag T. The heparin-binding (fibroblast) growth factor family of proteins. Annu Rev Biochem 1989; 58:575-606.

38. Basilico C, Moscatelli D. The FGF family of growth factors and oncogenes. Adv Cancer Res 1992; 59:115-165.

39. Miyamoto M, Naruo K, Seko C, Matsumoto S, Kondo T, Kurokawa T. Molecular cloning of a novel cytokine cDNA encoding the 9th member of the fibroblast growth factor family, which has a unique secretion property. Mol Cell Biol 1993; 13:4251-4259.

40. Weiner HL, Swain JL. Acidic fibroblast growth factor mRNA is expressed by cardiac myocytes in culture and the protein is localized to the extracellular matrix. Proc Natl Acad Sci USA 1989; 86:2683-2687.

41. Vlodavsky I, Fuks Z, Ishaimichaeli R, Bashkin P, Levi E, Korner G, Barshavit R, Klagsbrun M. Extracellular matrix-resident basic fibroblast growth factor—implication for the control of angiogenesis. J Cell Biochem 1991; 45:167-176.

42. Moscatelli D. Basic fibroblast growth factor (bFGF) dissociates rapidly from heparan sulfates but slowly from receptors—implications for mechanisms of bFGF release from pericellular matrix. J Biol Chem 1992; 267:25803-25809.

43. Casscells W, Speir E, Sasse J, Klagsburn M, Allen P, Lee M, Calvo B, Chiba M, Haggroth L, Folkman J, Epstein SE. Isolation, characterization, and localization of heparin-binding growth factors in the heart. J Clin Invest 1990; 85:434-445.

44. Kardami E, Fandrich RR. Basic fibroblast growth factor in atria and ventricles of the vertebrate heart. J Cell Biol 1989; 109:1865-1875.

45. Quinckler W, Maasberg M, Bernotat-Danielowski S, Luthe N, Sharma HS, Schaper W. Isolation of heparin-binding growth factors from bovine, porcine and canine hearts. Eur J Biochem 1989; 181:67-73.

46. Sasaki H, Hoshi H, Hong Y-M, Suzuki T, Kato T, Sasaki H, Saito M, Youki H, Karube K, Konno S, Onodera M, Saito T, Aoyagi S. Purification of acidic fibroblast growth factor from bovine heart and its localization in the cardiac myocytes. J Biol Chem 1989; 264:17606-17612.

47. Spirito P, Fu Y-M, Yu Z-X, Epstein SE, Casscells W. Immunohistochemical localization of basic and acidic fibroblast growth factors in the developing rat heart. Circulation 1991; 84:322-332.

48. Florkiewicz RZ, Sommer A. Human basic fibroblast growth factor gene encodes four polypeptides: three initiate translation from non-AUG codons. Proc Natl Acad Sci USA 1989; 86:3978-3981.

49. Liu L, Doble BW, Kardami E. Perinatal phenotype and hypothyroidism are associated with elevated levels of 21.5-kDa to 22-kDa basic fibroblast growth factor in cardiac ventricles. Dev Biol 1993; 157:507–516.

50. Kardami E, Padua RR, Pasumarthi KBS, Liu L, Doble BW, Davey SE, Cattini PA. Basic fibroblast growth factor in cardiac myocytes: expression and effects. In: Cummins P, ed. Growth Factors and the Cardiovascular System. Boston: Kluwer Academic Publishers, 1993:55–76.

51. Acland P, Dixon M, Peters G, Dickson C. Subcellular fate of the Int-2 oncoprotein is determined by choice of initiation codon. Nature 1990; 343:662–665.

52. Kiefer P, Acland P, Pappin D, Peters G, Dickson C. Competition between nuclear localization and secretory signals determines the subcellular fate of a single CUG-initiated form of FGF3. EMBO J 1994; 13:4126–4136.

53. Zhan X, Hu XG, Friedman S, Maciag T. Analysis of endogenous and exogenous nuclear translocation of fibroblast growth factor-1 in NIH 3T3 cells. Biochem Biophys Res Commun 1992; 188:982–991.

54. Imamura T, Engleka K, Zhan X, Tokita Y, Forough R, Roeder D, Jackson A, Maier JAM, Hla T, Maciag T. Recovery of mitogenic activity of a growth factor mutant with a nuclear translocation sequence. Science 1990; 249:1567–1570.

55. Parker TG, Chow KL, Schwartz RJ, Schneider MD. Positive and negative control of the skeletal alpha-actin promoter in cardiac muscle: a proximal serum response element is sufficient for induction by basic fibroblast growth factor (FGF) but not for inhibition by acidic FGF. J Biol Chem 1992; 267:3343–3350.

56. Baldin V, Roman AM, Bosc BI, Amalric F, Bouche G. Translocation of bFGF to the nucleus is G1 phase cell cycle specific in bovine aortic endothelial cells. EMBO J 1990; 9:1511–1517.

57. Hawker JR, Granger HJ. Internalized basic fibroblast growth factor translocates to nuclei of venular endothelial cells. Am J Physiol 1992; 262:H1525–H1537.

58. Klagsbrun M. Angiogenic factors: regulators of blood supply-side biology. New Biol 1991; 3:745–749.

59. Kardami E, Fandrich RR. Heparin-binding mitogen(s) in the heart: in search of origin and function. In: Kedes LH, Stockdale FE, ed. Cellular and Molecular Biology of Muscle Development. New York: Alan R Liss, 1989: 315–325.

60. Parlow MH, Bolender DL, Kokan-Moore NP, Lough J. Localization of bFGF-like proteins as punctate inclusions in the pre-septation myocardium of the chicken embryo. Dev Biol 1991; 146:139–147.

61. Joseph-Silverstein J, Consigli SA, Lyser KM, Ver Pault C. Basic fibroblast growth factor in the chick embryo: Immunolocalization to striated muscle cells and their precursors. J Cell Biol 1989; 108:2459–2466.

62. Fu Y, Spirito P, Yu ZX, Biro S, Sasse J, Lei J, Ferrans VJ, Epstein SE, Casscells W. Acidic fibroblast growth factor in the developing rat embryo. J Cell Biol 1991; 114:1261–1273.

63. Mason IJ, Fullerpace F, Smith R, Dickson C. FGF-7 (keratinocyte growth factor) expression during mouse development suggests roles in myogenesis, forebrain regionalisation and epithelial-mesenchymal interactions. Mech Develop 1994; 45:15–30.

64. deLapèyriere O, Ollendorff V, Planche J, Ott MO, Pizette S, Coulier F, Birnbaum D. Expression of the fgf6 gene is restricted to developing skeletal muscle in the mouse embryo. Development 1993; 118:601–611.

65. deLapèyriere O, Rosnet O, Benharroch D, Raybaud F, Marchetto S, Planche J, Galland F, Mattei MG. Structure, chromosome mapping and expression of the murine Fgf-6-gene. Oncogene 1990; 5:823–831.

66. Partanen J, Vainikka S, Alitalo K. Structural and functional specificity of FGF receptors. Philosoph Trans R Soc Lond [Biol] 1993; 340:297–303.

67. Johnson DE, Williams LT. Structural and functional diversity in the FGF receptor multigene family. Adv Cancer Res 1993; 60:1–41.

68. Jaye M, Schlessinger J, Dionne CA. Fibroblast growth factor receptor tyrosine kinases—molecular analysis and signal transduction. Biochim Biophys Acta 1992; 1135:185–199.

69. Hou JZ, Kan M, McKeehan K, McBride G, Adams P, McKeehan WL. Fibroblast growth factor receptors from liver vary in three structural domains. Science 1991; 251:665–668.

70. Dell KR, Williams LT. A novel form of fibroblast growth factor receptor-2: Alternative splicing of the 3rd immunoglobulin-like domain confers ligand binding specificity. J Biol Chem 1992; 267:21225–21229.

71. Chellaiah AT, McEwen DG, Werner S, Xu JS, Ornitz DM. Fibroblast growth factor receptor (FGFR)-3: Alternative splicing in immunoglobulin-like domain-III creates a receptor highly specific for acidic FGF/FGF-1. J Biol Chem 1994; 269:11620–11627.

72. Xu J, Matsuzaki K, McKeehan K, Wang F, Kan M, McKeehan W. Genomic structure and cloned cDNAs predict that four variants in the kinase domain of serine/threonine kinase receptors arise by alternative splicing and poly(A) addition. Proc Natl Acad Sci USA 1994; 91:7957–7961.

73. Duan DSR, Werner S, Williams LT. A naturally occurring secreted form of fibroblast growth factor (FGF) receptor-1 binds basic FGF in preference over acidic FGF. J Biol Chem 1992; 267:16076–16080.

74. Champion-Arnaud P, Ronsin C, Gilbert E, Gesnel MC, Houssaint E, Breathnach R. Multiple mRNAs code for proteins related to the BEK fibroblast growth factor receptor. Oncogene 1991; 6:979–987.

75. Burrus LW, Lueddecke BA, Zuber ME, Lieder KW, Olwin BB. Immunoaffinity purification and cDNA cloning of a putative receptor for acidic and basic fibroblast growth factors. J Cell Biochem Supp 1990; 14E: 71 (Abstr).

76. Kiefer MC, Stephans JC, Crawford K, Okino K, Barr PJ. Ligand-affinity cloning and structure of a cell surface heparan sulfate proteoglycan that binds basic fibroblast growth factor. Proc Natl Acad Sci USA 1990; 87:6985–6989.

77. Olwin BB, Hauschka SD. Fibroblast growth factor receptor levels decrease during chick embryogenesis. J Cell Biol 1990; 110:503–509.

78. Patstone G, Pasquale EB, Maher PA. Different members of the fibroblast growth factor receptor family are specific to distinct cell types in the developing chicken embryo. Dev Biol 1993; 155:107–123.

79. Jin Y, Pasumarthi KBS, Bock ME, Lytras A, Kardami E, Cattini PA. Cloning and expression of fibroblast growth factor receptor-1 isoforms in the mouse heart:

Evidence for isoform switching during heart development. J Mol Cell Cardiol 1994; 26:1449–1459.

80. Spivak-Kroizman T, Lemmon MA, Dikic I, Ladbury JE, Pinchasi D, Huang J, Jaye M, Crumley G, Schlessinger J, Lax I. Heparin-induced oligomerization of FGF molecules is responsible for FGF receptor dimerization, activation, and cell proliferation. Cell 1994; 79:1015–1024.

81. Springer BA, Pantoliano MW, Barbera FA, Gunyuzlu PL, Thompson LD, Herblin WF, Rosenfeld SA, Book GW. Identification and concerted function of two receptor binding surfaces on basic fibroblast growth factor required for mitogenesis. J Biol Chem 1994; 269:26879–26884.

82. Yayon A, Klagsbrun M, Esko JD, Leder P, Ornitz DM. Cell surface, heparin-like molecules are required for binding of basic fibroblast growth factor to its high-affinity receptor. Cell 1991; 64:841–848.

83. Rapraeger AC, Krufka A, Olwin BB. Requirement of heparan sulfate for bFGF-mediated fibroblast growth and myoblast differentiation. Science 1991; 252:1705–1708.

84. Olwin BB, Rapraeger A. Repression of myogenic differentiation of aFGF, bFGF, and K-FGF is dependent on cellular heparan sulfate. J Cell Biol 1992; 118:631–639.

85. Guimond S, Maccarana M, Olwin BB, Lindahl U, Rapraeger AC. Activating and inhibitory heparin sequences for FGF-2 (basic FGF)—distinct requirements for FGF-1, FGF-2, and FGF-4. J Biol Chem 1993; 268:23906–23914.

86. Walker A, Turnbull JE, Gallagher JT. Specific heparan sulfate saccharides mediate the activity of basic fibroblast growth factor. J Biol Chem 1994; 269:931–935.

87. Kan MK, Wang F, Xu JM, Crabb JW, Hou JZ, McKeehan WL. An essential heparin-binding domain in the fibroblast growth factor receptor kinase. Science 1993; 259:1918–1921.

88. Roghani M, Mansukhani A, Dellera P, Bellosta P, Basilico C, Rifkin DB, Moscatelli D. Heparin increases the affinity of basic fibroblast growth factor for its receptor but is not required for binding. J Biol Chem 1994; 269:3976–3984.

89. Mohammadi M, Dionne CA, Li W, Li N, Spivak T, Honegger AM, Jaye M, Schlessinger J. Point mutation in FGF receptor eliminates phosphatidylinositol hydrolysis without affecting mitogenesis. Nature 1992; 358:681–684.

90. Peters KG, Marie J, Wilson E, Ives HE, Escobedo J, Delrosario M, Mirda D, Williams LT. Point mutation of an FGF receptor abolishes phosphatidylinositol turnover and Ca^{2+} flux but not mitogenesis. Nature 1992; 358:678–681.

91. Muslin AJ, Peters KG, Williams LT. Direct activation of phospholipase c-gamma by fibroblast growth factor receptor is not required for mesoderm induction in Xenopus animal caps. Mol Cell Biol 1994; 14:3006–3012.

92. Vainikka S, Joukov V, Wennstrom S, Bergman M, Pelicci PG, Alitalo K. Signal transduction by fibroblast growth factor receptor-4 (FGFR-4) - comparison with FGFR-1. J Biol Chem 1994; 269:18320–18326.

93. Zhan X, Plourde C, Ku XG, Friesel R, Maciag T. Association of fibroblast growth factor receptor-1 with c- Src correlates with association between c-Src and cortactin. J Biol Chem 1994; 269:20221–20224.

94. MacNicol AM, Muslin AJ, Williams LT. Raf-1 kinase is essential for early Xenopus development and mediates the induction of mesoderm by FGF. Cell 1993; 73:571–583.

95. Wang JK, Gao GX, Goldfarb M. Fibroblast growth factor receptors have different signaling and mitogenic potentials. Mol Cell Biol 1994; 14:181–188.

96. Dull TJ, Gray A, Hayflick JS, Ullrich A, Insulin-like growth factor II precursor gene organization in relation to insulin gene family. Nature 1984; 310:777–781.

97. Bondy CA, Werner H, Roberts Jr CT, LeRoith D. Cellular pattern of insulin-like growth factor-I (IGF-I) and type I IGF receptor gene expression in early organogenesis: comparison with IGF-II gene expression. Mol Endocrinol 1990; 4:1386–1398.

98. Lee JE, Pintar J, Efstratiadis A. Pattern of the insulin-like growth factor II gene expression during early mouse embryogenesis. Development 1990; 110:151–159.

99. Baxter RC. Insulin-like growth factor binding proteins in the human circulation: a review. Horm Res 1994; 42:140–144.

100. Conover CA, Ronk M, Lombana F, Powell DR. Structural and biological characterization of bovine insulin-like growth factor binding protein-3. Endocrinology 1990; 127:2795–2803.

101. Blat C, Villaudy J, Binoux M. In vivo proteolysis of serum insulin-like growth factor (IGF) binding protein-3 results in increased availability of IGF to target cells. J Clin Invest 1994; 93:2286–2290.

102. Conover CA. Potentiation of insulin-like growth factor (IGF) action by IGF-binding protein-3: studies of underlying mechanism. Endocrinology 1992; 130:3191–3199.

103. Clemmons DR. IGF binding proteins and their functions. Mol Reprod Dev 1993; 35:368–375.

104. Rosenzweig SA, Oemar BS, Law NM, Shankavaram UT, Miller BS. Insulin like growth factor 1 receptor signal transduction to the nucleus. Adv Exp Med Biol 1993; 343:159–168.

105. Baserga R, Porcu P, Rubini M, Sell C. Cell cycle control by the IGF-1 receptor and its ligands. Adv Exp Med Biol 1993; 343:105–112.

106. Schumacher R, Mosthaf L, Schlessinger J, Brandenburg D, Ullrich A. Insulin and insulin-like growth factor-1 specificity is determined by distinct regions of their cognate receptors. J Biol Chem 1991; 266:19288–19295.

107. Lammers RA, Gray A, Schlessinger J, Ullrich A. Differential signalling potential of insulin- and IGF-1-receptor cytoplasmic domains. EMBO J 1989; 8:1369–1375.

108. Moxham CP, Jacobs S. Insulin/IGF-I receptor hybrids: a mechanism for increasing receptor diversity. J Cell Biochem 1992; 48:136–140.

109. Kato H, Faria TN, Stannard B, Roberts CT, Leroith D. Role of tyrosine kinase activity in signal transduction by the insulin-like growth factor-I (IGF-1) receptor—characterization of kinase deficient IGF-I receptors and the action of an IGF-I-mimetic antibody (alphaIR-3). J Biol Chem 1993; 268:2655–2661.

110. Kato H, Faria TN, Stannard B, Roberts Jr CT, LeRoith D. Essential role of tyrosine residues 1131, 1135, and 1136 of the insulin-like growth factor-I (IGF-

I) receptor in IGF-I action. Mol Endocrinol 1994; 8:40–50.

111. Hsu D, Knudson PE, Zapf A, Rolband GC, Olefsky JM. NPXY motif in the insulin-like growth factor-I response is required for efficient ligand-mediated receptor internalization and biological signaling. Endocrinology 1994; 134:744–750.

112. Treadway JL, Morrison BD, Soos MA, Siddle K, Olefsky J, Ullrich A, McClain DA, Pessin JE. Transdominant inhibition of tyrosine kinae activity in mutant insulin/insulin-like growth factor-I hybrid receptors. Proc Natl Acad Sci USA 1991; 88:214–218.

113. Sun XJ, Rothenberg P, Kahn CR, Backer JM, Araki E, Wilden PA, Cahill DA, Goldstein BJ, White MF. Structure of the insulin receptor substrate IRS-1 defines a unique signal transduction protein. Nature 1991; 352:73–77.

114. Nissley P, Kiess W, Sklar M. Developmental expression of the IGF-II/mannose 6-phosphate receptor. Mol Reprod Dev 1993; 35:408–413.

115. Rosenthal SM, Hsiao D, Silverman LA. An insulin-like growth Factor-II (IGF-II) analog with highly selective affinity for IGF-II receptors stimulates differentiation, but not IGF-I receptor down-regulation in muscle cells. Endocrinology 1994; 135:38–44.

116. Takahashi K, Murayama Y, Okamoto T, Yokota T, Ikezu T, Takashashi S, Giambarella U, Ogata E, Nishimoto I. Conversion of G-protein specificity of insulin-like growth factor-II/mannose 6-phosphate receptor by exchanging of a short region with beta-adrenergic receptor. Proc Natl Acad Sci USA 1993; 90:11772–11776.

117. Chuang LM, Myers MG, Seidner GA, Birnbaum MJ, White MF, Kahn CR. Insulin receptor substrate-1 mediates insulin and insulin-like growth factor-I-stimulated maturation of Xenopus oocytes. Proc Natl Acad Sci USA 1993; 90:5172–5175.

118. Sasaoka T, Langlois WJ, Leitner JW, Draznin B, Olefsky JM. The signaling pathway coupling epidermal growth factor receptors to activation of p21(ras). J Biol Chem 1994; 269:32621–32625.

119. Sasaoka T, Draznin B, Leitner JW, Langlois WJ, Olefsky JM. Shc is the predominant signaling molecule coupling insulin receptors to activation of guanine nucleotide releasing factor and p21 (Ras)-GTP formation. J Biol Chem 1994; 269:10734–10738.

120. Tamemoto H, Kadowaki T, Tobe K, Yagi T, Sakura H, Hayakawa T, Terauchi Y, Ueki K, Kaburagi K, Satoh S, Sekihara H, Yoshioka S, Horikoshi H, Furuta Y, Ikawa Y, Kasuga M, Yazaki Y, Aizawa S. Insulin resistance and growth retardation in mice lacking insulin receptor substrate-1. Nature 1994; 372:182–186.

121. Oemar BS, Law NM, Rosenzweig SA. Insulin-like growth factor-1 induces tyrosyl phosphorylation of nuclear proteins. J Biol Chem 1991; 266:24241–4.

122. Coppola D, Ferber A, Miura M, Sell C, Dambrosio C, Rubin R, Baserga R. A functional insulin-like growth factor I receptor is required for the mitogenic and transforming activities of the epidermal growth factor receptor. Mol Cell Biol 1994; 14:4588–4595.

123. Florini JR, Ewton DZ, Roof SL. Insulin-like growth factor-I stimulates terminal myogenic differentiation by induction of myogenin gene expression. Mol Endocrinol 1991; 5:718–724.

124. Quinn LS, Roh JS. Overexpression of the human type-1 insulin-like growth factor receptor in rat L6 myoblasts induces ligand-dependent cell proliferation and inhibition of differentiation. Exp Cell Res 1993; 208:504–508.

125. Werner H, Woloschak M, Adamo M, Shen-Orr Z, Roberts Jr CT, LeRoith D. Developmental regulation of the rat insulin-like growth factor I receptor gene. Proc Natl Acad Sci USA 1989; 86:7451–7455.

126. Armstrong FG, Hogg CO. Type-I insulin-like growth factor receptor gene expression in the chick. Developmental changes and the effect of selection for increased growth on the amount of receptor mRNA. J Mol Endocrinol 1994; 12:3–12.

127. Ballesteros M, Scott CD, Baxter RC. Developmental regulation of insulin-like growth factor-II/mannose 6-phosphate receptor mRNA in the rat. Biochem Biophys Res Commun 1990; 172:775–779.

128. Sklar MM, Thomas CL, Municchi G, Roberts CTJ, LeRoith D, Kiess W, Nissley P. Developmental expression of rat insulin-like growth factor-II/mannose 6-phosphate receptor messenger ribonucleic acid. Endocrinology 1992; 130:3484–3491.

129. Medema RH, Bos JL. The role of p21ras in receptor tyrosine kinase signaling. Crit Rev Oncogenesis 1993; 4:615–661.

130. Sadoshima J, Izumo S. Mechanical stretch rapidly activates multiple signal transduction pathways in cardiac myocytes: Potential involvement of an autocrine/paracrine mechanism. EMBO J 1993; 12:1681–1692.

131. Sadoshima J, Izumo S. Angiotensin II activates p21^{ras} by tyrosine kinase and protein kinase C-dependent mechanism in cardiac myocytes. Circulation 1993; 88:I-334 (Abstr).

132. Thorburn A, Thorburn J, Chen SY, Powers S, Shubeita HE, Feramisco JR, Chien KR. HRas-dependent pathways can activate morphological and genetic markers of cardiac muscle hypertrophy. J Biol Chem 1993; 268:2244–2249.

133. Thorburn J, McMahon M, Thorburn A. Raf-1 kinase activity is necessary and sufficient for gene expression changes but not sufficient for cellular morphology changes associated with cardiac myocyte hypertrophy. J Biol Chem 1994; 269:30580–30586.

134. Thorburn J, Frost JA, Thorburn A. Mitogen-activated protein kinases mediate changes in gene expression, but not cytoskeletal organization associated with cardiac muscle cell hypertrophy. J Cell Biol 1994; 126:1565–1572.

135. Nair AP, Hahn S, Banholzer R, Hirsch HH, Moroni C. Cyclosporin A inhibits growth of autocrine tumour cell lines by destabilizing interleukin-3 mRNA. Nature 1994; 369:239–242.

136. Normanno N, Selvam MP, Qi CF, Saeki T, Johnson G, Kim N, Ciardiello F, Shoyab M, Plowman G, Brandt R et al. Amphiregulin as an autocrine growth factor for c-Ha-ras- and c-erbB-2-transformed human mammary epithelial cells. Proc Natl Acad Sci USA 1994; 91:2790–2794.

137. Klein PS, Melton DA. Induction of mesoderm in *Xenopus laevis* embryos by translation initiation factor 4E. Science 1994; 265:803–806.

138. Hemmati-Brivanlou A, Melton DA. A truncated activin receptor inhibits meso-
     derm induction and formation of axial structures in Xenopus embryos. Nature
     1992; 359:609–614.
139. Abdellatif M, MacLellan WR, Schneider MD. p21 Ras as a governor of global
     gene expression. J Biol Chem 1994; 269:15423–15426.
140. Sakai N, Ogiso Y, Fujita H, Watari H, Koike T, Kuzumaki N. Induction of
     apoptosis by a dominant negative H-RAS mutant (116Y) in K562 cells. Exp Cell
     Res 1994 215:131–136.
141. Wang TW, Donahoe PK, Zervos AS. Specific interaction of type I receptors of
     the TGF-beta family with the immunophilin FKBP-12. Science 1994; 265:674–
     676.
142. Roscetti FW, Palladino MA. Transforming growth factor-beta and the immune
     system. Prog Growth Factor Res 1991; 3:159–175.
143. Gregory CR, Huie P, Billingham ME, Morris RE. Rapamycin inhibits arterial
     intimal thickening caused by both alloimmune and mechanical injury. Its effect
     on cellular, growth factor, and cytokine response in injured vessels.
     Transplanation 1993; 55:1409–1418.
144. Brillantes AB, Ondrias K, Scott A, Kobrinsky E, Ondriasov'a E, Moschella MC,
     Jayaraman T, Landers M, Ehrlich BE, Marks AR. Stabilization of calcium re-
     lease channel (ryanodine receptor) function by FK506-binding protein. Cell 1994;
     77:513–523.
144a. Charng M-J, Kinnunen P, Hawker J, Brand T, Schneider MD. FKBP-12 recog-
     nition is dispensable for signal generation by type I transforming growth factor-
     β receptors. J Biol Chem 1996; 271:22941–22944.
145. Schneider MD, Payne PA, Ueno H, Perryman MB, Roberts R. Dissociated ex-
     pression of c-myc and a fos-related competence gene during cardiac myogenesis.
     Mol Cell Biol 1986; 6:4140–4143.
146. Ueno H, Perryman MB, Roberts R, Schneider MD. Differentiation of cardiac
     myocytes following mitogen withdrawal exhibits three sequential stages of the
     ventricular growth response. J Cell Biol 1988; 107:1911–1918.
147. Brand T, MacLellan WR, Schneider MD. A dominant-negative receptor for type-
     beta transforming growth factors created by deletion of the kinase domain. J Biol
     Chem 1993; 268:11500–11503.
148. Shubeita HE, McDonough PM, Harris AN, Knowlton KU, Glembotski CC,
     Brown JH, and Chien KR. Endothelin induction of inositol phospholipid hydroly-
     sis, sarcomere assembly, and cardiac gene expression in ventricular myocytes.
     A paracrine mechanism for myocardial cell hypertrophy. J Biol Chem 1990;
     265:20555–20562.
149. Bishopric NH, Kedes L. Adrenergic regulation of the skeletal α-actin gene pro-
     moter during myocardial cell hypertrophy. Proc Natl Acad Sci USA 1991;
     88:2132–2136.
150. Kariya K, Karns LR, Simpson PC. An enhancer core element mediates stimu-
     lation of the rat beta-myosin heavy chain promoter by an alpha(1)-adrenergic ago-
     nist and activated beta-protein kinase-C in hypertrophy of cardiac myocytes. J Biol
     Chem 1994; 269:3775–3782.
151. Ransone LJ, Verma IM. Nuclear proto-oncogenes FOS and JUN. Annu Rev Cell
     Biol 1990; 6:539–557.

152. Forrest D, Curran T. Crossed signals: oncogenic transcription factors. Curr Opin Genet Dev 1992; 2:19–27.

153. Karin M. Signal transduction from the cell surface to the nucleus through the phosphorylation of transcription factors. Curr Opin Cell Biol 1994; 6:415–424.

154. Starksen NF, Simpson PC, Bishopric N, Coughlin SR, Lee WMF, Escobedo J, Williams LT. Cardiac myocyte hypertrophy is associated wtih c-myc protoncogene expression. Proc Natl Acad Sci USA 1986; 83:8348–8350.

155. Iwaki K, Sukhatme VP, Shubeita HE, Chien KR. Alpha- and beta-adrenergic stimulation induces distinct patterns of immediate early gene expression in neonatal rat myocardiaal cells. Fos/jun expression is associated with sarcomere assembly; Egr-1 induction is primarily an alpha 1-mediated response. J Biol Chem 1990; 265:13809–13817.

156. Black FM, Parker TG, Michael LH, Roberts R, Schneider MD. The c-*jun* and *jun*B proto-oncogenes are induced in myocardium by a hemodynamic load in vivo and fibroblast growth factors in vivo. J Cell Biochem 1991; 15C: 176(Abstr).

157. Sadoshima J, Izumo S. Molecular characterization of angiotensin II-induced hypertrophy of cardiac myocytes and hyperplasia of cardiac fibroblasts: Critical role of the AT1 receptor subtype. Circ Res 1993; 73:413–423.

158. Komuro I, Kaida T, Shibazaki Y, Kurabayashi M, Katoh Y, Hoh E, Takaku F, Yazaki Y. Stretching cardiac myocytes stimulates protoncogene expression. J Biol Chem 1990; 265:3595–3598.

159. Sadoshima J, Jahn L, Takahashi T, Kulik J, Izumo S. Molecular characterization of the stretch-induced adaptation of cultured cardiac cells: an in vitro model of load-induced cardiac hypertrophy. J Biol Chem 1992; 267:10551–10560.

160. Mulvagh SL, Michael LH, Perryman MB, Roberts R, Schneider MD. A hemodynamic load in vivo induces cardiac expression of the cellular oncogene, c-myc. Biochem Biophys Res Commun 1987; 147:627–636.

161. Izumo S, Nadal-Ginard B, Mahdavi V. Proto-oncogene induction and reprogramming of cardiac gene expression produced by pressure overload. Proc Natl Acad Sci USA 1988; 85:339–343.

162. Komuro M, Kurabayashi M, Takaku F, Yazaki Y. Expression of cellular oncogenes in the myocardium during the developmental stage and pressure-overload hypertrophy of the rat heart. Circ Res 1988; 62:1075–1079.

163. Rockman HA, Ross RS, Harris AN, Knowlton KU, Steinhelper ME, Field LJ, Ross J, Chien KR. Segregation of atrial-specific and inducible expression of an atrial natriuretic factor transgene in an invivo murine model of cardiac hypertrophy. Proc Natl Acad Sci USA 1991; 88:8277–8281.

164. Black FB, Packer SE, Parker TG, Michael LH, Roberts R, Schwartz RJ, Schneider MD. The vascular smooth muscle α-actin gene is reactivated during cardiac hypertrophy produced by load. J Clin Invest 1991; 88:1581–1588.

165. Brand T, Sharma HS, Schaper W. Expression of nuclear proto-oncogenes in isoproterenol-induced cardiac hypertrophy. J Mol Cell Cardiol 1993; 25:1325–1337.

166. Brand T, Sharma HS, Fleischmann KE, Duncker DJ, Mcfalls EO, Verdouw PD, Schaper W. Proto-oncogenes expression in porcine myocardium subjected to ischemia and reperfusion. Circ Res 1992; 71:1351–1360

167. Schunkert H, Jahn L, Izumo S, Apstein CS, Lorell BH. Localization and regu-

lation of c-fos and c-jun protooncogene induction by systolic wall stress in normal and hypertrophied rat hearts. Proc Natl Acad Sci USA 1991; 88:11480–
11484.

168. Schneider MD, Perryman MB, Payne PA, Spizz G, Roberts R, Olson EN. Autonomous expression of c-myc in BC_3H_1 cells partially inhibits but does not prevent myogenic differentiation. Mol Cell Biol 1987; 7:1973–1977.

169. Miner JH, Wold BJ. C-myc inhibition of myoD and myogenin-initiated myogenic
differentiation. Mol Cell Biol 1991; 11:2842–2851.

170. Lassar AB, Thayer MJ, Overell RW, Weintraub. Transformation by activated ras
or fas prevents myogenesis by inhibiting expression of MyoD1. Cell 1989;
58:659–667.

171. Li L, Chambard JC, Karin M, Olson EN. Fos and Jun repress transcriptional
activation by myogenin and MyoD: The amino terminus of Jun can mediate repression. Genes Dev 1992; 6:676–689.

172. Bishopric NH, Jayasena V, Webster KA. Positive regulation of the skeletal alpha-actin gene by fos and jun in cardiac myocytes. J Biol Chem 1992;
267:25535–25540.

173. Kovacic-Milivojevic B, Gardner DG. Divergent regulation of the human atrial
natriuretic peptide gene by c-jun and c-fos. Mol Cell Biol 1992; 12:292–301.

174. Goswami SK, Zarraga AM, Martin ME, Morgenstern D, Siddiqui MAQ. Fos-
mediated repression of cardiac myosin light chain-2 gene transcription. Cell Mol
Biol 1992; 38:49–58.

175. McBride K, Robitaille L, Tremblay S, Argentin S, Nemer M. *fos/jun* repression
of cardiac-specific transcription in quiescent and growth-stimulated myocytes is
targeted at a tissue-specific *cis* element. Mol Cell Biol 1993; 13:600–612.

176. Kim SJ, Angel P, Lafyatis R, Hattori K, Kim KY, Sporn MB, Karin M, Roberts AB. Autoinduction of transforming growth factor beta 1 is activated by the
AP-1 complex. Mol Cell Biol 1990; 10:1492–1497.

177. Lee ME, Dhadly MS, Ternizer DH, Clifford JA, Yoshizumi M, Quertermous T.
Regulation of endothelin-1 gene expression by Fos and Jun. J Biol Chem 1991;
266:19034–19039.

178. Jackson T, Allard MF, Sreenan CM, Doss LK, Bishop SP, Swain JL. The *c-myc*
proto-oncogene regulates cardiac development in transgenic mice. Mol Cell Biol
1990; 10:3709–3716.

179. Johnson RS, Vanlingen B, Papaioannou VE, Spiegelman BM. A null muation at
the c-jun locus causes embryonic lethality and retarded cell growth in culture.
Genes Dev 1993; 7:1309–1317.

180. Johnson RS, Spiegelman BM, Papaioannou V. Pleiotropic effects of a null mutation in the c-fos proto-oncogene. Cell 1992; 71:577–586.

181. Davis AC, Wims M, Spotts GD, Hann SR, Bradley A. A null c-myc mutation
causes lethality before 10.5 days of gestation in homozygotes and reduced fer-
tility in heterozygous female mice. Genes Dev 1993; 7:671–682.

182. Moens CB, Stanton BR, Parada LF, Rossant J. Defects in heart and lung development in compound heterozygotes for two different targeted mutations at the N-
myc locus. Development 1993; 119:485–499.

183. Kirshenbaum LA, MacLellan WR, Mazur W, French BA, Schneider MD. Highly efficient gene transfer to adult rat ventricular myocytes by recombinant adenovirus. J Clin Invest 1993; 92:381–387.

184. Rossi P, Karsenty G, Roberts AB, Roche NS, Sporn MB, de Crombrugghe B. A nuclear factor 1 binding site mediates the transcriptional activation of a type I collagen promoter by transforming growth factor-beta. Cell 1988; 52:405–414.

185. Brennan TJ, Edmondson DG, Li L, Olson EN. Transforming growth factor-beta represses the actions of myogenin through a mechanism independent of DNA binding. Proc Natl Acad Sci USA 1991; 88:3822–3826.

186. Li L, James G, Heller-Harrison R, Czech MP, Olson EN. FGF inactivates myogenic helix-loop-lelix proteins through phosphorylation of a conserved protein kinase-C site in their DNA-binding domains. Cell 1992; 71:1181–1194.

187. MacLellan WR, Lee TC, Schwartz RJ, Schneider MD. Transforming growth factor-beta response elements of the skeletal alpha-actin gene: combinatorial action of serum response factor, YY1, and the SV40 enhancer-binding protein, TEF-1. J Biol Chem 1994; 269:16754–16760.

188. Treisman R. The serum response element. Trends Biochem Sci 1992; 17:423–426.

189. Sadoshima J, Izumo S. Signal transduction pathways of angiotensin II-induced c-fos gene expression in cardiac myocytes in vitro: roles of phospholipid-derived second messengers. Circ Res 1993; 73:424–38.

190. Lee TC, Shi Y, Schwartz RJ. Displacement of BrdU-induced YY1 by serum response factor activates skeletal alpha-actin transcription in embryonic myoblasts. Proc Natl Acad Sci USA 1992; 89:9814–9818.

191. Taylor M, Treisman R, Garrett N, Mohun T. Muscle-specific (CArG) and serum-responsive (SRE) promoter elements are functionally interchangeable in Xenopus embryos and mouse fibroblasts. Development 1989; 106:67–78.

192. Tuil D, Clergue N, Montarras D, Pinset C, Kahn A, Phan DTF. CC Ar GG boxes, cis-acting elements with a dual specificity. Muscle-specific transcriptional activation and serum responsiveness. J Mol Biol 1990; 213:677–686.

193. Harvey RP, Lyons I, Li R, Parsons LM, Hartley L, Andrews J, Smith M. Targeted mutagenesis of the heart-expressed homeobox gene Nkx-2.5 results in abnormal heart development and embryonic lethality. J Cell Biochem 1994; 18D: 477 (Abstr).

194. Kariya K, Farrance IKG, Simpson PC. Transcriptional enhancer factor-1 in cardiac myocytes interacts with an α_1-adrenergic- and β-protein kinase-C-inducible element in the rat β-myosin heavy chain promoter. J Biol Chem 1993; 268:26658–26662.

195. Stewart AFR, Larkin SB, Farrance IKG, Mar JH, Hall DE, Ordahl CP. Muscle-enriched TEF-1 isoforms bind M-CAT elements from muscle-specific promoters and differentially activate transcription. J Biol Chem 1994; 269:3147–3150.

196. Kessler DS, Melton DA. Vertebrate embryonic induction: mesodermal and neural patterning. Science 1994; 266:596–604.

197. Muslin AJ, Williams LT. Well-defined growth factors promote cardiac development in axolotl mesodermal explants. Development 1991; 112:1095–1101.

198. Eisenberg CA, Bader DM. Establishment of a clonal cell line derived from cardiogenic mesoderm of the Japanese quail.

199. Komuro I, Fu YC, Izumo S. *Xenopus* cardiac specific homeobox-containing gene XCsx2, the earliest molecular marker for the precardiac mesoderm, is induced by the endoderm, bFGF, TGFβ, and *Xwnt*8 but not by activin. Circulation 1994; 90:I-634 (Abstr).

200. Logan M, Mohun T. Induction of cardiac muscle differentiation in isolated animal pole explants of Xenopus laevis embryos. Developmenet 1993; 118:865–875.

201. Zhou XL, Sasaki H, Lowe L, Hogan BLM, Kuehn MR. Nodal is a novel TGF-beta-like gene expressed in the mouse node during gastrulation. Nature 1993; 361:543–547.

202. Robbins J, Gulick J, Sanchez A, Howles P, Doetschman TC. Mouse embryonic stem cells express cardiac myosin heavy chain genes during development in vitro. J Biol Chem 1990; 265:11905–11909.

203. Miller-Hance WC, LaCorbiere M, Fuller SJ, Evans SM, Lyons G, Schmidt C, Robbins J, Chien KR. In vitro chamber specification during embryonic stem cell cardiogenesis: expression of the ventricular myosin light chain-2 gene is independent of heart tube formation. J Biol Chem 1993; 268:25244–25252.

204. van den Eijnden-van Raaij AJM, van Achterberg TAE, van der Kruijssen CMM, Piersma AH, Huylebroeck D, de Laat SW, Mummery CL. Differentiation of aggregated murine P19 embryonal carcinoma cells is induced by a novel visceral endoderm-specific FGF-like factor and inhibited by activin A. Mech Dev 1991; 33:157–166.

205. Slager HG, Vaninzen W, Freund E, van den Eijnden-vanRaaij AJM, Mummery CL. Transforming growth factor-beta in the early mouse embryo: implications for the regulation of muscle formation and implantation. Dev Genet 1993; 14:212–224.

206. Sugi Y, Sasse J, Lough J. Inhibition of precardiac mesoderm cell proliferation by antisense oligodeoxynucleotide complementary to fibroblast growth factor-2 (FGF-2). Dev Biol 1993; 157:28–37.

207. Deng C-X, Wynshaw-Boris A, Shen MM, Daugherty C, Ornitz DM, Leder P. Murine FGFR-1 is required for early postimplantation growth and axial organization. Genes Dev 1994; 8:3045–3057.

208. Yamaguchi TP, Harpal K, Henkmeyer M, Rossant J. *fgfr*-1 is required for embryonic growth and mesodermal patterning during mouse gastrulation. Genes Dev 1994; 8:3032–3044.

209. Liu JP, Baker J, Perkins AS, Robertson EJ, Efstratiadis A. Mice carrying null mutations of the genes encoding Insulin-like growth factor-I (Igf-1) and type-1 IGF receptor (Igf1r). Cell 1993; 75:59–72.

210. Powell-Braxton L, Hollingshead P, Wan C, Dowd M, Pitts-Meek S, Dalton D, Gillett N, Stewart TA. IGF-I is required for normal embryonic growth in mice. Genes Dev 1993; 7:2609–2617.

211. DeChiara TM, Robertson EJ, Efstratiadis A. Parental imprinting of the mouse insulin-like growth factor Ii gene. Cell 1991; 64:849–59.

212. Lau MMH, Stewart CEH, Liu Z, Bhatt H, Rotwein P, Stewart CL. Loss of the

imprinted IGF2-cation-independent mannose-6-phosphate receptor results in fetal overgrowth and perinatal lethality. Genes Dev 1994; 8:2953-2963.

213. Filson AJ, Louvi A, Efstratiadis A, Robertson EJ. Rescue of the T-Associated maternal effect in mice carrying null mutations in igf-2 and igf2r, 2 reciprocally imprinted genes. Development 1993; 118:731-736.

214. Ueno H, Colbert H, Escobedo JA, Williams LT. Inhibition of PDGF beta-receptor signal transduction by coexpression of a truncated receptor. Science 1991; 252:844-848.

215. Ueno H, Gunn M, Dell K, Tseng A, Williams L. A truncated form of fibroblast growth factor receptor-1 inhibits signal transduction by multiple types of fibroblast growth factor receptor. J Biol Chem 1992; 267:1470-1476.

216. Peters K, Werner S, Liao X, Wert S, Whitsett J, Williams L. Targeted expression of a dominant negative FGF receptor blocks branching morphogenesis and epithelial differentiation of the mouse lung. EMBO J 1994; 13:3296-3301.

217. Hemmati-Brivanlou A, Melton DA. Inhibition of activin receptor signaling promotes neuralization in Xenopus. Cell 1994; 77:273-281.

218. Mima T, Ueno H, Fischman DA, Williams LT, Mikawa T. FGF-receptor is required for in vivo cardiac myocyte proliferation at early embryonic stages of heart development. Proc Natl Acad Sci USA 1995; 92:467-471.

219. Amaya E, Musci TJ, Kirschner MW. Expression of a dominant negative mutant of the FGF receptor disrupts mesoderm formation in Xenopus embryos. Cell 1991; 66:257-290.

220. Werner S, Weinberg W, Liao X, Peters KG, Blessing M, Yuspa SH, Weiner RH, Williams LT. Targeted expression of a dominant-negative FGF receptor mutant in the epidermis of transgenic mice reveals a role of FGF in keratinocyte organization and differentiation. EMBO J 1993; 12:2635-2643.

221. Saint-Jeannet JP, Levi G, Girault JM, Koteliansky V, Thiery JP. Ventrolateral regionalization of Xenopus laevis mesoderm is characterized by the expression of alpha-smooth muscle actin. Development 1992; 115:1165-1173.

222. Rudnicki MA, Schnegelsberg PNJ, Stead RH, Braun T, Arnold HH, Jaenisch R. MyoD or myf-5 is required for the formation of skeletal muscle. Cell 1993; 75:1351-1359.

223. Fishman GI, Kaplan ML, Buttrick PM. Tetracycline-regulated cardiac gene expression in vivo. J Clin Invest 1994; 93:1864-1868.

224. Letterio JJ, Geiser AG, Kulkarni AB, Roche NS, Sporn MB, Roberts AB. Maternal rescue of transforming growth factor-beta 1 null mice. Science 1994; 264:1936-1938.

225. Slack JMW. The inducer that never was. Nature 1994; 369:279-280.

226. LaBonne C, Whitman M. Mesoderm induction by activin requires FGF-mediated intracellular signals. Development 1994; 120:463-472.

227. Cornell RA, Kimelman D. Activin-mediated mesoderm induction requires FGF. Development 1994; 120:452-462.

228. Komuro I, Katoh Y, Hoh E, Takaku F, Yazaki Y. Mechanisms of cardiac hypertrophy and injury: Possible role of protein kinase C activation. Jpn Circ J 1991; 55:1149-1157.

229. Villarreal FJ, Dillman WH. Cardiac hypertrophy-induced changers in mRNA levels for TGF-beta 1, fibronectin, and collagen. Am J Physiol 1992; 262:H1861–1866.

230. Takahashi NA, Calderone A, Izzo NJ, Maki TM, Marsh JD, Colucci WS. Hypertrophic stimuli induce transforming growth factor-beta(1) expression in rat ventricular myocytes. J Clin Invest 1994; 94:1470–1476.

231. Sakata Y. Tissue factors contributing to cardiac hypertrophy in cardiomyopathic hamsters (BIO14.6): Involvement of transforming growth factor-beta 1 and tissue renin-angiotensin system in the progression of cardiac hypertrophy. Hokkaido Igaku Zasshi 1993; 68:18–28.

232. Everett AD, Tufromcreddie A, Fisher A, Gomez RA. Angiotension receptor regulates cardiac hypertrophy and transforming growth factor-beta(1) expression. Hypertension 1994; 23:587–592.

233. Hanson MC, Fath KA, Alexander RW, de la Fontaine P. Induction of cardiac insulin-like growth factor 1 gene expression in pressure overload hypertrophy. Am J Med Sci 1993; 306:69–74.

234. Donohue TJ, Dworkin LD, Lango MN, Fliegner K, Lango RP, Benstein JA, Slater WR, Catanese VM. Induction of myocardial insulin-like growth factor-1 gene expression in left ventricular hypertrophy. Circulation 1994; 89:799–809.

235. Czerwinski SM, Novakofski J, Bechtel PJ. Is insulin-like growth factor gene expression modulated during cardiac hypertrophy. Med Sci Sports Exerc 1993; 25:495–500.

236. Russell-Jones DL, Leach RM, Ward JPT, Thomas CR. Insulin-like growth factor-I gene expression is increased in the right ventricular hypertrophy induced by chronic hypoxia in the rat. J Mol Endocrinol 1993; 10:99–102.

237. Adachi S, Ito H, Akimoto H, Tanaka M, Fujisaki H, Marumo F, Hiroe M. Insulin-like growth factor-II induces hypertrophy with increased expression of muscle specific genes in cultured rat cardiomyocytes. J Mol Cell Cardiol 1994; 26:789–795.

238. Tokola H, Salo K, Vuolteenaho O, Ruskoaho H. Basal and acidic fibroblast growth factor-induced atrial natriuretic peptide gene expression and secretion is inhibited by staurosporine. Eur J Pharmacol 1994; 267:195–206.

239. Ito H, Hiroe M, Hirata Y, Tsijino M, Adachi S, Shichiri M, Koike A, Nogami A, Marumo F. Insulin-like growth factor-I induces hypertrophy with enhanced expression of muscle specific genes in cultured rat cardiomyocytes. Circulation 1993; 87:1715–1721.

240. Komuro I, Katoh Y, Kaida T, Shibazaki Y, Kurabayashi M, Hoh E, Takaku F, Yazaki Y. Mechanical loading stimulates cell hypertrophy and specific gene expression in cultured rat cardiac myocytes: possible role of protein kinase C activation. J Biol Chem 1991; 266:1265–1268.

241. Sadoshima J, Xu YH, Slayter HS, Izumo S. Autocrine release of angiotensin-II mediates stretch-induced hypertrophy of cardiac myocytes in vitro. Cell 1993; 75:977–984.

242. Ruknudin A, Sachs F, Bustamante JO. Stretch-actived ion channels in tissue-cultured chick heart. Am J Physiol 1993; 264:H960–H972.

243. Toyozaki T, Hiroe M, Hasumi M, Horie T, Hosoda S, Tsushima T, Sekiguchi M. Insulin-like growth factor-I receptors in human cardiac myocytes and their relation to myocardial hypertrophy. Jpn Circ J 1993; 57:1120–1127.

244. Reiss K, Meggs LG, Li P, Olivetti G, Capasso JM, Anversa P. Upregulation of IGF1, IGF1-receptor, and late growth related genes in ventricular myocytes acutely after infarction in rats. J Cell Physiol 1994; 158:160–168.

245. Speir E, Tanner V, Gonzalez AM, Farris J, Baird A, Casscells W. Acidic and basic fibroblast growth factors in adult rat heart myocytes: localization, regulation in culture, and effects on DNA synthesis. Circ Res 1992; 71:251–259.

246. Donath MY, Zapf J, Eppenbergereberhardt M, Froesch ER, Eppenberger HM. Insulin-like growth factor I stimulates myofibril development and decreases smooth muscle alpha-actin of adult cardiomyocytes. Proc Natl Acad Sci USA 1994; 91:1686–1690.

247. Fuller SJ, Mynett JR, Sugden PH. Stimulation of cardiac protein synthesis by insulin-like growth factors. Biochem J 1992; 282:85–90.

248. Lange LG, Schreiner GF. Immune mechanisms of cardiac disease. N Engl J Med 1994; 330:1129–1135.

249. McCartney-Francis NL, Wahl SM. Transforming growth factor beta—a matter of life and death. J Leukocyte Biol 1994; 55:401–409.

250. Shull MM, Ormsby I, Kier AB, Pawlowski S, Diebold RJ, Yin MY, Allen R, Sidman C, Proetzel G, Calvin D, Annunziata N, Doetschman T. Targeted disruption of the mouse transforming growth factor-beta 1 gene results in multifocal inflammatory disease. Nature 1992; 359:693–699.

251. Kulkarni AB, Huh CG, Becker D, Geiser A, Lyght M, Flanders KC, Roberts AB, Sporn MB, Ward JM, Karlsson S. Transforming growth factor beta 1 null mutation in mice causes excessive inflammatory response and early death. Proc Natl Acad Sci USA 1993; 90:770–774.

252. Geiser AG, Letterio JJ, Kulkarni AB, Karlsson S, Roberts AB, Sporn MB. Transforming growth factor-beta1 (TGF-beta1) controls expression of major histocompatibility genes in the postnatal mouse: aberrant histocompatibility antigen expression in the pathogenesis of the TGF-beta1 null mouse phenotypes. Proc Natl Acad Sci USA 1993; 90:9944–9948.

253. Nepom GT, Erlich H. MHC class-II molecules and autoimmunity. Annu Rev Immunol 1991; 9:493–525.

254. Guardiola J, Maffei A. Control of MHC class II gene expression in autoimmune, infectious and neoplastic diseases. Crit Rev Immunol 1993; 13:247–68.

255. Milton AD, Fabre JW. Massive induction of donor-type class I and class II major histocompatibility complex antigens in rejecting cardiac allografts in the rat. J Exp Med 1985; 161:98–112.

256. Waltenberger J, Wanders A, Fellstrom B, Miyazono K, Heldin CH, Funa K. Induction of transforming growth factor-beta during cardiac allograft rejection. J Immunol 1993; 151:1147–1157.

257. Zhao XM, Frist WH, Yeoh TK, Miller GG. Expression of cytokine genes in human cardiac allografts: Correlation of IL-6 and transforming growth factor-beta (TGF-beta) with histological rejection. Clin Exp Immunol 1993; 93:448–451.

258. Raju GP, Belland SE, Eisen HJ. Prolongation of cardiac allograft survival with transforming growth factor-beta 1 in rats. Transplantation 1994; 58:392–396.

259. Wallick SC, Figari IS, Morris RE, Levinson AD, Palladino MA. Immunoregulatory role of transforming growth factor-beta (TGF-beta) in development of killer cells: comparison of active and latent TGF-beta-1. J Exp Med 1990; 172:1777–1784.

260. Carel JC, Schreiber RD, Falqui L, Lacy PE. Transforming growth factor beta decreases the immunogenicity of rat islet xenografts (rat to mouse) and prevents rejection in association with treatment of the recipient with a monoclonal antibody to interferon gamma. Proc Natl Acad Sci USA 1990; 87:1591–5.

261. Qin LH, Chavin KD, Ding YZ, Woodward JE, Favaro JP, Lin JX, Bromberg JS. Gene transfer for transplantation: prolongation of allograft survival with transforming growth factor-beta 1. Ann Surg 1994; 220:508–519.

262. Lefer AM, Ma XL, Weyrich AS, Scalia R. Mechanism of the cardioprotective effect of transforming growth factor beta 1 in feline myocardial ischemia and reperfusion. Proc Natl Acad Sci USA 1993; 90:1018–1022.

263. Heino J, Ignotz RA, Hemler ME, Crouse C, Massagué J. Regulation of cell adhesion receptors by transforming growth factor-beta. Concomitant regulation of integrins. J Biol Chem 1989; 264:380–8.

264. Gamble JR, Khewgoodall Y, Vadas MA. Transforming growth factor-beta inhibits E-selectin expression on human endothelial cells. J Immunol 1993; 150:4494–4503.

265. Isik FF, Valentine HA, McDonald TO, Baird A, Gordon D. Localization of bFGF in human transplant coronary atherosclerosis. Ann NY Acad Sci 1991; 638:487–8.

266. Zhao XM, Yeoh TK, Frist WH, Porterfield DL, Miller GG. Induction of acidic fibroblast growth factor and full-length platelet-derived growth factor expression in human cardiac allografts—analysis by PCR, in situ hybridization, and immunohistochemistry. Circulation 1994; 90:677–685.

267. Zhao XM, Frist WH, Yeoh TK, Miller GG. Modification of alternative messenger RNA splicing of fibroblast growth factor receptors in human cardiac allografts during rejection. J Clin Invest 1994; 94:992–1003.

268. Yokoyama T, Vaca L, Rossen RD, Durante W, Hazarika P, Mann DL. Cellular basis for the negative inotropic effects of tumor necrosis factor-alpha in the adult mammalian heart. J Clin Invest 1993; 92:2303–12.

269. Roberts AB, Vodovotz Y, Roche NS, Sporn MB, Nathan CF. Role of nitric oxide in antagonistic effects of transforming growth factor-beta and interleukin-1beta on the beating rate of cultured cardiac myocytes. Mol Endocrinol 1992; 6:1921–1930.

270. Gulick T, Chung MK, Pieper SJ, Lange LG, Schreiner GF. Interleukin 1 and tumor necrosis factor inhibit cardiac myocyte beta-adrenergic responsiveness. Proc Natl Acad Sci USA 1989; 86:6753–6757.

271. Vodovotz Y, Bogdan C, Paik J, Xie QW, Nathan C. Mechanisms of suppression of macrophage nitric oxide release by transforming growth factor-beta. J Exp Med 1993; 178:605–613.

272. Goureau O, Lepoivre M, Becquet F, Courtois Y. Differential regulation of inducible nitric oxide synthase by fibroblast growth factors and transforming growth factor beta in bovine retinal pigmented epithelial cells: inverse correlation with cellular proliferation. Proc Natl Acad Sci USA 1993; 90:4276–4280.

273. Lefer AM, Tsao P, Aoki N, Palladino MAJ. Mediation of cardioprotection by transforming growth factor-beta. Science 1990; 249:61–64.

274. Thompson NL, Bazoberry F, Speir EH, Casscells W, Ferrans VJ, Flanders KC, Kondaiah P, Geiser AG, Sporn MB. Transforming growth factor beta-1 in acute myocardial infarction in rats. Growth Factors 1988; 1:91–99.

275. Qian SW, Kondaiah P, Casscells W, Roberts AB, Sporn MB. A second messenger RNA species of transforming growth factor beta 1 in infarcted rat heart. Cell Regul 1991; 2:241–249.

276. Massagué J. The transforming growth factor-beta family. Annu Rev Cell Biol 1990; 6:597–641.

277. Chiba M, Sumida E, Sumida E, Oka N, Nakata M. The effect of hypoxia in basic FGF synthesis of cultured myocardial cells. Circulation 1991; 84:II–395 (Abstr).

278. Yanagisawa-Miwa A, Uchida Y, Nakamura F, Tomaru T, Kido H, Kamijo T, Sugimoto T, Kaji K, Utsuyama M, Kurashima C, Ito H. Salvage of infarcted myocardium by angiogenic action of basic fibroblast growth factor. Science 1992; 257:1401–1403.

279. Harada K, Grossman W, Friedman M, Edelman ER, Prasad PV, Keighley CS, Manning WJ, Sellke FW, Simons M. Basic fibroblast growth factor improves myocardial function in chronically ischemic porcine hearts. J Clin Invest 1994; 94:623–630.

280. Sellke FW, Yang SY, Friedman M, Harada K, Edelman ER, Grossman W, Simons M. Basic FGF enhances endothelium-dependent relaxation of the collateral-perfused coronary microcirculation. Am J Physiol 1994; 267:H1303–1311.

281. Unger EF, Banai S, Shou MT, Lazarous DF, Jaklitsch MT, Scheinowitz M, Correa R, Klingbeil C, Epstein SE. Basic fibroblast growth factor enhances myocardial collateral flow in a canine model. Am J Physiol 1994; 266:H1588–H1595.

282. Ladoux A, Frelin C. Hypoxia is a strong inducer of vascular endothelial growth factor messenger RNA expression in the heart. Biochem Biophys Res Commun 1993; 195:1005–1010.

283. Cambien F, Poirier O, Lecerf L, Evans A, Cambou JP, Arveiler D, Luc G, Bard JM, Bara L, Ricard S, et al. Deletion polymorphism in the gene for angiotensin-converting enzyme is a potent risk factor for myocardial infarction. Nature 1992; 359:641–644.

284. Grainger DJ, Kemp PR, Liu AC, Lawn RM, Metcalfe JC. Activation of transforming growth factor-beta is inhibited in transgenic apolipoprotein(a) mice. Nature 1994; 370:460–462.

285. Grainger DJ, Kemp PR, Witchell CM, Weissberg PL, Metcalfe JC. Transforming growth factor beta decreases the rate of proliferation of rat vascular smooth muscle cells by extending the g(2) phase of the cell cycle and delays the rise in cyclic AMP before entry into m phase. Biochem J 1994; 299:227–235.

286. Grainger DJ, Kemp PR, Metcalfe JC, Liu AC, Lawn RM, Williams NR, Grace AA, Schofield PM, Chauhan A. The serum concentration of active transforming growth factor-β is severely depressed in advanced atherosclerosis. Nature Med 1995; 1:74–79.

287. Hanks SE, Quinn AM, Hunter T. The protein kinase family: conserved features and deduced phylogeny of the catalytic domain. Science 1988; 241:42–52.

16

Gene Therapy and the Vessel Wall

Jonathan D. Marmur
Mount Sinai School of Medicine
New York, New York

Major advances in the fields of recombinant DNA technology, cell biology, and percutaneous angioplasty have established the scientific and technical basis for the transfer of genetic information to the vessel wall (1). Although gene therapy was initially proposed as a means to treat inherited disorders, whereby transfer of a normal copy of a single defective gene would prevent the development of disease, the majority of current and planned human gene therapy trials have been developed to treat acquired diseases. The concept of gene therapy at present encompasses the transfer of genetic information using genetically modified cells, chromosomes, portions of genes, or nucleic acids in a variety of forms (e.g., viral vectors, DNA oligonucleotides, RNA ribozymes), for therapeutic intent (2). Thus, in its broadest sense, gene therapy may be defined as the genetic-based treatment of inherited and acquired diseases.

RATIONALE FOR GENE THERAPY

As initially proposed by Anderson (3, 4), certain criteria must be met to rationally base a therapeutic strategy on gene transfer. First, the genes involved in the disorder must be identified and characterized so that there is at least a partial understanding of the disease process on a genetic basis. Second, because gene therapy represents a novel and relatively untested form of pharmacology, it is associated with potential risks that are justifiable only in the context of a patient population for which no effective alternative therapy exists. Indeed, the rationale for the US Food and Drug Administration (FDA), National Institutes of Health (NIH) Recombinant DNA Advisory Committee (RAC)-approved vascular gene therapy trial for the treatment of patients with critical peripheral arterial insufficiency was based in part on the poor prognosis of these patients and on the virtual absence of effective medical therapy (5). Finally, the design of a gene therapy trial must provide both scientific and clinical data in order to evaluate gene transfer efficiency, to validate preclinical animal data, and to acquire safety and efficacy data for clearly defined clinical endpoints (2).

These criteria suggest that a variety of cardiovascular disorders, such as restenosis after percutaneous coronary arterial stenting and coronary arteriopathy associated with cardiac transplantation, may be potential targets for gene therapy. However, several problems related to the delivery, integration, and regulation of the therapeutic gene constitute an obstacle to the broader application of the concepts of gene therapy. Further advances in the application of gene therapy to human vascular disease will depend on advances in the methods of gene delivery to the targeted cell; the achievement of stable gene expression at a defined level within the target cell; and the design of vectors that are not deleterious to the patient or to the public health.

VESSEL WALL AS A TARGET FOR MOLECULAR GENETIC INTERVENTION

Despite the high prevalence of cardiovascular disease, disorders of the vascular system have been represented to date in only a small proportion of the approved human gene therapy protocols (6). This may be due to the availability of effective medical and surgical therapies for many of the common cardiovascular pathologies, such as hypertension and atherosclerosis. However, in light of recent advances in the understanding of the molecular biology of the cardiovascular system (7), the time may now be appropriate for the introduction of gene therapy to the management of a broad array of vasculopathies. As outlined by Dzau et al. (8), these vasculopathies are potential candidates for either systemic or local gene therapy (Table 1).

With respect to local gene therapy, features of the vessel wall may favor and others may impede the development of effective strategies to deliver exogenous genetic material. Favorable characteristics include the accessibility of a large portion of the vascular tree to catheter-based delivery devices, the relative simplicity of the vessel wall architecture and paucity of cell types, and the availability of a plethora of both simple and sophisticated technologies (e.g.,

Table 1   Vascular Diseases Potentially Amenable to Gene Therapy

Therapy and Disease	Example of Target Gene
Systemic gene therapy	
Atherosclerosis	High-density lipoprotein
Hypercoagulable states	Tissue plasminogen activator
Local gene therapy	
Restenosis after angioplasty	Cell cycle regulatory gene
Transplant rejection	Leukocyte adhesion molecule
Transplant vasculopathy	Cytokine
Angiogenesis	Vascular endothelial growth factor
Thrombosis	Tissue factor
Aortic aneurysms	Protease inhibitor

Source: Adapted from Ref. 8.

quantitative angiography, intravascular ultrasound, and angioscopy) to assess the effects of an intervention. Unfavorable characteristics include the slow replication rate of endothelial and vascular smooth muscle cells that may render the vessel wall impenetrable to vectors such as retroviruses that require cell division for successful gene transduction. In addition, unlike other cell types such as hepatocytes (9) and airway epithelium (10), vascular endothelium and smooth muscle do not appear to be particularly well suited for receptor-mediated cell-specific gene delivery.

EX VIVO CELL-MEDIATED VS. DIRECT GENE TRANSFER

To overcome the obstacles to gene delivery inherent to the arterial wall, initial studies utilized a cell-mediated approach in which cultured vascular cells were transduced ex vivo and then introduced to the vessel wall via a double balloon catheter (1). As reviewed by Nabel et al. (11), an advantage of cell mediated gene transfer is that the effects of gene transfer in a particular cell type can be evaluated (e.g., endothelial vs. smooth muscle cell). Disadvantages include the requirement for syngeneic cell lines and the transfection of cells in culture that necessitates a time delay between cell harvest and implantation. Despite these technical difficulties, ex vivo gene transfer has been demonstrated in several animal models, including seeding of genetically modified endothelial or vascular smooth muscle cells on canine prosthetic grafts (12) and denuded porcine (13) and rat arteries (14), as well as seeding of stents with sheep endothelial cells (15), and seeding of autologous transduced endothelial cells onto rat skeletal muscle capillaries (16).

The direct introduction of genetic material into the vessel wall represents a conceptually attractive alternative to the instillation of genetically altered cells and has been demonstrated in a number of animal models using a variety of gene transfer vectors. These studies demonstrate that the degree of gene transfer (transfection efficiency) and the stability of gene expression over time is influenced in large part by the nature of the gene transfer vector (e.g., retroviral vs. adenoviral). Thus, much of the work in the field of gene therapy has focused on the development of gene transfer vectors.

GENE TRANSFER VECTORS

The development of technology to transfer genetic material into the vessel wall of living animals has broad implications for the study and treatment of cardiovascular disorders, including the opportunity to study the effects of gene expression in various physiological and pathological states that cannot be readily modeled in tissue culture (17). The transfer of genes into the vascular cells of adult animals has been achieved using a variety of vectors (Table 2), including viral vectors (retrovirus, adenovirus, adenoassociated virus) and nonviral vectors (cationic liposomes, receptor-mediated molecular conjugates, and "naked" DNA gel delivery systems) (18).

Recombinant viral vectors exploit the mechanisms that viruses have evolved to achieve efficient gene transfer. The common strategy for the design of these vectors involves the replacement of elements of the parent viral genome that are essential for replication with heterologous DNA sequences such that the recombinant virion is capable of effective transfer of the insert gene but incapable of replication. Using this basic paradigm, a variety of DNA and RNA viruses have been used in gene therapy applications.

Retroviruses

Retroviral vectors were the first viral vectors to be used for in vivo arterial gene transfer studies (1). An understanding of the retroviral life cycle and the ability to manipulate the viral genome has allowed the development of gene transfer vectors that utilize the efficient gene transfer capability of the retrovirus (19). A mature retrovirus comprises an inner core enclosed in a phospholipid envelope. The envelope is a phospholipid bilayer derived from the plasma membrane of the virus-producing cell and is covered with glycoproteins that appear as surface projections on electron microscopy. The retroviral core consists of an icosahedral protein shell, the capsid, which contains two copies of the positive sense viral mRNA gene including 5' cap and 3' poly (A) structures (20). Also contained within the capsid are the virally encoded protease, reverse transcriptase, and integrase enzymes. The structure of the proviral form of a typical retrovirus, the Moloney murine leukemia virus (MoMLV), and the retroviral vector gene transfer system are illustrated in Figure 1.

Table 2 Gene Transfer Vectors

Vector (Number of Clinical Trials as of 8/95)	DNA-Carrying Capacity (kb)	In Vivo Efficiency	Integration	Duration of Expression	Advantages	Disadvantages
Retrovirus (76)	7	Low	High	Months	Extensive experience in clinical trials; easy to manufacture; appears to be safe	Need for active cell replication; potential risk for insertional mutagenesis; risk of viral replication
Adenovirus (15)	8	High	Low	Weeks	Able to concentrate to high titers; can infect nonreplicating cells; possibly targetable	Presence of adenoviral genes may stimulate intense inflammatory response; risk of viral replication
Adenoassociated virus (1)	5	Low	High	Months	Nonpathogenic (ubiquitous in humans); less risk of insertional mutagenesis (potential for site specific integration); can infect nonreplicating cells	Difficult to manufacture at high titers; lack of information on long-term consequences of integration and gene expression from the AAV provirus
Liposomes (12)	>30	Low	Low	Weeks to months	No risk of vector replication; no size constraints; minimal toxicity	Inefficient for in vivo gene delivery
Receptor-mediated molecular conjugates (0)	>30	Low–moderate	Low	Weeks to months	Potential for targeting specific tissues; ability to deliver protein as well as DNA in the complex	Limited to tissues with suitable receptors

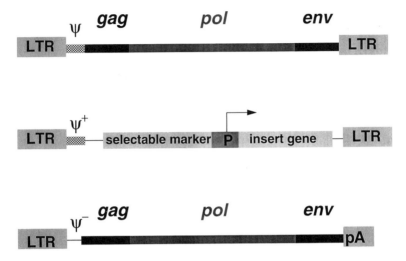

Figure 1 Retroviral gene delivery system. Shown schematically are the structure of the proviral form of a typical retrovirus (MoMLV), a retroviral vector, and a packaging cell line genome. The *cis*-acting elements of the retrovirus provirus are the long terminal repeat (LTR), which mediates transcription initiation and termination; the encapsidation signal (ψ); and signals necessary for reverse transcription (located between LTR and structural genes; not shown). The retroviral protein coding regions are *gag* (which yield virion core proteins); *pol* (which yield reverse transcriptase, integrase, and viral protease), and *env* (which yield the viral envelope glycoproteins). The retroviral vector retains the *cis*-acting elements of the provirus, but the structural genes are replaced with a gene insert containing a gene of interest, often in combination with a promoter (p) and a gene encoding for a selectable marker. The ψ+ symbol indicates the extended packaging signal, which encompasses part of the *gag* gene. A typical packaging cell genome retains the structural genes, deletes the packaging element (ψ–), and alters the remaining *cis*-acting elements in an attempt to lessen the homology to the vector and thereby diminish the potential for recombination to generate replication-competent virus. (Modified from Ref. 21.)

Retroviral-mediated gene transfer is dependent on a two-component system: the packaging cell line and the viral vector. The packaging cell contains a retroviral genome from which the signals responsible for packaging or encapsidation of the viral genome (referred to as "psi"; ψ) have been deleted (21). The packaging cell line is capable of producing all the proteins needed for viral replication, but is incapable of creating an infectious particle because the signal for packaging the viral genome into the capsid is lacking (designated as ψ–). Thus, the packaging cell produces empty noninfectious viral capsids. In order to fill these empty retroviral particles with a therapeutic or marker gene of interest, a genetically engineered retroviral genome known as a retroviral vector is introduced into the packaging cell line. The retroviral vector is the complement to the packaging cell genome: all the normal viral protein-coding sequences have been replaced by an insert gene, but the encapsidation and replication signals have been retained (Fig. 1). A packaging cell line containing a retroviral vector is known as a producer cell line. The producer cell will assemble retroviral particles that contain the gene insert from the retroviral vector; because this genome is lacking retroviral genes essential to replication, the produced virions will be replication-deficient, a desired safety feature. The amount of genetic material that can be inserted efficiently into the retroviral vector is approximately 7 kb of DNA, which is usually enough to code for one large protein or several small proteins.

Upon addition of the retroviral particles to a culture of cells, the viral particle binds to the cell, the retroviral vector enters the cell, and the vector sequence is subsequently integrated into the host cell genome. Because the retroviral vector is lacking several genes needed for replication this transfer procedure is termed *transduction* to differentiate it from *infection*, which is reserved for replication-competent viruses (21). Following integration of the retroviral vector, its internal sequences are expressed, resulting in the expression of a novel RNA molecule and the protein in the transduced cell. Integration into the target cell genome confers the potential for stable long-term gene expression, but is associated with the risk of insertional mutagenesis (22).

The advantages of retroviral vectors include the ability to infect a wide range of cell types in vitro, the integration of genetic material transported by the vector into the target cell genome, the lack of toxicity of these viruses in transduced cells, and the lack of vector spread or production of viral proteins after transduction. These properties have been exploited successfully in a number of human gene therapy protocols involving ex vivo modification of target cells followed by reimplantation of the genetically modified cells (23).

Despite these advantages, a number of features may limit the utility of retroviral vectors vis-à-vis the vasculature. A characteristic feature of retroviruses is that replication of target cells is necessary for proviral integration (24). This presents a major limitation for direct arterial retroviral gene transfer because vasculature cells have a low proliferation rate in vivo (25). Moreover, murine retroviral vectors are rapidly inactivated by human complement (26) and therefore may be unsuitable for direct gene delivery to human tissues in vivo. Finally, standard retroviruses are produced in relatively low titer because replication-deficient viruses are collected as supernatants from the producer cell line and cannot be concentrated. This has important implications for in vivo gene delivery in which efficient gene transfer requires a high multiplicity of infection (moi; i.e., the number of infectious particles per target cell). Strategies to overcome these limitations include the use of producer cell lines as delivery vehicles and attempts to alter the lability and tropism of the vector through genetic engineering of the glycoproteins (env) on the lipid envelope of the retroviral particle (27).

Adenoviruses as Vectors

Early studies using retroviral vectors and liposomes for arterial gene transfer reported low efficiencies, generally <1% of vascular cells in vivo (28–31). Because adenoviral vectors transfer genes efficiently in a broad spectrum of eukaryotic cells, more recent studies have investigated the utility of the adenovirus as a vector for gene transfer to the vessel wall (32–34). Wild-type adenoviruses target primarily the epithelial cell and produce clinical illnesses that are usually mild and rarely life-threatening. The basic structure of the adenovirus is a nonenveloped icosahedral (20 facets and 12 vertices) protein capsid enclosing an inner DNA-protein core. The double-stranded linear DNA genome is 36 kb and is bordered at each extremity by a 100–140 base-pair-long redundancy, the inverted terminal repeat (ITR). Adjacent to the left ITR are located several specific sequences that direct the packaging of the viral genome into preformed capsids (35). Like retroviruses, the requirement for these encapsidation signals (ψ) makes virion assembly specific and precludes entry of cellular DNA into empty adenoviral capsids.

The adenoviral genome is functionally classified into two major noncontiguous overlapping regions, early (E1-E4) and late (L1-L5), based on the time of transcription after infection. The E1 region encodes a transactivator believed to be required for the expression of all other viral gene products as well as for viral replication (36). Replication-incompetent vectors based on adenovirus have as a common construction technique deletion of E1 and replacement of this essential region of the viral genome with the promoter/gene cassette of interest (37) (Fig. 2). The E3 region encodes viral proteins that regulate immunosurveillance in vivo. Because this region is not essential for viral replication, it may be deleted to create space for larger exogenous gene inserts. Stocks of recombinant virus can then be grown in specialized cell lines that have been previously transfected with portions of the adenoviral genome and selected for continual expression of the required E1 genes. The commonly used human 293 cell line contains the left 14% of the adenovirus type 5 genome, including the E1 region, and can serve as a source of the E1 proteins in the assembly of viral vector particles (38). Viral stock propagated in 293 cells can be generated routinely to high titers, approximately 10^{10}–10^{12} particles per ml.

The adenoviral vector system possesses a number of favorable characteristics. Unlike retroviruses, adenoviruses infect both replicating and nonreplicating cells, including terminally differentiated cells. In addition, adenoviral vectors are not inactivated by human complement and are stable in vivo, per-

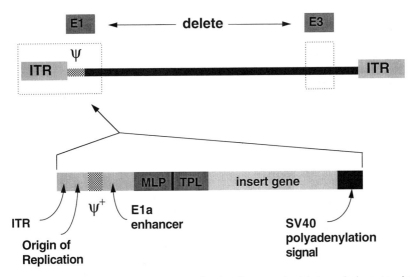

Figure 2 Typical cassette for a replication-incompetent adenoviral vector. In the adenoviral genome (top) there is a deletion in the E1 region to render the virus incapable of replication and a deletion in the E3 region to provide additional space for the insert gene. The cassette (bottom) is inserted into the left end of the construct and contains the 5′ ITR, the adenovirus origin of replication, the encapsidation signal (ψ+), the E1a enhancer upstream from the major late promoter (MLP) that drives the inserted gene, and the tripartite leader sequences (TPL; included to increase the efficiency of translation), followed by the foreign cDNA and a polyadenylation signal from the SV40 virus. (Modified from Ref. 37.)

mitting direct gene delivery in a variety of contexts (36), including the arterial wall (34). After entry into the target cell nucleus, adenoviral DNA sequences remain in an extrachromosomal form and rarely integrate into the host cell chromosome, thereby diminishing the likelihood of insertional mutagenesis and dysregulation of cellular genes. Arteries infected with adenoviral vectors achieve higher levels of reporter gene expression with transduction efficiencies 10–100-fold higher than those reported for retroviral and liposome vectors (18, 32, 39, 40).

Despite these advantages there are limitations to currently available adenoviral vectors. In several models, adenoviral-mediated gene expression is transient and an inflammatory reaction is detectable in target tissues (41, 42). These problems also apply to the vascular system; in most studies arterial reporter gene expression is diminished or undetectable by 28 days (18, 32, 43). The lack of persistent gene expression may be due to the development of an immune response to adenoviral proteins and/or acute adenovirus-associated tissue toxicity, as demonstrated by medial smooth muscle loss and neutrophilic infiltrates (44). Adenovirus based strategies to achieve arterial gene transfer may also be limited by the apparent impermeability of the endothelial layer to this vector, thereby necessitating mechanical disruption of the intima prior to gene transfer that is targeting medial smooth muscle (34). Finally, each of the approximately 20 serotypes of human adenovirus may generate neutralizing antibody, potentially limiting the possibility of repeated administration of a particular vector.

Adenoassociated Viruses as Vectors

Another viral vector that has been used in human gene therapy trials is the adenoassociated virus (AAV). AAV is a single-stranded DNA virus, and a member of the parvovirus family (45). Unlike the adenovirus, it is not associated with known pathology in humans or animals, despite high levels of silent infection in vivo. Adenoassociated viruses are described as replication-defective because either adenovirus or herpesvirus (defined in this setting as helper virus) is needed to provide adjunctive helper function to establish viral replication and complete an AAV life-cycle (46). The defective nature of AAV may be a useful feature for gene therapy where replication and spread of the virus vector is not desirable. The defective nature of AAV does not represent an impediment to the gene-transferring capacities of recombinant adenoassociated virions; it has been demonstrated that both wild-type and recombinant AAV integrate into the host genome efficiently and establish a latent infection in the absence of the helper virus (47). Transduction of a variety of primary human cells has been reported, including hepatocytes (48), bronchial epithelial cells (49), and peripheral blood mononuclear cells (50). The wild-type virus efficiently integrates into the host genome and usually does so preferentially in a small region of chromosome 19 (51–53). Such site-specific integration could diminish the likelihood of insertional mutagenesis, which is a major concern of gene therapy when one is using viruses that integrate into the genome.

A characteristic of AAV that makes it attractive for targeting the vasculature is the ability of recombinant virus to infect and result in gene expression in nondividing cells (54, 55). Recombinant virus is produced by replacing AAV genes (Rep and cap) with recombinant genes flanked only by the 125 base AAV inverted terminal repeat sequences (ITRs) (Fig. 3). Recombinant genes are packaged into infectious viral particles when a helper plasmid is cotransfected in the producer cell in the presence of a helper adenovirus (47). The helper plasmid contains all of the replication (Rep) and capsid (cap) genes of AAV, but no AAV ITRs and therefore is not packaged into the AAV particle. Because the helper and recombinant plasmids have no genetic homology, homologous recombination does not occur. This results in the production of replication

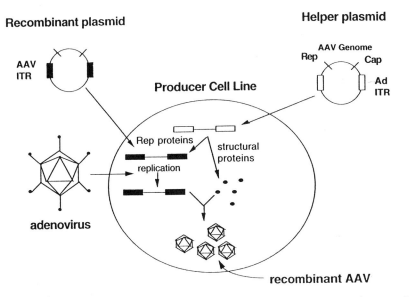

Figure 3 Generation of helper-free recombinant AAV. The producer cell is cotransfected with a helper plasmid providing the replication (Rep) and capsid (Cap) genes flanked by the adenoviral (Ad) ITR, and a recombinant AAV plasmid containing the gene of interest flanked by the AAV ITRs. The cotransfection with adenovirus provides the necessary conditions for replication and packaging. (Modified from Ref. 37.)

incompetent recombinant virus without the potential for generation of wild-type virus, which is a desirable safety feature. A potential disadvantage of the AAV system is the limiting packaging capability of the virion of 5 kb (45). However, when targeting the media of elastic arteries, the small size of AAV (18–26 nm) relative to adenovirus (65–80 nm) (45) may represent an advantage. Penetration of particles from the lumen into the media of these arteries varies as a function of particle size (56). Theoretically, the small size of AAV may allow it to penetrate the subendothelium and reach the media without the need for mechanical disruption of the intima prior to infection.

NONVIRAL GENE TRANSFER VECTORS

Although viruses constitute highly efficient gene transfer vehicles, the risks, costs, and limitations associated with recombinant viral vectors have led investigators to develop a variety of synthetic chemical nonviral vector systems. To mediate gene transfer effectively, these systems must overcome the same cellular barriers encountered by viruses: transport across the cell membrane, transfer from cytoplasm to nucleus, and persistence within the host cell nucleus (57). Recombinant viral vectors take advantage of the mechanisms that viruses have evolved to facilitate each of these steps. Because synthetic vectors require analogous mechanisms to achieve gene transfer, the development of nonviral vectors initially focused on methods to achieve effective eukaryotic membrane transition (57). These methods have involved encapsulation of DNA into lipid membrane vesicles (liposomes) that fuse with the target cell membrane, or precipitation of DNA into particles that are taken up by endocytosis.

Liposomes

Liposomes are artificial lipid bilayers that deliver nucleic acid to cells through fusion with cell membranes or via receptor-mediated endocytosis (58). The lipid bilayer may have a neutral or positively charged (cationic) surface. Cationic liposomes condense spontaneously with negatively charged DNA to form liposome–polynucleotide complexes. After entering the cell, these complexes are partially degraded in lysosomes, and the portion of plasmid DNA released in the cytoplasm translocates to the nucleus via unknown mechanisms, where it remains in an extrachromosomal location (59). Advantages of liposomes include the ease of preparation, the lack of viral sequences that may pose a safety hazard, and the absence of any DNA/RNA size constraint in vector construction. Disadvantages include low efficiency of gene transduction and the transience of gene expression. These limitations may be minimized by chemical modification of the liposome; for example, complexing the heat-inactivated hemagglutinating virus of Japan with cationic liposomes improves transfection efficiency of the vessel wall in vivo (60). The proliferative state of the cell population targeted by cationic liposomes also appears to affect in vivo arterial transfection efficiency. Balloon dilatation of rabbit iliac artery prior to gene transfer increases liposome-mediated gene delivery, presumably due to the resultant intimal smooth muscle cell proliferation (61).

Molecular Conjugates

To exploit more specifically endogenous cellular transport mechanisms, molecular conjugate vectors have been designed that enter the cell via targeted receptor-mediated endocytosis (62). Receptor-mediated endocytosis is a process that utilizes internalization pathways that can operate with high efficiency; for example, the iron transport protein transferrin can be imported in the order of thousands of molecules per minute per cell (63). Molecular conjugates designed to exploit these mechanisms consist of two functional domains: a DNA-binding domain to transport the DNA as part of the vector complex and a ligand domain to target a cellular receptor that allows entry of the complex via a specific receptor-mediated endocytic pathway. Reversible noncovalent binding of the DNA to the complex is achieved using a polycationic amine, such as poly(L)lysine, which is covalently linked to a ligand, such as transferrin, that targets a specific cellular receptor. Examples of targeted cells include hepatocytes, using the asiologlycoprotein receptor (64), and cells of the hematopoietic system, using the transferrin receptor (65). Molecular conjugate vectors share many of the advantages inherent in DNA–liposome complexes, plus the potential for highly targeted gene delivery. However, vectors based on this approach appear to be less efficient than recombinant viral vectors for the transfer of genetic material in vivo (66).

ANTISENSE OLIGONUCLEOTIDES TO "KNOCK OUT" GENE EXPRESSION IN VIVO

In most human gene therapy trials, the objective is to generate high levels of a particular protein to produce a desired therapeutic effect. An alternative gene therapy approach is to block the production or function of a protein that plays a critical role in disease pathogenesis. To block or "knock out" the synthesis of a protein, investigators have used antisense oligonucleotides: short pieces of RNA or DNA that are complementary to specific sequences of a target gene (67). Antisense therapeutics exploit the specificity of nucleic acid base pairing, and take advantage of the natural tendency of DNA and RNA to bind complementary strands in solution. By constructing an oligonucleotide with a sequence that is complementary to the target gene, antisense technology may be used to inhibit gene expression at several potential sites along the information flow from DNA to protein: (a) at the level of transcription, by triple helix formation with uncoiled DNA or by hybridization to nascent RNA; (b) at the level of RNA splicing through hybridization at intron–exon junctions; and (c) at the level of translation, through the inhibition of the binding of initiation factors, inhibition of the assembly of ribosomal subunits at the start codon, or inhibition of ribosome sliding along the coding sequences of the mRNA.

Ribozymes as an Alternative to Antisense Oligonucleotides

Despite their conceptual elegance, antisense oligonucleotides may have limited efficacy (68). Inhibition of vascular gene expression by these molecules may be constrained by a number of variables including the stability of the oligonucleotide in vivo, the ability of the oligonucleotide to enter and be retained by the target cell, and the ability of the oligonucleotide to interact in a non-sequence-specific manner with other molecules, such as charged glycosaminoglycans present in the connective tissue of the vessel wall. As an alternative to the use of antisense oligonucleotides, strategies have been developed based on the use of ribozymes, which are short catalytic RNAs possessing specific endoribonuclease activity (69, 70).

Ribozymes exist in several forms and are classified on the basis of their primary and presumed secondary structures. The best-characterized type of ribozyme is the hammerhead, found in vivo in certain plant viruses (71). In nature, these enzymes cleave intramolecularly (i.e., in *cis*) and cut 3' to the sequence GUC. However, with the appropriate manipulations, they can be made to cut intermolecularly (i.e., in *trans*), and the cleavage site can be NUX (where N is any base and X is A, C, or U) (72). Hammerhead ribozymes contain two separable functions: a catalytic core region containing several conserved bases, which cleaves the target RNA; and flanking regions, which, by nucleic acid complementarity, direct the ribozyme core to a specific target site. Thus, by attaching the core to sequences complementary to those flanking the target site GUC, ribozymes can be designed to specifically cleave almost any target RNA molecule (73). A major advantage of ribozymes is that unlike antisense oligonucleotides, in which one molecule has the capacity to neutralize only one mRNA molecule, a single ribozyme is able to destroy a large number of mRNA molecules (i.e., antisense oligonucleotides are stoichiometric and ribozymes are catalytic). In vitro, it has been estimated that some ribozymes cleave an RNA molecule every 2 min (73).

VASCULAR DISEASES AND ANIMAL MODELS OF GENE THERAPY

Using the vectors described above, both ex vivo and direct in vivo gene transfer into vascular endothelial and smooth muscle cells have been performed in several animal models of vascular disease. Pathophysiological processes involving the vessel wall that have been targeted for molecular intervention include restenosis after percutaneous revascularization (angioplasty), thrombosis associated with vascular implants and injury, and chronic arterial insufficiency associated with an inadequate development of a collateral circulation (i.e., lack of compensatory angiogenesis).

Restenosis after Angioplasty

Percutaneous transluminal coronary angioplasty (PTCA) is a common procedure for the treatment of myocardial ischemia secondary to atherosclerosis. Recurrent stenosis after successful PTCA, or restenosis, occurs in up to 50% of patients within 6 months and is the most significant impediment to the long-term success of the procedure (74). The multiple causative factors that have been implicated in restenosis may be segregated into two broad categories: recoil and intimal hyperplasia. Recoil occurs acutely (over 5–10 min) due to the elastic properties of the artery, and subacutely (over 1–3 weeks) due to constrictive vascular remodeling, a predominantly adventitial process (75). Both acute elastic recoil and subacute vascular remodeling may be effectively treated with mechanical devices, such as intraluminal stents (76). Stents appear to reduce dramatically the rate of restenosis, particularly when they are deployed with high-pressure balloon inflation that results in complete circumferential expansion. However, even in vessels ideally suited for stenting, a restenosis rate of ~10% at 6 months poststenting can be anticipated (77). The predominant mechanism underling restenosis in stented vessels, and an important contributing factor to restenosis after PTCA without stenting, is intimal hyperplasia.

Intimal hyperplasia represents a fundamental response to vascular injury. It is the final histological expression of a variety of molecular and cellular pathways involving thrombosis, inflammation, and smooth muscle cell migration, proliferation, and secretion of extracellular matrix. Attempts to inhibit this process using prolonged infusions of specific antibodies against individual antigens have been only partially successful, or have had no effect (78, 79). Inhibiting the interaction between a single growth factor and its receptor may not significantly alter the overall response to injury because there is a redundancy of pathways mediating the healing response to injury. An alternative strategy to inhibit smooth muscle cell proliferation derives from the observation that cell-cycle-regulatory genes constitute a final common pathway for all growth factors. Inhibition of these genes (e.g., c-*myb*, c-*myc*) using locally delivered antisense oligonucleotides has been reported to inhibit intimal hyperplasia in vivo (80–82). A more recent gene therapy approach to suppress smooth muscle cell proliferation after injury is the delivery and subsequent overexpression of a gene that encodes a local diffusible inhibitor of cellular replication, such as nitric oxide (83). Local delivery of vascular endothelial growth factor (VEGF) has also been reported to inhibit intimal hyperplasia, presumably by accelerating endothelial regeneration (84). It has been hypothesized that the endothelium exerts a negative regulatory effect on smooth muscle cell growth. Other approaches to smooth muscle cell growth inhibition include the use of recombinant chimeric toxins (85) and the delivery of a gene (e.g., herpes virus thymidine kinase) that can convert an innocuous drug (e.g., ganciclovir) to a toxic metabolite (33).

Thrombosis Associated with Vascular Implants and Injury

The demonstration that site-specific gene transfer to the vascular endothelium is feasible has stimulated the development of genetic strategies to prevent thrombosis that may complicate spontaneous or iatrogenic atherosclerotic plaque disruption, as well as thrombosis that may be associated with implanted vascular devices. To test the hypothesis that increased endothelial cell expression of an antithrombotic or fibrinolytic gene reduces thrombus formation in vivo, Dichek et al. (86) transduced cultured baboon endothelial cells with a retroviral vector carrying the human cDNA for tissue plasminogen activator (t-PA). These cells were seeded onto collagen-coated vascular grafts that were interposed in exteriorized arteriovenous femoral shunts. By measuring [^{111}In]platelet deposition and [^{125}I]fibrin accumulation, a focal antithrombotic effect, apparently due to local enhancement of thrombolysis, was demonstrated in vivo. Thus, the strategy of delivering genetically modified endothelial cells that overexpress antithrombotic molecules may be useful for the prevention of thrombotic closure of implanted cardiovascular devices or iatrogenically denuded vessels following PTCA.

Chronic Arterial Insufficiency and Therapeutic Angiogenesis

Arterial insufficiency of the heart, brain, and limb may result in disabling angina pectoris, myocardial infarction, stroke, claudication, and gangrene of the extremities. In many patients, surgical or percutaneous endoluminal revascularization of these vascular beds may fail or may not be feasible due to diffuse and severe large vessel disease, the lack of a suitable conduit for arterial reconstruction, the presence of small vessel disease, or a concomitant illness that renders the risk of surgical intervention prohibitive.

Angiogenesis, the process through which new blood vessels are formed (87), may play an important role in the neovascularization of ischemic tissue. Over the last decade, a number of factors involved in the control of blood vessel generation and growth have been identified. The isolation and purification of these factors have led to the notion of therapeutic angiogenesis (88), by which the growth of new capillaries and collateral vessels into an ischemic territory is stimulated by the administration of angiogenic peptides. This therapeutic strategy constitutes a form of medical revascularization that may provide an option for patients whose vasculopathy is not amenable to conventional surgical or percutaneous endoluminal approaches.

The cloning of genes that encode angiogenic factors and the development of systems to deliver plasmid DNA into the vessel wall raise the possibility of gene therapy to promote neovascularization into tissues suffering arterial insufficiency. The first National Institutes of Health RAC/FDA-approved gene therapy protocol for human vascular disease is for the treatment of peripheral vascular disease, in which the cDNA encoding the angiogenic peptide VEGF is delivered to the vessel wall using "naked" plasmid DNA loaded onto a hydrogel-coated balloon catheter (5). Approval for this study was based on the demonstrated efficacy of locally delivered VEGF cDNA in a rabbit hindlimb ischemia model (89), the lack of effective medical alternatives, and the poor prognosis for patients with chronic critical leg ischemia.

Table 3 Gene Therapy: Analogies with Traditional Therapies

Gene Therapy	Analogous Traditional Therapy
Antisense oligonucleotides and ribozymes	Drug design based on ligand-receptor interaction (e.g., β-blockade)
Transient gene expression (e.g., exogenous mRNA)	Protein replacement therapy (e.g., insulin)
Permanent exogenous gene integration into the genome of the patient	Surgery: permanent alteration of tissue

CONCLUSION

Gene therapy is a novel and rapidly advancing field in cardiovascular medicine. Progress in molecular and cellular biology has made the transfer of genetic material to the vessel wall possible using a variety of vectors and delivery strategies. These techniques provide the means with which either to produce proteins not normally present or to "knock out" the production of proteins normally synthesized by the cellular elements of the vasculature. Although gene therapy is radical, there are aspects that are analogous to traditional medicine (90) (Table 3). Several challenges remain before gene therapy can be broadly applied to cardiovascular disorders, including issues related to the efficiency, stability, cost, and safety of gene transfer.

REFERENCES

1. Nabel EG, Plautz G, Boyce FM, Stanley JC, Nabel GJ. Recombinant gene expression in vivo within endothelial cells of the arterial wall. Science 1989; 244:1342–1344.
2. Curiel DT, Pilewski JM, Albelda SM. Gene therapy approaches for inherited and acquired lung diseases. Am J Respir Cell Mol Biol 1996; 14:1–18.
3. Anderson WF. Prospects for human gene therapy. Science 1984; 226:401–409.
4. Anderson WF. Human gene therapy. Science 1992; 256:808–813.
5. Isner JM, Walsh K, Symes J, Pieczek A, Takeshita S, Lowry J, Rossow S, Rosenfield K, Weir L, Brogi E, Schainfeld R. Arterial gene therapy for therapeutic angiogenesis in patients with peripheral artery disease. Circulation 1995; 91:2687–2692.
6. Sobel RE, Scanlon KJ. Clinical protocols. Cancer Gene Ther 1995; 2:137–145.
7. Dzau VJ, Gibbons GH, Cooke JP, Omoigui N. Vascular biology and medicine in the 1990s: scope, concepts, potential, and perspectives. Circulation 1993; 87:705–719.
8. Dzau VJ, Gibbons GH, Morishita R, Pratt RE. New perspectives in hypertension research. Hypertension 1994; 23:1132–1140.
9. Chang AGY, Wu GY. Gene therapy: applications to the treatment of gastrointestinal and liver diseases. Gastroenterology 1994; 106:1076–1084.

10. Gao L, Wagner E, Cotten M, Argarwal S, Harris C, Romer R, Miller L, Hu PC, Curiel D. Direct in vivo gene transfer to airway epithelium employing adenovirus-polylysine-DNA complexes. Hum Gene Ther 1993; 4:17–24.
11. Nabel EG, Pompili VJ, Plautz GE, Nabel GJ. Gene transfer and vascular disease. Cardiovasc Res 1994; 28:445–455.
12. Wilson JM, Birinyi LK, Salomon RN, Libby P, Callow AD, Mulligan RC. Implantation of vascular grafts lined with genetically modified endothelial cells. Science 1989; 244:1344–1346.
13. Plautz G, Nabel EG, Nabel GJ. Introduction of vascular smooth muscle cells expressing recombinant genes in vitro. Circulation 1991; 83:578–583.
14. Lynch CM, Clowes MM, Osborne WR, Clowes AW, Miller AD. Long-term expression of human adenosine deaminase in vascular smooth muscle cells of rats: a model for gene therapy. Proc Natl Acad Sci USA 1992; 89:1138–1142.
15. Dichek DA, Neville RF, Zwiebel JA, Freeman SM, Leon MB, Anderson WF. Seeding of intravascular shunts with genetically engineered endothelial cells. Circulation 1989; 80:1347–1353.
16. Messina LM, Podrazik RM, Whitehill TA, Ekhterae D, Brothers TE, Wilson JM, Burkel WE, Stanley JC. Adhesion and incorporation of lacZ-transduced endothelial cells into the intact capillary wall in the rat. Proc Natl Acad Sci USA 1992; 89:12018–12022.
17. Buttrick PM, Kaplan ML, Kitsis RN, Leinwand LA. Distinct behavior of cardiac myosin heavy chain gene constructs in vivo. Discordance with in vitro results. Circ Res 1993; 72:1211–1217.
18. Nabel EG. Gene therapy for cardiovascular disease. Circulation 1995; 91:541–548.
19. Miller AD. Retroviral vectors. Curr Top Microbiol Immunol 1992; 158:1–24.
20. Vile RG, Russell SJ. Retroviruses as vectors. Br Med Bull 1995; 51:12–30.
21. Morgan RA, Anderson WF. Human gene therapy. Annu Rev Biochem 1993; 62:191–217.
22. Cone RD, Mulligan RC. High-efficiency gene transfer into mammalian cells: generation of helper-free recombinant retrovirus with broad mammalian host range. Proc Natl Acad Sci USA 1984; 81:6349–6353.
23. Grossman M, Raper SE, Kozarsky K, Stein EA, Engelhardt JF, Muller D, Lupien PJ, Wilson JM. Successful ex vivo gene therapy directed to liver in a patient with familial hypercholesterolaemia. Nat Genet 1994; 6:335–341.
24. Miller DG, Adam MA, Miller AD. Gene transfer by retrovirus vectors occurs only in cells that are actively replicating at the time of infection. Mol Cell Biol 1990; 10:4239–4242.
25. Clowes AW, Reidy MA, Clowes MM. Kinetics of cellular proliferation after arterial injury. I. Smooth muscle growth in the absence of endothelium. Lab Invest 1983; 49:327–333.
26. Welsh RM, Cooper NR, Jensen FC, Oldstone MBA. Human serum lyses RNA tumour viruses. Nature 1975; 257:612–614.
27. Miller N, Vile R. Targeted vectors for gene therapy. FASEB J 1995; 9:190–199.
28. Nabel EG, Plautz G, Nabel G. Site-specific gene expression in vivo by direct gene transfer into the vessel wall. Science 1990; 249:1285–1288.

29. Lim CS, Chapman GD, Gammon RS, Muhlestein JB, Bauman RP, Stack RS, Swain JL. Direct in vivo gene transfer into the coronary and peripheral vasculatures of the intact dog. Circulation 1991; 83:2007–2011.

30. Leclerc G, Gal D, Takeshita S, Nikol S, Weir L, Isner JM. Percutaneous arterial gene transfer in a rabbit model. J Clin Invest 1992; 90:936–944.

31. Flugelman MY, Jaklitsch MT, Neewman KD, Casscells W, Bratthauer GL, Dichek DA. Low level in vivo gene transfer into the arterial wall through a perforated balloon catheter. Circulation 1992; 85:1110–1117.

32. Lee SW, Trapnell BC, Rade JJ, Virmani R, Dichek DA. In vivo adenoviral vector-mediated gene transfer into balloon-injured rat carotid arteries. Circ Res 1993; 73:797–807.

33. Ohno T, Gordon D, San H, Pompili VJ, Imperiale MJ, Nabel GJ, Nabel EG. Gene therapy for vascular smooth muscle cell proliferation after arterial injury. Science 1994; 265:781–784.

34. Willard JE, Landau C, Glamann B, Burns D, Jessen ME, Pirwitz MJ, Gerard RD, Meidell RS. Genetic modification of the vessel wall. Comparison of surgical and catheter-based techniques for delivery of adenovirus. Circulation 1994; 89:2190–2197.

35. Hearing P, Samulski RJ, Wishart WL, Shenk T. Identification of a repeated sequence element required for efficient encapsidation of the adenovirus type 5 chromosome. J Virol 1987; 61:2555–2558.

36. Nevins JR. Mechanism of activation of early viral transcription by the adenovirus E1A gene product. Cell 1981; 26:213–220.

37. Nienhuis AW, Walsh CE, Liu J. Viruses as therapeutic gene transfer vectors. In: Young NS, ed. Viruses and the Bone Marrow. New York: Marcel Dekker, 1993:353–414.

38. Graham FL, Smiley J, Russell WC, Nairn R. Characteristics of a human cell line transformed by DNA from human adenovirus type 5. J Gen Virol 1977; 36:59–72.

39. Lemarchand P, Jones M, Yamada I, Crystal RG. In vivo gene transfer and expression in normal uninjured blood vessels using replication-deficient recombinant adenovirus vectors. Circ Res 1993; 72:1132–1138.

40. Guzman RJ, Lemarchand P, Crystal RG, Epstein SE, Finkel T. Efficient and selective adenovirus-mediated gene transfer into vascular neointima. Circulation 1993; 88:2838–2848.

41. Simon RH, Engelhardt JF, Yang Y, Zepeda M, Weber-Pendleton S, Grossman M, Wilson JM. Adenovirus-mediated transfer of the CFTR gene to lung of non-human primates: toxicity study. Hum Gene Ther 1993; 4:771–780.

42. Gerard RD, Herz J. Adenovirus-mediated low density lipoprotein receptor gene transfer accelerates cholesterol clearance in normal mice. Proc Natl Acad Sci USA 1993; 90:2812–2816.

43. Barr E, Carroll J, Kalynych AM, Tripathy SK, Kozarsky K, Wilson JM, Leiden JM. Efficient catheter-mediated gene transfer into the heart using replication-defective adenovirus. Gene Ther 1994; 1:51–58.

44. Schulick AH, Newman KD, Virmani R, Dichek DA. In vivo gene transfer into injured carotid arteries. Optimization and evaluation of acute toxicity. Circulation 1995; 91:2407–2414.

45. Berns KI. Parvovirus replication. Microbiol Rev 1990; 54:316–329.

46. Berns KI, Bohenzky RA. Adeno-associated viruses: an update. Adv Vir Res 1994; 32:243–306.

47. Samulsksi RJ, Chang LS, Shenk T. Helper-free stocks of recombinant adeno-associated viruses: normal integration does not require viral gene expression. J Virol 1989; 63:3822–3828.

48. Muzyczka N. Use of adeno-associated virus as a general transduction vector for mammalian cells. Curr Topic Microbiol Immunol 1992; 158:97–129.

49. Flotte TR, Solow R, Owens RA, et al. Gene expression from adeno-associated virus vectors in airway epithelial cells. Am J Respir Cell Mol Biol 1992; 7:349–356.

50. Philip R, Brunette E, Kilinski L, Murugesh D, McNally MA, Ucar K, Rosenblatt J, Okarma TB, Lebkowski JS. Efficient and sustained gene expression in primary T lymphocytes and primary and cultured tumor cells mediated by adeno-associated virus plasmid DNA complexed to cationic liposomes. Mol Cell Biol 1994; 14:2411–2418.

51. Kotin RM, Siniscalco M, Samulski RJ, Zhu XD, Hunter L, Laughlin CA, McLaughlin S, Muzyczka N, Rocchi M, K.I. Berns KI. Site-specific integration by adeno-associated virus. Proc Natl Acad Sci USA 1990; 87:2211–2215.

52. Kotin RM, Menninger JC, Ward DC, Berns KI. Mapping and direct visualization of a region-specific viral DNA integration site on chromosome 19q13-qter. Genomics 1991; 10:831–834.

53. Samulski RJ, Zhu X, Xiao X, Brook JD, Housman DE, Epstein N, Hunter LA. Targeted integration of adeno-associated virus (AAV) into human chromosome 19. EMBO J 1991; 10:3941–3950.

54. Flotte TR, Afione SA, Zeitlin PL. Adeno-associated virus vector gene expression occurs in nondividing cells in the absence of vector DNA integration. Am J Respir Cell Mol Biol 1994; 11:517–521.

55. Podsakoff G, Wong KK Jr, Chatterjee S. Efficient gene transfer into nondividing cells by adeno-associated virus-based vectors. J Virol 1994; 68:5656–5666.

56. Rome JJ, Shayani V, Flugelman MY, Newman KD, Farb A, Virmani R, Dichek D. Anatomic barriers influence the distribution of an in vivo gene transfer into the arterial wall. modeling with microscopic tracer particles and verification with a recombinant adenoviral vector. Arterioscler Thromb 1995; 14:148–161.

57. Curiel DT. Gene transfer mediated by adenovirus-polylysine-DNA complexes. In: Vos J-MH, ed. Viruses in Human Gene Therapy. Durham, NC: Carolina Academic Press, 1995:179–212.

58. Felgner PL, Gladek TR, Holm M, Roman R, Chan HW, Wenz M, Northrop JP, Ringold GM, Danielsen M. Lipofection: a highly efficient, lipid-mediated DNA-transfection procedure. Proc Natl Acad Sci USA 1987; 84:7413–7417.

59. Malone RW, Felgner PL, Verma IM. Lipofectin mediated RNA transfection. Proc Natl Acad Sci USA 1989; 86:6077–6081.

60. Morishita R, Gibbons GH, Kaneda Y, Ogihara T, Dzau VJ. Novel and effective gene transfer technique for study of vascular renin angiotensin system. J Clin Invest 1993; 91:2580–2585.

61. Takeshita S, Gal D, Leclerc J, Pickering JG, Riessen R, Weir L, Isner JM. Increased gene expression after liposome-mediated arterial gene transfer associated with intimal smooth muscle cell proliferation. J Clin Invest 1994; 93:652–661.

62. Cotten M, Wagner E. Non-viral approaches to gene therapy. Curr Opin Biotechnol 1993; 4:705–710.

63. Thortenson K, Romslo I. The role of transferrin in the mechanism of cellular iron uptake. Biochem J 1990; 271:1–10.

64. Wu GY, Wu CH. Receptor-mediated gene delivery and expression in vivo. J Biol Chem 1988; 263:14621–14624.

65. Huebers H, Finch C. The physiology of transferrin and transferrin receptors. Physiol Rev 1987; 67:520–582.

66. Curiel DT. High efficiency gene transfer employing adenovirus-polylysine-DNA complexes. Nat Immun 1994; 13:141–164.

67. Milligan JF, Jones RJ, Froehler BC, Matteucci MD. Development of antisense therapeutics. Implications for cancer gene therapy. Ann NY Acad Sci 1994; 716:228–241.

68. Stein CA, Cheung Y-C. Antisense oligonucleotides as therapeutic agents—is the bullet really magic? Science 1993; 261:1004–1012.

69. Cech TR. The chemistry of self-splicing RNA and RNA enzymes. Science 1987; 236:1532–1539.

70. Pyle AM. Ribozymes: a distinct class of metalloenzymes. Science 1993; 261:709–714.

71. Buzayan JM, Gerlach WL, Bruening G. Satellite tobacco ringspot virus RNA: a subset of the RNA sequence is sufficient for autolytic processing. Proc Natl Acad Sci USA 1986; 83:8859–8862.

72. Ruffner DE, Stormo GD, Uhlenbeck OC. Sequence requirements of the hammerhead RNA self-cleavage reaction. Biochemistry 1990; 29:10695–10702.

73. Uhlenbeck OC. A small catalytic oligoribonucleotide. Nature 1987; 328:596–600.

74. Nobuyoshi M, Kimura T, Nosaka H, Mioka S, Ueno K, Yokoi H, Hamasaki N, Horiuchi H, Ohishi H. Restenosis after successful percutaneous transluminal coronary angioplasty: serial angiographic follow-up of 229 patients. J Am Coll Cardiol 1988; 12:616–23.

75. Anderson HR, Maeng M, Thorwest M, Falk E. Remodeling rather than neointimal formation explains luminal narrowing after deep vessel wall injury. Circulation 1996; 93:1716–1724.

76. Haude M, Erbel R, Issa H, Meyer J. Quantitative analysis of elastic recoil after balloon angioplasty and after intracoronary implantation of balloon-expandable Palmaz-Schatz stents. J Am Coll Cardiol 1993; 21:26–34.

77. Serruys PW. Benestent-II pilot study: 6 months follow-up of phase 1, 2, and 3. (abstract). Circulation 1995; 92:I-542.

78. Ferns GAA, Raines EW, Sprugel KH, Motani AS, Reidy MA, Ross R. Inhibition of neointimal smooth muscle accumulation after angioplasty by an antibody to

PDGF. Science 1991; 253:1129–1132.

79. Lindner V, Reidy MA. Proliferation of smooth muscle cells after vascular injury is inhibited by an antibody against basic fibroblast growth factor. Proc Natl Acad Sci USA 1991; 88:3739–3743.

80. Simons E, Edelman ER, DeKeyser J, Langer R, Rosenberg RD. Antisense c-*myb* oligonucleotides inhibit intimal arterial smooth muscle cell accumulation in vivo. Nature 1992; 359:67–70.

81. Morishita R, Gibbons GH, Ellison KE, Nakajima M, Zhang L, Kaneda Y, Ogihara T, Dzau VJ. Single intraluminal delivery of antisense cdc3 kinase and proliferating-cell nuclear antigen oligonucleotides results in chronic inhibition of neointimal hyperplasia. Proc Natl Acad Sci USA 1993; 90:8474–8478.

82. Shi Y, Fard A, Galeo A, Hutchinson HG, Vermani P, Dodge GR, Hall DJ, Shaheen F, Zalewski A. Transcatheter delivery of c-myc antisense oligomers reduces neointimal formation in a porcine model of coronary artery balloon injury. Circulation 1994; 90:944–951.

83. von der Leyden HE, Gibbons GH, Morishita R, Lewis NP, Zhang L, Nakajima M, Kaneda Y, Cooke JP, Dzau VJ. Gene therapy inhibiting neointimal vascular lesion: in vivo transfer of endothelial cell nitric oxide synthase gene. Proc Natl Acad Sci USA 1995; 92:1137–1141.

84. Asahara T, Bauters C, Pastore C, Kearney M, Rossow S, Bunting S, Ferrara N, Symes JF, Isner JM. Local delivery of vascular endothelial growth factor accelerates reendothelialization and attenuates intimal hyperplasia in balloon-injured rat carotid artery. Circulation 1995; 91:2793–2801.

85. Casscells W, Lappi DA, Olwin BB, Wai C, Siegman M, Speir EH, Sasse J, Baird A. Elimination of smooth muscle cells in experimental restenosis: targeting of fibroblast growth factor receptors. Proc Natl Acad Sci USA 1992; 89:7159–7163.

86. Dichek DA, Anderson J, Kelly AB, Hanson SR, Harker LA. Enhanced in vivo antithrombotic effects of endothelial cells expressing recombinant plasminogen activators transduced with retroviral vectors. Circulation 1996; 93:301–309.

87. Folkman J, Shing Y. Angiogenesis. J Biol Chem 1992; 267:10931–10934.

88. Höckel M, Schlenger K, Doctrow S, Kissel T, Vaupel P. Therapeutic angiogenesis. Arch Surg 1993; 128:423–429.

89. Takeshita S, Weir L, Zheng LP, Chen D, Riessen R, Bauters C, Symes JF, Ferrara N, Isner JM. Therapeutic angiogenesis following arterial gene transfer of vascular endothelial growth factor in a rabbit model of hindlimb ischemia. Proc Natl Acad Sci USA 1995. In press.

90. Wolff JA, Lederberg J. An early history of gene transfer and therapy. Hum Genet Ther 1994; 5:469–480.

17

The Extracellular Matrix and Smooth Muscle Cell Migration

**Andrea S. Weintraub and
Mark B. Taubman**
*Mount Sinai School of Medicine
New York, New York*

Intimal hyperplasia, the characteristic lesion of atherosclerosis, is the result of a wound-healing response that occurs in injured blood vessels (1–3). The initial inflammatory phase is characterized by platelet aggregation, thrombus formation, and leukocyte infiltration (4–9). The influx of monocytes and neutrophils provides a rich source of growth factors, cytokines, and proteolytic enzymes within the injured vessel wall. The presence of these soluble factors, in turn, facilitates the eventual chemoattraction and recruitment of vascular smooth muscle cells (VSMCs), fibroblasts, and other cellular components involved in arterial remodeling, to the site of injury (10–15). During the granulation phase, VSMCs modulate from a quiescent contractile phenotype to a proliferative state characterized by rapid cell division, with concomitant migration from the tunica media into the intima (16–27). In the final phase, there is exuberant secretion of extracellular matrix (ECM) by neointimal VSMCs, which results in progressive expansion of the lesion (28–32). In human coronary arteries, this may ultimately lead to symptomatic vessel stenosis. Balloon angioplasty of occlusive coronary lesions is frequently followed by late intimal hyperplasia with symptomatic restenosis (33–35).

VSMC MIGRATION

VSMC migration is an obligatory component of vessel organization and remodeling during normal angiogenesis and under pathological conditions. VSMCs, the predominant cell type in the arterial wall, are affixed to ECM components and, in so doing, both provide structural support to the vessel and contribute to the maintenance of vascular tone. In order for VSMC relocation into the expanding neointima as response to injury, there must be a finely controlled balance between VSMC adhesion to and detachment from the surrounding ECM framework.

In Vitro Cell Migration Assays

Cell movement occurs as either a directed or a random event (3) and can be evaluated in monolayer (two-dimensional [2D]) or three-dimensional (3D) culture systems. Many two-dimensional assessments of VSMC chemotaxis have been performed using a modified Boyden chamber assay (36–38). VSMCs grown in monolayer on plastic culture dishes are trypsinized and resuspended to a set density (Fig. 1). Aliquots of cells are plated into the upper wells, and the migration factor of interest is added into the lower wells, with a polycarbonate filter of the appropriate pore size interposed between the two chambers. After the desired incubation period, cell migration is ascertained by removing the nonmigrated cells from the upper surface of the filter, and fixing, staining, and counting the cells on the lower surface of the filter. Analysis of the data can determine whether the VSMC response to a given agent is chemotaxic (directional migration) or chemokinetic (random movement) (39). Technical limitations of this assay include cell loss during staining, inadvertent selection of nonrepresentative areas for cell counting, and subjective counting errors (38). More important is that the modified Boyden chamber is a nonphysiological milieu for the study of cell migration. Therefore, data generated from this type of assay may have limited applicability to in vivo cellular events.

The circular outgrowth assay (Fig. 2) described by Clyman et al. (40) is another mechanism for studying VSMC chemotaxis in two dimensions. The 96-well upper chamber of a Minifold filtration apparatus is used to coat different ligands onto an uncharged polystyrene filter, with a perforated stainless steel screen interposed as a barrier between the substrate-coated filter and the upper chamber (40). VSMC suspensions are then placed in the wells of the upper chamber and allowed to attach to the substrate-coated sheet. The screen is then removed, leaving distinct circular areas of cells adherent to the membrane,

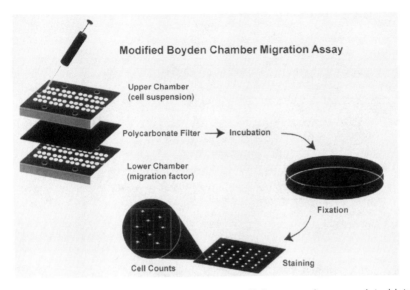

Figure 1 Modified Boyden chamber assay. Cell suspensions are plated into the upper chamber wells and the migration factor of interest is added into the lower chamber wells, with a polycarbonate filter interposed between the chambers. Cell migration is determined by fixation, staining, and counting cells on the lower surface of the filter.

and serum-supplemented medium is added to the upper chamber. The cells are permitted to migrate out on top of the substrate-coated sheet, and then fixed and stained after the desired interval. Migration rate is determined as the increase in the diameter of the circular area covered by the cells over time (40).

In "wound and scrape" cell migration experiments (Fig. 3), confluent cell monolayers are fractured with a razor blade and then removed from one side of the wound (41–42). The plates are then treated with the migration agent of interest and, after the designated time, cells are fixed in paraformaldehyde. The cells that have migrated into the scraped area can then be counted using an ocular grid opposing the original wound line (41).

Stainless-steel, silicon, or Teflon "fences" (Fig. 4) have been used to compartmentalize plastic tissue culture plates into inner and outer zones (43–45). Plates are coated with the migration substrate of interest, and cells are seeded at a preset density into the inner region and grown to confluence. The partition is removed, and the cells, now released from contact inhibition, are capable of chemotaxis towards the substrate. Migration is measured as the outgrowth distance of the cells from the fence (44). One obvious advantage of this

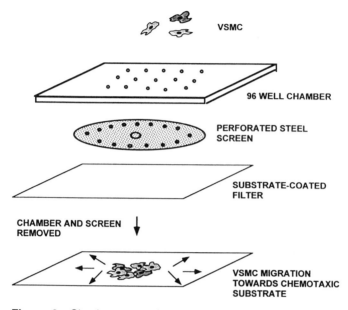

Figure 2 Circular outgrowth assay. Cell suspensions are plated into the upper chamber wells. A perforated stainless steel screen is interposed as a barrier between the upper chamber and a substrate-coated polystyrene filter. After the screen is removed, there are discrete circular areas of cells that can migrate along the substrate-coated filter.

technique over the "wound and scrape" assay is that upon removal of the template, cell migration begins at a preset uninjured origin.

Despite the usefulness of two-dimensional culture systems and plastic monolayer migration experiments, these assays cannot provide the full picture of VSMC mobility and adhesion, which occurs in vivo in three dimensions. 3D collagen gels have therefore been utilized to simulate better the in vivo environment of VSMCs (46–48). Artificial matrices differ from native connective tissue in the collagen composition, the presence of other extracellular matrix components, and in the 3D structural composition of fibrillar materials. The use of type I collagen gels has distinct advantages over two-dimensional models. Type I collagen is a major constituent of the extracellular matrix of VSMCs in vivo and VSMCs adhere rapidly to and invade into collagen gels in three dimensions, as they do in vivo. In addition, the gels more closely resemble the in vivo state by allowing greater cell-to-cell and cell-to-substrate communication during invasion. The use of gels also allows for studying changes in VSMC morphology which are apparent in three dimensions, but not in monolayer culture. The gels are prepared in standard plastic culture plates using a com-

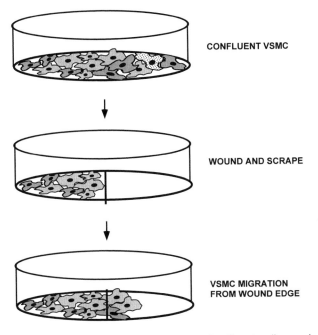

CONFLUENT VSMC

WOUND AND SCRAPE

VSMC MIGRATION
FROM WOUND EDGE

Figure 3 Wound and scrape assay. Confluent cell monolayers are fractured with a razor blade and scraped from one side of the wound. After incubation with the migration factor of interest, cells that have migrated from the wounded edge into the scraped area are counted.

mercially available solution of type I rat tail collagen mixed with M199 culture media, adjusted to pH 7.4, and polymerized at 37°C (47–48). VSMC suspensions can be seeded at known concentrations either onto the surface of the gels, or sandwiched between two gel layers (48–50). Nodules of VSMCs form after cells are seeded on the gel surface, whereas VSMCs grown between gel layers orient themselves in concentric circles at the gel periphery (51). Therefore, VSMC migration into the gel can be determined either by counting the number of cells on and below the gel surface using phase-contrast microscopy (48), or by measurement of gel contraction (51, 52)

Both endothelial cells (53–56) and VSMCs (57) grown on type I collagen gels exhibit substantially different behaviors than those cultured on plastic monolayers. Ziegler et al. (56) demonstrated a striking decrease in endothelial cell growth (determined by [³H]thymidine incorporation) on 3D collagen gels compared to cell growth on a plastic monolayer. We have shown that VSMC lines deficient in the extracellular matrix protein osteopontin display decreased adhesion and invasion of 3D collagen gels compared to control VSMCs,

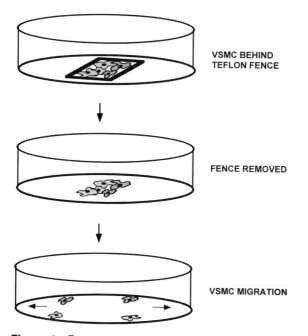

Figure 4 Fence migration assay. Monolayer culture plates are precoated with the migration factor of interest and compartmentalized into inner and outer zones by the addition of a Teflon fence. Cells are seeded into the inner zone and grown to confluence, after which the fence is removed. Migration is measured as outgrowth from the fence.

whereas these cell lines have morphologies, plating, and growth characteristics indistinguishable from normal VSMCs on plastic monolayers after standard cell culture conditions (57). These data underscore the usefulness and importance of a 3D culture system in revealing information about VSMC mobility and adhesion beyond what standard two-dimensional cultures can provide. However, even the most sophisticated in vitro model is only a "best guess," because cultured cells are still in an unnatural environment relative to their indigenous tissue and have been subject to multiple manipulations (58).

In Vivo Cell Migration Assays

Balloon injury of rat and rabbit carotid and aortic arteries has been widely used as an in vivo model for examining changes in the vessel wall associated with atherosclerosis (2, 59–60). This can be performed as a single or double arterial injury. In the double injury model initially described in rabbits (61–62), a second balloon injury is performed 2 weeks after the initial injury in the presence of a substantial neointima. The double injury model is associated with a rapid and exuberant production of ECM and an enhanced proliferative and migratory response (63). Since coronary balloon angioplasty in humans is performed on atherosclerotic vessels with abundant neointima, double injury experiments may provide a more representative model of human angioplasty.

Following arterial injury, it is necessary to differentiate between VSMC proliferation in the intima and VSMC migration into the intima. Measurement of VSMC proliferation can be determined using either [^{3}H]thymidine or bromodeoxyuridine labeling. To label all VSMCs undergoing DNA synthesis during the 24 h period preceding measurement, the experimental animal receives injections of thymidine-methyl-^{3}H at specified intervals prior to sacrifice (24) and the vessel of interest is harvested and fixed by immersion in the same solution. Tissue sections are dipped in emulsion and stored for several weeks before developing. The level of DNA synthesis is expressed as the percentage of cells exhibiting radiolabeling. The obvious drawback to this approach is the requisite use of significant amounts of radioactivity and the generation of radioactive waste material. As an alternative, bromodeoxyuridine (BrdU), a thymidine analogue, can be injected into the animal prior to sacrifice, and immunostaining with a monoclonal antibody directed against BrdU can be performed on tissue sections of the vessel (24, 64). The BrdU index (number of BrdU-VSMC nuclei/total number of VSMC nuclei) can then be determined.

To quantify VSMC migration in vivo, balloon-injured rat carotid arteries can be removed following fixation, opened longitudinally, and pinned out on Teflon cards (65–66). Dehydrated specimens are then coated with gold/palladium and examined by light or scanning electron microscopy. The total area of the specimen as well as the area occupied by intimal VSMCs can be determined by counting squares of an overlying ruled grid (66). VSMCs are not found in the intimal layer of normal rat carotid arteries (67, 68); therefore, all neointimal VSMCs have either migrated to the intima from the tunica media or are progeny of these medially derived VSMCs. In order to differentiate between the two, an assessment of neointimal proliferation using [^{3}H]thymidine labeling is performed in both the intima and the media at an earlier time point. If there is a paucity of DNA synthesis in the media, but a neointima develops, these neointimal VSMCs must have their origin as medial VSMCs that have migrated. Expansion of the neointima, then, is a result of both continued medial VSMC migration and neointimal VSMC proliferation.

MODULATION OF VSMC MIGRATION:
AGONISTS AND INHIBITORS

Many agents have been implicated in the regulation of VSMC migration, both in vitro and in vivo following balloon arterial injury of experimental animals.

Among these are platelet-derived growth factor (PDGF), basic fibroblast growth factor (bFGF), transforming growth factor β (TGFβ), α-thrombin, and heparin.

Among its many functions, PDGF has been implicated as an important migration element for VSMCs (12, 66, 69–71). Primate AB and BB isoforms of PDGF have been shown to induce VSMC migration in a modified Boyden chamber assay (70). In similar Boyden chamber assays, PDGF-AA inhibits the VSMC migration induced by PDGF-AB, PDGF-BB, fibronectin (72), and smooth muscle cell-derived migration factor (SDMF, 72). Stautosporine, a protein kinase C inhibitor, reverses PDGF-AA-inhibited VSMC migration in a modified Boyden chamber (70).

In vitro, VSMC migration is regulated by phenotypic state: proliferating VSMCs migrate well toward PDGF, while contractile cells have a significantly inhibited migratory response to PDGF, in a modified Boyden chamber (73). This inhibition is overcome by incubation with the calcium ionophore ionomycin. In light of this calcium responsiveness, Pauly et al. (73) explored possible differences in activation of the calcium-sensitive enzyme CaM kinase II. Using incorporation of radioactive phosphate during autophosphorylation as an assay of CaM kinase II activation, it was demonstrated that in quiescent cells PDGF failed to activate CaM kinase II (73).

In vivo, the administration of anti-PDGF antibodies has been recently shown to inhibit significantly neointimal VSMC accumulation in rat carotid arteries after balloon injury (12, 66). Antibody infusion before and after arterial deendothelialization decreased the thickness and cellular content of the neointima (12). Thrombocytopenic rats had decreased VSMC migration following balloon injury, presumably as a result of decreased endogenous levels of PDGF (66). Continuous administration of PDGF-BB to rats following arterial filament loop catheter injury caused a 15-fold increase in the size of the neointima; [^{3}H]thymidine labeling studies suggested that this PDGF-stimulated neointimal expansion was the result of VSMC migration and not proliferation (10).

bFGF has been previously implicated as a key agent in VSMC proliferation in vivo following balloon injury of rat carotid arteries (13) but was not chemotactic for VSMCs in a modified Boyden chamber (12, 69). It was recently suggested that bFGF is a significant mediator of VSMC migration in vivo (66). In an elegant series of experiments, Jackson et al. (66) injured rat carotid arteries, either with a balloon catheter or with a monofilament loop to create a gentle endothelial denudation. Balloon injury resulted in significantly greater VSMC accumulation in the neointima as determined by in vivo scanning electron microscopy. Furthermore, the administration of bFGF to experimental animals injured by gentle denudation resulted in a 15-fold increase in VSMC migration. Animals that received serial infusions of anti-bFGF antibody following balloon carotid injury had 80% fewer VSMCs migrate into the intima than control animals that received nonimmune IgG (66). The authors speculated that bFGF and PDGF may both be required for VSMC migration after injury, with bFGF activating the necessary proteolytic enzymes and PDGF supplying the chemotaxic signal (66).

TGFβ can either stimulate or inhibit VSMC proliferation in vitro; the effect appears dependent on the culture conditions (44, 74–75). Human venous VSMCs did not migrate in response to TGFβ over a wide range of doses in a stainless steel fence in vitro migration assay (76). TGFβ also inhibited the VSMC migration induced by PDGF and bFGF (76). The authors speculated that in in vivo following vascular injury, TGFβ may actually ameliorate the effects of PDGF and bFGF, and thus help arrest the development of intimal hyperplasia (76).

α-Thrombin induces both migration and proliferation of bovine and human aortic VSMCs in a modified Boyden chamber, and requires a functionally intact thrombin active site (38). Using metabolic labeling and immunoprecipitation, and flow cytometry, α-thrombin has also been shown to stimulate VSMC synthesis of the urokinase receptor. The induction of this receptor is a component of cell migration and invasion in tissue remodeling and tumor metastasis, presumably through enhancement of cell surface proteolytic activity (38, 77). Low-molecular-weight and standard heparin inhibit serum-induced baboon aortic VSMC migration in a Boyden chamber, but not PDGF-induced migration (78). In an in vivo baboon balloon injury model, there were no significant differences in intimal lesion size between experimental animals who received low-molecular-weight heparin or saline (78).

VSMC INTERACTIONS WITH THE ECM

Uninjured cultured human VSMCs show stable expression of both collagenous (types I, III, IV, V, and VI collagens) and noncollagenous gene products (79–80). The atherosclerotic lesion is composed of neointimal VSMCs surrounded by an expansive collagen, elastin, and proteoglycan-rich ECM (Table 1) (32). Interstitial collagens (types I and III) are the major plaque components, with type IV collagen forming the thick basement membrane layers surrounding the plaque VSMCs (81–83). Three important families of proteoglycans are present in the matrix of the vessel wall: heparan sulfates (HSPGs), which are positioned on cell membranes; chondroitin sulfates (CSPGs), located in the interstitial matrix; and dermatan sulfate proteoglycans (DSPGs), at the periphery of collagen fibrils (3). VSMCs synthesize primarily CSPGs and DSPGs (32, 84).

Early in the development of the atherosclerotic plaque, there is an increase in proteoglycan content, which later decreases with lesion progression. Com-

Table 1 Components of the Extracellular Matrix in the Vessel Wall

Matrix Component	Location in Normal Vessel	Location in Injured Vessel	References
Collagens			
Interstitial (types I and III)	Media	Media, plaque	79–83
Type IV	Media	Media, basement membrane around plaque	80–82
Proteoglycans			
Heparin sulfates	Cell membranes	Neointima (decreased in plaque)	3, 78, 85–90
Chondroitin sulfates	Interstitial matrix	Neointima (increased in plaque)	3, 32, 84–85, 87, 89, 91
Dermatan sulfates	Periphery of collagen fibrils, adventitia	Neointima (increased in plaque)	3, 32, 84–85, 92–98
Adhesive proteins			
Fibronectin	Soluble, matrix	Soluble, matrix	39–40, 99, 107–109
Vitronectin	Soluble, matrix	Soluble, matrix	39–40, 99, 107–109
Laminin	Matrix	Matrix	99, 109, 121
Counteradhesive proteins			
Tenascin	Matrix	Matrix	110, 112, 115–119, 129
Thrombospondin	Matrix	Matrix	110, 113–115, 120
Laminin	Matrix	Matrix	99, 109, 121
SPARC (osteonectin)	Matrix	Matrix	115

mon plaque findings are increases in DSPG and CSPG, with decreases in HSPG and hyaluronic acid (85). HSPG and heparin are associated with inhibition of VSMC migration (78, 86–87). Heparin also decreases collagen and elastin synthesis, and increases CSPG and HSPG synthesis in the neointima (87, 89). The decreased levels of HSPG in the mature plaque may therefore favor VSMC movement into the neointima (85).

Balloon injury of rat carotid arteries induces the accumulation of mRNA for the HSPGs perlecan, syndecan, and ryudocen, the CSPG versican, the DSPG biglycan, type I procollagen, and tropoelastin (87). Perlecan (87, 90), syndecan (87), ryudocen (87), and versican (87, 91) have all been localized, by immunocytological techniques, to the developing neointima. The induction of these matrix protein genes peaks at approximately 2 weeks after balloon injury (87), which is concomitant with the expansion of the neointimal lesion. Decorin, a DSPG present only in the adventitia of normal human aortas, and strikingly absent from the medial and intimal layers (92), may participate in the regulation of collagen fibrillogenesis (93). Decorin is induced by interleukin-1 (94) and downregulated by TGFβ (95–98). Using immunostaining techniques, plaque ECM stains strongly for biglycan and decorin, which colocalize with collagen types I and III, and interstitial collagen, respectively (92). In contrast, restenotic lesions are characterized by patchy biglycan and nearly absent decorin staining (92). The data of Riessen et al. (92) suggest that the key matrix features of the restenotic lesions are collagen, biglycan, and decorin, and that biglycan and decorin are not components of the basement membrane. The authors speculate that decorin may be a characteristic of nonproliferative mature connective tissue, whereas biglycan may be involved in the remodeling of proliferative matrix components (92).

Migrating VSMCs bind to adhesive ECM proteins to form complexes of cytoskeletal and membrane proteins (99). Dialogue between VSMC and the ECM components is mediated through cell surface receptors that can recognize specific matrix elements. Integrins are a class of heterodimeric, membrane-spanning glycoproteins (100–105) that harmonize events in the ECM and the cytoskeleton (106). A key function of integrins in the vasculature is purported to be the transduction of intercellular signals modulating cell–cell and cell–matrix adhesion, interactions that are essential for the maintenance of normal vessel architecture and for arterial remodeling (100, 106–107). Fibronectin and vitronectin are adhesive matrix glycoproteins synthesized by endothelial cells, VSMCs, monocyte/macrophages, and platelets (108), that can interact with VSMC αvβ3 integrin receptors, and induce VSMC migration in a modified Boyden chamber in a dose-dependent fashion comparable to that induced by PDGF-BB (107, 109). These glycoproteins are present as circulating plasma elements and are also present in the vessel wall. The elevated levels of fibronectin and vitronectin present in atherosclerotic lesions (39, 107, 108) may facilitate VSMC recruitment to the neointima.

Mobility of VSMC within the adhesive surface of the vessel wall requires the expression of specialized matrix proteins with counteradhesive properties (110) as well as matrix-degrading proteases (111) and new cell surface matrix receptors. This is necessary to facilitate the cell rounding and partial detachment from underlying basement membranes that are preludes to cell migration. Tenascin (110, 112), thrombospondin (110, 113, 114), and SPARC (115) are examples of counteradhesive matrix glycoproteins whose expression are linked to cell surface events that promote cell movement, regulate cell adhesion, and therefore modulate tissue repair. The counteradhesive effects of tenascin may be due to a direct steric blockade of fibronectin-integrin binding or, alternatively, to the activation of a receptor-mediated signaling pathway with consequent disruption of focal adhesions (110, 116–119). Similar cell–matrix disunion occurs via the heparin-binding motif of thrombospondin (110, 120). Laminin, a major structural component of basement membranes, has been shown to have both adhesive and antiadhesive domains, and in ductus arteriosus VSMC, interferes with VSMC adhesion to other matrix components and causes a decrease in the number of focal contacts to type I collagen (121).

The ECM, therefore, does not merely function as an inert structural support, but plays an important role in the migratory and proliferative responses of VSMC (64, 122). Studies of VSMC cultured in three-dimensional collagen gels have established that matrix composition profoundly influences cell shape, growth, and migration (46–48, 51, 123). For example, increases in the concentration of fibronectin, hyaluronan, and hyaluronan binding protein contribute to enhanced migration of ductus arteriosus VSMC through 3D gels (48). Treatment of ductal VSMCs with CSPG induces shedding of an elastin-binding protein essential for VSMC attachment to elastin-coated surfaces, a critical event in the detachment of VSMC from the anchoring matrix as a first step in migration (124). In turn, VSMCs are likely to play an important role in determining the composition of their surrounding extracellular environment by secreting matrix and matrix-degrading proteins, including collagen (89, 123, 125–127), elastin (128), tenascin (110, 129), clusterin (130), thrombospondin (110, 113, 114), fibrillin (131), collagenase (132), gelatinase (133), and other matrix metalloproteinases (134).

VASCULAR REMODELING: THE ROLE OF MATRIX METALLOPROTEINASES

In order for VSMCs to relocate from the media to the intima following vascular injury, they must digest their surrounding substrate (135). Matrix metalloproteinases (MMPs) are a family of metal-dependent enzymes, including interstitial collagenases, gelatinases, and stromelysins, that selectively digest components of the extracellular matrix (Table 2) (136). Interstitial collagenase (MMP-1) cleaves helical collagen fibrils that are resistant to hydrolysis by most other proteases (136), producing fragments susceptible to digestion by gelatinases (137). The 72 kD gelatinase (MMP-2) specifically digests non-fibrillar collagens typically found in basement membranes, and invasive behavior of transformed cells correlates with high levels of MMP-2 expression (138). The 92 kD gelatinase (MMP-9), in addition to nonfibrillar collagens, can also digest proteoglycans and elastin (137). The stromelysins (MMP-3) are the most versatile MMP that can degrade a variety of extracellular matrix components (including proteoglycans, fibronectin, laminin, and elastin), as well as activate the zymogen forms of other MMPs (139–141).

Normal VSMCs constitutively secrete MMP-2, as well as endogenous tissue inhibitors of MMP, known as TIMP-1 and 2 (137). The TIMPs inhibit both the proteolytic activation and the activity of all MMPs (136). Injured VSMCs, such as those found in fibrous margins of atherosclerotic plaques, have increased expression of MMP-1, MMP-3, and MMP-9 (136); macrophage foam cells within these lesions constitutively express MMP-1 and MMP-3 (142). Cytokine (IL-1 and TNF-α) stimulated VSMCs have enhanced expression of MMP-1, MMP-3, and MMP-9, and therefore, possess the capacity to resorb all of their surrounding ECM framework as a prelude to migration (136, 137). Heparin inhibits the induction of MMP-1, MMP-3, and MMP-9 mRNA and protein by phorbol esters; this effect is not observed for MMP-2 or TIMP-1 and is thought to be mediated by protein kinase C (143).

VSMC phenotype directly influences MMP expression. Expression of MMP-2 mRNA and protein levels is suppressed in contractile VSMCs, while levels of endogenous TIMP are enhanced; MMP activity in synthetic VSMCs is 30 times that seen in quiescent cells (134). This may account, in part, for the noninvasive, sedentary behavior of quiescent VSMCs in the uninjured artery, which predictably shifts to a more mobile phenotype following injury (134). Thus, VSMC secretion of matrix-degrading proteases permits VSMC migration through the ECM into the developing neointima where ongoing proliferation can occur.

In a rat model of carotid balloon injury, Clowes et al. (24) anticipated a 36% increase in VSMC mass by 12 weeks postinjury, from the level of proliferative activity these cells demonstrated. Since total VSMC number at 12 weeks was identical to the cell number at 2 weeks postinjury, it was assumed that the discrepant VSMC mass was a result of cell death (24). Pathologists have traditionally described two types of cell death: necrosis and apoptosis. In morphological terms, necrosis pertains to irreversible cell swelling with inevitable lysis resulting from a catastrophic environmental insult (144). Apoptosis involves cytoplasmic shrinkage, nuclear disintegration, cell surface blebbing, and

Table 2 Metalloproteinases in the Vessel Wall

Protease	Site of Action	References
Interstitial collagenase (MMP-1)	Helical collagen fibrils	136
72 kDa Gelatinase (MMP-2)	Basement membrane nonfibrillar collagen	137, 138
92 kDa Gelatinase (MMP-9)	Nonfibrillar collagen, proteoglycans, elastin	137
Stromelysins (MMP-3)	Proteoglycans, fibronectin, laminin, elastin, zymogen forms of other MMPs	139–141

eventual extrusion of cellular organelles as compact apoptotic bodies, without generating an inflammatory response (144). Apoptosis implies a form of programmed cell death, which suggests activation of a genetically encoded mechanism for cell suicide. For a detailed discussion of VSMC apoptosis in atherosclerosis, which is beyond the scope of this chapter, the reader is referred to other excellent reviews (145–151).

OSTEOPONTIN AND VSMC

Osteopontin (OPN) is an extracellular matrix glycoprotein that contains an RGD-binding motif capable of interaction with integrins (152). Originally isolated from bone, OPN has been localized in an array of tissues, including kidney, sensory epithelium of the embryonic ear, placenta, decidua, lung, and neural tissue, and is secreted by a variety of mammalian fibroblast and epithelial tumor cells (153–157). OPN has recently been identified in VSMCs using differential screening techniques employing two novel strategies (158–161).

OPN mRNA levels are increased following aortic balloon injury (159); in situ hybridization localizes OPN mRNA to the injured media and nascent neointima (159, 162–164). OPN promotes VSMC spreading and is chemotactic for VSMC in a modified Boyden chamber (165, 166). This migration is inhibited by a monoclonal antibody that recognizes the β3 integrin subunit (167). Most recently, Liaw et al. (167) have shown that in addition to αvβ3 integrins, both αvβ5 and αvβ1 are also OPN receptors, mediating cell adhesion and spreading, but not migration.

To establish further the role of OPN in migration, rat aortic VSMCs were infected with recombinant retroviruses containing OPN antisense cDNA constructs to create 10 cell lines stably underexpressing OPN (57). All control VSMC lines (infected with either the OPN-sense construct [n = 15] or the empty vector [n = 10]) displayed normal adhesion and invasion in a three dimensional (3D) collagen gel culture system, whereas eight of 10 clones infected with the OPN-antisense construct did not adhere to or invade these gels normally. Representative photomicrographs of the infected VSMC lines and uninfected control VSMCs in 3D collagen gels are shown in Figure 5. In monolayer culture, all VSMC lines studied had typical VSMC morphology and demonstrated the same rate of growth. In contrast, when plated onto 3D gels, uninfected VSMCs and VSMCs harboring the empty vector quickly attached to and invaded the gel to form latticelike networks throughout the matrix. Most sense clones invaded and formed cell connections indistinguishable from the controls. In contrast, the majority of antisense-infected clones failed to adhere to or invade the gels or to form networks, even at late time points. Exogenous OPN restored the ability of the antisense clones to adhere, spread, and invade the collagen gels, in a dose dependent fashion (Fig. 5). Adhesion and invasion

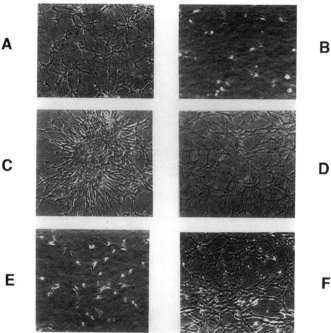

Figure 5 Light micrographs of VSMC clones in three-dimensional (3D) collagen gels. VSMC were plated at a density of 5×10^4 on the surface of 3D collagen gels. Representative photographs corresponding to planes within the gel matrix were taken 24 h after seeding. (A) VSMC infected with empty vector. (B) VSMC infected with antisense OPN mRNA. (C) VSMC infected with sense OPN mRNA. (D) Normal VSMC. (E) OPN antisense clone plated with 50 ng/ml exogenous OPN. (F) Restoration of VSMC adhesion and invasion with 400 ng/ml exogenous OPN.

of normal VSMCs on collagen gels were blocked in the presence of a neutralizing goat polyclonal antibody against rat VSMC-derived OPN (166) in a dose-dependent fashion.

RNA blot analysis demonstrated high levels of OPN antisense mRNA in the nonmigrating antisense clones; no antisense mRNA was detected in untransfected VSMCs or VSMCs transfected with retroviruses containing OPN in the sense orientation or with the empty vector (57). Antisense OPN clones likewise had lower OPN protein levels than the controls following agonist stimulation.

To determine the mechanism underlying the failure of antisense clones to invade collagen gels, VSMC adhesion and spreading were examined during the initial hours after seeding. On light microscopic examination, 30 min after seeding, apparently equal numbers of antisense cells and control VSMCs were present on the surface of the gel. By the end of the first hour, however, approximately half of the antisense cells were sloughed from the cell surface into the overlying media. Within 3 h, the control cells had begun to spread and invade the surface of the gel while the majority of the antisense cells had failed to remain adherent to the gel surface. The data suggest that while the antisense VSMCs initially adhered to the surface of the gel, they failed to spread or invade the matrix; thus, inhibition of OPN did not prevent the initial attachment of VSMCs to the gel. One hypothesis is that the primary defect in the antisense lines may be a failure to spread or invade into the gel substance, resulting in an inability to maintain attachment. In this regard, it has been proposed by Meredith et al. (168) that the failure of cells to properly attach to and migrate into matrix may lead to programmed cell death.

INTERVENTIONS TO INHIBIT VSMC MIGRATION

Elucidation of the mechanisms regulating VSMC migration may be pivotal in designing therapeutic strategies to attenuate the sequelae of this process: intimal hyperplasia with plaque formation and coronary restenosis. The ability to devise nontoxic synthetic mimics that inhibit VSMC migration in human VSMCs portends possible therapeutic options for ameliorating vessel restenosis following balloon angioplasty of human coronary arteries. A variety of synthetic analogues known to have inhibitory effects on vessel restenosis after balloon injury in experimental animal models have recently been evaluated specifically for their effects on VSMC migration.

Angiopeptin (AP), an analogue of the peptide hormone somatostatin, inhibits migration of rat aortic VSMCs in response to type I collagen in a Boyden chamber assay, by interfering with the requisite cell signaling mediated through a G_i-dependent pathway, ostensibly by blocking adenylyl cyclase and cyclic AMP accumulation (169). β-Cyclodextrin tetradecasulfate, an orally active synthetic heparin analogue, inhibits migration of human coronary VSMCs in both Boyden chamber and linear under agarose migration assays (170).

2-Bromomethyl-5-chlorobenzene sulfonylphthalimide (SCH 13929) is a low-molecular-weight, orally active PDGF antagonist that inhibits PDGF-stimulated VSMC migration in vitro in a modified Boyden chamber (171). In an in vivo rat carotid balloon injury model, oral administration of SCH 13929 decreased the size of the intimal lesions compared to controls (171). Given the data of Ferns et al. (12), which showed a significant decrease in neointimal size with the administration of anti-PDGF antibody following balloon injury, it is not surprising that a different mechanism of PDGF inhibition could ameliorate restenosis in an animal model.

Carvedilol is a competitive β- and α1-adrenergic antagonist that in high doses can also function as a calcium channel antagonist and an antioxidant (172–175). In a modified Boyden chamber assay, carvedilol blocked PDGF-induced VSMC chemotaxis in a concentration-dependent fashion (176). Pretreatment with carvedilol also decreased neointima formation following balloon angioplasty of rat carotid arteries (176).

Rapamycin, a macrolide antibiotic, has recently been shown to inhibit both human and rat VSMC proliferation by blocking cell cycle progression at the G1/S transition (177). This inhibition of cell proliferation is associated with decreases in cell cycle kinase activity and a reduction in the phosphorylation of retinoblastoma protein. The antiproliferative properties of rapamycin are mediated through binding to the cytosolic receptor, FKBP12 (177). FKPB12 is a highly conserved protein that is expressed in many cells and tissues, and catalyzes the *cis–trans* isomerization of peptidyl-prolyl amide bonds of peptides (178–181); both rapamycin and the immunosuppressive agent FK506 inhibit this rotamase activity. In addition to its effects on cell growth, rapamycin has a concentration-dependent inhibitory effect on PDGF-BB-induced rat and human aortic VSMC migration, as assayed in a modified Boyden chamber (182). In contrast, FK506 (1–500 ng/ml) has no effect on PDGF-induced VSMC migration. The effect of rapamycin is competitively inhibited by molar excesses of FK506, indicating that the inhibition of migration by rapamycin was mediated by the binding to FKBP12, since both rapamycin and FK506 share the same cytosolic receptor. Studies in animal models have demonstrated that rapamycin retards the development of accelerated arteriosclerosis after cardiac transplantation and restenosis following mechanical injury (183–184). Most notably, rapamycin markedly inhibits the development of intimal hyperplasia in response to balloon injury of pig coronary arteries (185). It remains to be determined to what extent the effects of rapamycin are due to inhibition of migration or proliferation. However, rapamycin may be an important therapeutic tool for inhibiting intimal hyperplasia.

CONCLUSIONS

Neointimal lesions are the end result of VSMC migration and ECM synthesis following arterial injury. This process of vessel remodeling involves a complex orchestration of cellular events including secretion of soluble mediators of VSMC migration, balanced synthesis/degradation of the ECM through the expression of adhesive and counteradhesive matrix proteins as well as matrix metalloproteinases, VSMC migration, and the programmed cell death of selected VSMC populations. Coordination of these intricate processes involves the interaction of numerous growth factors and cytokines. The interruption of this cascade of events at multiple sites may represent key therapeutic tools to block abnormal VSMC migration and thus ameliorate the development of intimal hyperplasia.

REFERENCES

1. Ross R. The pathogenesis of atherosclerosis—an update. N Engl J Med 1985; 314:488–500.
2. Ross R. The pathogenesis of atherosclerosis: a perspective for the 1990s. Nature 1993; 362:801–809.
3. Davies MG, Hagen PO. Pathobiology of intimal hyperplasia. Br J Surg 1994; 81:1254–1269.
4. Wilentz JR, Sanborn TA, Haudenschild CC, Valeri CR, Ryan TJ, Faxon DP. Platelet accumulation in experimental angioplasty: time course and relation to vascular injury. Circulation 1987; 75:636–642.
5. Marmur JD, Taubman MB, Fuster V. Pathophysiology of restenosis: the role of platelets and thrombin. J Vasc Med Biol 1993; 4:55–63.
6. Fingerle J, Johnson R, Clowes AW, Majesky MW, Reidy MA. Role of platelets in smooth muscle cell proliferation and migration after vascular injury in rat carotid artery. Proc Natl Acad Sci USA 1989; 86:8412–8416.
7. Tanaka H, Sukhova GK, Swanson SJ. Sustained activation of vascular cells and leukocytes in the rabbit aorta after balloon injury. Circulation 1993; 88:1788–1803.
8. Lucas JF III, Makhoul RG, Cole CW, Mikat E, McCann RL, Hagen PO. Mononuclear cells adhere to sites of vascular balloon catheter injury. Curr Surg 1986; 43:112–115.
9. Kaplan AV, Leung LL, Leung WH, Grant GW, McDougall IR, Fischell TA. Roles of thrombin and platelet membrane glycoprotein IIb/IIIa in platelet-subendothelial deposition after angioplasty in an ex vivo whole arterial model. Circulation 1991; 84:1270–1288.
10. Jawien A, Bowen-Pope DF, Lindner V, Schwartz SM, Clowes AW. Platelet-derived growth factor promotes smooth muscle cell migration and intimal thickening in a rat model of balloon angioplasty. J Clin Invest 1992; 89:507–511.
11. Taubman MB, Rollins BJ, Poon M, Marmur J, Green RS, Berk BC, BC, Nadal-Ginard B. JE mRNA accumulates rapidly in aortic injury and in PDGF-stimulated vascular smooth muscle cells. Circ Res 1992; 70:314–325.
12. Ferns GAA, Raines EW, Sprugel KH, Motani AS, Reidy MA, Ross R. Inhibition of neointimal smooth muscle accumulation after angioplasty by an antibody to PDGF. Science 1991; 253:1129–1132.
13. Lindner V, Lappi DA, Baird A, Majack RA, Reidy MA. Role of basic fibroblast growth factor in vascular lesion formation. Circ Res 1991; 68:106–113.
14. Jackson CL, Reidy MA. Basic fibroblast growth factor: its role in the control of smooth muscle cell migration. Am J Pathol 1993; 143:1024–1031.
15. Miano JM, Tota RR, Vlasic N, Danishefsky KJ, Stemerman MB. Early proto-oncogene expression in rat aortic smooth muscle cells following endothelial removal. Am J Pathol 1990; 137:761–765.

16. Spaet TH, Stemerman MB, Veith FJ, Lejnieks I. Intimal injury and regrowth in the rabbit aorta: medial smooth muscle cells as a source of neointima. Circ Res 1975; 36:58–70.

17. Webster WS, Bishop SP, Geer JC. Experimental aortic intimal thickening: morphology and source of intimal cells. Am J Pathol 1974; 76:245–264.

18. Hassler O. The origin of cells constituting arterial intimal thickening: an experimental autoradiographic study with the use of ^{3}H-thymidine. Lab Invest 1970; 22:286–293.

19. Chamley-Campbell J, Campbell GR, Ross R. The smooth muscle cell in culture. Physiol Rev 1979; 59:1–61.

20. Campbell GR, Campbell JH. The phenotypes of smooth muscle expressed in human atheroma. In: Lee KT, Onodera K, Tanakta K, eds. Atl II: Recent Progress in Atherosclerosis Research. New York: New York Academy of Sciences, 1990:143–158.

21. Chamley-Campbell JH, Campbell GR. What controls smooth-muscle phenotype? Atherosclerosis 1981; 40:347–357.

22. Chamley-Campbell J, Campbell GR, Ross R. Phenotype-dependent response of cultured aortic smooth muscle to serum mitogens. J Cell Biol 1981; 89:379–383.

23. Thyberg J, Hedin U, Sjolund M, Palmberg L, Bottger BA. Regulation of differentiated properties and proliferation of arterial smooth muscle cells. Arteriosclerosis 1990; 10:966–990.

24. Clowes AW, Reidy MA, Clowes MM. Kinetics of cellular proliferation after arterial injury, I: smooth muscle growth in the absence of endothelium. Lab Invest 1983; 49:327–333.

25. Clowes AW, Schwartz SM. Significance of quiescent smooth muscle migration in the injured rat carotid artery. Circ Res 1985; 56:139–145.

26. Grunwald J, Haudenschild CC. Intimal injury in vivo activates vascular smooth muscle cell migration and explant outgrowth in vitro. Arteriosclerosis 1984; 4:183–188.

27. Casscells W. Migration of smooth muscle and endothelial cells: critical events in restenosis. Circulation 1992; 86:723–729.

28. Nikkari ST, Wight TN, Clowes AW. Smooth muscle cell (SMC) expression of extracellular matrix (ECM) genes after arterial injury. FASEB J 1993; 7:A791.

29. Li Z, Alavi M, Wasty F, Ismail N, Moore S. Collagen biosynthesis by neointimal smooth muscle cells in vitro. FASEB J 1993; 7:A798.

30. Majack RA, Cook SC, Bornstein P. Platelet-derived growth factor and heparin-like glycosaminoglycans regulate thrombospondin synthesis and deposition in the matrix by smooth muscle cells. J Cell Biol 1985; 105:1059–1070.

31. Asunda V, Cowan K, Matzura D, Wagner W, Dreher KL. Characterization of extracellular matrix proteoglycan transcripts expressed by vascular smooth muscle cells. Eur J Cell Biol 1990; 52:98–104.

32. Wight TN. Cell biology of arterial proteoglycans. Arteriosclerosis 1989; 9:1–20.

33. Nobuyoshi M, Kimura T, Nosaka H. Restenosis after successful percutaneous transluminal coronary angioplasty: serial angiographic follow-up of 229 patients. J Am Coll Cardiol 1988; 12:616–622.

34. Leimgruber PP, Roubin GS, Hollman J. Restenosis after successful coronary angioplasty in patients with single vessel disease. Circulation 1986; 73:710–717.

35. Mata LA, Bosch X, David PR, Rapols HJ, Corcos T, Bourassa MG. Clinical and angiographic assessment to 6 months after double vessel percutaneous angioplasty. J Am Coll Cardiol 1985; 6:1239–1244.

36. Falk W, Goodwin RH, Leonard EJ. J Immunol Methods 1980; 33:239–247.

37. Capsoni F, Minonzio F, Ongari AM, Zanussi C. A new, simplified single-filter assay for in vitro evaluation of chemotaxis of ^{51}Cr-labeled polymorphonuclear leukocytes. J Immunol Methods 1989; 120:125–131.

38. Noda-Heiny H, Sobel BE. Vascular smooth muscle cell migration mediated by thrombin and urokinase receptor. Am J Physiol 1995; 268:C1195–C1201.

39. Naito M, Hayashi T, Funaki C, Kuzuya M, Asai K, Yamada K, Kuzuya F. Vitronectin-induced haptoaxis of vascular smooth muscle cells in vitro. Exp Cell Res 1991; 194:154–156.

40. Clyman RI, Mauray F, Kramer RH. β1 and β3 integrins have different roles in adhesion and migration of vascular smooth muscle cells on extracellular matrix. Exp Cell Res 1992; 200:272–284.

41. Irving JA, Lala PK. Functional role of cell surface integrins on human tropho-blast cell migration: regulation by TGF-β, IGF-II, and IGFBP-1. Exp Cell Res 1995; 217:419–427.

42. Pepper MS, Ferrera N, Orci L, Montesano R. Leukemia inhibitory factor (LIF) inhibits angiogenesis in vitro. J Cell Sci 1995; 108:73–83.

43. Pratt BM, Harris AS, Morrow JS, Madri JA. Mechanisms of cytoskeletal regulation: modulation of aortic endothelial cell spectrin by the extracellular matrix. Am J Pathol 1984; 117:349–354.

44. Merwin JR, Newman W, Beall LD, Tucker A, Madri J. Vascular cells respond differentially to transforming growth factors beta$_1$ and beta$_2$ in vitro. Am J Pathol 1991; 138:37–51.

45. Augustin-Voss HG, Pauli BU. Quantitative analysis of autocrine regulated, matrix-induced, and tumor cell-stimulated endothelial cell migration using a silicon template compartmentalization technique. Exp Cell Res 1992; 198:221–227.

46. Delvos V, Gajdusek C, Sage H, Harker LA, Schwartz SM. Interactions of vascular wall cells with collagen gels. Lab Invest 1982; 46:61–72.

47. Wren FE, Schor AM, Schor SL, Grant ME. Modulation of smooth muscle cell behavior by platelet-derived factors and the extracellular matrix. J Cell Physiol 1986; 127:297–302.

48. Boudreau N, Turley E, Rabinovitch M. Fibronectin, hyaluronan, and a hyaluronan binding protein contribute to increased ductus arteriosus smooth muscle cell migration. Dev Biol 1991; 143:235–247.

49. Karst W, Merker HJ. The differentiation behavior of MDCK cells grown on matrix components and collagen gels. Cell Differ Dev 1988; 22:211–234.

50. Lilja S, Merker HJ, Ghaida J. The influence of matrix components on the morphological differentiation of a proliferating hepatocyte line from liver of newborn mice. Histol Histopathol 1988; 3:249–262.

51. Akita M, Murata E, Kaneko K, Ghaida J, Merker HJ. Cell shape and arrange-

ment of cultured aortic smooth muscle cells grown on collagen gels. Cell Tissue Res 1993; 274:91–95.

52. Thie M, Schlumberger W, Semich R, Rauterberg J, Robenek H. Aortic smooth muscle cells in collagen lattice culture: effects on ultrastructure, proliferation, and collagen synthesis. Eur J Cell Biol 1991; 55:295–304.

53. Allen TD, Schor SL, Schor AM. An ultrastructural review of collagen gels: a model system for cell-matrix, cell-basement membrane, and cell-cell interactions. Scanning Electron Microsc 1984; 1984(I):375–390.

54. Gospodarowicz D, CR III. The extracellular matrix and the control of proliferation of vascular endothelial cells. J Clin Invest 1980; 65:1351–1364.

55. Macarak EJ, Howard PS. Adhesion of endothelial cells to extracellular matirx proteins. J Cell Physiol 1983; 116:76–83.

56. Ziegler T, Alexander RW, Nerem RM. An endothelial cell–smooth muscle cell co-culture model for use in the investigation of flow effects on vascular biology. Ann Biomed Eng 1995; 23:216–225.

57. Weintraub AS, Giachelli CM, Krauss RS, Almeida M, Taubman MB. Autocrine secretion of osteopontin by vascular smooth muscle cells regulates their adhesion to collagen gels. Am J Pathol 1996; 149:259–272.

58. Freshney RI. Culture of Animal Cells: a Manual of Basic Techniques, 2nd ed. New York: Alan R. Liss, 1987.

59. Clowes AW, Clowes MM, Fingerle J, Reidy MA. Regulation of smooth muscle cell growth in injured artery. J Cardiovasc Pharmacol 1989; 14(suppl 6):S12–S15.

60. Schwartz SM, Heimark RL, Majesky MW. Developmental mechanisms underlying pathology of arteries. Physiol Rev 1990; 70:1177–1209.

61. Groves HM, Kinlough-Rathbone RL, Richardson M, Jorgensen J, Moore S, Mustard JF. Thrombin generation and fibrin formation following injury to rabbit neointima. Studies of vessel wall reactivity and platelet survival. Lab Invest 1982; 46:605–612.

62. Richardson M, Kinlough-Rathbone RL, Groves HM, Jorgensen J, Mustard JF, Moore S. Ultrastructural changes in re-endothelialized and non-endothelialized rabbit aortic neo-intima following re-injury with a balloon catheter. Br J Exp Pathol 1984; 64:597–611.

63. Fyfe BS, Marmur JD, Rossikhina M, Mendlowitz M, Thiruvikraman SV, Gargiulo N, Guha A, Nemerson Y, Taubman MB. Rat aortic double injury is associated with fibrin deposition in the setting of enhanced tissue factor activation and early neointimal proliferation. In revision.

64. Strauss BH, Chisholm RJ, Keeley FW, Gotliev AI, Logan RA, Armstrong PW. Extracellular matrix remodeling after balloon angioplasty injury in a rabbit model of restenosis. Circ Res 1994; 75:650–658.

65. Jackson CL, Reidy MA. The role of plasminogen activation in smooth muscle cell migration after arterial injury. Ann NY Acad Sci 1992; 667:141–150.

66. Jackson CL, Raines EW, Ross R, Reidy MA. Role of endogenous platelet-derived growth factor in arterial smooth muscle cell migration after balloon catheter injury. Arterioscler Thromb 1993; 13:1218–1226.

67. Reidy MR, Schwartz SM. Endothelial regeneration, III: time course of intimal

changes after small defined injury to rat aortic endothelium. Lab Invest 1981; 44:301–308.

68. Tada T, Reidy MA. Endothelial regeneration, IX: arterial injury followed by rapid endothelial repair induces smooth-muscle-cell proliferation but not intimal thickening. Am J Pathol 1987; 129:429–433.

69. Grotendorst GR, Chang T, Seppa HEJ, Kleinman HK, Martin GR. Platelet-derived growth factor is a chemoattractant for vascular smooth muscle cells. J Cell Physiol 1982; 113:261–266.

70. Koyama N, Morisaki N, Saito Y, Yoshida S. Regulatory effects of platelet-derived growth factor-AA homodimer on migration of vascular smooth muscle cells. J Biol Chem 1992; 32:22806–22812.

71. Koster R, Windstetter U, Uberfuhr P, Baumann G, Nikol S, Hofling B. Enhanced migratory activity of vascular smooth muscle cells with high expression of platelet-derived growth factor A and B. Angiology 1995; 46:99–106.

72. Koyama N, Koshikawa T, Morisaki N, Saito Y, Yoshida S. Secretion of a potent new migration factor for smooth muscle cells (SMC) by cultured SMC. Atherosclerosis 1991; 86:219–226.

73. Pauly RR, Bilato C, Sollott SJ, Monticone R, Kelly PT, Lakatta EG, Crow MT. Role of calcium/calmodulin-dependent protein kinase II in the regulation of vascular smooth muscle cell migration. Circulation 1995; 91:1107–1115.

74. Majack RA. Beta-type transforming growth factor specifies organizational behavior in vascular smooth muscle cell cultures. J Cell Biol 1987; 105:465–471.

75. Battegay EJ, Raines EW, Seifert RA, Bowen-Pope DF, Ross R. TGF-beta induces bimodal proliferation of connective tissue cells via complex control of an autocrine PDGF loop. Cell 1990; 63:515–524.

76. Mii S, Ware JA, Kent KC. Transforming growth factor-beta inhibits human vascular smooth muscle cell growth and migration. Surgery 1993; 114:464–470.

77. Blasi F. Fibrinolytic tests and extravascular proteolysis. Urokinase and urokinase receptor: a paracrine/autocrine system regulating cell migration and invasiveness. Fibrinolysis 1993; 7:17–23.

78. Geary RL, Koyama N, Wang TW, Vergel S, Clowes AW. Failure of heparin to inhibit intimal hyperplasia in injured balloon arteries. Circ 1995; 91:2972–2981.

79. Tan EML, Glassberg E, Olsen DR, Noveral JP, Unger GA, Peltonen J, Chu ML, Levine E, Sollberg S. Extracellular matrix gene expression by human endothelial and smooth muscle cells. Matrix 1991; 11:380–387.

80. Sharifi BG, LaFleur DW, Pirola CJ, Forrester JS, Fagin JA. Angiotensin II regulates tenascin gene expression in vascular smooth muscle cells. J Biol Chem 1992; 267:23910–23915.

81. McCullagh KG, Duance VC, Bishop KA. The distribution of collagen types I, III, and V (AB) in normal and atherosclerotic human aorta. J Pathol 1980; 130:45–55.

82. Katsuda S, Okada Y, Minamoto T, Oda Y, Matsui Y, Nakanishi I. Collagens in human atherosclerosis: immunohistochemical analysis using collagen type-specific antibodies. Arterioscler Thromb 1992; 12:494–502.

83. Murata K, Motoyama T, Kotake C. Collagen types in various layers of the hu-

man aorta and their changes with the atherosclerotic process. Atherosclerosis 1986; 60:251–262.

84. Jarvelainen HT, Kinsella MG, Wight TN, Sandell LJ. Differential expression of small chondroitin/dermatan sulfate proteoglycans, PG-I/biglycan and PG-II/decorin, by vascular smooth muscle cells and endothelial cells in culture. J Biol Chem 1991; 266:17640.

85. Wasty F, Alavi MZ, Moore S. Distribution of glycosaminoglycans in the intima of human aortas: changes in atherosclerosis and diabetes mellitus. Diabetologia 1993; 36:316–322.

86. Majack RA, Clowes AW. Inhibition of vascular smooth muscle cell migration by heparin-like glycosaminoglycans. J Cell Physiol 1984; 118:253–256.

87. Nikkari ST, Jarvelainen HT, Wight TN, Ferguson M, Clowes AW. Smooth muscle cell expression of extracellular matrix genes after arterial injury. Am J Pathol 1994; 144:1348–1356.

88. Clowes AW, Clowes MM. Kinetics of cellular proliferation after arterial injury. II. Inhibition of smooth muscle growth by heparin. Lab Invest 1985; 52:611–616.

89. Snow AD, Bolender RP, Wight TN, Clowes AW. Heparin modulates the composition of the extracellular matrix domain surrounding arterial smooth muscle cells. Am J Pathol 1990; 137:313–330.

90. Clowes AW, Clowes MM, Gown AM, Wight TN. Localization of proteoheparan sulfate in rat aorta. Histochemistry 1984; 80:379–384.

91. Lark MW, Yeo TK, Mar H, Lara S, Hellstrom KE, Wight TN. Arterial chondroitin sulfate proteoglycan: localization with a monoclonal antibody. J Histochem Cytochem 1988; 36:1211–1221.

92. Riessen R, Isner JM, Blessing E, Loushin C, Nikol S, Wight TN. Regional differences in the distribution of the proteoglycans biglycan and decorin in the extracellular matrix of atherosclerotic and restenotic human coronary arteries. Am J Pathol 1994; 144:962–974.

93. Vogel KG, Paulsson M, Heinegard D. Specific inhibition of type I and type II collagen fibrillogenesis by the small proteoglycan of tendon. Biochem J 1984; 223:587–595.

94. Edwards IJ, Xu H, Wright MJ, Wagner WD. Interleukin-1 upregulates decorin production by arterial smooth muscle cells. Arterioscler Thromb 1994; 14:1032–1039.

95. Kahari VM, Larjava H, Vitto J. Differential regulation of extracellular matrix proteoglycan expression. J Biol Chem 1991; 266:10608–10615.

96. Vogel KG, Hernandez DJ. The effects of transforming growth factor-β and serum on proteoglycan synthesis by tendon fibrocartilage. Eur J Cell Biol 1992; 59:304–313.

97. Schonherr E, Jarvalainen HT, Kinsella MG, Sandell LJ, Wight TN. Platelet-derived growth factor and transforming growth factor-β1 differentially affect the synthesis of biglycan and decorin by monkey arterial smooth muscle cells. Arterioscler Thromb 1993; 13:1026–1036.

98. Border WA and Ruoslahti E. Transforming growth factor-β in disease: the dark side of tissue repair. J Clin Invest 1992; 90:1–7.

99. Burridge K, Fath K, Kelly T, Nuckolls G, Turner C. Focal adhesions: transmembrane junctions between the extracellular matrix and the cytoskeleton. Annu Rev Cell Biol 1988; 4:487–452.

100. Juliano RL and Haskill S. Signal transduction from extracellular matrix. J Cell Biol 1993; 120:577–585.

101. Dustin ML and Springer TA. Role of lymphocyte adhesion receptors in transient cell interactions and cell locomotion. Annu Rev Immunol 1991; 60:155–190.

102. Hemler ME. VLA proteins in the integrin family: structures, functions, and their role in leukocytes. Annu Rev Immunol 1990; 8:365–400.

103. McDonald JA. Receptors for extracellular matrix components. Am J Physiol 1989; 257:L331–337.

104. Ruoslahti E. Integrins. J Clin Invest 1991; 87:1–5.

105. Hynes RO. Integrins: versatility, modulation, and signaling in cell adhesion. Cell 1992; 69:11–25.

106. Luscinskas FW, Lawler J. Integrins as dynamic regulators of vascular function. FASEB J 1994; 8:929–938.

107. Brown SL, Lundgren CH, Nordt T, Fujii S. Stimulation of migration of human aortic smooth muscle cells by vitronectin: implications for atherosclerosis. Cardiovasc Res 1994; 28:1815–1820.

108. Raines EW, Ross R. Smooth muscle cells and the pathogenesis of the lesions of atherosclerosis. Br Heart J 1993; 69:S30–S37.

109. Clyman RI, McDonald KA, Kramer RH. Integrin receptors on aortic smooth muscle cells mediate adhesion to fibronectin, laminin, and collagen. Circ Res 1990; 67:175–186.

110. Majesky MW. Neointima formation after acute vascular injury: role of counteradhesive extracellular matrix proteins. Texas Heart Inst J 1994; 21:78–85.

111. Clowes AW, Clowes MM, Au YP, Reidy MA, Belin D. Smooth muscle cells express urokinase during mitogenesis and tissue-type plasminogen activator during migration in injured rat carotid artery. Circ Res 1990; 67:61–67.

112. Hedin U, Holm J, Hansson GK. Induction of tenascin in rat arterial injury: relationship to altered smooth muscle cell phenotype. Am J Pathol 1991; 139:649–656.

113. Raugi GJ, Mullen JS, Bark DH, Okada T, Mayberg MR. Thrombospondin deposition in rat carotid artery injury. Am J Pathol 1990; 137:179–185.

114. RayChaudhury A, Frazier WA, D'Amore PA. Comparison of normal and tumorigenic endothelial cells: differences in thrombospondin production and responses to transforming growth factor-beta. J Cell Sci 1994; 107:39–46.

115. Sage EH, Bornstein P. Extracellular matrix proteins that modulate cell-matrix interactions: SPARC, tenascin, and thrombospondin. J Biol Chem 1991; 266:14831–14834.

116. Prieto AL, Anderson-Fisone C, Crossin KL. Characterization of multiple adhesion and counteradhesive domains in the extracellular matrix protein cytotactin. J Cell Biol 1992; 119:663–678.

117. Aukhil I, Joshi P, Yan Y, Erickson HP. Cell- and heparin-binding domains of

the hexabrachion arm identified by tenascin expression proteins. J Biol Chem 1993; 268:2542–2553.

118.   Murphy-Ullrich JE, Lightner VA, Aukhil I, Yan YZ. Focal adhesion integrity is downregulated by the alternatively spliced domain of human tenascin. J Cell Biol 1991; 115:1127–1136.

119.   Lightner VA, Erickson HP. Binding of hexabrachion (tenascin) to the extracellular matrix and substratum and its effect on cell adhesion. J Cell Sci 1990; 95:263–277.

120.   Murphy-Ullrich JE, Hook M. Thrombospondin modulates focal adhesions in endothelial cells. J Cell Biol 1989; 109:1309–1319.

121.   Clyman RI, Tannenbaum J, Chen YQ, Cooper D, Yurchenco PD, Kramer RH, Waleh NS. Ductus arteriosus smooth muscle cell migration on collagen: dependence on laminin and its receptors. J Cell Sci 1994; 107:1007–1018.

122.   Schor SL. Cell proliferation and migration on collagen substrata in vitro. J Cell Sci 1980; 41:159–175.

123.   Madri JA, Bell L, Marx M, Merwin JR, Basson C, Printz C. Effects of soluble factors and extracellular matrix components on vascular cell behavior in vitro and in vivo: models of de-endothelialization and repair. J Cell Biochem 1991; 45:123–130.

124.   Hinek A, Boyle J, Rabinovitch M. Vascular smooth muscle cell detachment from elastin and migration through elastic laminae is promoted by chondroitin sulfate-induced "shedding" of the 67-kDa cell surface elastin binding protein. Exp Cell Res 1992; 203:344–353.

125.   Majesky MW, Lindner V, Twardzik DR, Schwartz SM, Reidy MA. Production of transforming growth factor beta-1 during repair of arterial injury. J Clin Invest 1991; 88:904–910.

126.   Madri JA, Marx M. Matrix composition, organization, and soluble factors: modulators of microvascular cell differentiation in vitro. Kidney Int 1992; 41:560–565.

127.   Thie M, Harrach B, Schonherr E, Kresse H, Robenek H, Rauterberg J. Responsiveness of aortic smooth cells to soluble growth mediators is influenced by cell-matrix contact. Arteioscler Thromb 1993; 13:994–1004.

128.   Hinek A, Rabinovitch M. 67-kD elastin-binding protein is a protective "companion" of extracellular insoluble elastin and intracellular tropoelastin. J Cell Biol 1994; 126:563–574.

129.   Hedin U, Holm J, Hansson GK. Induction of tenascin in rat arterial injury: relationship to altered smooth muscle cell phenotype. Am J Pathol 1991; 139:649–656.

130.   Thomas-Salgar S, Millis AJT. Clusterin expression in differentiating smooth muscle cells. J Biol Chem 1994; 269:17879–17885.

131.   Ramirez R, Pereira L, Zhang H, Lee B. The fibrillin-Marfan syndrome connection. Bio Essays 1993; 15:1–6.

132.   Yanagi, Sasaguri HY, Sugama K, Morimatsu M, Nagase H. Production of tissue collagenase (matrix metalloproteinase I) by human aortic smooth muscle cells in response to platelet-derived growth factor. Atherosclerosis 1991; 91:207–216.

133. Galis ZS, Muszynski M, Sukhova GK, Simon-Morrisey E, Unemori EN, Lark MW, Amento E, Libby P. Cytokine-stimulated human vascular smooth muscle cells synthesize a complement of enzymes required for extracellular matrix digestion. Circ Res 1994; 75:181–189.

134. Pauly RR, Passaniti A, Bilato C, Monticone R, Cheng L, Papadopoulos N, Gluzband YA, Smith L, Weinstein C, Lakatta EG, Crow MT. Migration of cultured vascular smooth muscle cells through a basement membrane barrier requires type IV collagenase activity and is inhibited by cellular differentiation. Circ Res 1994; 75:41–54.

135. Sperti G, Van Leeuwen RTJ, Quax PHA, Maseri A, Kluft C. Cultured rat aortic vascular smooth muscle cells digest naturally produced extracellular matrix: involvement of plasminogen-dependent and plasminogen-independent pathways. Circ Res 1992; 71:385–392.

136. Galis ZS, Muszynski M, Sukhova GK, Simon-Morrisey E, Libby P. Enhanced expression of vascular matrix metalloproteinases induced in vitro by cytokines and in regions of human atherosclerotic lesions. Ann NY Acad Sci 1995; 748:501–507.

137. Galis ZS, Sukhova GK, Lark MW, Libby P. Increased expression of matrix metalloproteinases and matrix degrading activity in vulnerable regions of human atherosclerotic plaques. J Clin Invest 1994; 94:2493–2503.

138. Liotta LA, Tryggvason K, Garbisa S, Hart I, Foltz CM, Shafie S. Metastatic potential correlates with enzymatic degradation of basement membrane collagen. Nature 1980; 284:67–68.

139. Chin JR, Murphy G, Werb Z. Stromelysin, a connective tissue degrading metalloendopeptidase secreted by stimulated rabbit synovial fibroblasts in parallel with collagenase: biosynthesis, isolation, characterization, and substrates. J Biol Chem 1985; 260:12367–12376.

140. Murphy G, Reynolds JJ, Werb Z. Biosynthesis of tissue inhibitor of metalloproteinases by human fibroblasts in culture: stimulation by 12-0-tetradecanoylphorbol 13-acetate and interleukin-1 in parallel with collagenase. J Biol Chem 260:3079–3083.

141. Ogata Y, Enghild JJ, Nagase H. Matix metalloproteinase 3 (stromelysin) activates the precursor for the human matrix metalloproteinase 9. J Biol Chem 1992; 267:3581–3584.

142. Galis ZS, Sukhova GK, Kranzhofer R, Clark S, Libby P. Macrophage foam cells from experimental atheroma constitutively produce matrix-degrading proteinases. Proc Natl Acad Sci 1995; 92:402–406.

143. Kenagy RD, Nikkari ST, Welgus HG, Clowes AW. Heparin inhibits the induction of three matrix metalloproteinases (stromelysin, 92-kD gelatinase, and collagenase). J Clin Invest 1994; 93:1987–1993.

144. Wyllie AH, Kerr JFR, Currie AR. Cell death: the significance of apoptosis. Int Rev Cytol 1980; 68:251–306.

145. Bennett MR, Evans GI, Schwartz SM. Apoptosis of human vascular smooth muscle cells derived from normal vessels and coronary atherosclerotic plaques. J Clin Invest 1995; 95:2266–2274.

146. Geng YJ and Libby P. Evidence for apoptosis in advanced human atheroma. Am J Pathol 1995; 147:251–266.

147. Han DKM, Haudenschild CC, Hong MK, Tinkle BT, Leon MB, Liau G. Evidence for apoptosis in human atherogenesis and in a rat vascular injury model. Am J Pathol 1995; 147:267–277.

148. Isner JM, Kearney M, Bortman S, Passieri J. Apoptosis in human atherosclerosis and restenosis. Circ 1995; 91:2703–2711.

149. Bochaton-Piallet ML, Gabbiani F, Redard M, Desmouliere A, Gabbiani G. Apoptosis participates in cellularity regulation during rat aortic intimal thickening. Am J Pathol 1995; 146:1059–1064.

150. Bennett MR, Evans GI, Schwartz SM. Apoptosis of rat vascular smooth muscle cells is regulated by p53-dependent and -independent pathways. Circ Res 1995; 77:266–273.

151. Schwartz SM, Bennett MR. Death by any other name. Am J Pathol 1995; 147:229–234.

152. Oldberg A, Franzen A, Heinegard A A. Cloning and sequence analysis of rat bone sialoprotein (osteopontin) cDNA reveals an ARG-GLY-ASP binding sequence. Proc Natl Acad Sci USA 1986; 83:8819–8823.

153. Nomura S, Wills AJ, Edwards DR, Heath JK, and Hogan BLM. Developmental expression of 2AR (osteopontin) and SPARC (osteonectin) RNA as revealed by in situ hybridization. J Cell Biol 1988; 106:441–450.

154. Denhardt DT and Guo X. Osteopontin: a protein with diverse functions. FASEB J 1993; 7:1475–1482.

155. Senger DR, Perruzzi CA, Gracey CF, Papadopoulos A, Tenen DG. Secreted phosphoproteins associated with neoplastic transformation: close homology with plasma proteins cleaved during blood coagulation. Cancer Res 1988; 48:5770–5774.

156. Senger DR, Perruzzi CA, Papadopoulos A. Elevated expression of secreted phosphoprotein I (osteopontin, 2AR) as a consequence of neoplastic transformation. Anticancer Res 1989; 9:1291–1300.

157. Gardner HAR, Berse B, Senger DR. Specific reduction in osteopontin synthesis by antisense RNA inhibits the tumorgenicity of transformed Rat1 fibroblasts. Oncogene 1994; 9:2321–2326.

158. Giachelli CM, Bae N, Lombardi D, Majesky M, Schwartz S. Molecular cloning and characterization of 2B7, a rat mRNA which distinguishes smooth muscle cell phenotypes in vitro and is identical to osteopontin (secreted phosphoprotein I, 2AR). Biochem Biophys Res Comm 1991; 177:867–873.

159. Giachelli CM, Bae N, Almeida M, Denhardt DT, Alpers CE, Schwartz SM. Osteopontin is elevated during neointima formation in rat arteries and is a novel component of human atherosclerotic plaques. J Clin Invest 1993; 92:1686–1696.

160. Wax SD, Rosenfield CL, Taubman MB. Identification of a novel PDGF-responsive gene in vascular smooth muscle cells. J Biol Chem 1994; 269:13041–13047.

161. Green RS, Lieb ME, Weintraub AS, Gacheru SN, Rosenfield CL, Shah S, Kagan HM, Taubman MB. Identification of lysyl oxidase and other platelet-derived growth factor-inducible genes in vascular smooth muscle cells by differential screening. Lab Invest 1995; 73:476–482.

162. Fitzpatrick LA, Severson A, Edwards WD, Ingram RT. Diffuse calcification in human coronary arteries: association of osteopontin with atherosclerosis. J Clin Invest 1994; 94:1597–1604.

163. O'Brien ER, Garvin MR, Stewart DK, Hinohara T, Simpson JB, Schwartz SM, Giachelli CM. Osteopontin is synthesized by macrophages, smooth muscle, and endothelial cells in primary and restenotic human coronary atherosclerotic plaques. Arterioscler Thromb 1994; 14:1648–1656.

164. Ikeda T, Shirasawa T, Esaki Y, Hirokawa K. Osteopontin mRNA is expressed by smooth muscle-derived foam cells in human atherosclerotic lesions of the aorta. J Clin Invest 1993; 92:2814–2820.

165. Liaw L, Almeida M, Hart CE, Schwartz SM, Giachelli CM. Osteopontin promotes vascular cell adhesion and spreading and its chemotactic for smooth muscle cells in vitro. Circulation Res 1994; 74:214–224.

166. Yue TL, McKenna PJ, Ohlstein EH, Farach-Carson MC, Butler WT, Johanson K, McDevitt P, Feuerstein GZ, Stadel JM. Osteopontin-stimulated vascular smooth muscle cell migration is mediated by b3 integrin. Exp Cell Res 1994; 214:459–464.

167. Liaw L, Skinner MP, Raines EW, Ross R, Cheresh DA, Schwartz SM, Giachelli CM. The adhesive and migratory effects of osteopontin are mediated via distinct cell surface integrins. J Clin Invest 1995; 95:713–724.

168. Meredith JE, Fazeli B, Schwartz MA. The extracellular matrix as a cell survival factor. Mol Biol Cell 1993; 4:953–961.

169. Mooradian DL, Feranades B, Diglio CA, Lester BR. Angiopeptin (BIM23014C) inhibits vascular smooth cell migration in vitro through a G-protein-mediated pathway and is associated with inhibition of adenylyl cyclase and cyclic AMP accumulation. J Cardiovasc Pharmacol 1995; 25:611–618.

170. Okada SS, Kuo A, Muttreja MJ, Hozakowska E, Weisz PB, Barnathan ES. Inhibition of human vascular smooth muscle cell migration and proliferation by β-cyclodextrin tetradecasulfate. J Pharmacol Exp Ther 1995; 273:948–954.

171. Mullins DE, Hamud F, Reim R, Davis HR. Inhibition of PDGF-stimulated biological activity in vitro and of intimal lesion formation in vivo by 2-bromomethyl-5-chlorobenzene sulfonylphthalimide. Arterioscler Thromb 1994; 14:1047–1055.

172. Willette RN, Sauermelch CF, Ruffolo RR Jr. Local cutaneous hemodynamic effects of carvedilol and labetalol in the anesthetized rat. Eur J Pharmacol 1990; 176:237–240.

173. Nichols AJ, Gellai M, Ruffolo RR Jr. Studies on the mechanism of arterial vasodilation produced by the novel antihypertensive agent carvedilol. Fundam Clin Pharmacol 1991; 5:25–38.

174. Ruffolo RR Jr, Gellai M, Hieble JP, Willette RN, Nichols AJ. The pharmacokinetics of carvedilol. Eur J Clin Pharmacol 1990; 38:S82–S88.

175. Yue TL, Cheng H, Lysko PG, McKenna PJ, Feuerstein R, Gu J, Lysko KA, Davis LL, Feuerstein G. J Pharmacol Exp Ther 1992; 263:92–98.

176. Ohlstein EH, Douglas SA, Sung CP, Yue TL, Louden C, Arleth A, Poste G, Ruffolo RR Jr, Feuerstein GZ. Cardvedilol, a cardiovascular drug, prevents vascular smooth muscle cell proliferation, migration, and neointimal formation following vascular injury. Proc Natl Acad Sci USA 1993; 90:6189–6193.

177. Marx SO, Jayaraman T, Go LO, Marks AR. Rapamycin-FKBP inhibits cell cycle regulators of proliferation in vascular smooth muscle cells. Circ Res 1995; 76:412–417.

178. Nelson PA, Lippke JA, Murcko MA, Rosborough SL, Peattie DA. cDNA encoding murine FK506-binding protein (FKBP): nucleotide and deduced amino acid sequences. Gene 1991; 109:255–258.

179. Sewell TJ, Lam E, Martin MM, Leszyk J, Weidner J, Calaycay J, Griffin P, Williams H, Hung S, Cryan J, Sigal NH, Wiederrecht GJ. Inhibition of calcineurin by a novel GK-506-binding protein. J Biol Chem 1994; 269:21094–21102.

180. Standaert RF, Galat A, Verdine G, Schreiber SL. Molecular cloning and overexpression of the human FK506-binding protein FKBP. Nature 1990; 346:671–674.

181. Hendrickson BA, Zhang W, Craig RJ, Jin YJ, Bierer BE, Burakoff S, DiLella AG. Structural organization of the genes encoding human and murine FK506-binding protein (FKBP) 13 and comparison to FKBP1. Gene 1993; 134:271–275.

182. Poon M, Marx SO, Taubman MB, Marks AW. Rapamycin inhibits vascular smooth muscle cell migration. Circulation 1995; 92:1–298.

183. Wu G, Cramer D, Chapman F, Cajulis E, Wang H, Starzl T, Makowka L, L. FK 506 inhibits the development of transplant arteriosclerosis. Transplant Proc 1991; 23:3272–3274.

184. Gregory C, Huie P, Billingham M, Morris R. Rapamycin inhibits arterial intimal thickening caused by both alloimmune and mechanical injury. Transplantation 1993; 55:1409–1418.

185. Gallo R, Padurean A, Chesebro JH, Fallon JT, Fuster V, Marks AR, Badimon JJ. Rapamycin (Sirolimus) reduces luminal narrowing after balloon angioplasty in porcine coronary arteries. J Am Coll Cardiol 1996; 27(suppl A):(abstr) 939–948.

18

Microfibril Pathology and Cardiovascular Manifestations in Marfan Syndrome

Lygia V. Pereira
Universidade de São Paulo
São Paulo, Brazil

Hui Zhang
Long Island College Hospital
Brooklyn, New York

Francesco Ramirez
Mount Sinai School of Medicine
New York, New York

Heritable disorders of the connective tissue have been usually classified as "... a clinically heterogeneous group of conditions characterized by weakness of the body supporting structures resulting from metabolic dysfunction of extracellular matrix components" (1). Recent findings have expanded this definition to include gene products that play broad regulatory roles in connective tissue morphogenesis. However, most of the information regarding connective tissue pathology is still being gathered from the study of extracellular matrix (ECM) components, mainly the collagens. Indeed, collagenopathies have been instrumental in defining the general criteria of how dominant negative mutations exert their effects on extracellular aggregates. They have also provided some insight into the pleiotropic consequences of the defects and possible relationship with more common disorders. The lessons derived from the study of the collagenopathies are now being transferred to conditions caused by mutations in matrix components responsible for the formation of morphologically, chemically, and functionally distinct supramolecular aggregates.

Among the macromolecules on which investigative effort has recently focused is fibrillin: one of the major building blocks of elastic fibers. The renewed attention was spurred by the discovery that fibrillin mutations are the cause of Marfan syndrome (MFS). Recognized as a clinical entity since the last century, MFS is often used as a paradigm of more common cardiovascular conditions, in particular of dissecting aortic aneurysm. It follows that an in depth knowledge of MFS is expected to advance our understanding of cardiovascular pathophysiology. Aside from improving diagnosis of the disorder, the delineation of the genetic lesion in MFS has already stimulated a new wave of research interest in elastogenesis, and the role of the ECM in cardiovascular function.

ELASTIC FIBERS AND MICROFIBRILS

The physiological requirements of tissues such as lung, skin, and blood vessels require the ability to stretch and recoil. This elastic property is provided by elastic fibers present in the ECM of these tissues. Elastic fibers consist of two morphologically distinct components: a core of cross-linked elastin and a microfibrillar sheet around it (2–4).

The formation of mature elastic fibers takes place during embryogenesis, and continues up to early childhood. Thereafter, it can be only stimulated locally by injury. During elastogenesis, microfibrils are first deposited into the ECM where they form a scaffold that apparently directs the subsequent deposition of elastin (3). This stepwise process is best exemplified in the tunica media of the aorta, where rings of microfibrils are first seen during embryogenesis and before elastin deposition. Although the physical relationship between microfibrils and elastin is virtually unknown, recent findings have shed some light on elastin metabolism and the assembly and maintenance of the elastic fiber (5–8). Intracellular binding of precursor tropoelastin to a 67 kDa protein [elastin-binding protein (EBP)] apparently prevents premature self-aggregation and proteolysis during its passage through the secretory pathways. Furthermore, EBP seems to remain bound to the secreted tropoelastin molecule. This seems to result in the participation of the EBP in the initial phase of elastic fiber assembly and its subsequent trapping within it. Should this scenario be proven correct, the presence of EBP in mature elastic fibers might also prevent proteolysis of insoluble elastin and extend the longevity of this matrix structure in aorta and elastic cartilage (6).

In addition to guiding elastogenesis, microfibrils have a strictly structural function in the ECM (9). As such, they form a fibrous aggregate that links elastin to other matrix components; for instance, microfibrils serve as a bridge between elastin bundles and the basement membrane at the dermal/epidermal junction. Microfibrils are also found devoid of any elastin in nonelastic tissues, where they appear to serve an anchoring function. For example, microfibrils link the lenses to the ciliary body of the eye.

Only a few of the microfibrillar components have been characterized so far, chiefly because these extracellular aggregates are highly insoluble. For the same reason, it is likely that only a fraction of all microfibrillar constituents have been hitherto identified using the available means of analysis. Immunobiochemical experiments have established the close association between microfibrils and a 31 kDa protein: microfibril-associated glycoprotein (MAGP) (10). Cloning experiments, on the other hand, have inferred the primary structure of MAGP and identified within it a cluster of cysteines that may mediate covalent interactions between molecules (10). Another microfibrillar component identified biochemically is emilin (elastin microfibril interface located protein); this 115 kDa protein was originally isolated from aortic tissues where it seems to appear just prior to elastin deposition (11, 12). The same approach has identified a 36 kDa glycoprotein with restricted expression to elastin-associated microfibrils on the adventitia (13). Identification of the ubiquously expressed 32 kDa associated microfibril protein (AMP) relied on screening an expression library with ocular zonule protein antisera (14). Both strategies were instrumental in isolating and eventually characterizing the fibrillin proteins (15–19). Additional components associated or interacting with the microfibrils are the enzyme lysyl oxidase and the structural proteins vitronectin, amyloid P, versican, and proteoglycans (20–23).

FIBRILLIN PROTEINS

The fibrillin protein was first purified from the medium of human fibroblast cell cultures using monoclonal antibodies raised against a microfibrillar extract (15). This and subsequent biochemical analyses established that this 350 kDa glycoprotein is the major building block of microfibrils. Subsequent cloning experiments elucidated the complete primary structure of this protein (17–19, 24). They also provided conclusive evidence for a causal association between fibrillin mutations and MFS (25). Finally, they led to the serendipitous discovery of a second fibrillin gene linked to an MFS-like condition, congenital contractural arachondactyly (CCA) (16, 18).

Despite previous evidence, the fibrillins are now known to represent a small family of structurally related proteins. Two members of the fibrillin protein family have been identified so far and fully characterized, fibrillin-1 (the protein responsible for MFS) and fibrillin-2 (the product of the gene linked to CCA). There is also a less-characterized fibrillin-like protein (FLP) (26). Fibrillins-1 and -2 are strikingly similar; consequently their structure will be described together as an exemplification of the general characteristics of the fibrillin family.

Fibrillin consists of five structurally distinct regions A, B, C, D, and E (Fig. 1) (17). Two of these regions, B and D, are composed of a series of consecutive cysteine-rich modules. The most abundant of these modules exhibits close homology to the epidermal growth factor (EGF) protein motif. The hallmark of the EGF motif is the presence of six characteristically spaced cysteines forming intramolecular disulfide bonds in the following order: C_1-C_3, C_2-C_4, and C_5-C_6 (27, 28). This stabilization of the molecule results in a triple-stranded β-sheet configuration (Fig. 1). Most of the EGF motifs of fibrillin contain the additional consensus sequence (D, [D/N], N, and Y/F) that identifies them with a particular subclass of EGF motifs, notably those that bind calcium (Fig. 1) (29). In other polypeptides, calcium-binding EGF motifs (EGF-cb) mediate noncovalent interactions between proteins (29, 30). Since the majority of fibrillin consists of EGF-cb repeats, there is great opportunity for a variety of noncovalent interactions among the fibrillins and between them and other microfibrillar components. Furthermore, the spacing between the last cysteine of an EGF-cb motif and the first cysteine of the next one is constant throughout region D. This conserved spacing may allow consecutive EGF-cb motifs to form a longer common β-sheet, and act as single functional units (Fig. 1). Thus the

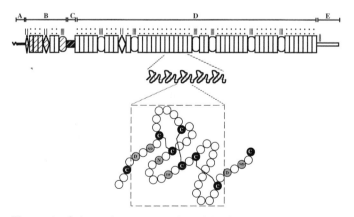

Figure 1   Schematic representation of the fibrillin protein (top) with the folding of an EGF-cb repeat (bottom) and a theoretical multirepeat unit (middle). Colons above the protein signify putative noncovalent interaction; bars indicate potential disulfide bridges.

primary structure of fibrillin can potentially facilitate folding of individual molecules or multirepeat domains, as well as networking between them.

The stretches of consecutive EGF-cb motifs in region D are flanked by another class of cysteine-rich motif (Fig. 1). These motifs are homologous to the eight-cysteine motif present in the transforming growth factor-β1 binding protein (TGFbp) (31). Characteristic of the TGFbp motif is a cluster of three consecutive cysteine residues that can potentially form interchain disulfide bonds. These sequences may therefore further and more strongly stabilize the noncovalent interactions mediated by the EGF-cb repeats. They may also define the boundaries of a functional unit consisting of several EGF-cb repeats. The third kind of cysteine-rich motif present in fibrillin is repeated only twice in the molecule. This motif, apparently unique to fibrillin and thus named Fib-motif, contains two consecutive cysteines that may also be free to interact covalently with other molecules.

The shorter cysteine-rich region of fibrillin (region B) is composed of modules reminiscent of the TGFbp and Fib motifs. Therefore, region B contains a relatively high concentration of cysteine residues that can be potentially available for interchain bonding. Both the amino and carboxy ends of fibrillin (regions A and E) consist of unique sequences. Region A is highly basic, whereas region E is relatively rich in lysines and contains two potential interchain disulfide bonds. In addition, fibrillin contains putative glycosylation sites and cell-attachment signals. The last region of fibrillin, region C, separates the two cysteine-rich sequences (Fig. 1). It also gives a separate identity to each of the two fibrillins since it is mostly made of prolines in fibrillin-1 and of glycines in fibrillin-2. This distinctive feature may also confer functional specificity on each fibrillin molecule.

FIBRILLIN GENES

The two fibrillin genes are called FBN1 and FBN2 and are located on chromosomes 15 and 5, respectively (18). Both of them are highly fragmented with an approximate ratio of noncoding to coding sequences of 10:1. The structure of the FBN1 gene has been fully characterized and thus it serves as the prototype for the entire gene family (17). The exon organization of the 110 kb gene reflects the modular arrangement of the protein, i.e., most of the cysteine-rich modules in regions B and D are encoded by single exons. As a result, fibrillin is encoded by 65 exons that are organized in a "cassette type" structure (Fig. 2A). This type of modular arrangement was first described in the collagen genes, where numerous 54 bp exons, or multiples of it, code for the long Gly-X-Y domain (32, 33). Analogous to the postulated evolution of the collagen genes from the 54 bp exon, the modular arrangement of fibrillin suggests that it may also have arose by duplications of an ancestral EGF-like coding unit (17).

(A)

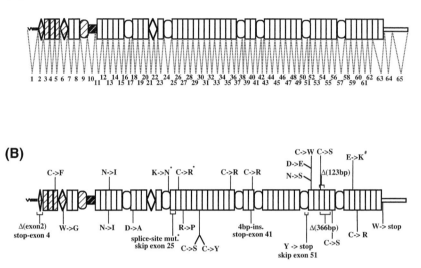

Figure 2 (A) Relationship between the sequence of the fibrillin protein and the exon organization of the gene. (B) Summary of the nature and location of fibrillin mutations in patients with MFS.

Another interesting feature of the fibrillin gene is that each of the cysteine-rich repeat-coding exons begins and ends with in-phase split codons. Aside from corroborating the way it evolved, such characteristic implies that mutations deleting any of these exons will keep intact the reading frame of the resulting transcript and give rise to shortened products. Finally, preliminary data indicate that the FBN2 gene presents the same genomic organization as FBN1 (18). This in turn implies that the fibrillin gene originated from a common multiexon structure.

MICROFIBRIL ASSEMBLY

Microfibrils appear under the electron microscope as thread-like filaments, regularly beaded in longitudinal sections and tubular in cross-sections (34, 35). Rotary shadowing analysis of these beaded fibers indicated that six to eight linear arms are attached to each globular domain. Similar analysis of purified fibrillin monomers revealed flexible linear molecules, most likely the constituents of the aforementioned arms (36). Subsequent immunolabeling experiments using monoclonal antibodies against fibrillin provided the first model for the organization of fibrillin molecules in the microfibrils (Fig. 3) (37). Based on the constant periodicity of antibodies binding, a head-to-tail assembly of fibrillin

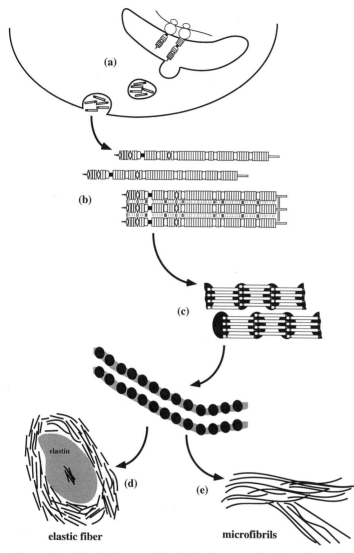

Figure 3 Microfibril assembly. Following secretion from the cell (a), fibrillin monomers polymerize (b) and interact with other polymers and ECM components (c) to give rise to bead-on-a-string profiles that either associate with elastin in the elastic fiber (d) or form structural networks by themselves (e).

monomers was proposed with one fibrillin length between every two beads. For this to occur, the fibrillin molecules must be precisely aligned with one another and assembled in parallel. Additional evidence also indicates that the most amino portion of fibrillin is embedded in the globular bead. Thus, it is conceivable that the amino-terminus of fibrillin represents the site of interaction between the heads and the tails of consecutive molecules (37).

How does this assembly model correlate with the primary structure of fibrillin? At this time, we can only speculate about it using several lines of circumstantial evidence; with this reservation in mind, in Figure 3 is presented a hypothetical model for microfibril assembly. Fibrillin is secreted from cells as a monomer, which is then rapidly incorporated into disulfide-bonded aggregates (38). These are the nucleus upon which microfibrils are built. Fibrillin monomers may interact with one another noncovalently via the EGF-cb motifs; indeed, calcium has been shown to be necessary for the integrity of microfibrils in culture (39). The interactions are held more tightly together, probably through the disulfide bonds provided by the TGFbp and Fib motifs. In addition, the free cysteines at the amino and carboxy termini of fibrillin may also form covalent links between fibrillin monomers, and between them and other components. The latter interaction may well occur in the domain visualized at the electron microscope as the globular bead. These series of complex interactions may in turn be favored by the proline/glycine-rich segment and/or by the bending of this portion of the molecule (16, 17).

Are microfibrils heteropolymers composed of both fibrillins-1 and -2, or are they made of only one of the two fibrillins? Recent work has begun to address this question by looking at fibrillin distribution (16). A similar distribution of fibrillins-1 and -2 is detected in many tissues. However, hyaline cartilage seems to be composed of fibrillin-1 and not fibrillin-2, whereas the opposite occurs in elastic cartilage. Another difference in the localization of the fibrillins is found in the aortic wall. While fibrillin-1 is present throughout the wall, fibrillin-2 seems to be restricted to the elastic media. In general, there is a preferential localization of fibrillin-2 to areas of the matrix rich in elastin. In addition to the differential spatial arrangements, the fibrillins display distinct temporal pattern of expression (40). During mouse embryogenesis, fibrillin-2 is produced transiently and earlier than fibrillin-1. These differences indicate spatiotemporal heterogeneity of microfibrils and, consequently, distinct contributions of the fibrillins to the assembly and maintenance of the elastic network. This postulate is in turn consistent with the different pathologies to which the two genes have been linked (18, 41).

FIBRILLIN PATHOGENESIS

MFS is a systemic disorder of connective tissue inherited as an autosomal dominant trait (1). The major manifestations of the disease affect the skeletal, ocular, and cardiovascular organ systems. Abnormalities in the cardiovascular system include mitral valve prolapse, regurgitation, aortic dilatation, and dissection; the last manifestation is the leading cause of death of patients with MFS (42).

Dilatation of the aorta is present in the majority of children and adults with MFS, and it can affect anywhere along the course of the vessel. Dissection usually occurs in the adult after the aortic root dilates more than 5–6 cm at the sinuses of Valsalva. In contrast, the same correlation is not well established in the child. In both cases, however, other factors should be considered, such as family history (if available), body surface area, and dilatation rate. In terms of clinical management, the most widely accepted approach is the use of β-adrenergic blockade to slow the rate of dilatation. Ultimately, however, corrective surgery with replacement of the aortic root is required to counteract progression of the disease.

For several years, MFS has been the subject of intensive investigations that can be broadly classified into two phases. The first one was mostly focused on the characterization of the clinical and genetic features of MFS; the second one focused on the elucidation of the genetic defect. In the late 1980s investigators began to postulate a causal relationship between the pleiotropic manifestations of MFS and structural alterations in the microfibrils, and fibrillin is particular. This hypothesis was immediately, albeit indirectly, supported by a rapid succession of immunohistological, biochemical, and genetic studies (18, 19, 38, 43, 44). When regarded collectively, this body of work paved the way to the first identification of a fibrillin mutation in MFS (25). The discovery of the "MFS gene" did in turn spur a new wave of interest in ECM physiopathology, sustained by inferential evidence gathered from fibrillin mutations in MFS.

With the exception of two known cases, each MFS family has a private gene defect (25). This is probably due to the relatively low reproductive fitness of patients with MFS caused by the early morbidity and mortality of this disease. There is also no "hot-spot" for mutations in FBN1, since different mutations have been found distributed along the entire length of the gene (Fig. 2B). This observation may reflect the functional importance of all the structurally distinct regions of the fibrillin protein. In most cases there is no obvious correlation between phenotype and genotype; as a result, the severity of the phenotype cannot currently be predicted on the basis of the nature and location of the mutation. There is, however, emerging evidence suggesting that mutations clustered within the middle of region D are associated with the most severe form of the disease, the so-called neonatal MFS (45).

The fibrillin mutations identified so far can be classified into two general groups (Fig. 2B). The first consists of missense mutations that alter residues of the EGF-cb consensus sequence (45–49). These changes are believed to affect the folding and/or the calcium binding ability of the EGF-cb repeat. It can also be argued that altering a single EGF-cb repeat may have the "domino effect" of disrupting the function of the whole multirepeat unit (17). It remains, however, to be clarified precisely the result of these kinds of mutations on the assembly and function of the microfibrils, and how they relate to MFS pathogenesis. Studies of fibrillin synthesis and processing in cell culture are beginning to shed some light on this matter (39). The data indicate that substitutions of cysteine residues in the EGF-cb repeats lead to delay in secretion, and to reduced deposition of fibrillin into the matrix. In contrast, mutations altering residues of the calcium-binding consensus seem to impair fibrillin incorporation into the ECM. Thus, while correct folding of the EGF-cb repeats may be critical to normal intracellular trafficking, calcium binding seems to be required only for the incorporation of fibrillin into the matrix. One could envision two ways of how these alterations may act. First, they may impair intermolecular interactions; second, or concomitantly, they may increase the susceptibility to proteolysis.

The second group of mutations comprises those generating shortened forms of fibrillin (48, 50–52). They include genomic deletions causing the loss of multiple cysteine-rich repeats, frame-shifts and nonsense mutations leading to truncated carboxy-termini, and splice site mutations that cause exon skipping and the loss of an internal repeat. These mutations are believed to act in the same general manner: by disrupting the postulated alignment of fibrillin monomers. This may in turn have two consequences: it may damage the functional integrity of the microfibrils, and it may render the fibers more susceptible to degradation.

The third kind of mutation has raised the interesting issue of whether microfibril formation is also susceptible to a gene dosage effect. A recent report described an FBN1 allele with a frame-shift mutation whose level of expression is only 6% of normal (48, 50). The patient carrying this nearly null allele has a mild variation of the MFS phenotype. The authors proposed that the patient's mild phenotype may be accounted for by the reduced amount of mutant fibrillin monomers, which may in turn allow preferential interaction among normal molecules during microfibil assembly (50). In the same report, the authors also described a patient with severe MFS and a different mutation producing 16% the normal level of transcripts. Taken at face value, the results seem to suggest that the relative ratio between mutant and normal monomers determine the threshold above which full-blown MFS is manifested.

The clinical variability of MFS and the heterogeneity of the fibrillin mutations have so far precluded the development of accurate presymptomatic means to diagnose this disorder. Linkage analysis can be still employed in well-documented cases of familial MFS. The combined informative value of four intragenic markers has significantly improved diagnosis of familial MFS (53). This is of great importance, particularly in view of the possibility of intrafamilial variability, which results in individuals carrying the same mutation and yet presenting different phenotypes with regard to age of onset, affected tissues, and severity of manifestations (47, 54). Genetic background in the form of "modifiers" influencing the expression of a given mutation is probably responsible for the clinical variability of MFS.

FIBRILLINOPATHIES

Aside from MFS, genetic linkage studies first, and mutational analyses later, have connected the FBN1 gene with an MFS-related condition: ectopia lentis (EL) (18, 41, 45, 55). Both familial and isolate EL overlap with MFS in the ocular manifestations and, to a much lesser extent, the skeletal presentation. The major feature that differentiates the two conditions is the absence of cardiovascular involvement in patients with EL. Albeit with difficulty, differential diagnosis can therefore separate these overlapping phenotypes into clinically distinct entities. As for the lack of genotype/phenotype correlation in MFS, there is also no apparent explanation for why fibrillin-1 mutations in EL have no effect on the cardiovascular system (55). A similar, but not identical, consideration applies to the finding of genetic linkage between CCA and FBN2 (18, 41).

As already mentioned, the expression of the two fibrillin genes has been compared in human tissues and, more recently, during mouse embryogenesis (16, 40). The data revealed differential patterns of gene expression consistent with the notion of spatiotemporal heterogeneity of seemingly identical microfibrils. These observations and the diversity of the pathologies associated with the two gene products strongly suggest distinct functions of the two proteins.

Before the discovery of fibrillin-2, it was often argued that microfibrils play at least two roles in elastogenesis. The first is to direct elastic fiber assembly, and the second is to confer biomechanical properties to the mature product. The different pathologies and expression patterns could be interpreted as suggesting that each of the fibrillins plays predominantly one of the two postulated roles: fibrillin-1 the structural role and fibrillin-2 the regulatory function. Assuming that this hypothesis is correct, one could then argue that fibrillin-2 mutations are more deleterious than those of fibrillin-1, because they deprive the developing organ of a critical matrix component. This argument would also predict that patients with CCA represent the milder end in the spectrum of fibrillin-2 mutations. For example, these individuals might carry mutations affecting the level of gene expression rather than protein structure. Although solely based on inferential evidence, the hypothesis is consistent with the lower incidence of CCA compared to MFS; this is a testable hypothesis and one very much in the minds of investigators.

Along these lines, there is increasing interest in understanding the diversified manifestations of the fibrillinopathies, particularly those regarding the cardiovascular system. Consonant with the hypothesized diversification of fibrillin functions, the progressive weakening of the aortic wall in MFS patients exemplifies the load-bearing structural function of fibrillin-1 in the adventitia. The near absence of fibrillin-2 in this segment of the aorta is likewise consistent with the absence of dissecting aneurysms in patients with CCA.

CONCLUSION

The work briefly outlined here has concluded the search for the genetic lesion, the second phase of MFS research. As such, it has also opened the next investigative phase, which is likely to focus on the establishment of genotype–phenotype correlations. Major goals of future research will include elucidation of the full pathogenesis of the disorder, including the origins of pleiotropy and clinical variability, and the development of novel therapeutic approaches to ameliorate, or even eliminate, the clinical burden of MFS. Although a great deal can still be learned from the characterization of naturally occurring mutations, these goals will be probably best served by the generation of animal models for MFS.

Transgenic technology can be used for the development of a mouse model for MFS. For example, the introduction of a mutant allele producing a truncated form of fibrillin into the pronuclei of mouse fertilized eggs may reproduce the human clinical phenotype in the transgenic animals. As an alternative, the more sophisticated approach of homologous recombination in embryonic stem cells could be used to target specific regions of the protein. The strategy could also ascertain the contribution of qualitative and quantitative changes in fibrillin to the development and survival of the mice. In both cases, the animals would be invaluable tools to study MFS variability by allowing us to examine the same mutation in different inbred strains. Aside from elucidating the precise contribution of a genetic background, these mice will also provide the means to characterize the "modifier" genes. Finally, they will allow investigators to dissect the contribution of each fibrillin to microfibril assembly and elastogenesis. It will also be possible to assign specific roles to other microfibrillar components of unknown function or those yet to be discovered.

The development of animal models for MFS other than mice will lead to a better appreciation of different parameters for conventional medical therapies, including dosage, time of initiation, and route of administration of agents that slow the rate of aortic root dilatation. Novel gene therapy strategies may also be evaluated in animals. According to the dominant negative model for the pathogenesis of fibrillin, inactivation of the mutant transcripts should enable the formation of normal microfibers, and thus the attenuation of the MFS phenotype. This may be accomplished by ribozimes or antisense oligonucleotides targeted to specific transcripts.

In conclusion, the impressive progress made during the past few years in MFS research has brought the role of the ECM in morphogenesis and organs' function to a wider appreciation than before. We are already witnessing some benefit from these recent achievements in the form of an increased understanding of the etiopathology of the disorder, and of more efficient means for presymptomatic and prenatal diagnosis. We have briefly outlined here the challenges ahead, which will be undoubtedly undertaken with the same tenacity and effort as those that brought today's accomplishments.

NOTE ADDED IN PROOF

While this manuscript was in preparation, a direct causal relationship between CCA and mutations in FBN2 was established in two patients (56). The missense mutations cause the substitution of cisteine residues in EGF-cb repeats located in the region that corresponds to the so-called neonatal segment of fibrillin-1. Another important development has been the creation of a mouse line that replicates the cardiovascular phenotypes of MFS (57).

ACKNOWLEDGMENT

The authors thank L. Apelis for typing the manuscript. This is article 179 from the Brookdale Center for Molecular Biology at the Mount Sinai School of Medicine in New York City.

REFERENCES

1. McKusick V. Heritable Disorders of Connective Tissue, 1st Ed. St. Louis: CV Mosby, 1956.
2. Karrer HE, Cox J. Electron microscope study of developing chick embryo aorta. J Ultrastruct Res 1961; 4:420–454.
3. Greenlee TK, et al. The fine structure of elastic fibers. J Cell Biol 1966; 30:59–71.
4. Fahrenbach WH, et al. Ultrastructural studies on early elastogenesis. Anat Rec 1966; 155:563–576.
5. Hinek A, et al. The elastin receptor: a galactosidase-binding protein. Science 1988; 239:1534–1541.
6. Hinek A, Rabinovitch M. 67-kD elastin-binding protein is a protective "companion" to extracellular insoluble elastin and intracellular tropoelastin. J Cell Biol 1994; 126:563–574.
7. Mecham RP, et al. Elastin binds to a multifunctional 67 kD peripheral membrane protein. Biochemistry 1983; 28:3716–3722.
8. Mecham RP, et al. 67 kD elastin binding protein is homologous to the tumor cell 67 kD laminin receptor. J Biol Chem 1989; 264:16652–16657.

9. Mecham RP, Hauser JE. The Elastic Fiber. In: Hay ED, ed. Cell Biology of the Extracellular Matrix, 2nd ed. New York, Plenum Publishing, 1992:79–109.
10. Gibson MA, et al. Complementary DNA cloning establishes microfibril-associated glycoprotein (MAPG) to be a discrete component of the elastin-associated microfibrils. J Biol Chem 1991; 266:7596–7601.
11. Bressan GM, et al. Isolation and characterization of a 115,000-dalton matrix-associated glycoprotein from chick aorta. J Biol Chem 1983; 258:13262–13267.
12. Bressan GM, et al. Emilin, a component of elastic fibers preferentially located at the elastin-microfibrils interface. J Cell Biol 1993; 121:201–212.
13. Kobayashi R, et al. Isolation and characterization of a new 36-kDA microfibril-associated glycoprotein from porcine aorta. J Biol Chem 1989; 264:17437–17444.
14. Horrigan SK, et al. Characterization of an associated microfibril protein through recombinant DNA techniques. J Biol Chem 1992; 267:10087–10095.
15. Sakai LY, et al. Fibrillin, a new 350-kD glycoprotein, is a component of extracellular microfibrils. J Cell Biol 1986; 103:2499–2509.
16. Zhang H, et al. Structure and expression of fibrillin-2, a novel microfibrillar component preferentially located in elastic matrices. J Cell Biol 1994; 124:855–863.
17. Pereira L, et al. Genomic organization of the sequence coding for fibrillin, the defective gene product in Marfan syndrome. Hum Mol Genet 1993; 2:961–968.
18. Lee B, et al. Linkage of Marfan syndrome and a phenotypically related disorder to two fibrillin genes. Nature 1991; 352:330–334.
19. Maslen CL, et al. Partial sequence of a candidate gene for the Marfan syndrome. Nature 1991; 352:334–337.
20. Zimmerman DR, et al. Versican is expressed in the proliferating zone in the epidermis and in association with the elastic network of the dermis. J Cell Biol 1994; 124:817–825.
21. Dahlback K, et al. Immunohistochemical demonstration of age-related deposition of vitronectin (S-protein of complement) and terminal complement complex on dermal elastic fibers. Invest Dermatol 1989; 93:727–733.
22. Baccarani-Contri M, et al. Immunocytochemical localization of proteoglycans within normal elastic fibers. Eur J Cell Biol 1990; 53:305–312.
23. Breathnach SM, et al. Amyloid P component is located on elastic fiber microfibrils in normal human tissue. Nature 1991; 293:652–654.
24. Corson GM, et al. Fibrillin binds calcium and is coded by cDNAs that reveal a multidomain structure and alternatively spliced exons at the 5' end. Genomics 1993; 17:476–484.
25. Dietz HC, et al. Marfan syndrome caused by a recurrent de novo missense mutation in the fibrillin gene. Nature 1991; 352:337–339.
26. Mecham RP, Davis E. Elastic fiber structure and assembly. In: Yurchenco PD, Birk DE, Mecham RP, eds. Extracellular Matrix Assembly and Structure. New York: Academic Press, 1994:281–341.
27. Davis C. The many faces of epidermal growth factor repeats. New Biologist 1990; 2:410–419.
28. Cooke RM, et al. The solution structure of human epidermal growth factor. Nature 1987; 327:339–341.

29. Handford PA, et al. The first EGF-like domain from human factor IX contains a high affinity calcium binding site. EMBO J 1990; 9:475–480.

30. Rebay I, et al. Specific EGF repeats of Notch mediate interactions with Delta and Serrate: implications for Notch as a multifunctional receptor. Cell 1991; 67:687–699.

31. Kanzaki T, et al. TGF-β1 binding protein: a component of the large latent complex of TGF-β1 with multiple repeat sequences.

32. Vuorio E, de Crombrugghe B. The family of collagen genes. Annu Rev Biochem 1990; 59:837–872.

33. Yamada Y, et al. The collagen gene: evidence for its evolutionary assembly by amplification of a DNA segment containing an exon of 54 bp. Cell 1980; 22:887–892.

34. Keene DR, et al. Extraction of extendable beaded structures and their identification as fibrillin-containing extracellular matrix microfibrils. J Histochem Cytochem 1991; 39:441–449.

35. Ren ZX, et al. An analysis by rotary shadowing of the structure of the mammalian vitreous humor and zonular apparatus. J Struct Biol 1991; 106:57–63.

36. Maddox BK, et al. Connective tissue microfibrils: isolation and characterization of three large pepsin-resistant domains of fibrillin. J Biol Chem 1989; 264:21381–21385.

37. Sakai LY, et al. Purification and partial characterization of fibrillin, a cysteine-rich structural component of connective tissue microfibrils. J Biol Chem 1991; 266:14763–14770.

38. McGookey-Milewicz D, et al. Marfan syndrome: defective synthesis, secretion and extracellular matrix formation of fibrillin by cultured dermal fibroblasts. J Clin Invest 1992; 89:79–86.

39. Ayoama T, et al. Missense mutations impair intracellular processing of fibrillin and microfibril assembly in Marfan syndrome. Hum Mol Genet 1993; 2:2135–2140.

40. Zhang H. Cloning and characterization of fibrillin 2, a new extracellular matrix protein. Ph.D. dissertation, City University of New York, New York, NY, 1994.

41. Tsipouras P, et al. Linkage of Marfan syndrome, dominant ectopia lentis and congenital contractural arachnodactyl to the fibrillin genes on chromosomes 15 and 5. N Engl J Med 1992; 326:905–909.

42. McKusick V. The cardiovascular aspects of Marfan's syndrome: a heritable disorder of connective tissue. Circulation 1955; 11:321–342.

43. Hollister DW, et al. Marfan syndrome:immunohistologic abnormalities of the elastin-associated microfibrillar fiber system. N Engl J Med 1990; 323:152–159.

44. Kainulainen K, et al. Location of chromosome 15 of the gene defect causing Marfan syndrome. N Engl J Med 1990; 323:935–939.

45. Kainulainen K, et al. Mutations in the fibrillin gene responsible for dominant ectopia lentis and neonatal Marfan syndrome. Nature Genet 1994; 6:64–69.

46. Dietz HC, et al. Clustering of fibrillin (FBN1) missense mutations in Marfan syndrome patients at cysteine residues in the EGF-like domains. Human Mutations 1992; 1:366–374.

47. Dietz HC, et al. Marfan phenotype variability in a family segregating a missense mutation in the EGF-like motif of the fibrillin gene. J Clin Invest 1992; 89:1674–1680.

48. Dietz HC, et al. Four novel FBN1 mutations: significance for mutant transcript level and EGF-like domain calcium binding in the pathogenesis of Marfan syndrome. Genomics 1993; 17:468–475.

49. Hewett DR, et al. A novel fibrillin mutation in the Marfan syndrome which could disrupt calcium binding of the epidermal growth factor-like module. Hum Mol Genet 1993; 2:475–477.

50. Dietz HC, et al. The skipping of constitutive exons in vivo induced by nonsense mutation. Science 1993; 254:680–683.

51. Godfrey M, et al. Prenatal diagnosis and a donor splice site mutation in fibrillin in a family with Marfan syndrome. Am J Hum Genet 1993; 53:472–480.

52. Kainulainen K, et al. Two mutations in Marfan syndrome resulting in truncated polypeptide chains of fibrillin. Proc Natl Acad Sci USA 1992; 88:5917–5921.

53. Pereira L, et al. Diagnosis of Marfan syndrome: a molecular approach for stratification of cardiovascular risk within families. N Engl J Med 1994; 331:148–153.

54. Pyeritz RE, McKusick VA. The Marfan syndrome: diagnosis and management. N Engl J Med 1979; 300:772–777.

55. Lonnqvist L, et al. A novel mutation of the fibrillin gene causing ectopia lentis. Genomics 1994; 19:573–576.

56. Putnam EA, et al. Fibrillin-2 (FBN2) mutations result in the Marfan-like disorder, congenital contractural arachnodactyly. Nat Gen 1995; 11:456–458.

57. Pereira L, et al. Mouse model for genetically predisposed aneurysm delineates the mechanism behind vascular dissection. Manuscript submitted.

19

The Role of Tissue Factor in Arterial Thrombosis and Atherosclerosis

Mark B. Taubman
Mount Sinai School of Medicine
New York, New York

Thrombosis plays an integral role in the development and progression of symptomatic atherosclerosis. Thrombosis occurs spontaneously in the setting of acute coronary syndromes, such as myocardial infarction, unstable angina, and sudden death (1,2). Thrombosis also occurs as a complication of vessel manipulation, such as that accompanying arterial bypass surgery, balloon angioplasty, atherectomy, or coronary artery stenting (3-5).

Thrombus likely plays two roles in the atherosclerotic process. In some instances, it can cause total occlusion of the vessel lumen, leading to ischemia or infarction of the downstream tissues. The efficacy of thrombolytic therapy in the treatment of acute myocardial infarction (reviewed in 6) is testimony to the importance of thrombotic occlusion in the causes of this disease and has justified the use of the term *coronary thrombosis* by an earlier generation to designate a heart attack. Even under conditions in which the thrombus is not occlusive, it can provide substantial bulk that can cause partial obstruction or serve as a nidus for the propagation of the atherosclerotic lesion.

In addition to its obstructive properties, thrombus is also thought to play a role in the more insidious progression of atherosclerosis. Thrombus is comprised of platelets, fibrin, and the proteins necessary to generate fibrin. Other components, including white blood cells and secretory proteins, are often trapped within the propagating thrombus. Activated platelets release a variety of growth factors such as platelet-derived growth factor (PDGF), and cytokines that have been implicated in vascular smooth muscle cell (VSMC) proliferation and migration (7,8). Arteries of rats made thrombocytopenic with antiplatelet antibodies failed to develop intimal hyperplasia, suggesting that platelet products were necessary (9). PDGF is a potent SMC mitogen (10) and an SMC chemoattractant (11). Antibodies against PDGF have been shown to attenuate intimal hyperplasia following experimental balloon arterial injury (12).

Clotting factors produced during the development of the thrombus also have direct effects on SMC. α-Thrombin is a growth agonist for VSMC (13) and induces in VSMC many of the same transmembrane signals as PDGF, including phospholipase C-mediated phosphoinositide hydrolysis and activation of Na^+–H^+ exchange (14,15). α-Thrombin also induces in VSMC many of the same "immediate early" genes as PDGF, including the protoncogenes c-*fos* and c-*myc*, the chemoattractant gro/*KC* (14,16), and tissue factor (17). Thus, α-thrombin generated during thrombus formation may play an important role in the subsequent intimal hyperplasia by stimulating SMC growth. Recently, factor X/Xa was reported to be mitogenic for rat VSMC (18) and, in a preliminary study, an inhibitor of factor Xa blocked restenosis after balloon angioplasty of rabbit femoral arteries (19).

CHRONIC ATHEROSCLEROSIS AND THROMBUS FORMATION

As noted above, thrombus is an important component of the mature atherosclerotic plaque. In addition, acute thrombosis is often the final event leading to catastrophic arterial occlusion. The steps leading to acute thrombosis are not fully understood. Plaque rupture is thought to play a major role (1,2,20). Plaque rupture often involves "soft" lipid-rich lesions that appear nonobstructive on coronary angiography. The rupture may occur at fissures in the plaque and may expose circulating blood to thrombogenic proteins located within the plaque. In some acute coronary events, plaque rupture is not thought to play a significant role (1,2,20). Instead, thrombosis appears to occur in the setting of a severely stenotic vessel dominated by a heavily calcified, "stable" plaque. We assume that the surface of this stenotic plaque predisposes to thrombotic events. In addition, rheological factors associated with progressive stenosis and increased shear stress may induce mediators of thrombosis on the cells near the luminar surface.

The thrombogenicity of human atherosclerotic lesions has been studied by Badimon and co-workers using an ex vivo perfusion system in which plaque components (normal intima, fatty streak, fibrolipid and sclerotic plaques, and lipid-rich atheromatous core with cholesterol crystals) were placed in a perfusion chamber (21) and exposed to circulating blood at high shear rate conditions. Thrombus formation, determined morphologically, and deposition of radiolabeled platelets were then examined. Using this system, the lipid-rich core, often exposed during plaque rupture, was found to be the most thrombogenic (22–24).

VESSEL INJURY AND THROMBUS FORMATION

Thrombus formation is commonly associated with acute arterial injury. This is seen clinically with all interventional procedures designed at reducing human coronary stenosis, including percutaneous transluminal coronary angioplasty (PTCA), directional coronary atherectomy (DCA), and, most recently, coronary artery stenting (3–5). Acute thrombosis can result in rapid and total occlusion of the vessel lumen. This can largely be prevented by the use of platelet inhibitors, anticoagulants, and antithrombins (25). Such treatments, while effective in preventing occlusive thrombosis, do not abolish the deposition of smaller, nonocclusive mural thrombi (26,27).

Thrombus formation after vessel injury involves adherence of platelets to the subendothelium and activation of the coagulation cascade by exposure of circulating clotting factors to procoagulant factors within the vessel wall. Platelets and coagulation are intimately connected. Fibrin and platelet deposition occur in close proximity (28,29) and platelet adhesion precedes fibrin deposition in most models of injury (see below). Platelets amplify coagulation by providing calcium and phospholipid membranes that are essential components of the prothrombinase complex; this amplification has been estimated at five to six orders of magnitude (reviewed in 30). In turn, coagulation contributes to platelet activation through the generation of thrombin, which is a potent activator of platelets in vivo (31).

The relative contributions of platelet and fibrin deposition to thrombus formation vary with the degree of injury, the type of vessel (carotid, femoral, aorta, or coronary), the state of the vessel prior to injury (normal, cholesterol-fed, previously injured), and the species. In the pig carotid balloon injury model, superficial injury, defined as endothelial denudation and no medial injury, is associated with platelet deposition but no fibrin generation. Deeper injury, defined by the presence of a medial tear, results in marked platelet accumulation and fibrin generation, even in the presence of high doses of the anticoagulant heparin (32). Unlike the porcine model, balloon injury to normal rodent arteries has not been reported to result in fibrin deposition, even in those cases in which medial smooth muscle injury has been documented (33–35). In normal rabbit aorta, endothelial denudation with a balloon catheter results within 10 min in the deposition of a diffuse monolayer of platelets with no associated fibrin formation (33,35). Similar findings have been reported in the rat carotid injury model (34).

In contrast to that found using normal arteries, fibrin deposition is seen when previously injured rabbit arteries, possessing a neointima, are subjected to a second injury (33,35,36). Using scanning and transmission electron microscopy, abundant fibrin formation was detected in areas of damaged smooth muscle and exposed connective tissue within 30 min of the reinjury (35). Platelet deposition was also more dense than after an initial injury and platelets were enmeshed in the fibrin to form fibrin–platelet microthrombi. Two observations suggested that in contrast to platelet deposition on the exposed subendothelium of normal arteries, the mechanism responsible for platelet accumulation on the injured neointima involved activation of the coagulation cascade. First, aggregates of platelets seen on injured neointima were associated with fibrin (35,36). Second, treatment of rabbits with intravenous heparin reduced platelet accumulation on injured neointima by approximately 50% (36), but had no effect on platelet deposition on the subendothelium. We have recently examined fibrin deposition in rat aortic and carotid arteries using a similar double-injury model, in which animals were subjected to a second balloon injury 2 weeks after the initial injury (37). Fibrin deposition was not seen at any time following single injury, but as present on teh liminal surface following the second injury. Microthrombi were also noted on the luminal surface within 1 h of the second injury.

COAGULATION CASCADE AND THROMBOSIS

As noted above, clinically important thrombosis requires the deposition of platelets and activation of the coagulation cascade. Until recently, the platelet has held center stage in regulating intraarterial thrombosis. This chapter will focus on recent studies implicating the coagulation cascade, and tissue factor in particular, in the thrombotic complications associated with chronic atherosclerosis and acute vessel injury.

TISSUE FACTOR

Tissue factor (TF) is a low-molecular-weight glycoprotein that initiates the extrinsic clotting cascade and has been widely considered the major regulator of coagulation and hemostasis (38–40). Unlike other coagulation factors, which circulate through the blood, TF is located on the plasma membrane and is not normally found in the circulation. Human TF consists of three domains: a short cytoplasmic domain of 19 residues, a single transmembrane domain of 23 residues, and a large extracellular domain of 219 residues. In addition, there is a 32 residue aminoterminal leader sequence that is cleaved to produce the mature molecule. A schematic diagram of the coagulation cascade is shown in Figure 1. TF binds to factor VII/VIIa, and the resulting complex acts as a catalyst for the conversion of factors IX and X to IXa and Xa respectively, triggering the clotting cascade. This ultimately leads to the generation of thrombin, which in turn cleaves fibrinogen to fibrin, the major ingredient of the thrombus. The crystal structures of both TF (41) and the TF/VIIa complex (42) have recently been reported.

TF IN ATHEROSCLEROTIC PLAQUES

The distribution of TF in the arterial wall is not uniform. TF mRNA and antigen are easily detectable by in situ hybridization and immunohistochemistry in the adventitia of normal human coronary arteries, internal mammary arteries, and aortas (43,44). In contrast, TF mRNA and antigen are undetectable in normal vascular endothelium. TF mRNA has been demonstrated at low levels in the media of coronary and internal mammary arteries, whereas TF antigen

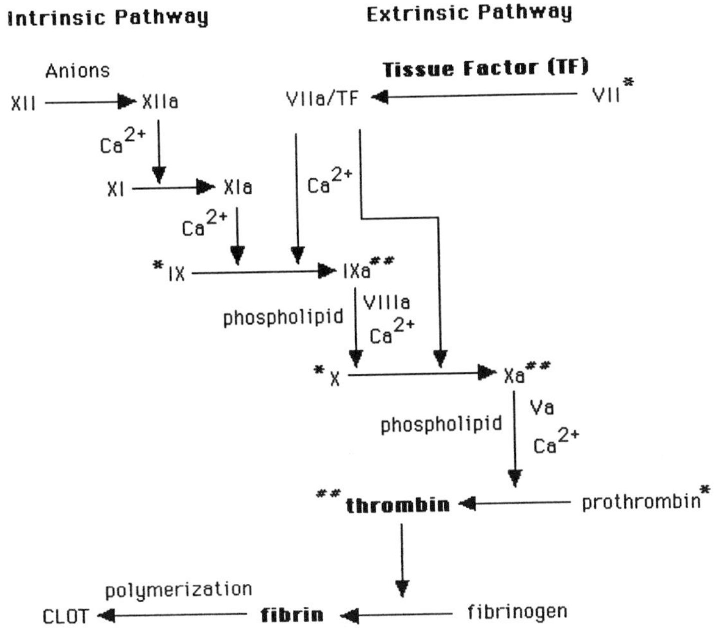

Figure 1 Schematic diagram of the coagulation cascade. Classic view of the coagulation cascade shows components of the intrinsic and extrinsic pathways. *, Vitamin K-dependent clotting factors, sensitive to coumadin. ##, Heparin-sensitive clotting factors. The roles of bolded factors are discussed in detail in the text. Feedback mechanisms are not included for the sake of simplicity.

has been either undetectable or found at low levels in the same vessels (43,44). TF has also been examined in atherosclerotic plaques from carotid endarterectomy specimens (44). TF mRNA and protein were absent from the endothelium, but were identified in mesenchymal-like intimal cells (presumably VSMC) as well as in foam cells and monocytes adjacent to cholesterol clefts, and in the extracellular matrix.

The availability of DCA has provided a rich source of specimens from human coronary atheromas. Using immunohistochemical techniques, Annex and co-workers (45) found TF antigen present in 33% of de novo lesions (n = 43) and in 6% of restenotic lesion (n = 18) from DCA specimens. We have recently examined procoagulant activity in 63 DCA specimens using a quantitative TF-specific activity assay (46). Significant TF activity was detected in 25 of 32 (78%) nonhomogenized and 28 of 31 (90%) homogenized specimens, yielding an overall detection rate of 53 of 63 (84%). Immunohistochemistry with a polyclonal antihuman TF antibody was performed on specimens from 50 of the 63 lesions studied with the TF activity assay. TF antigen was detected in 43 lesions (86%), and was expressed in cellular and acellular areas of the plaque (Fig. 2). Histologically defined thrombus was present in 19 of the 43 lesions with detectable TF antigen and in none of the seven lesions without detectable TF antigen (19 of 43 vs. 0 of 7; p < 0.02). TF antigen was undetectable by immunohistochemistry in 4 of 13 (31%) restenotic lesions and in

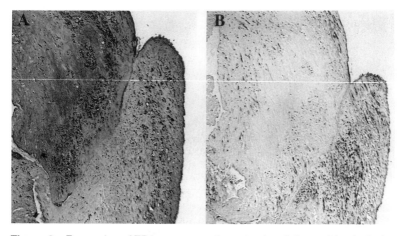

Figure 2 Expression of TF in coronary atherectomies. Adjacent histological sections of a human coronary atherectomy specimen stained with polyclonal anti-TF antibody (A) and antismooth muscle cell α actin antibody (B). TF is localized extracellularly and intracellularly, in smooth muscle cells (peroxidase-DAB, counterstained with hematoxylin; original magnification × 100). (Courtesy Dr. John T. Fallon, Mount Sinai School of Medicine, New York, NY.)

3 of 37 de novo lesions (8%; $p < 0.05$). The higher detection rate in our series of DCA specimens may relate to differences in the sensitivity of the anti-human TF antibody or to differences in the patient populations. These factors may also account for the apparently more diffuse immunohistochemical localization of TF antigen than with those previously reported (44,45).

In the above atherectomy study, some specimens with predominantly extracellular staining on immunohistochemistry demonstrated high levels of TF procoagulant activity. Because of the danger of drawing conclusions based on studies on small fragments of atherectomies, we examined TF expression in atherosclerotic human coronary and carotid arteries. Studies involved the use of antibodies to TF as well as a recently developed, highly sensitive binding assay employing digoxigenin-labeled factors VIIa and X (47). TF was detected in all (50) atherosclerotic plaques using either technique. Of particular note was the intense staining of the lipid-rich core (Fig. 3). TF staining and digoxigenin-

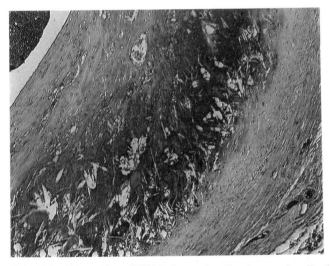

Figure 3 Expression of TF in atherosclerotic plaques: localization to lipid-rich core. AHA type IV atherosclerotic plaque in the left anterior decending coronary artery from a patient who died following an acute myocardial infarction. This routinely processed histological section was stained for digoxigenin after incubation with digoxigenin-labeled human recombinant factor VIIa. Binding of labeled factor VIIa to TF is particularly prominent in the lipid-rich core of the plaque. Staining is also present in the adventitia, in cells surrounding the lipid-rich core (macrophages), in cells of the fibrous cap (smooth muscle cells and macrophages), in the extracellular fibrous matrix of the fibrous cap, and in smooth muscle cells of the media (peroxidase-DAB, counterstained with hematoxylin; original magnification × 25). (Courtesy Dr. John T. Fallon, Mount Sinai School of Medicine, New York, NY.)

labeled VIIa binding were also noted in macrophages surrounding the lipid-rich core and in plaque VSMC. Staining was also noted in relatively acellular, fibrotic regions of advanced plaques. The arterial media showed staining of only rare VSMC. The endothelium overlying the plaque also stained for TF. The finding of abundant TF in the lipid-rich core is consistent with studies described above using the ex vivo perfusion chamber (23).

The causes of TF in the lipid-rich core and in the extracellular matrix of acellular, fibrotic regions remain to be determined. Based on immunohisto-chemical evidence, it is likely that the macrophage is responsible for the bulk of this TF. These studies, in conjunction with the activity assays described above, raise the possibility that the extracellular TF is released from cells in a functional and stable state. The shedding of TF from the plasma membrane in vesicles has been reported (48). As an alternative, active TF may be released during cell death. Whatever the cause, these studies suggest that rupture of lipidrich plaques presents active TF to circulating blood and may be directly responsible for acute thrombosis accompanying plaque rupture. In addition, acute interventions, such as PTCA, DCA, or intracoronary stenting, may expose previously sequestered TF to circulating blood in a fashion analogous to spontaneous plaque rupture.

TF IN VESSEL INJURY

In addition to exposure of previously synthesized TF, vessel injury may also induce de novo TF synthesis. As noted above, TF is not present in normal endothelium or VSMC, although it is always found in the adventitia. The presence of TF in the adventitia allows for rapid hemostasis in the event of external injury to the blood vessel and presumably is necessary to prevent serious hemorrhage from potentially minor wounds. Recent studies have suggested that arterial injury induces TF in VSMC (49). Rat aortas were harvested after balloon injury, and the media and adventitia separated using collagenase digestion and microscopic dissection. In uninjured aortic media, TF mRNA was undetectable by RNA blot hybridization. Two hours after balloon injury TF mRNA levels increased markedly; return to near baseline levels occurred at 24 h. In situ hybridization detected TF mRNA in the adventitia but not in the media or endothelium of uninjured aorta. Two hours after balloon dilatation, a marked induction of TF mRNA was observed in the adventitia and media. With use of a functional clotting assay, TF procoagulant activity was detected at low levels in uninjured rat aortic media and rose by $\approx$10-fold 2h after balloon dilatation; return to baseline occurred within 4 days (Fig. 4). Rat aortic double injury, as described above, caused a more rapid (15 min vs. 2 h) and more pronounced ($\approx$3fold greater than after single injury) induction of TF activity in intimal/media homogenates (37). The rapid and more pronounced TF induction

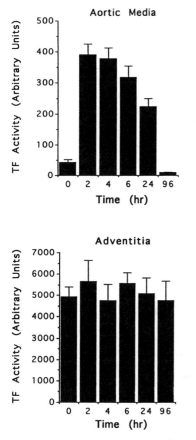

Figure 4 TF activity in rat aortic media and adventitia after arterial injury. Bars represent the level of TF activity in uninjured (time 0) and balloon-injured rat aortic tissue harvsted at various times (h) after arterial injury. Pure medial and adventitial preparations were separated by collagenase treatment, followed by fine microscopic dissection. Each bar represents the mean ± SEM of measurements performed in six rats. Units correspond to the amount of factor Xa generated and are expressed as total activity per milligram of protein. (From Ref. 49.)

following double injury may be responsible in part for the fibrin deposition noted in this model, but not in single-injury models.

Induction of TF in the arterial wall has also been reported in rabbit (50, 51) and porcine (52) models of arterial injury. In these models also the induction of TF has been seen in the VSMC near the luminal border. The role of TF induction in acute injury remains to be determined. However, in nine rabbits subjected to arterial injury and mechanical stenosis, antibodies to TF were shown to inhibit the variations in cyclical flow (50). These variations are thought to result in part from cycles of thrombus formation and dislodgement, suggesting that inhibition of TF reduces thrombosis after arterial injury. A similar antibody was used to inhibit thrombus formation in a rabbit femoral artery eversion graft preparation in four of five animals (53). In a different approach, an active-site inactivated factor VIIa (DEGR-VIIa) and tissue factor pathway inhibitor (TFPI, see below) each inhibited angiographic restenosis and intimal hyperplasia in an atherosclerotic rabbit balloon injury model (54). While these studies were small and not designed to identify the source(s) of TF in these models, they do suggest that the presence of TF activity at the site of injury is important in either the initiation or maintenance of thrombosis.

CELLULAR REGULATION OF TF

The above studies provide two mechanisms by which TF regulates thrombosis: exposure of TF by plaque rupture or acute interventions and de novo synthesis of TF in response to injury. These studies have also implicated macrophages, VSMC, and perhaps endothelial cells as sources of TF in the vessel wall. While the agents responsible for TF induction in vivo remain to be determined, considerable information exists as to the regulation of TF in cell culture.

In endothelial cell culture, TF mRNA and/or procoagulant activity is induced by phorbol esters (55,56), tumor necrosis factor (55,57,58), endotoxin (56,59), interleukin-1 (60,61), and α-thrombin (62). Similar results have been found in monocytes, where TF mRNA and/or procoagulant activity is stimulated by the above agents as well as a variety of mediators of inflammation and antigen-specific cellular immune responses (reviewed in 39). In mouse fibroblasts, TF has been found to be a member of the class of "immediate early" genes induced by serum and growth factors, including PDGF, fibroblast growth factor (FGF), and transforming growth factor β (63,64).

In human monocytes, the primary TF mRNA transcript is 2.2 kB and has a short half-life (45–90 min; 55,65). Under most circumstances, the induction of TF gene expression by agonists in fibroblasts (63), monocytes (65), and endothelial cells (55,56) occurs principally at the level of transcription, as determined by nuclear runoff assays. In addition, analysis done in the presence of the transcription inhibitor actinomycin D has suggested that increases in TF mRNA stability are also partly responsible for agonist-induced accumulation of TF mRNA (55) and, in some cases (e.g., lipopolysaccharide stimulation of TF in human umbilical vein endothelial cells and monocytes; 39,56), is the predominant mechanism. As is the case with other "immediate early" genes, TF is superinducible in the presence of protein synthesis inhibitors, such as cycloheximide (39,63).

The presence of TF procoagulant activity in cultured VSMC was initially reported by Maynard and co-workers (48). We examined the regulation of TF gene expression in cultured rat aortic VSMC (17). TF mRNA and procoagulant activity were found to be rapidly and markedly induced ($\approx$10-fold) in early- and late-passaged rat aortic VSMC by serum, PDGF, epidermal growth factor, angiotensin II, and α-thrombin (17). The induction of TF mRNA by these agents was dependent upon mobilization of intracellular Ca^{2+}, but not by influx of extracellular Ca^{2+}. In contrast to other growth factor-responsive genes, downregulation of protein kinase C activity by prolonged treatment with phorbol esters failed to block agonist-mediated TF induction. We have recently extended these studies to human aortic and coronary artery VSMC (66). Serum, PDGF, and α-thrombin induced TF mRNA and protein in both cell types. A 30 min exposure to these agonists was sufficient for the induction of TF mRNA and protein. Nuclear runoff analyses demonstrated that PDGF-induced TF transcription occurred within 30 min. Of note, PDGF AA, which is induced in the vessel wall by injury (12,67), was a potent agonist for TF, suggesting a novel function for this isoform as a procoagulant.

TF GENE REGULATION

Mackman and co-workers have cloned and sequenced the human (68) and mouse TF genes (69). The human gene is 12.4 kb in length and contains 6 exons. There is a single major transcription start site 26 bp downstream from a TATA consensus promoter element. Analysis of the nucleotide sequence for the 2106 bp upstream of the transcription start site has revealed consensus binding sites for AP1, NFκB, Sp1, and Egr-1. The mouse TF gene (69) displays a high degree of conservation with the human (85%) in the upstream region immediately flanking the promoter.

The regulation of the human TF promoter has been extensively studied and shown to involve a number of different elements, working either cooperatively or singly, depending upon the agonist used. Basal promoter activity in COS-7 cells was unchanged by deletions from −2106 to −384. The region between −383 and −279 bp appeared to contain a repressor element (70). Deletion of the region between −278 and −112 suggested that the minimal TF promoter contained three Sp1 sites and spanned a region between −111 and +14 bp. Studies performed in HeLa cells confirmed this and demonstrated that mutations of the Sp1 sites reduced promoter activity, suggesting that the three Sp1 sites controlled basal TF expression (71). This region also contained a serum response region (SRR) that did not contain the serum response element (SRE) previously identified in other immediate early genes, such as c-*fos*, and thus was likely to be novel. Deletional analysis and mutagenesis of single binding sites within this region failed to abolish induction by serum or phorbol esters, suggesting that several elements might act cooperatively (71). In contrast to the response of the human promoter to serum, the response to lipopolysaccharide in THP-1 monocytes and endothelial cells required the cooperative activity of two AP1 sites and the NFκB site between -227 and -172 bp (72,73). These results demonstrate that the regulation of TF transcription is complex and involves a variety of elements, some of which may be novel. The reader is directed to work by Mackman (74) for a more detailed review of studies involving the human TF promoter and, in particular, the regulation of the NFκB binding site.

FIBRINOLYTIC SYSTEM

Although this chapter focuses on the potential role of TF in atherosclerosis and thrombosis, the fibrinolytic system undoubtedly plays a role in balancing, if not offsetting, the effects of increased TF production in the vessel wall. This is underscored by the success of activators of fibrinolysis (tissue plasminogen activator, streptokinase, urokinase) in revascularization in the setting of acute myocardial infarction (reviewed in 6). A general scheme of the fibrinolytic system is shown in Figure 5. Fibrinolysis requires the generation of plasmin from plasminogen, an inactive proenzyme. The active plasmin degrades fibrin, as well as other extracellular matrix proteins. Two naturally occurring plasminogen activators have been identified, tissue-type plasminogen activator (tPA) and urokinase-type plasminogen activator (uPA). The reader is directed to several recent reviews for detailed information concerning the molecular biology of the fibrinolytic system (75,76).

Plasminogen activator inhibitor (PAI-1) is a rapid and irreversible inhibitor of both tPA and uPA (77). By inhibiting fibrinolytic activity, PAI-1 may augment the effects of TF expression and contribute to the development of thrombosis. Increased plasma levels of PAI-1 in humans have been associated with an increased risk of thrombosis, myocardial infarction, and unstable angina (77–81). In addition, transgenic mice overexpressing the human PAI-1 gene develop peripheral thrombi (82).

Like TF, the expression of PAI-1 is limited in normal vessels; PAI-1 mRNA has been found predominantly in endothelial cells (77). In contrast, PAI-1 mRNA has been detected by in situ hybridization in the intimal VSMC and adventitial arterioles of atherosclerotic arteries (77,83). In some studies, a wider distribution of PAI-1-containing cells, including endothelial cells, macrophages, and intimal and medial VSMC has been reported in atherosclerotic vessels (84,85). Like TF, PAI-1 is regulated in endothelial cells (86,87), VSMC (88), and macrophages (89). Of note, α-thrombin, a potent stimulator of TF in VSMC, also stimulates PAI-1 in VSMC (90,91). Therefore, thrombin may be

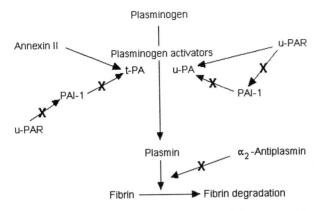

Figure 5 Schematic diagram of the fibrinolytic system. Diagram shows major components: →, activation; ✗, inhibition. Fibrin is degraded by plasmin, which is generated from plasminogen to plasminogen activators (t-PA and u-PA). Plasminogen activator inhibitor (PAI-1) inhibits both types of plasminogen activators. The u-PA receptor (u-PAR) is membrane bound and complexes with PAI-1 to inhibit its activity. u-PAR also stimulates u-PA. α-antiplasmin inhibits plasmin activity directly. Annexin II stimulates t-PA.

part of two procoagulant feedback loops, potentiating the synthesis of TF and PAI-1.

In addition to PAI-1, a second inhibitor, PAI-2 also occurs naturally (92). PAI-2 is found largely as an intracellular protein. Therefore, its role in regulating thrombosis is unclear. It is certainly possible that under conditions of cell injury PAI-2 is released into the extracellular matrix and can contribute to inhibiting fibrinolysis. The reader is referred to a review by Bachmann (93) on the molecular biology and expression of PAI-2.

TISSUE FACTOR PATHWAY INHIBITOR

Tissue factor pathway inhibitor (TFPI) is an endogenous inhibitor or TF-induced coagulation (94–96). TFPI directly inhibits factor Xa and, as a result, produces feedback inhibition of the factor VIIa/TF complex (97). TFPI appears to be made predominantly by endothelial cells (98,99) and circulates in the blood at relatively low concentrations (1–2 nM). TFPI is highly bound to lipoproteins, particularly low-density lipoprotein (LDL). While it is likely that circulating levels of TFPI modulate the effect of TF, it remains to be determined to what degree this occurs and whether local regulation of TFPI is important in mediating intrarterial thrombosis. Exogenously administered TFPI has been shown to inhibit venous thrombosis in rabbits (100) and to attenuate stenosis in balloon-injured hyperlipidemic pigs (101). The reader is directed to an article by Broze (102) for a detailed review of TFPI.

CONCLUSIONS AND THERAPEUTIC IMPLICATIONS

Thrombosis is a critical component of atherosclerosis, where it plays a role not only in acute occlusive events leading to ischemia, infarction, and death but also in providing a milieu conducive to the progression of the atherosclerotic plaque. Large thrombi consist of platelets and fibrin, the latter generated by a cascade of events initiated by TF, a highly regulated protein. The fibrinolytic system, as well as endogenous inhibitors of TF, modulate the activity of TF and under most conditions may prevent intraarterial fibrin deposition. In the setting of plaque rupture, in severely stenotic vessels, or in the presence of acute injury to atherosclerotic arteries, the exposure and/or synthesis of TF, in conjunction with acute platelet deposition, are likely to produce a clinically important thrombosis.

A number of strategies have been employed to inhibit thrombosis in the setting of acute obstruction or during iatrogenic vessel injury. The use of fibronolytics has been particularly helpful in the early phases of acute myocardial infarction or peripheral vascular occlusions (reviewed in 6), where flow can be restored to a majority of vessels and infarct size reduced. Considerable attention has focused on the use of antiplatelet agents in a variety of settings. Aspirin, in particular, has been shown to be beneficial in decreasing the incidence of stroke and postmyocardial infarction coronary events (see 103–106). This has led to the widespread use of aspirin in populations considered to be prone to atherosclerosis and has lent support to the notion that platelet accumulation is a critical feature in the progression of atherosclerotic disease. Aspirin is widely used in the setting of acute coronary syndromes and as adjunctive therapy for PTCA, DCA, and stenting. Further support for the role of platelets in acute vessel injury has been provided by studies employing inhibitors of the platelet receptor GIIb/IIIa (reviewed in 107). These initial studies (108,109) have suggested that inhibition of platelet binding at the time of PTCA not only inhibits acute thrombotic events but also decreases restenosis, once again implicating the thrombus in the progression of atherosclerotic disease.

In contrast to approaches designed at stimulating fibrinolysis or inhibiting platelet adhesion, a variety of approaches have targeted components of the coagulation cascade. Heparin has been the treatment of choice to inhibit the propagation of thrombus and has been the mainstay for treating deep venous thrombosis, acute pulmonary embolism, and acute thromboembolic events. More recent studies have focused on the use of low-molecular-weight heparins, because of the potential for easier dosing, longer half-life, and less bleeding. These studies have been summarized recently (110,111). The role of heparin in coronary thrombosis has been less clear. Heparin is widely used in the settings of unstable angina and as an adjunct to thrombolytic therapy in acute myocardial infarction, where it is thought that inhibition of thrombus propagation is critical. While heparin therapy has been credited with limiting the incidence of acute occlusion following acute coronary interventions, it has not been successful in inhibiting late restenosis. This may be due in part to the inability of heparin to prevent microthrombi (31), which may provide growth factors and cytokines that stimulate the restenotic process, or to the fact that TF expression is still elevated in the cells of the vessel wall after the cessation of heparin administration.

Oral anticoagulants, coumadin and warfarin, have been used for the chronic treatment of thromboembolic disease, venous thromboembolism, and pulmonary embolism, much as heparin has been used for the acute treatment of these diseases (reviewed in 112–114). The role of oral anticoagulants in unstable angina and myocardial infarction remains to be determined. A variety of trials underway (summarized in 112) should help clarify the use of these agents, alone or in combination with antiplatelet agents, in the treatment of diseases attributed to arterial thrombosis.

Considerable attention has been given to targeting thrombin as a way of inhibiting thrombosis, in part because it is the final step in generating fibrin and because thrombin itself is an agonist for smooth muscle cell proliferation and migration. Thus, antithrombins may have two distinct effects on inhibiting the atherosclerotic process. These agents include naturally occurring antithrombins, synthetic peptides, and chemical analogs. Hirudin, the most widely studied antithrombin, was originally cloned from the leech and shown to bind tightly to thrombin, blocking its action both as a procoagulant and as a direct cellular agonist (115,116). Hirudin blocks thrombus formation in porcine (31,117) and primate (118) models of arterial injury. In the porcine model, hirudin appears more effective than heparin in reducing microthrombi. A number of clinical trials are being conducted to examine the role of hirudin and its analogs, such as hirulog, in unstable angina, myocardial infarction, and restenosis. One problem that has been faced by many of these studies has been high levels of bleeding, necessitating reduction of dosage. The use of antithrombins and the design of new agents have recently been reviewed (119–121). One particularly intriguing approach to inhibiting thrombin is the use of aptamers: oligonucleotides which act directly on proteins. Several of these aptamers have been shown to bind specifically to thrombin and to reduce arterial platelet formation (122,123).

As the initiation of coagulation and the resultant synthesis of thrombin, TF has emerged as a potential target for inhibiting thrombosis and the progression of atherosclerosis. As noted above, TFPI is currently under clinical investigation as an anticoagulant and its effects on intimal hyperplasia in animal models are being studied. Direct factor Xa inhibitors, such as tick anticoagulant peptide (TAP) and leech anticoagulant peptide (ATS), are also under investigation (124,125). The recent crystallization of TF and the TF/VIIa should provide important new insights into the design of molecules for directly inhibiting TF. It thus appear highly likely that the multipronged approaches at inhibiting thrombosis will prove fruitful and will contribute immeasurably to the treatment and progression in knowledge of atherosclerotic disease.

REFERENCES

1. Fuster V, Badimon L, Badimon JJ, Chesebro JH. The pathogenesis of coronary artery disease and the acute coronary syndromes. N Engl J Med 1992; 326:242–250.
2. Fuster V, Badimon L, Badimon JJ, Chesebro JH. The pathogenesis of coronary artery disease and the acute coronary syndromes. N Engl J Med 1992; 326:310–318.
3. Losordo DW, Rosenfield K, Pieczek A, Baker K, Harding M, Isner JM. How does angioplasty work?: serial analysis of human iliac arteries using intravascular ultrasound. Circulation 1992; 86:1845–1858.
4. Nath FC, Muller DW, Ellis SG, Rosenchein U, Chapekis A, Quain L, Zimmerman C, Topol EJ. Thrombosis of a flexible coil coronary stent: frequency, predictors and clinical outcome. J Am Coll Cardiol 1993; 21:622–627.
5. Carrozza JP Jr, Baim DS. Complications of directional coronary atherectomy: incidence, causes, and management. Am J Cardiol 1993; 72:47E–54E.
6. Marder VJ. Thrombolytic therapy: overview of results in major vascular occlusions. Thromb Haemost 1995; 74:101–105.
7. Ross R. The pathogenesis of atherosclerosis: a perspective for the 1990s. Nature 1993; 362:801–809.
8. Schwartz SM, Heimark RL, Majesky MW. Developmental mechanisms underlying pathology of arteries. Physiol Rev 1990; 70:1177–1209.
9. Fingerle J, Johnson R, Clowes AW, Majesky MW, Reidy MA. Role of platelets in smooth muscle cell proliferation and migration after vascular injury in rat carotid artery. Proc Natl Acad Sci USA 1989; 86:8412–8416.
10. Seifert R, Schwartz S, Bowen-Pope D. Developmentally regulated production of platelet-derived growth factor-like molecules. Nature 1984; 311:669–671.
11. Grotendorst GR, Chang T, Seppae HEJ, Kleinman HK, Martin GR. Platelet-derived growth factor is a chemoattractant for vascular smooth muscle cells. J Cell Physiol 1981; 113:261–266.
12. Ferns GAA, Raines EW, Sprugel KH, Motani AS, Reidy MA, Ross R. Inhibition of neointimal smooth muscle accumulation after angioplasty by an antibody to PDGF. Science 1991; 253:1129–1132.
13. Huang CL, Ives HE. Growth inhibition by protein kinase C late in mitogenesis. Nature 1987; 329:849–850.
14. Berk BC, Taubman MB, Cragoe Jr EJ, Fenton II JW, Griendling KK. Throm-

bin signal transduction mechanisms in vascular smooth muscle cells. J Biol Chem 1990; 265:17334–17340.

15. Berk BC, Taubman MB, Griendling KK, Cragoe Jr EJ, Fenton II JW, Brock TA. Thrombin-stimulated events in cultured vascular smooth-muscle cells. Biochem J 1991; 274:799–805.

16. Marmur JD, Poon M, Rossikhina M, Taubman MB. The induction of PDGF-responsive genes in vascular smooth muscle: implications for the early response to vessel injury. Circulation 1992; 86:III-53–60.

17. Taubman MB, Marmur JD, Rosenfield CL, Guha A, Nichtberger S, Nemerson Y. Agonist-mediated tissue factor expression in cultured vascular smooth muscle cells: role of Ca^{2+} mobilization and protein kinase C activation. J Clin Invest 1993; 91:547–552.

18. Gasic GP, Arenas CP, Gasic TB, Gasic GJ. Coagulation factors X, Xa, and protein S as potent mitogens of cultured aortic smooth muscle cells. Proc Natl Acad Sci USA 1992; 89:2317–2320.

19. Ragosta M, Gimple LW, Haber HL, Dunwiddie CT, Vlasuk GP, Rowers ER, Sarembock IJ. Effectiveness of specific Factor Xa inhibition on restenosis following balloon angioplasty in rabbits. J Am Coll Cardiol 1992; 19:164A.

20. Davies MJ, Thomas AC. Plaque fissuring- the cause of acute myocardial infarction, sudden ischaemic death, and crescendo angina. Br Heart J 1985; 53:363–373.

21. Badimon L, Badimon JJ, Galvez A, Chesebro J, Fuster V. Influence of arterial damage and wall shear rate on platelet deposition. Arteriosclerosis 1986; 6:312–320.

22. Mailhac A, Badimon JJ, Fallon JT, Fernandez-Ortiz A, Meyer B, Chesebro JH, Fuster V, Badimon L. Effect of an eccentric severe stenosis on fibrin(ogen) deposition on severely damaged vessel wall in arterial thrombosis. Relative contribution of fibrin(ogen) and platelets. Circulation 1994; 90:988–996.

23. Fernandez-Ortiz A, Badimon JJ, Falk E, Fuster V, Meyer B, Mailhac A, Weng D, Shah PK, Badimon L. Characterization of the relative thrombogenicity of atherosclerotic plaque components: implications for consequences of plaque rupture. J Am Coll Cardiol 1994; 23:1562–1569.

24. Badimon JJ, Weng D, Chesebro HJ, Fuster V, Badimon L. Platelet deposition induced by severely damaged vessel wall is inhibited by a boroarginine synthetic peptide with antithrombin activity. Thromb Haemost 1994; 71:511–516.

25. Schwartz L, Bourassa MG, Lesperance J, Aldridge HE, Kazim F, Salvatori VA, Henderson M, Bonan R, David PR. Aspirin and dipyridamole in the prevention of restenosis after percutaneous transluminal coronary angioplasty. N Eng J Med 1988; 318:1714–1719.

26. Uchida Y, Hasegawa K, Kawamura K, Shibuya I. Angioscopic observation of the coronary luminal changes induced by percutaneous transluminal coronary angioplasty. Am Heart J 1989; 117:769–776.

27. Johnson DE, Hinohara T, Selmon MR, Braden LJ, Simpson JB. Primary peripheral arterial stenoses and restenoses excised by transluminal atherectomy: a histopathologic study. J Am Coll Cardiol 1990; 15:419–425.

28. Weiss HJ, Turitto VT, Baumgartner HR. Role of shear rate and platelets in promoting fibrin formation on rabbit subendothelium. Studies utilizing patients with quantitative and qualitative platelet defects. J Clin Invest 1986; 78:1072–1082.

29. Weiss HJ, Lages B. Studies of thromboxane B2, platelet factor 4, and fibrinopeptide A in bleeding-time blood of patients deficient in von Willebrand factor, platelet glycoprotein Ib and IIb-IIIa, and storage granules. Blood 1993; 82:481–490.

30. Walsh PN. Platelet-coagulant protein interactions. In: Colman RW, Hirsh J, Marder VJ, Salzman EW, eds. Hemostasis and Thrombosis: Basic Principles and Clinical Practice, 3rd ed. Philadelphia: J.B. Lippincott, 1994:629–651.

31. Heras M, Chesebro JH, Penny WJ, Bailey KR, Badimon L, Fuster V. Effects of thrombin inhibition on the development of acute platelet thrombus deposition during angioplasty in pigs. Heparin versus recombinant hirudin, a specific thrombin inhibitor. Circulation 1989; 79:657–665.

32. Steele PM, Chesebro JH, Stanson AW, Holmes D, Badimon L, Fuster V. Balloon angioplasty. Natural history of the pathophysiological response to injury in a pig model. Circ Res 1985; 57:105–112.

33. Stemerman MB. Thrombogenesis of the rabbit arterial plaque. An electron microscope study. Am J Path 1973; 81:15–42.

34. Clowes AW, Reidy MA, Clowes MM. Kinetics of cellular proliferation after arterial injury. Lab Invest 1983; 49:327–333.

35. Richardson M, Kinlough-Rathbone RL, Groves HM, Jorgensen J, Mustard JF, Moore S. Ultrastructural changes in re-endothelialized and non-endothelialized rabbit aortic neo-intima following re-injury with a balloon catheter. Br J Exp Pathol 1984; 64:597–611.

36. Groves HM, Kinlough-Rathbone RL, Richardson M, Jorgensen J, Moore S, Mustard JF. Thrombin generation and fibrin formation following injury to rabbit neointima. Studies of vessel wall reactivity and platelet survival. Lab Invest 1982; 46:605–612.

37. Fyfe BS, Marmur JD, Rossikhina M, Mendlowitz M, Thiruvikraman SV, Gargiulo N, Guha A, Fallon JT, Nemerson Y, Taubman MB. Rat aortic double injury is associated with fibrin deposition accompanying enhanced tissue factor activation and early neointimal proliferation. Submitted to Arter Thromb Vasc Biol.

38. Nemerson Y. Tissue factor and hemostasis. Blood 1988; 71:1–8.

39. Edgington TS, Mackman N, Brand K, Ruf W. The structural biology of expression and function of tissue factor. Thromb Haemost 1991; 66:67–79.

40. Rapaport SI, Rao LVM. The tissue factor pathway: how it has become a "prima ballerina." Thromb Haemost 1995; 74:7–17.

41. Harlos K, Martin DM, O'Brien DP, Jones EY, Stuart DI, Polikarpov I, Miller A, Tuddenham EG, Boys CW. Crystal structure of the extracellular region of human tissue factor. Nature 1994; 370:662–666.

42. Banner DW, D'Arcy A, Chene C, Winkler FK, Guha A, Konigsberg WH, Nemerson Y, Kirchhofer D. The crystal structure of the complex of blood coagulation factor VIIa with soluble tissue factor. Nature 1996; 380:41–46.

43. Drake TA, Morrissey JH, Edgington TS. Selective cellular expression of tissue factor in human tissues. Am J Pathol 1989; 134:1087–1097.

44. Wilcox JN, Smith KM, Schwartz SM, Gordon D. Localization of tissue factor in the normal vessel wall and in the atherosclerotic plaque. Proc Natl Acad Sci USA 1989; 86:2839–2843.

45. Annex BH, Denning SM, Channon KM, Sketch MH Jr, Stack RS, Morrissey JH, Peters KG. Differential expression of tissue factor protein in directional atherectomy specimens from patients with stable and unstable coronary syndromes. Circulation 1995; 91:619–622.

46. Marmur JD, Thiruvikraman SV, Fyfe BS, Guha A, Sharma SK, Ambrose JA, Fallon JT, Nemerson Y, Taubman MB. The identification of active tissue factor in human coronary atheroma. Circulation 1996; 94:1226–1232.

47. Thiruvikraman SV, Guha A, Roboz J, Taubman MB, Nemerson Y, Fallon JT. In situ localization of tissue factor in human atherosclerotic plaques by binding of digoxigenin labeled factors VIIa and X. Lab Invest 1996; 75:451–461.

48. Maynard JR, Heckman CA, Pitlick FA, Nemerson Y. Association of tissue factor activity with the surface of cultured cells. J Clin Invest 1975; 55:814–824.

49. Marmur JD, Rossikhina M, Guha A, Fyfe B, Friedrich V, Mendlowitz M, Nemerson Y, Taubman MB. Tissue factor is rapidly induced in arterial smooth muscle after balloon injury. J Clin Invest 1993; 91:2253–2259.

50. Pawashe AB, Golino P, Ambrosis G, Migliaccio F, Ragni M, Pascucci I, Chiariello M, Bach R, Garen A, Konigsberg WK, Ezekowitz MD. A monoclonal antibody against rabbit tissue factor inhibits thrombus formation in stenotic injured rabbit carotid arteries. Circ Res 1994; 74:56–63.

51. Speidel CM, Eisenberg PR, Ruf W, Edgington TS, Abendschein DR. Tissue factor mediates prolonged procoagulant activity on the luminal surface of balloon-injured aortas in rabbits. Circulation 1995; 92:3323–3330.

52. Gallo R, Fallon JT, Toschi V, Gertz SD, Padurean A, Nemerson Y, Chesebro J, Fuster V, Badimon JJ. Bi-phasic increase of tissue factor activity after angioplasty in porcine coronary arteries. Circulation 1995; 92:1–354.

53. Jang IK, Gold HK, Leinbach RC, Fallon JT, Collen D, and Wilcox JN. Antithrombotic effect of a monoclonal antibody against tissue factor in a rabbit model of platelet-activated arterial thrombosis. Arterioscler Thromb 1992; 12:948–954.

54. Jang Y, Guzman LA, Lincoff AM, Gottsauner-Wolf M, Forudi F, Hart CE, Courtman DW, Ezban M, Ellis SG, Topol EJ. Influence of blockade at specific levels of the coagulation cascade on restenosis in a rabbit atherosclerotic femoral artery injury model. Circulation 1995; 92:3041–3050.

55. Scarpati EM, Sadler JE. Regulation of endothelial cell coagulatn properties. J Biol Chem 1989; 264:20705–20713.

56. Crossman DC, Carr DP, Tuddenham EGD, Pearson JD, McVey JH. Regulation of tissue factor mRNA in human endothelial cells in response to endotoxin or phorbol este. J Biol Chem 1990; 265:9782–9787.

57. Nawroth PP, Stern DM. Modulation of endothelial cell hemostatic properties by tumor necrosis factor. J Exp Med 1986; 163:740–745.

58. Conway EM, Bach R, Rosenberg RD, Konigsberg WH. Tumor necrosis factor

enhances expression of tissue factor mRNA in endothelial cells. Thromb Res 1989; 53:231–241.

59. Moore KL, Andreoli SP, Esmon NL, Esmon CT, Bang NU. Endotoxin enhances tissue factor and suppresses thrombomodulin expression of human vascular endothelium in vitro. J Clin Invest 1987; 79:124–130.

60. Bevilacqua MP, Pober JS, Majeau GR, Cotran RS, Gimbrone Jr MA. Interleukin-1 (IL-1) induces biosynthesis and cell surface expression of procoagulant activity in human vascular endothelial cells. J Exp Med 1984; 160:618–623.

61. Nawroth PP, Handley DA, Esmon CT, Stern DM. Interleukin 1 induces endothelial cell procoagulant while suppressing cell-surface anticoagulant activity. Proc Natl Acad Sci USA 1986; 83:3460–3464.

62. Brox JH, Osterud B, Bjrklid E, Fenton II JW. Production and availability of thromboplastin in endothelial cells: the effects of thrombin, endotoxin and platelets. Br J Haematol 1984; 57:239–246.

63. Hartzell S, Ryder K, Lanahan A, Kau LF, Nathans D. A growth-factor responsive gene of murine Blab/c 3T3 cells encodes a protein homologous to a human tissue factor. Mol Cell Biol 1989; 9:2567–2573.

64. Bloem LJ, Chen L, Konigsberg WH, and Bach R. Serum stimulation of quiescent human fibroblasts induces the synthesis of tissue factor mRNA followed by the appearance of tissue factor antigen and procoagulant activity. J Cell Physiol 1989; 139:418–423.

65. Gregory SA, Morrissey JH, Edgington TS. Regulation of tissue factor gene expression in the monocyte procoagulant response to endotoxin. Mol Cell Biol 1989; 9:2752–2755.

66. Schecter AD, Fallon JT, Thiruvikraman SV, Taby O, Rosenfield CL, Rossikhina M, Nemerson Y, Taubman MB. Delayed surface expression of active tissue factor in human arterial smooth muslce cells determined by a novel in situ activity assay. Circulation 92:1–804.

67. Kraiss LW, Raines EW, Wilcox J, Seifert RA, Barrett TB, Kirkman TR, Hart CE, Bowen-Pope DF, Ross R, Clowes AW, Kraiss LJ. Regional expression of platelet-derived growth factor and its receptors in a primate graft model of vessel wall assembly. J Clin Invest 1993; 92:338–348.

68. Mackman N, Morrissey JH, Fowler B, Edgington TS. Complete sequence of the human tissue factor gene, a highly regulated cellular receptor that initiates the coagulation protease cascade. Biochemistry 1989; 28:1755–1762.

69. Mackman N, Imes S, Maske WH, Taylor B, Lusis AJ, Drake TA. Structure of the murine tissue factor gene: chromosome location and conservation of regulatory elements in the promoter. Arterioscler Thromb 1992; 12:474–483.

70. Mackman N, Fowler BJ, Edgington TS, Morrissey JH. Functional analysis of the human tissue factor promoter and induction by serum. Proc Natl Acad Sci USA 1990; 87:2254–2258.

71. Cui MZ, Parry GCN, Edgington TS, Mackman N. Regulation of tissue factor gene expression in epithelial cells Induction by serum and phrobol 12-myristate 13-acetate. Arterioscler Thromb 1994; 14:807–814.

72. Mackman N, Brand K, Edgington TS. Lipopolysaccharide-mediated transcriptional activation of the human tissue factor gene in THP-1 monocytic cells requires both activator protein 1 and nuclear factor kB binding sites. J Exp Med 1991; 174:1517–1526.

73. Parry GC, Mackman N. Transcriptional regulation of tissue factor expression in human endothelial cells. Arterioscler Thromb 1995; 13:1711–1717.

74. Mackman N. Regulation of the tissue factor gene. FASEB J 1995; 9:883–889.

75. Collen D, Lijnen HR. Molecular basis of fibronolysis, as relevant for thrombolytic therapy. Thromb Haemost 1995; 74:167–171.

76. Verstraete M. The fibrinolytic system: from petri dishes to genetic engineering. Thromb Haemost 1995; 74:25–35.

77. Loskutoff DJ, Sawdey M, Keeton M, Schneiderman J. Regulation of PAI-1 gene expression in vivo. Thromb Haemost 1993; 70:135–137.

78. Juhan-Vague I, Alessi MC. Plasminogen activator inhibitor 1 and atherothrombosis. Thromb Haemost 1993; 70:138–143.

79. Krishnamurti CC, Carr F, Hassett MA, Young GD, Alving BM. Plasminogen activator inhibitor: a regulator of ancrod-induced fibrin deposition in rabbits. Blood 1987; 69:798–803.

80. Barbash GI, Hod H, Roth A, Miller HI, Rath S, Harzhahav Y, Modan M, Zivelin A, Laniado S, Seligsohn U. Correlation of baseline plasminogen activator inhibitor activity with patency of the infarct artery after thrombolytic therapy in acute myocardial infarction. Am J Cardiol 1989; 64:1231–1235.

81. Vaughan DE, Declerck PJ, Van Houtte E, De Mol M, Collen D. Reactivated recombinant plasminogen activator inhibitor 1 (rPAI-1) effectively prevents thrombolysis in vivo. Thromb Haemost 1992; 68:60–63.

82. Erickson LA, Fici GJ, Lund JE, Boyle TP, Polites HG, Marotti KR. Development of venous occlusions in mice transgenic for the plasminogen activator inhibitor 1 gene. Nature 1990; 346:74–76.

83. Schneiderman J, Sawdey MS, Keeton MR, Bordin GM, Bernstein EF, Dilley RB, Loskutoff DJ. Increased type I plasminogen activator inhibitor gene expression in atherosclerotic human arteries. Proc Natl Acad Sci USA 1992; 89:6998–7002.

84. Lupu F, Bergonzelli GE, Heim DA, Cousin E, Genton CY, Bachman F. Localization oand production of plasminogen activator inhibitor-1 in human healthy and atherosclerotic arteries. Arterioscler Thromb 1993; 13:1090–1100.

85. Chomiki N, Henry M, Alessi MC, Anfosso F, Juhan-Vague I. Plasminogen activator inhibitor-1 expression in human liver and healthy or atherosclerotic vessel walls. Thomb Haemost 1994; 72:44–53.

86. Aznar JA, Estelles A, Tormo G, Sapena P, Tormo V, Blanchn S, Espana F. Plasminogen activiator inhibitor activity and other fibrinolytic variables in patients with coronary artery disease. Br Heart J 1988; 59:535–541.

87. Etingin OR, Hajjar DP, Hajjar KA, Harpel PC, Nachman RL. Lipoprotein(a) regulates PAI-1 expression in endothelial cells. J Biol Chem 1991; 266:2459–2465.

88. Olofsson BO, Dahlen G, Nilsson TK. Evidence for increased levels of plasminogen activator inhibitor and tissue plasminogen activator in plasma of patients

with angiographically verified coronary artery disease. Eur Heart J 1989; 10:77–82.

89. Tipping PG, Davenport P, Gallicchil M, Filonzi EL, Apostolopoulos J, Wojta J. Atheromatous plaque macrophages produce plasminogen activator inhibitor type-1 and stimulate its production by endothelial cells and vascular smooth muscle cells. Am J Pathol 1993; 143:875–885.

90. Wojta J, Gallicchio M, Zoellner H, Hufnagl P, Last K, Filonzi EL, Binder BR, Hamilton JA, McGrath K. Thrombin stimulates expression of tissue-type plasminogen activator and plasminogen activator inhibitor type 1 in cultured human vascular smooth muscle cells. Thromb Haemost 1993; 70:469–474.

91. Noda-Heiny H, Fujii S, Sobel BE. Induction of vascular smooth muscle cell expression of plasminogen activator inhibitor-1 by thrombin. Circ Res 1993; 72:36–43.

92. Kruithof EKO, Vassalli JD, Schleuning WD, Mattaliano RJ, Bachmann F. Purification and characterization of plasminogen activator inhibitor from the histocytic lymphoma cell line U-937. J Biol Chem 1986; 261:11207–11213.

93. Bachmann F. The enigma PAI-2. Gene expression, evolutionary and functional aspects. Thromb Haemost 1995; 74:172–179.

94. Broze Jr GJ, Miletich JP. Isolation of the tissue factor inhibitor produced by HepG2 hepatoma cells. Proc Natl Acad Sci USA 1987; 84:1886–1890.

95. Rao LVM, Rapaport SI. Studies on the mechanism of inactivation of the extrinsic pathway of coagulation. Blood 1987; 69:645–651.

96. Broze Jr GJ, Girard TG, Novotny WF. Regulation of coagulation by a multivalent Kunitz-type inhibitor. Biochemistry 1990; 29:7539–7546.

97. Broze Jr GJ, Warrren LA, Novotny WF, Higuchi DA, Girard TG, Miletich JP. The lipoprotein-associated coagulation inhibitor that inhibits the factor VII-tissue factor complex also inhibits factor Xa: insight into its possible mechanism of action. Blood 1988; 71:335–343.

98. Bajaj MS, Kuppuswamy MN, Saito H, Spitzer SG, Bajaj SP. Cultured normal human hepatocytes do not synthesize lipoprotein-associated coagulation inhibitor: evidence that endothelium is the principal site of its synthesis. Proc Natl Acad Sci USA 1990; 87:8869–8873.

99. Werling RW, Zacharski LR, Kisiel W, Bajaj SP, Memoli VA, Rousseau SM. Distribution of tissue factor pathway inhibitor in normal and malignant human tissues. Thromb Haemost 1993; 69:366–369.

100. Holst J, Lindblad B, Bergqvist D, Nordfang O, Ostergaard PB, Petersen JG, Nielsen G, Hedner U. Antithrombotic effect of recombinant truncated tissue factor pathway inhibitor (TFPI1-161) in experimental venous thrombosis—a comparison with low molecular weight heparin. Thromb Haemost 1994; 71:214—219.

101. Oltrana L, Speidel CM, Recchia D, Abendschein DR. Inhibition of tissue factor-mediated thrombosis markedly attenuates stenosis after balloon-induced arterial injury in hyperlipidemic minipigs. Circulation 1994; 90:I–344.

102. Broze Jr GJ. Tissue factor pathway inhibitor. Thromb Haemost 1995; 74:90–93.

103. Fuster V, Dyken ML, Vokonas PS, Hennekens C. Aspirin as a therapeutic agent in cardiovascular disease. Circulation 1993; 87:659–675.

104. Goodnight SH. Antiplatelet therapy with aspirin: from clinical trials to practice. Thromb Haemost 1995; 74:401–415.
105. Underwood MJ, More RS. The aspirin papers. Br Med J 1994; 308:71–72.
106. Antiplatelet Trialists' Collaboration. Collaborative overview of randomised trials of antiplatelet therapy. I: prevention of death, myocardical infarction, and stroke by prolonged antiplatelet therapy in various categories of patients. Br Med J 1994; 308:81–106.
107. Coller BS, Anderson K, Weisman HF. New antiplatelet agents: platelet GPIIb/IIIa antagonists. Thromb Haemost 1995; 74:302–308.
108. EPIC Investigators. Use of a monoclonal antibody directed against the platelet glycoprotein IIb/IIIa receptor in high-risk coronary angioplasty. Am J Cardiol 1992; 330:956–961.
109. Topol EJ, Califf RM, Weisman HF, Ellis SG, Tcheng JE, Worley S, Ivanhoe R, George BS, Fintel D, Weston M, Sigmon K, Anderson KM, Lee KL, Willerson JT. Randomised trial of coronary intervention with antibody against platelet IIb/IIIa integrin for reduction of clinical restenosis: results at six months. Lancet 1994; 343:881–886.
110. Hirsh J, Siragusa S, Cosmi V, Ginsberg JS. Low molecular weight heparins (LMWH) in the treatment of patients with acute venous thromboembolism. Thromb Haemost 1995; 74:360–363.
111. Kakkar VV. Effectiveness and safety of low molecular weight heparins (LMWH) in the prevention of venous thromboembolism VTE). Thromb Haemost 1995; 74:364–368.
112. Altman R, Rouvier J, Gurfinkel E. Oral anticoagulant treatment with and without aspirin. Thromb Haemost 1995; 74:506–510.
113. Ansell JE. Oral anticoagulant therapy—50 years later. Arch Intern Med 1993; 153:586–596.
114. Hirsh J. Oral anticoagulant drugs. N Engl J Med 1991; 324:1865–1875.
115. Stone SR, Hofsteenge J. Kinetics of the inhibition of thrombin by hirudin. Biochem 1986; 25:4622–4628.
116. Markwardt F. Pharmacological approaches to thrombin regulation. Ann NY Acad Sci 1986; 485:204–214.
117. Heras M, Chesebro JH, Webster MWI, Mruk JS, Grill DE, Penny WJ, Bowie EJM, Badimon L, and Fuster V. Hirudin, heparin, and placebo during deep arterial injury in the pig: the in vivo role of thrombin in platelet-mediated thrombosis. Circulation 1991; 82:1476–1484.
118. Kelly AB, Marzec UM, Krupski W, Bass A, Cadroy Y, Hanson SR, Harker LA. Hirudin interruption of heparin-resistant arterial thrombus formation in baboons. Blood 1991; 77:1006–1012.
119. Callas D, Fareed J. Comparative pharmacology of site directed antithrombin agents. Implication in drug development. Thromb Haemost 1995; 74:473–481.
120. Turpie AGG, Weitz JI, Hirsch J. Advances in antithrombotic therapy: novel agents. Thromb Haemost 1995; 74:565–571.
121. Harker L, Hanson SR, Kelly AB. Antithrombotic benefits and hemorrhagic risks of direct thrombin antagonists. Thromb Haemost 1995; 74:4646–472.

122. Bock LC, Griffin LC, Latham JA, Vermaas EH, Toole JJ. Selection of single stranded DNA molecules that bind and inhibit human thrombin. Nature 1992; 355:564–566.

123. Li WX, Kaplan AV, Grant GW, Toole JJ, Leung LLK. A novel nucleotide-based thrombin inhibitor inhibits clot-bound thrombin and reduces arterial platelet thrombus formation. Blood 1994; 83:677–682.

124. Waxman L, Smith DE, Arcuri KE, Vlasuk GP. Tick anticoagulant peptide (TAP) is a novel inhibitor of blood coagulation factor Xa. Science 1990; 248:593–596.

125. Dunwiddie CT, Thornberry N, Bull H, Sardana M, Friedman P, Jacobs J, Simpson E. Antistasin, a leech-derived inhibitor of factor Xa: kinetic analysis of enayme inhibition and identification of the reactive site. J Biol Chem 1989; 264:16694–16699.

20

Regulation of the Production of Lipoproteins Containing Apolipoprotein B

Edward A. Fisher
Mount Sinai School of Medicine
New York, New York

Lipoproteins are macromolecular complexes that serve to transport water-insoluble lipids, such as triglycerides, cholesterol, and cholesteryl esters, in the plasma. The protein components of lipoproteins are mainly synthesized by the liver and intestine and are termed apoproteins (or, apolipoproteins [apo]). These include the well-known molecules apoAI and apoB, which are the major proteins of high- and low-density lipoproteins (HDL, LDL), respectively. The lipids are derived from both exogenous (dietary) and endogenous (primarily from hepatic synthesis) sources.

Although much at the molecular and physiological levels remains to be discovered about lipoprotein metabolism, a strong and consistent finding in epidemiological studies has been the positive correlation between the risk of coronary artery disease (CAD) and the plasma levels of either LDL-cholesterol (LDL-C) or apoB (e.g., see [1]). It is tempting to attribute this association to the simple fact that apoB is an integral component of LDL, the lipoprotein particle containing the bulk of cholesterol in the plasma, but statistical analysis has shown that the risk of CAD associated with the plasma level of apoB can be independent of LDL-C (2).

471

This direct relevance of apoB to CAD has been a strong stimulus for studies of the synthesis of apoB and its assembly into lipoprotein particles promoting atherosclerosis. Aided by powerful technological advances in cell and molecular biology, significant inroads into understanding apoB metabolism have been made. A review of the current state of knowledge in this area will first be preceded by a brief summary of lipoprotein metabolism to provide the context for the subsequent information.

REVIEW OF LIPOPROTEIN METABOLISM

Lipoprotein metabolism can be conveniently classified into two processes: those that involve the exogenous or endogenous lipids. A schematic diagram of this division is shown in Figure 1. The exogenous lipids are those derived from dietary sources, such as the cholesterol and fats (triglycerides) in food. The endogenous lipids are those synthesized by the liver and secreted as part of a lipoprotein particle. The processing of exogenous lipids begins in the intestinal lumen. Free cholesterol and lipid esters (such as triglycerides and cholesteryl esters) become complexed with bile acids to form mixed micelles. The lipid esters are hydrolyzed by pancreatic lipases and the resulting free cholesterol and free fatty acids are then absorbed by enterocytes. In the enterocyte, there is reesterification to form cholesteryl esters and triglycerides, which then associate with apoproteins (particularly apoB, the apoAs, and the apoCs) to form lipoprotein particles called chylomicrons, which on a dry weight basis are over 80% triglyceride (Table 1). The chylomicrons are secreted into the intestinal lymph and enter the systemic circulation by way of the thoracic duct. When the chylomicrons encounter lipoprotein lipase (LpL) bound to the endothelial surfaces of the capillary beds of muscle (including cardiac) and fat tissue, the triglycerides are hydrolyzed and the fatty acids enter the muscle cells or adipocytes, where they provide a direct energy source in muscle and a storage form of energy (after reesterification to triglyceride) in adipocytes. The remnant chylomicron, now depleted in triglyceride and relatively enriched in cholesteryl ester, can undergo a number of subsequent fates, including (a) removal from the plasma by the liver (as shown in Fig. 1), via the low-density lipoprotein receptor and low-density lipoprotein receptor-related protein, with the participation of cell-surface heparin sulfate proteoglycans (HSPGs) (3); or (b) entrapment in the subintimal space of arterial tissue and uptake by macrophages and smooth muscle cells (not shown in Fig. 1; reviewed in [4]). This possibility has led to the hypothesis that atherogenesis, a hallmark of which is the accumulation of cellular cholesteryl esters, has a postprandial component mediated by lipid delivery to macrophages and smooth muscle cells of the arterial wall by chylomicron remnants (4,5).

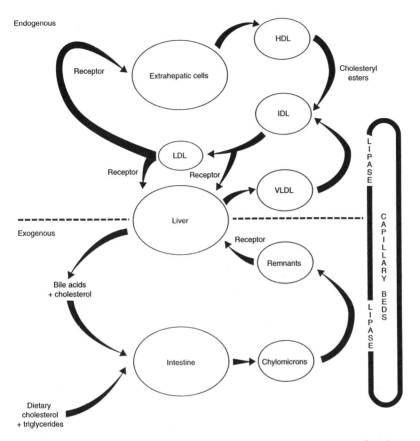

Figure 1 Human lipoprotein metabolism. Pathways for the transport of endogenous and exogenous lipids are summarized, emphasizing the central role of the liver. The details are described in the text. (Adapted from Ref. 62.)

Lipids synthesized by the liver (endogenous pathway) are assembled with apoproteins (particularly apoB) to form very-low-density lipoprotein (VLDL) particles, which are secreted into the space of Disse where they enter the circulation. There are a number of parallels between chylomicron and VLDL metabolism: VLDL are triglyceride rich (Table 1) and are acted on by endothelium-bound LpL to form remnant particles, shown in Figure 1 as IDL (intermediate-density lipoproteins). VLDL remnants can likewise be taken up by hepatic and nonhepatic cells, including those in vascular tissue. In addition, VLDL remnants can undergo an additional process: conversion to LDL, a process discussed later on. Note that under normal circumstances although the bulk

Table 1 Composition of the Lipoprotein Types in Percentage Dry Weight

	Chylomicrons	VLDL	LDL	HDL
Lipid constituents				
Unesterified cholesterol	1–3	4–8	6–8	3–5
Phospholipid	3–6	15–20	18–24	26–32
Esterified cholesterol	2–4	16–22	45–50	15–20
Triglyceride	80–95	45–65	4–8	2–7
Protein constituents				
Total protein	1–2	6–10	18–22	45–55
Apoproteins[a]				
AI	Major	Minor	Minor	Major
AII	Major	Minor	Minor	Major
AIV	Minor	Minor	Minor	Minor
B	Major	Major	Major	Minor
CI	Major	Major	Minor	Minor
CII	Major	Major	Minor	Minor
CIII	Major	Major	Minor	Minor
D	Unknown	Minor	Minor	Minor
E	Minor	Major	Minor	Minor

[a]Major refers to apoproteins making up 5% or more of total protein.
Source: Based on Refs. 39 and 62.

of plasma apoB is derived from the liver, LDL is not directly produced by the liver but is the end product of VLDL metabolism. In some pathological conditions, such as familial combined hyperlipidemia (FCHL), a genetic condition predisposing to premature CAD (6), there is some evidence for direct hepatic production of LDL-apoB as well as overproduction of VLDL-apoB (7, 8).

The other major lipid/lipoprotein pathway shown in Figure 1 involves HDL and has been termed *reverse cholesterol transport*. This refers to the presumed ability of HDL to accept cellular cholesterol from peripheral tissues and to transfer it to the liver either directly (by interacting with hepatic cells) or indirectly (by transferring cholesterol via cholesteryl ester transfer protein [CETP] to VLDL, IDL, or LDL particles that are eventually taken up by hepatic cells). The liver can then eliminate this cholesterol by direct secretion into the bile or by converting it to bile acids, which are then secreted. A recent finding with potential importance to the molecular mechanisms by which HDL interacts with cells is the report of an HDL-binding receptor, SR-B1, which turns out to be a member of the "scavenger receptor" family (the prototype of which is expressed in macrophages and binds native and modified apoB-containing lipoproteins) (9). SR-B1 is expressed mainly in liver, ovary, and adrenal gland. Intensive studies are in progress to define its physiological roles in both reverse cholesterol transport and the delivery of cholesterol as substrate for the steroidogenic pathways.

A simple generalization, then, is that apoB-containing lipoproteins serve as net suppliers of cholesterol from the diet and liver *to* most peripheral cells, with the undesirable potential to promote the cellular accumulation of cholesteryl esters, while HDL serves as a net carrier of cholesterol *away* from most peripheral cells to the liver, with the desirable potential to promote the elimination of cholesterol in bile. Thus, LDL-C and HDL-C have been dubbed *bad* and *good*, respectively, to reflect the direction the cholesterol is taking with regard to peripheral tissues. This directionality of cholesterol transport is thought to be the biological basis for the well-known positive and negative associations with the risk of CAD of LDL-C and HDL-C, respectively.

MOLECULAR BIOLOGY OF APOPROTEIN B

Gene and Transcription

ApoB is encoded by a gene of approximately 43 kbp located on chromosome 2. There are 29 exons and 28 introns, and the mature mRNA transcript is over 14 kb long. Tissue-specific expression in the liver and small intestine is primarily controlled by the interaction of multiple *trans*-acting proteins with DNA sequences between –128 and –52 (in reference to transcription start). The *trans*-acting factors include those found to be generally important (in that they are involved in the transcriptional regulation of many genes expressed in liver or intestine), such as C/EBP, or CCAAT enhancer-binding protein (10–12), as well as those with more specific regulatory effects (such as apolipoprotein factor-type 1 [AF-1;10]). There is also a more distal (–2 to –3 kb) "reducer" element, to which binds the *trans*-acting factor ARP-1, a negative regulator of apoAI transcription (13).

The above information was primarily obtained by the standard approach of transiently expressing in human hepatocarcinoma cells (HepG2) chimeric DNA fragments containing putative apoB promoter/enhancer sequences ligated to a reporter, such as chloramphenicol acyltransferase (CAT). By taking another approach, that of examining the chromatin structure of the apoB gene in HepG2 cells, regions within introns potentially involved in transcriptional regulation were identified. Subsequent testing of these regions in vitro, similar to the methods used above, led to the discovery and mapping of positive enhancer elements in introns 2 and 3 (14,15).

Most relevant to this chapter is the fact that in the majority of studies with animal and cell culture models, apoB transcriptional activity in either the liver or intestine is not particularly responsive to metabolic perturbations that significantly change the secretion of apoB-lipoproteins (16,17).

ApoB mRNA Processing

Certainly the most fascinating aspect of apoB gene expression is the tissue-specific editing of apoB mRNA (18,19). In this nuclear process, the C at position 6666 (of the over 14 kb transcript) is deaminated so that a CAA (glutamine) codon is converted to a UAA (translational stop) codon. This process in humans is confined to the small intestine, which explains why the apoB species associated with chylomicrons is shorter (dubbed apoB48 because it is 48% of full-length apoB) than the species synthesized by liver (dubbed apoB100 because it is 100% of full length). There are 4536 and 2152 amino acids in apoB100 and apoB48, respectively.

In all mammals examined to date, apoB48 is the predominant intestinal form, but in some animal species, such as the rat and mouse, there is also significant editing activity in liver, so that VLDL with either apoB48 or apoB100 is secreted. Only those VLDL with apoB100, however, are converted to LDL, so that hepatic editing activity is presently viewed as antiatherogenic by reducing the fraction of VLDL with apoB100, thereby decreasing the substrate for conversion to LDL.

The molecular basis of the editing process is under active investigation (20,21). The apoB mRNA *cis*-acting sequence surrounding the C at 6666 that confers specificity of the process has been narrowed down to the 26 base region 6662–6687 (22,23), which contains a "mooring" sequence in the 3'-portion. The mooring sequence is thought to be the site to which bind one or more *trans*-acting protein factors involved in the deamination. Three proteins related to editing have been purified. One is the cytidine deaminase that catalyzes the C to U conversion. It was initially called p27 (because it is approximately 27 kD) and is now referred to as apobec-1 (24). The other two are proteins of approximately 44 and 60 kD (p44, p60), which have no deaminase activity (25). Since apobec-1 does not bind particularly well to apoB mRNA, a simple model (Fig. 2) is that p44 and/or p60 bind to the mooring sequence and then through protein–protein interaction with apobec-1 the deaminating activity is positioned properly to act on the C at position 6666. There may well be other proteins besides p44 and p60 with functions "auxiliary" to that of apobec-1, based on a number of in vitro reconstitution experiments (26). Based on the HepG2 cell model, apparently human liver has some of these auxiliary factors but does not edit the apoB message because apobec-1 is not expressed (27). One way theorized to reduce LDL production in humans would be to express apobec-1 by liver-specific gene therapy.

ApoB mRNA Translation

Using the HepG2 model system, the time needed to translate the full-length message into apoB100 is approximately 14 min (28). The HepG2 apoB mRNA

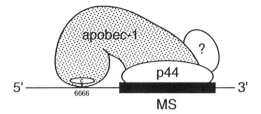

Figure 2 Model of apoB mRNA editing. The cytosine (C) at position 6666 is deaminated by apobec-1. Current information indicates that apobec-1 is properly positioned by protein–protein interactions with auxiliary proteins such as p44, p60, and others (?) that are bound to the mooring sequence (MS).

is relatively stable, with a half-life of approximately 16 h (29). In primary rat hepatocytes, the apoB mRNA is also relatively stable, with half lives for both the edited and unedited messages in excess of 9 h (Wang and Fisher, unpublished results).

The apoB mRNA in the actively translating pool (i.e., associated with ribosomes) is part of a polysome complex with unusual structural features as observed in ultracentrifugal sedimentation analysis of extracts derived from liver (rat, rabbit) and hepatic cells (HepG2, rat McA-RH7777) (30). The functional significance of these features is not known, but they may be involved in targeting apoB mRNA to areas of the endoplasmic reticulum (ER) specialized for the synthesis of apoB and its assembly into lipoproteins.

As noted earlier, apoB transcription (as assessed typically by apoB mRNA abundance) is not particularly responsive to metabolic perturbations and apoB mRNA is quite stable, but there are situations in which the synthesis or secretion of apoB varies. This implies the possibility of translational and posttranslational regulation of apoB metabolism. There is limited information available about translational regulation. The most complete study has been done in rats made diabetic by injection with streptozotocin (31). In spite of unchanged apoB mRNA levels in the livers of the diabetic animals, the synthetic rate of hepatic apoB was approximately one-third of that in the livers of control animals.

Translational control is exerted mainly at two steps: the initiation of the ribosomal-mRNA complex and the elongation of the nascent peptide. The percentage of apoB mRNA associated with ribosomes was equivalent in diabetic and control livers, implying that initiation was not affected. In contrast, the elongation rate of the nascent apoB protein was significantly slower in the diabetic group, based on measurements of the ribosomal half-transit times. It is known that a number of elongation factors are sensitive to modifications, such as phosphorylation, which, in turn, may have been altered in the diabetic state.

POSTTRANSLATIONAL REGULATION OF APOB PRODUCTION

The following section will discuss information thought to be primarily relevant to hepatic apoB metabolism. Although aspects of apoB metabolism are undoubtedly similar in liver and intestine, there is a much smaller body of information concerning the synthesis of intestinal apoB and its assembly into chylomicrons, for both historical and technical reasons. First, the liver has long been a focus for study because it is the source of the bulk of plasma apoB and, as indicated in Figure 1, it occupies a central position in the production and clearance of apoB-lipoproteins. Second, there is a relative deficiency of appropriate or convenient intestinal cell culture models. The interested reader is referred to a recent review (32) for a summary of current knowledge of intestinal apoB metabolism and chylomicron formation.

A diagrammatic representation of hepatic VLDL assembly is given in Figure 3. This model is based on the work of many investigators, whose contributions are summarized in a number of recent reviews (e.g., 16,17,33–35). Either cotranslationally or shortly after, nascent apoB associates with lipids, the bulk of which are triglycerides, but that also includes cholesteryl esters and phospholipids. These lipids are synthesized mainly by enzyme systems associated with the smooth ER and they must be transferred within the aqueous en-

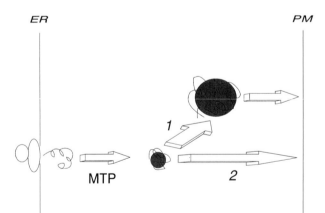

Figure 3 Assembly of apoB-lipoproteins in mammalian liver cells. ApoB mRNA is translated on ribosomes bound to the ER membrane. There is cotranslational complexing with lipids transferred by MTP to form a dense primordial lipoprotein. Arrow 1 indicates further lipidation and assembly with other apoproteins to form the mature lipoprotein particles secreted across the plasma membrane (PM). Arrow 2 indicates that in species that have hepatic apoB mRNA editing activity, such as rat and mouse, a fraction of the primordial lipoprotein particles containing apoB48 are not further lipidated, but are secreted as dense particles.

vironment of the ER lumen to apoB. This transfer is mediated by the microsomal triglyceride transfer protein (MTP). Despite its name, MTP can transfer all three lipid classes to apoB. The essential importance of MTP to apoB-lipoprotein assembly has been demonstrated by recent reports that MTP mutations underlie the genetic disease abetalipoproteinemia, which is characterized by the inability of the liver and the intestine to secrete VLDL and chylomicrons, respectively (36,37). The result of the initial MTP-mediated lipid transfer is a "primordial", relatively dense, lipoprotein containing one molecule of apoB. In subsequent steps, there is further addition of lipids and other VLDL components, such as apoE (but no more apoB), in processes that may not depend on MTP activity. Although primordial lipoprotein particles are formed in the ER, some of the full maturation of VLDL extends into the Golgi apparatus (33). Note in Figure 3 that some of the primordial apoB48-lipoproteins made in rodent liver are not further lipidated. Instead, they are secreted as particles significantly denser than VLDL.

Based on the above model, there are two simple ways in which the hepatic production of VLDL can be varied. One is by the composition of the lipoprotein particles; the other is by the number of particles. For example, the sucrose feeding of rats increases hepatic triglyceride (TG) synthesis and the VLDL that is secreted is enriched in that lipid (i.e., plasma VLDL-TG levels rise). A human equivalent of this phenomenon may be in persons with carbohydrate-sensitive type IV hyperlipidemia, characterized by hypertriglyceridemia responsive to reduction in dietary carbohydrate (38). Thus, the production of apoB can be independent of the lipids (mainly TG) associated with VLDL.

The other mode of regulating VLDL production (by varying particle number) has received considerable attention since this involves change in the hepatic secretion of the apoB that ultimately enters the LDL-apoB plasma pool, the size of which is correlated with CAD risk, as noted in the opening of this chapter. The central importance of apoB to VLDL metabolism is borne out by the fact that of the apoproteins associated with VLDL (Table 1) only apoB is absolutely required for VLDL secretion (39). Thus, apoB is both a prime determinant and an index of the number of VLDL particles secreted by the liver.

Although some evidence for regulating apoB secretion at the level of translation was cited earlier, the bulk of the data indicate that apoB secretion is primarily regulated at the posttranslational level by presecretory degradation. In other words, if the amount of apoB newly synthesized by a liver cell is compared to that secreted, there is a net loss of apoB. Depending on the experimental conditions and the model system employed, the degradation can remove from the secretory pathway as little as 10–20% (primary rat [40–42] or human hepatocytes [43] maintained in normal medium) to almost 90% (HepG2 cells deprived of fatty acids [44]) of the apoB, thereby decreasing apoB-containing lipoprotein production correspondingly. ApoB degradation can be further modulated, for example, by providing hepatic cells with insulin, n-3 fatty acids, or inhibitors of MTP. Despite the fact that these diverse treatments all promote apoB degradation, what is becoming increasingly clear is that various metabolic perturbations may exert their effects at different steps in the itinerary of an apoB molecule through the secretory pathway. Two steps having particular relevance to the degradation of apoB are reviewed below.

Regulation at the Translocational Level

ApoB degradation may be regulated as early as the translocation of the nascent protein across the membrane of the ER. Work primarily from the laboratory of Lingappa (45,46) has indicated that apoB may have domains containing *stop-pause* sequences, which result in a frequently interrupted threading of the protein into the ER lumen. This would likely facilitate the almost immediate association of critical domains of apoB with lipids as the nascent protein enters the ER environment (47). Apparently, if this initial complex is not rapidly formed, apoB conformation is not stabilized and degradation quickly ensues.

There is some controversy about the stop-pause hypothesis (see [48], for example), with opposing data supporting the hypothesis that the observed "jerky" nature of the threading of nascent apoB is not intrinsic to the translocation process, but reflects traditional "stuttering" due to the secondary structure of the apoB mRNA in certain regions. Nevertheless, the stop-pause hypothesis is more compatible with the finding of many groups (49–51) that a large fraction of newly synthesized apoB in liver cells appears to be on the cytosolic side of the ER membrane.

The above scenario suggests that the mechanism by which inhibition of MTP activity by mutations (i.e., abetalipoproteinemia) or pharmacological agents (under development in the pharmaceutical industry) decreases apoB secretion is an induction of degradation. The inability to transfer lipids to nascent, partially translocated, apoB would result in a prolonged translocational pause and the maintenance of a significant fraction of apoB on the cytosolic surface of the ER, subject to attack by proteases. Furthermore, the conformation of the partially translocated apoB that entered the ER lumen would not be stabilized and would be susceptible to ER-associated proteases. This model is supported by a number of studies in which apoB cDNAs were expressed in cell types that either contained or lacked MTP activity (52–54). In cells lacking MTP activity, apoB translocation was not successfully completed and the bulk of the newly synthesized apoB was degraded.

Regulation by Interference with Lipid Assembly

As noted above, if lipid is not transferred rapidly to an apoB molecule, degradation ensues. Besides the MTP-related studies, in which lipids may be available but cannot be transferred, there are also studies in which MTP activity is normal, but lipid synthesis is manipulated to make VLDL components such as triglyceride, cholesterol/cholesteryl ester, and phospholipid limiting (44,55,56). Although there is some controversy as to which lipid component plays the most important role in VLDL assembly, with most investigators favoring triglycerides, since it is the most abundant component (Table 1), the severe restriction of any of the lipids needed to form a VLDL particle has resulted in decreased apoB secretion, explainable by increased degradation in cases investigated by pulse-chase labeling techniques.

Given the information on apoB translocation, it would seem that the apoB degradation induced by lipid deprivation would occur at an early point in lipoprotein assembly. It is surprising that this has not always been found to be the case. For example, in the HepG2 system, restriction of triglyceride synthesis by depriving the cells of exogenous fatty acids does result in extremely rapid degradation of apoB (approximately 80% within 20 min [44]), so that in the deprived cells the ER content of apoB is quite low compared to that in the sufficient cells. In contrast, limiting phosphatidylcholine synthesis by making rat hepatocytes deficient in choline also promotes apoB degradation, but the ER levels of apoB in the deficient and sufficient cells are the same, implying that there is a post-ER process (57).

Not all of the metabolic factors that increase apoB degradation have been studied in sufficient detail to conclude exactly when and where in the secretory pathway they exert their effects, but of those that have been studied in depth, some clearly operate early (e.g., MTP inhibition, decreased triglyceride synthesis) and some later (e.g., choline deficiency and the provision of n-3 fatty acids). This suggests that the many steps involved in lipoprotein assembly, which requires multiple types of molecules (apoproteins, triglycerides, etc.) and two organelles (ER and Golgi), may afford numerous opportunities for metabolic factors and pharmacological agents to disrupt VLDL assembly and promote apoB degradation.

ApoB degradation, therefore, may occur before, during, or after a number of steps in the lipoprotein assembly/secretion process. Furthermore, if there has been sufficient maturation of the particles by the time degradation occurs, the secretion of other components of the nascent VLDL particle, such as the lipids and other apoproteins, will also be reduced. A diagram summarizing the relationships among apoB synthesis, VLDL assembly, and apoB degradation is shown in Figure 4. Note that the molecular nature of the degradative process

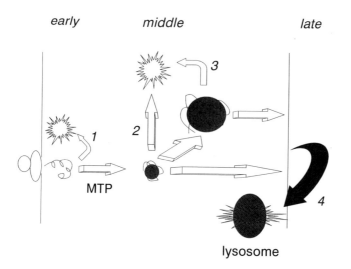

Figure 4   Relationship between hepatic apoB degradation and lipoprotein assembly. The basic scheme in Figure 3 is extended to show opportunities for apoB degradation during different points of the assembly process. Arrow 1 indicates that if MTP activity is inhibited or there is insufficient lipid for MTP to transfer to nascent apoB, the primordial lipoprotein may not form and apoB is rapidly degraded (as depicted by the explosive symbol). Arrow 2 indicates that if the pathway for the further processing of primordial lipoproteins is not completed, the immature particles may be shunted to degradation. Arrow 3 indicates that even after relatively complete maturation of a lipoprotein particle, there may be an identifiable feature, such as the acyl chain composition of the associated lipids, that can target it to degradation. Arrow 4 indicates the "reuptake" pathway for newly secreted lipoproteins, in which particles that encounter LDL receptors or specific proteoglycans on the cell surface before they can diffuse away are endocytosed and degraded in the lysosome. Thus, degradation occurring at early, middle, and late points in the itinerary of an apoB-lipoprotein constitute a "triple threat" to its ultimate appearance in the plasma.

is not indicated in Figure 4 nor discussed above. Only very preliminary data are available concerning the protease(s) degrading apoB in any of the model systems and metabolic treatments cited above. Lysosomal inhibitors, such as chloroquine, do not prevent apoB degradation of the type discussed above, but, in general, the agent ALLN does. Unfortunately, ALLN inhibits a wide variety of enzyme systems, such as the cysteine proteases and calpains, and it is too nonspecific an agent to identify either the major sites of apoB degradation or the particular protease or proteases involved. Studies underway in a number of laboratories are attempting to accomplish these important identifications.

Postsecretory Control

The above two sections are concerned with the presecretory control of hepatic apoB production. At least two postsecretory pathways can also influence plasma levels of apoB.

The first occurs at the cell surface. All cells have surrounding them an unstirred water layer that serves to retard diffusion of molecules away from the surface. It was shown that a fraction of the apoB-containing lipoproteins newly secreted by HepG2 cells could encounter an LDL receptor before diffusing away from the cell surface and be taken up by receptor-mediated endocytosis. This apoB would then be degraded in the lysosome and factors that upregulated hepatic LDL receptor activity would lead to an apparent net decrease in the production of apoB (58). This work was extended to show that another class of cell-surface molecules, the heparin sulfate proteoglycans (HSPG), could also serve to "capture" newly secreted apoB-containing lipoproteins (59). The clinical relevance of these findings in vitro is not established, but compatible with the reuptake process is the finding that hepatic overproduction of apoB in some individuals with FCHL can be reduced by treatment with agents that increase LDL receptor activity, such as the HMGCoA reductase inhibitors (7,8).

The other postsecretory process with the potential to regulate plasma levels of apoB is the conversion of VLDL remnants to LDL. Although the number and nature of the steps that accomplish this conversion are not well understood, it is thought to be achieved in the extracellular environment. Thus, variations in VLDL composition (to make it a better or worse substrate for enzymes, such as hepatic lipase, and other factors mediating the conversion) and in the activity of hepatic receptors that remove VLDL remnants from the circulation (such as the LDL receptor and possibly LRP), thereby removing convertible substrate from plasma, are thought to play important roles in determining the net amount of LDL produced from VLDL.

In abetalipoproteinemia, an experiment of nature provided insight into the role of MTP in the assembly of VLDL and chylomicrons. The understanding of the conversion of VLDL to LDL may likewise be served by the study of genetic variation. A large kindred has been reported in which some family members who have LDL receptor mutations are protected from hypercholesterolemia because of an inheritable decrease in the production of LDL. This genetic trait does not map to the known lipoprotein transport/processing genes, and most likely represents a mutation in a previously unknown factor critical in the conversion of VLDL to LDL (60). Work is underway to identify the molecular basis of the defect in this family. Accomplishing this goal will undoubtedly contribute to both fundamental knowledge and the development of novel therapeutic strategies to lower plasma LDL levels.

CONCLUSION: RELEVANCE TO HUMAN ATHEROGENESIS

The relationship between apoB-containing lipoproteins and atherogenesis is *direct*: they serve to deliver the cholesteryl esters that accumulate in the cells of the vascular wall. This direct relationship is consistent with the reproducible and strong epidemiological observations that plasma levels of apoB or LDL-C are correlated with CAD risk and the clinical observations that the accelerated atherogenesis in FH and FCHL is correlated with elevated plasma levels of apoB-lipoproteins. Not reviewed in this article are important *indirect* roles of apoB-lipoproteins: their ability to influence adversely signal transduction, cellular proliferation, and thrombosis in vascular tissue in ways that serve to promote lesion formation.

Not surprising, then, is that it is generally considered beneficial to reduce the plasma levels of apoB-lipoproteins. One well-known way is to increase their removal from plasma by the administration of HMGCoA reductase inhibitors, thereby increasing LDL receptor activity. Another strategy would be to lower the production of the apoB-lipoproteins. Niacin exerts, at least in part, its hypolipidemic effects in this manner, and preliminary evidence regarding MTP inhibitors indicate that they have the potential to do the same.

The exact mechanisms by which these agents decrease apoB production are not well understood. Given the evidence summarized in this chapter about the pivotal relationship between degradation and net production of apoB, many therapeutic agents, already in use or yet to be developed, may operate through this relationship. A more complete understanding of the ways in which different perturbations and treatments promote apoB degradation would be expected to reveal critical and regulatable steps of apoB-lipoprotein assembly and secretion, which could then be manipulated to decrease the level of atherogenic particles and retard the development of CAD in high-risk patients.

ACKNOWLEDGMENTS

I thank the researchers in my laboratory who through the years have contributed to the data and concepts presented in this article: Xiaoli Chen, Emma Kummrow, Deborah Mitchell, Charlotte Veloski, Hongxing Wang, and Shuyun Zhang. I also thank faculty colleagues, who, through collaborations and discussions, have also enriched my understanding of apoB metabolism: Fred Goldberg, Mahmood Hussain, Haris Jamil, Julian Marsh, Janet and Charles Sparks, Zemin Yao, and Kevin Jon Williams. Also appreciated is the editorial assistance of Jill Feltheimer Fisher.

Research from the author's laboratory was supported by grants from the National Institutes of Health (HL22633), the Howard Heinz Endowment, Council for Tobacco Research, and the W.W. Smith Charitable Trust.

REFERENCES

1. Anderson KM, Castelli WP, Levy D. Cholesterol and mortality: 30 years of follow-up from the Framingham Study. JAMA 1987; 257:2176-2180.
2. Breslow JL. Human apolipoprotein molecular biology and genetic variation. Annu Rev Biochem 1985; 54:699-727.
3. Ji Z-S, Fazio S, Lee Y-L, Mahley RW. Secretion-capture role for apolipoprotein E in remnant lipoprotein metabolism involving cell surface heparan sulfate proteoglycans. J Biol Chem 1994; 269:2764-2772.
4. Williams KJ, Tabas I. The response-to-retention hypothesis of early atherogenesis. Arterioscler Thromb 1995; 15:551-561.
5. Zilversmit DB. Atherogenesis: a post-prandial phenomenon. Circulation 1979; 60:473-485.
6. Goldstein JL, Schrott HG, Hazzard WR, Bierman EL, Motulsky AG. Hyperlipidemia in coronary heart disease. II. Genetic analysis of lipid levels in 176 families and delineation of a new inherited disorder, combined hyperlipidemia. J Clin Invest 1973; 52:1544-1568.
7. Arad Y, Ramakrishnan R, Ginsberg HN. Effects of lovastatin therapy on VLDL triglyceride metabolism in subjects with combined hyperlipidemia: evidence for reduced assembly and secretion of triglyceride-like lipoproteins. Metabolism 1992; 41:487-493.
8. Cortner JA, Bennett MJ, Le NA, Coates PM. The effect of lovastatin on VLDL apolipoprotein B production by the liver in familial combined hyperlipidemia. J Inher Metab Dis 1993; 16:127-134.
9. Acton S, Rigotti A, Landsculz KT, Xu S, Hobbs HH, Krieger M. Identification of scavenger receptor SR-BI as a high density lipoprotein receptor. Science 1996; 271:518-520.
10. Metzger S, Leff T, Breslow JL. Nuclear factors AF-1 and C/EBP bind to the human apoB gene promoter and modulate its transcriptional activity in hepatic cells. J Biol Chem 1990; 265:9978-9983.
11. Kardassis D, Zannis VI, Cladaras C. Organization of the regulatory elements and nuclear activities participating in the transcription of the human apolipoprotein B gene. J Biol Chem 1992; 267:2622-2632.
12. Carlsson P, Eriksson P, Bjursell G. Two nuclear proteins bind to the major positive element of the apolipoprotein B gene promoter. Gene 1990; 94:295-301.
13. Ladias JA, Karathanasis SK. Regulation of the apolipoprotein AI gene by ARP-1, a novel member of the steroid receptor superfamily. Science 1991; 251:561-565.
14. Levy-Wilson B, Fortier C. The limits of the DNase I-sensitive domain of the human apolipoprotein B gene coincide with the locations of chromosomal anchorage loops and define the 5' and 3' boundaries of the gene. J Biol Chem 1989; 264:21196-21204.
15. Levy-Wilson B, Fortier C, Blackhart BD, McCarthy BJ. DNase I- and micrococcal nuclease-hypersensitive sites in the human apolipoprotein B gene are tissue specific. Mol Cell Biol 1988; 8:71-80.

16. Yao Z, McLeod RS. Synthesis and secretion of hepatic apolipoprotein B-containing lipoproteins. Biochim Biophys Acta 1994; 1212:152–166.

17. Sparks JD, Sparks CE. Insulin regulation of triacylglycerol-rich lipoprotein synthesis and secretion. Biochim Biophys Acta 1994; 1215:9–32.

18. Chen SH, Habib G, Yang CY, Gu ZW, Lee BR, Weng SA, Silberman SR, Cai SJ, Deslypere JP, Rosseneu M, Gotto AM Jr, Li WH, Chan L. Apolipoprotein B-48 is the product of a messenger RNA with an organ-specific in-frame stop codon. Science 1987; 238:363–366.

19. Powell LM, Wallis SC, Pease RJ, Edwards YH, Knott TJ, Scott J. A novel form of tissue-specific RNA processing produces apolipoprotein-B48 in intestine. Cell 1987; 50:831–840.

20. Smith HC. Apolipoprotein B mRNA editing: the sequence to the event. Semin Cell Biol 1993; 4:267–278.

21. Chan L, Seeburg PH. RNA editing. Sci Med 1995; 68–80.

22. Shah RR, Knott TJ, Legros JE, Navaratnam N, Greeve JC, Scott J. Sequence requirements for the editing of apolipoprotein B mRNA. J Biol Chem 1991; 266:16301–16304.

23. Backus JW, Smith HC. Apolipoprotein B mRNA sequences 3' of the editing site are necessary and sufficient for editing and editosome assembly. Nucleic Acids Res 1991; 19:6781–6786.

24. Teng B, Burant CF, Davidson NO. Molecular cloning of an apolipoprotein B messenger RNA editing protein. Science 1993; 260:1816–1820.

25. Navaratnam N, Shah R, Patel D, Fay V, Scott J. Apolipoprotein B mRNA editing is associated with UV crosslinking of proteins to the editing site. Proc Natl Acad Sci USA 1993; 90:222–226.

26. Yamanaka S, Poksay KS, Balestra ME, Zeng GQ, Innerarity TL. Cloning and mutagenesis of the rabbit apoB mRNA editing protein. A zinc motif is essential for catalytic activity, and noncatalytic auxiliary factor(s) of the editing complex are widely distributed. J Biol Chem 1994; 269:21725–21734.

27. Giannoni F, Bonen DK, Funahashi T, Hadjiagapiou C, Burant CF, Davidson NO. Complementation of apolipoprotein B mRNA editing by human liver accompanied by secretion of apolipoprotein B48. J Biol Chem 1994; 269:5932–5936.

28. Boström K, Wettesten M, Borén J, Bondjers G, Wiklund O, Olofsson S-O. Pulse-chase studies of the synthesis and intracellular transport of apolipoprotein B-100 in HepG2 cells. J Biol Chem 1986; 261:13800–13806.

29. Pullinger CR, North JD, Teng BB, Rifici VA, Ronhild de Brito AE, Scott J. The apolipoprotein B gene is constitutively expressed in HepG2 cells: regulation of secretion by oleic acid, albumin, and insulin, and measurement of the mRNA half-life. J Lipid Res 1989; 30:1065–1077.

30. Chen X, Sparks JD, Yao Z, Fisher EA. Hepatic polysomes that contain apoprotein B mRNA have unusual physical properties. J Biol Chem 1993; 268:21007–21013.

31. Sparks JD, Zolfaghari R, Sparks CE, Smith HC, Fisher EA. Impaired hepatic apolipoprotein B and E translation in streptozotocin diabetic rats. J Clin Invest 1992; 89:1418–1430.

32. Hussain MM, Kancha RK, Zhou Z, Luchoomun J, Zu H, Bakillah A. Chylomi-

cron assembly and catabolism: role of apolipoproteins and receptors. Biochem Biophys Acta 1996; in press.

33. Vance JE, Vance DE. Lipoprotein assembly and secretion by hepatocytes. Annu Rev Nutr 1990; 10:337–356.

34. Innerarity TL, Borén J, Yamanaka S, Olofsson S-O. Biosynthesis of apolipoprotein B48-containing lipoproteins. J Biol Chem 1996; 271:2353–2356.

35. Dixon JL, Ginsberg HN. Regulation of hepatic secretion of apolipoprotein B-containing lipoproteins: information obtained from cultured liver cells. J Lipid Res 1993; 34:167–177.

36. Wetterau JR, Aggerbeck LP, Bouma ME, Eisenberg C, Munck A, Hermier M, Schmitz J, Gay G, Rader DJ, Gregg RE. Absence of microsomal triglyceride transfer protein in individuals with abetalipoproteinemia. Science 1993; 258:999–1001.

37. Sharp D, Blinderman L, Combs KA, Kienzle B, Ricci B, Wager-Smith K, Gill CM, Turck CW, Bouma M-E, Rader DJ, Aggerbeck LP, Gregg RE, Gordon DA, Wetterau JR. Cloning and gene defects in microsomal triglyceride transfer protein associated with abetalipoproteinaemia. Nature 1993; 365:65–69.

38. Jacobson MS. Atherosclerosis Prevention. Chur, Switzerland: Harwood Academic Publishers, 1991:42–44.

39. Gotto AM Jr, Pownall HJ, Havel RJ. Introduction to the plasma lipoproteins. Methods Enzymol 1986; 128:1–41.

40. Borchardt RA, Davis RA. Intrahepatic assembly of very low density lipoproteins. J Biol Chem 1987; 262:16394–16402.

41. Sparks JD, Sparks CE. Insulin modulation of hepatic synthesis and secretion of apolipoprotein B by rat hepatocytes. J Biol Chem 1990; 265:8854–8862.

42. Wang H, Chen X, Fisher EA. N-3 fatty acids stimulate intracellular degradation of apoprotein B in rat hepatocytes. J Clin Invest 1993; 91:1380–1389.

43. Edelstein C, Davidson NO, Scanu AM. Oleate stimulates the formation of triglyceride-rich particles containing apoB100-apo(a) in long-term primary cultures of human hepatocytes. Chem Phys Lipids 1994; 67/68:135–143.

44. Dixon JL, Furukawa S, Ginsberg HN. Oleate stimulates secretion of apolipoprotein B-containing lipoproteins from HepG2 cells by inhibiting early intracellular degradation of apolipoprotein B. J Biol Chem 1991; 266:5080–5086.

45. Chuck SL, Yao Z, Blackhart BD, McCarthy BJ, Lingappa VR. New variation on the translocation of proteins during early biogenesis of apolipoprotein B. Nature 1990; 346:382–385.

46. Chuck SL, Lingappa VR. Pause transfer: a topogenic sequence in apolipoprotein B mediates stopping and restarting of translocation. Cell 1992; 68:9–21.

47. Borén J, Rustaeus S, Olofsson S-O. Studies on the assembly of apolipoprotein B100 and B48-containing very low density lipoproteins in McA-RH7777 cells. J Biol Chem 1994; 41:25879–25888.

48. Pease RJ, Harrison GB, Scott J. Cotranslocational insertion of apolipoprotein B into the inner leaflet of the endoplasmic reticulum. Nature 1991; 353:448–450.

49. Davis RA, Thrift RN, Wu CC, Howell KE. Apolipoprotein B is both integrated into and translocated across the endoplasmic reticulum membrane. J Biol Chem 1990; 265:10005–10011.

50. Dixon JL, Du X. Differential immunocytochemical localization of epitopes of apolipoprotein B in the secretory pathway. Circulation 1995; 92:I-165 (abstr).

51. Boren J, Rustaeus S, Wettesten M, Andersson M, Wiklund A, Olofsson SO. Influence of triacylglycerol biosynthesis rate on the assembly of apoB100-containing lipoproteins in HepG2 cells. Arterioscler Thromb 1993; 13:1743–1754.

52. Thrift RN, Drisko J, Dueland S, Trawick JD, Davis RA. Translocation of apolipoprotein B across the endoplasmic reticulum is blocked in a nonhepatic cell line. Proc Natl Acad Sci USA 1992; 89:9161–9165.

53. Leiper JM, Bayliss JD, Pease RJ, Brett DJ, Scott J, Shoulders CC. Microsomal triglyceride transfer protein, the abetalipoproteinemia gene product, mediates the secretion of apolipoprotein B-containing lipoproteins from heterologous cells. J Biol Chem 1994; 269:21951–21954.

54. Gordon DA, Jamil H, Sharp D, Mullaney D, Yao Z, Gregg RE, Wetterau J. Secretion of apolipoprotein B-containing lipoproteins from HeLa cells is dependent on expression of the microsomal triglyceride transfer protein and is regulated by lipid availability. Proc Natl Acad Sci USA 1994; 91:7628–7632.

55. Yao Z, Vance DE. The active synthesis of phosphatidylcholine is required for very low density lipoprotein secretion from rat hepatocytes. J Biol Chem 1988; 263:2998–3004.

56. Cianflone KM, Yasruel Z, Rodriguez MA, Vas D, Sniderman AD. Regulation of apoB secretion from HepG2 cells: evidence for a critical role for cholesteryl ester synthesis in the response to a fatty acid challenge. J Lipid Res 1990; 31:2045–2055.

57. Verkade HJ, Fast DG, Rusiñol AE, Scraba DG, Vance DE. Impaired biosynthesis of phosphatidylcholine causes a decrease in the number of very low density lipoprotein particles in the Golgi but not in the endoplasmic reticulum of rat liver. J Biol Chem 1993; 268:24990–24996.

58. Williams KJ, Brocia RW, Fisher EA. The unstirred water layer as a site of control of apolipoprotein B secretion. J Biol Chem 1990; 265:16741–16744.

59. Williams KJ, Fless GM, Petrie KA, Snyder ML, Brocia RW, Swenson TL. Mechanisms by which lipoprotein lipase alters cellular metabolism of lipoprotein (a), low density lipoprotein, and nascent lipoproteins. J Biol Chem 1992; 267:13284–13292.

60. Vega GL, Hobbs HH, Grundy SM. Low density lipoprotein kinetics in a family having defective low density lipoprotein receptors in which hypercholesterolemia is suppressed. Arterioscler Thromb 1991; 11:578–585.

61. Gotto AM. Clinician's Manual on Hyperlipidemia. London: Science Press, 1991:6–8.

62. Scriver CR, Beaudet AL, Sly WS, Valle D. The Metabolic Basis of Inherited Disease. New York: McGraw-Hill, 1995:1839.

21

Platelets and Cardiovascular Disease

**Christine M. Grimaldi and
Deborah L. French**
*Mount Sinai School of Medicine
New York, New York*

Platelets play a key role in the development of the thrombotic complications of atherosclerotic cardiovascular disease. The primary role of platelets is to form thrombi at sites of vessel injury. In hemostasis and in the disease state, the formation of platelet aggregates on altered vascular surfaces are primarily responsible for the development of normal and pathological thrombi. The events associated with platelet thrombus formation include: (1) adherence of platelets to the site of vessel damage, (2) platelet shape change and release of granule contents, (3) activation-dependent binding of adhesive glycoproteins, and (4) fibrinogen- or von Willebrand factor–mediated platelet-platelet interactions that result in aggregate formation (1). Platelet adhesion and aggregation are mediated by a variety of platelet adhesion receptors (2–4). This chapter will discuss the biology of platelet function focusing on the biochemistry and function of platelet adhesion receptors. The platelet specific receptor, glycoprotein (GP) IIb/IIIa, will be emphasized and the recent advancements in the treatment of thrombotic vascular disease using anti-GPIIb/IIIa therapy will be discussed.

PLATELET ADHESION RECEPTORS

Membrane receptors expressed on the platelet surface are responsible for platelet adhesion to the subendothelial matrix and platelet aggregation at the site of the vascular injury. These receptors play key roles in initiating both physiological hemostasis and pathological thrombosis. The platelet adhesion receptors that will be discussed in this chapter are members of the integrin (5,6) and leucine-rich motif (4,7) families (Table 1).

Integrin Family of Receptors

The term integrin was coined by Richard Hynes in 1987 (5) to name a family of membrane receptors that integrated the cellular cytoskeleton with components of the extracellular matrix (ECM). These are the major receptors by which cells attach to the ECM. In addition, some integrin receptors mediate important cell-to-cell adhesion events (6) and some function in protein trafficking (8). These receptors are heterodimeric transmembrane molecules comprised of noncovalently associated α- and β-chains. Currently, 8 different β-chains and 14 different α-chains have been identified (5,6). Combinations of these polypeptide chains form up to 20 different receptors that are subgrouped according to their β-chains, designated β_1–β_8 (Fig. 1). Some β-chains can combine with multiple α-chains (e.g., $\alpha_1\beta_1$, $\alpha_2\beta_1$, $\alpha_3\beta_1$) and some α-chains can combine with multiple β-chains (e.g., $\alpha_v\beta_1$, $\alpha_v\beta_3$, $\alpha_v\beta_5$), but random association of all chains does not occur and some chains cannot interact with each other (e.g., $\alpha_{IIb}\beta_1$). Most cells express several integrin receptors and different types of cells express different repertoires of heterodimers.

Platelets express receptors from the β_1 and β_3 integrin subgroups. The β_1 integrin receptors are the largest subgroup of receptors and are expressed on most cells. These receptors mediate binding to ECM proteins including collagens, laminin, fibronectin, vitronectin, as well as the vascular cell adhesion molecule (VCAM-1). Platelets express three β_1 integrin receptors that can be utilized for platelet adhesion to the subendothelial matrix. These receptors and their ligands are $\alpha_2\beta_1$ (GPIa/IIa), which binds collagen; $\alpha_5\beta_1$ (GPIc*/IIa), which is the classic fibronectin receptor; and $\alpha_6\beta_1$ (GPIc/IIa), which binds laminin. Platelets express both members of the β_3 (GPIIIa) subgroup (9), in which the β_3 subunit associates with α_{IIb} (GPIIb) to form the $\alpha_{IIb}\beta_3$(GPIIb/IIIa) receptor (10) and with α_v to form the classic receptor for vitronectin, $\alpha_v\beta_3$ (11). The β_3 (GPIIIa) subunit is widely expressed in many cell types, but in normal tissue the expression of the α_{IIb} (GPIIb) subunit is restricted to the megakaryocyte cell lineage making the GPIIb/IIIa receptor platelet specific. The $\alpha_v\beta_3$ vitronectin receptor is expressed on endothelial cells, smooth muscle cells, osteoclasts, platelets, and a variety of normal and malignant cultured cells. The

Table 1 Platelet Receptors in Adhesion and Aggregation

Receptor family	Receptor names	Ligand(s)	Function	Surface number
Integrin	$\alpha_{IIb}\beta_3$, GPIIb/IIIa, CD41/CD61	Fibrinogen, von Willebrand factor, Fibronectin, Vitronectin	Aggregation and adhesion	80,000
	$\alpha_v\beta_3$, Vitronectin receptor, CD51/CD61	Vitronectin, Fibrinogen, Fibronectin, von Willebrand factor	Adhesion	50–100
	$\alpha_2\beta_1$, VLA-2, GPIa/IIa, CD49a/CD29	Collagen	Adhesion	< 1,000
	$\alpha_5\beta_1$, VLA-5, GPIc/IIa, CD49e/CD29	Fibronectin	Adhesion	< 1,000
	$\alpha_6\beta_1$, VLA-6, GPIc'/GPIIa, CD49f/CD29	Laminin	Adhesion	< 1,000
Leucine-rich motif	GPIb/IX, CD42b/CD42a	von Willebrand factor	Adhesion	25,000

GP = glycoprotein; CD = cluster determinant; VLA = very late antigen. Modified from Ref. 143.

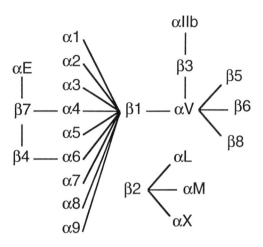

Figure 1   The integrin family of receptors. Integrin receptors are expressed as non-covalently associated, calcium-dependent heterodimers comprised of different α and β subunits. To date, 14 different α subunits and 8 different β subunits have been identified. A repertoire of more than 20 integrin receptors is generated by the combination of different α chains with a single β chain, and different β chains with a single α chain. (Reproduced from The Journal of Clinical Investigation 1991; 87:1–5 by copyright permission of the American Society for Clinical Investigation.)

amino acid sequences of the α_v and α_{IIb} subunits are homologous (6), and both the GPIIb/IIIa and vitronectin receptors exhibit promiscuous binding to fibrinogen, fibronectin, vitronectin, and von Willebrand factor (10,11). The GPIIb/IIIa complex is abundantly expressed on the platelet surface ($\sim 80,00$ molecules per platelet) (12), which probably arose due to the need for efficient and rapid platelet aggregation to arrest hemorrhage, whereas only 50–100 vitronectin receptors are expressed on the surface of platelets (13). Even though the β_3 integrins share similar ligand specificities, the vitronectin receptor probably does not play a major role in platelet physiology because so few receptors are expressed on the platelet surface.

Leucine-Rich Family of Receptors

Platelets express another receptor complex designated GPIb-IX, which mediates rapid attachment of unstimulated platelets to the subendothelial ECM of damaged vessels via recognition of von Willebrand factor (14). This event usually occurs under high shear conditions found in the microcirculation. The individual subunits of the receptor complex belong to the "leucine-rich family" of glycoproteins (7). The GPIb subunit is comprised of two covalently associated chains, a large α-chain of M_r 145,000 and a small β-chain of M_r 22,000.

This subunit is noncovalently associated with GPIX (M_r of 17,000) on the platelet surface and some, but not all of these complexes have been shown to associate with another glycoprotein of unknown function, GPV (M_r of 82,000) (15). GPIbα contains seven tandem leucine-rich repeats of 24 amino acids, GPIbβ and GPIX each contain a single leucine-rich sequence, and GPV contains as many as 15 leucine-rich sequences (14,15). The exact function of the leucine-rich regions is not known, but interactions that may affect structure and function of the receptor have been suggested (14). The binding site for von Willebrand factor has been localized to sites within the amino terminal end of the GPIbα chain (14).

PLATELET GPIIb/IIIa ($\alpha_{IIb}\beta_3$) RECEPTOR

GPIIb/IIIa was among the first receptors to be identified in the integrin family (16) and has served as a prototype for this family of receptors because of its early isolation (17) and the critical role of this receptor in response to thrombogenic stimuli (10). This receptor is important in platelet physiology and mediates interaction of activated platelets with ligands, including fibrinogen, von Willebrand factor, vitronectin, and fibronectin (10).

Biochemistry and Structure

The structural characteristics and functional domains of the GPIIb and GPIIIa polypeptides have been extensively studied (Fig. 2). Glycoprotein IIb is a 1008 amino acid polypeptide with an M_r of $\sim 140,000$ (1,10). Upon complete reduction of disulfide bonds, two GPIIb polypeptide chains are generated, designated GPIIbα (GPIIb heavy chain) (M_r 120,000) and GPIIbβ (GPIIb light chain) (M_r 23,000). These chains are covalently linked by a single disulfide bond (18). The GPIIbα chain is extracellular, and the GPIIbβ chain contains a small extracellular region, a single transmembrane-spanning domain, and a cytoplasmic tail consisting of 20 amino acids (19). Glycoprotein IIb is heavily glycosylated containing both N- and O-linked oligosaccharides (20). Four calcium-binding domains have been identified on GPIIbα that have homology to the calcium-binding motifs of calmodulin (21). These sites do not appear to be essential for heterodimer assembly but are required for transport of the assembled GPIIb/IIIa complex from the endoplasmic reticulum (ER) to the Golgi apparatus (22–25). Calcium ions are required for maintenance of the GPIIb/IIIa heterodimer and for optimal fibrinogen binding (26,27).

Glycoprotein IIIa is expressed as a 762 amino acid polypeptide with an M_r of $\sim 95,000$ under nonreducing conditions and $\sim 110,000$ under reducing conditions (1,10). As with GPIIb, GPIIIa has a large extracellular domain, a single

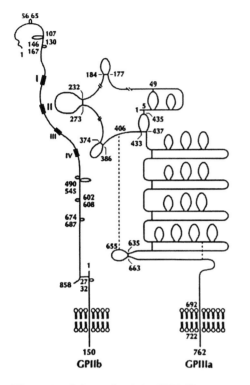

Figure 2 Schematic of the GPIIb/IIIa receptor. The GPIIb and GPIIIa polypeptides form the noncovalently associated GPIIb/IIIa receptor. Mature GPIIb has an M_r of 140,000 and is comprised of the BPIIbα (M_r 120,000) and GPIIbβ (M_r 23,000) subunits that are covalently linked via a single disulfide bond. Four regions with partial homology to the divalent cation binding motifs of calmodulin have been identified on the GPIIbα subunit (I–IV). GPIIIa is expressed as a single polypeptide chain with an M_r of 95,000. The GPIIb and GPIIIa polypeptides each contain a large extracellular domain, a single transmembrane spanning domain, and a short cytoplasmic tail. (Modified from Ref. 111.)

transmembrane-spanning domain, ad a cytoplasmic tail comprised of 41 amino acids. One striking feature of all β-subunits in the integrin family is the presence of highly conserved cysteine-rich regions (5,6). Glycoprotein IIIa contains 56 cysteines that form 28 disulfide bonds. Based on the complex disulfide-bond pattern proposed by Calvete et al. (28), GPIIIa can be subdivided into four separate domains: the proteinase-resistant N-terminal domain (amino acids 1–62); the adhesive protein-binding domain (amino acids 101–422); the cysteine-rich, proteinase-resistant core (amino acids 423–622); and the carboxyl-terminal domain consisting of the remaining residues in the extracellular, trans-membrane, and cytoplasmic domains. The cysteine-rich proteinase-resistant core appears to have no functional role in complex formation or fibrinogen binding, since a recombinant truncated GPIIIa fragment, devoid of this core region, forms stable heterodimers with GPIIb that are functional and bind fibrinogen (29). A putative metal-binding domain has been identified within the amino terminal region of the GPIIIa subunit (30). A site in this region bears resemblance to the metal ion-dependent adhesion sites in the leukocyte β_2 subgroup α subunits which contain an extra sequence of ~ 200 amino acids designated an I- or A-domain (5,6). This domain has unique Mg^{2+} binding properties and crystallization studies have demonstrated the contribution of this domain in ligand binding (31).

Biosynthesis of the GPIIb/IIIa Complex

The cDNA sequence for GPIIb was determined from RNA isolated from human erythroleukemia cells (HEL) (19) and the sequence for GPIIIa was determined from RNA isolated from HEL and endothelial cells (32,33). The full-length genomic sequences of GPIIb (34) and GPIIIa (35) have been determined and interestingly both genes are located on chromosome 17. The GPIIb gene spans ~ 17.2 kilobases (kb) and contains 30 exons (34), and the GPIIIa gene spans ~ 46 kb and contains 14 exons (35).

The biosynthetic and processing events required for the assembly of GPIIb/IIIa complexes have been studied in megakaryocytes (36), megakaryocytic cell lines (37), and transfected COS cells (38,39). Each gene is separately transcribed, in which GPIIb (~ 3.3 kb) and GPIIIa (~ 3.6 kb) transcripts are translated into nascent polypeptide chains (39). GPIIb is initially expressed as a single polypeptide precursor molecule of $M_r \sim 140,000$, designated proGPIIb, and GPIIIa is synthesized as a single molecule of $M_r \sim 95,000$ (40). Appropriate assembly and maturation of the GPIIb/IIIa complex only occur if both proteins are expressed and properly folded (36-40). Uncomplexed GPIIb and GPIIIa polypeptides are retained in the ER and eventually degraded. Properly assembled GPIIb/IIIa complexes are transported to the Golgi apparatus where proteolytic cleavage of proGPIIb is thought to be mediated by the serine proteinase furin or a furin-like protease (41). ProGPIIb undergoes proteolytic cleavage at arginine 859 (42), resulting in the generation of the $M_r \sim 120,000$ GPIIbα-chain and $M_r \sim 23,000$ GPIIbβ-chain that are covalently linked by a preformed intrachain disulfide bond (18). The analysis of metabolically labeled megakaryocytes and HEL cells demonstrated that expression of the mature, fully processed GPIIb/IIIa complex occurs within 4–5 hours and the half-life of uncomplexed single chains is approximately 8 hours (39). Once maturation of the GPIIb/IIIa complex is complete, the receptor is expressed on the cell surface in an "inactive" or "low affinity" conformation that requires activation for exposure of the ligand-recognition sites (43).

BIOLOGY OF PLATELET FUNCTION

Under normal circumstances, circulating platelets are in an inactive state and do not interact with the intact layer of endothelial cells that line the blood vessel wall. Tissue injury results in the exposure of subendothelial ECM proteins, such as collagen and von Willebrand factor, which are then made accessible to platelets. Rapid attachment of platelets to the subendothelium is mediated primarily through the GPIb receptor via the recognition of von Willebrand factor (14). Following adhesion of platelets to the subendothelium, a series of physiologic events occur that results in platelet activation (1,10). Activated platelets change shape from discs to irregular spiney spheres and components of the α-granules and dense bodies, such as calcium and the agonists adenosine diphosphate (ADP) and serotonin, are released. The agonist thromboxane A_2 is synthesized by platelets from arachidonic acid released from membrane phospholipids, and is released. During platelet activation, GPIIb/IIIa undergoes a conformational change that exposes ligand-recognition sites for soluble fibrinogen, fibronectin von Willebrand factor, and vitronectin. Despite the multiple ligand specificities exhibited by GPIIb/IIIa, the interactions that occur between GPIIb/IIIa and fibrinogen are by far the most important for the formation of in vitro platelet aggregates as detected by aggregometry (44). Under ex vivo flow, von Willebrand factor appears to play a more important role in platelet aggregation (45). A question that still requires resolution is the determination of the ligands that are most important in vivo.

Structure of Fibrinogen

Fibrinogen-mediated platelet aggregation plays a critical role in in vitro platelet aggregation and probably makes a major contribution to formation of a primary hemostatic plug at the site of vascular injury. The platelet aggregate also provides a surface for catalyzing the coagulation cascade, resulting in the formation of fibrin, which reinforces the initial thrombus (46,47). Fibrinogen is composed of three nonidentical subunits designated Aα, Bβ, and γ that are assembled as disulfide-linked heterodimers ($a\alpha_2B\beta_2\gamma_2$) with an M_r of $\sim 340,000$ (Fig. 3) (48,49). Each subunit is separately encoded by different genes located on chromosome 4 (50). Since the subunits of fibrinogen are arranged as dimers, the multivalent binding of fibrinogen to GPIIb/IIIa receptors on two adjacent platelets bridges between them (51), resulting in the growth of a platelet plug or thrombus.

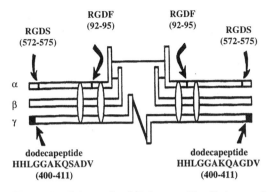

Figure 3 Schematic of fibrinogen. The fibrinogen heterodimer is composed of three nonidentical subunits designated Aα, Bβ, and γ. The Aα chain of fibrinogen contains two RGD-containing sequences; the amino terminus RGDF sequence is located between residues 92 and 95 and the carboxyl terminus RGDS sequence is located between residues 572 and 575. The dodecapeptide sequence, histidine–histidine–leucine–glycine–glycine–alanine–lysine–glutamine–alanine–glycine–aspartic acid–valine (HHLGGAKQAGDV) is located at the carboxyl terminus of the γ chain between residues 400 and 411. (Modified from Ref. 145.)

During coagulation, the fibrinogen is converted to fibrin by the enzyme thrombin. The Aα and Bβ subunits of fibrinogen are cleaved by thrombin to generate fibrin monomers, which spontaneously polymerize (52). The fibrin clot is strengthened by the crosslinking of fibrin by the transglutaminase factor XIII (53). The fibrinolytic enzyme plasmin, which is important for the dissolution of fibrin clots in vivo, degrades fibrin and fibrinogen into a number of fragments (54). The fibrinogen fragments produced by plasmin-degradation are designated X, Y, D, and E, and the generation of these fragments has been useful in the identification of regions of fibrinogen that interact with specific regions of GPIIIb/IIIa.

Fibrinogen and GPIIb/IIIa Recognition Sequences

Functional regions on GPIIb/IIIa and fibrinogen have been identified that appear to be important for fibrinogen-mediated platelet aggregation. Three recognition sequences of fibrinogen that have the potential to interact with GPIIb/IIIa include: a dodecapeptide sequence located at the extreme carboxyl terminus of the fibrinogen γ-chain (residues 400–411) (55), an arginine–glycine–aspartic acid–phenylalanine (RGDF) sequence located at the amino terminal region of the Aα-chain (residues 95–98) (56), and an arginine–glycine–aspartic acid–serine (RGDS) sequence located at the carboxyl terminus of the Aα-chain (residues 572–575) (56).

The docapeptide recognition sequence was identified from binding studies preformed using cyanogen bromide-generated fragments of the fibrinogen γ-chain. Initially, a 27 residue fragment located in the carboxyl-terminus of the fibrinogen γ-chain was identified that specifically bound to platelets (57). A smaller cleavage product of this fragment generated by staphylococcal protease restricted this region to a pentadecapeptide sequence (γ-chain residues 397–411) (58). Synthetic peptides generated from the pentadecapeptide sequence demonstrated that the minimal sequence required to inhibit ^{125}I-labeled fibrinogen binding to platelets effectively corresponded to residues 400–411 of the γ-chain (55). The minimal functional unit of the dodecapeptide sequence that can mediate partial inhibition is the lysine–glutamine–alanine–glycine–aspartic acid–valine (KQAGDV) sequence. The dodecapeptide sequence is exclusively expressed in fibrinogen and is not present in the other adhesive ligands that interact with GPIIb/IIIa.

The RGD recognition sequence was originally identified by fibroblast adhesion studies in the ECM protein fibronectin (59). RGD containing peptides corresponding to the two RGD sequences at residues 95–98 (RGDF) and 572–575 (RGDS) in the Aα chain of fibrinogen, have been shown to specifically bind to platelets and inhibit agonist-induced platelet aggregation (60). RGD containing peptides have also been shown to block the binding of platelets to soluble and immobilized fibrinogen (61–63). Since fibronectin, vitronectin, and von Willebrand factor contain RGD sequences, the promiscuous binding exhibited by GPIIb/IIIa is attributed to the recognition of this tripeptide sequence (64). Numerous studies have been performed to characterize the binding of GPIIb/IIIa to the RGD sequence. The ability of the RGD sequence to interact with resting and activated platelets was assessed with RGD peptides immobilized to polyacrylonitrile beads by variable numbers of glycine residues ([G_{1-19}]-RGDF) (65). The interaction of the RGD beads with activated platelets, resting platelets, and platelets that were inhibited with prostaglandin E_1 (PGE_1) improved as the length of the flexible glycine arm increased. Conversely, RGD beads containing only three glycine residues preferentially bound to activated platelets as opposed to resting or PGE_1-treated platelets (65). These data suggest that accessibility of the RGD sequence is an important factor for recognition of adhesive ligands.

Fibrinogen-binding Sites on GPIIb/IIIa

Binding sites for the fibrinogen γ chain dodecapeptide sequence have been identified on GPIIb/IIa. GPIIb residues 296–314 (66) and GPIIIa residues 274–368 (67) have been implicated as binding sites. Synthetic peptides and recombinant fragments corresponding to these regions inhibit soluble fibrinogen binding to GPIIb/IIIa and platelet aggregation. The binding of soluble fibrinogen to these sites on GPIIb/IIIa is inhibited by the addition of dodecapaptide or RGD-containing peptides. In addition to recognition of the fibrinogen dodecapeptide sequence, regions of the GPIIb/IIIa receptor that recognize the RGD sequence have also been identified. A region of GPIIIa including residues 109–171 was identified by chemical and photoaffinity cross-linking studies (68). A GPIIIa Asp119Trp point mutation, identified from a patient with Glanzmann thrombasthenia, impairs the ligand-binding function of GPIIb/IIIa (30). The binding of fibrinogen, fibronectin, and von Willebrand factor to the patient's platelets was negligible (69), and a lysate prepared from transiently transfected CHO cells expressing the Asp119Trp mutant GPIIb/IIIa receptor was unable to bind to an RGD-agarose affinity column (30). Another site between residues 212 and 222 of GPIIIa has also been shown to be important for ligand binding (70,71). Platelets from patients with Glanzmann thrombasthenia containing Arg214Trp, Arg214Gln, and Arg216Gln mutations in GPIIIa expressed surface receptors that were unable to bind soluble fibrinogen (72–75). Transfection studies of the Arg214Trp mutant demonstrated that cells expressing the mutant receptor did not adhere to immobilized fibrinogen (72). This region does not contain an RGD-binding site and has been proposed as a site involved in the maintenance of the tertiary structure of the neighboring RGD-binding site (76). Since the fine structure of the GPIIb/IIIa complex has not been determined by crystallography, the crucial residues involved in ligand binding have not been established.

PROPOSED MODELS FOR PLATELET AGGREGATION

An early model for platelet aggregation suggested that the two fibrinogen RGD-sites and γ-chain dodecapeptide sequence were required for multivalent binding to GPIIb/IIIa receptors (77). Examination of activated platelets by electron microscopy, however showed that the γ-chains of fibrinogen were accessible for interaction with GPIIb/IIIa receptors whereas the RGD sites in the Aα-chains of fibrinogen appeared to be inaccessible for binding (51). The use of an alternatively spliced form of fibrinogen, in which the dodecapeptide sequence is disrupted, showed that the dodecapeptide sequence was necessary for GPIIb/IIIa binding of soluble fibrinogen and platelet aggregation (78–80). Since this molecule contained two intact RGD sequences at residues 95–98 and 572–575 in the Aα-chain, these results suggested that these sites may not play a critical role in platelet adhesion and aggregation.

Unlike the binding of fibrinogen, the binding of fibronectin, von Willebrand factor, and vitronectin to GPIIb/IIIa is mediated by the RGD-recognition sequences (81). The identification of an RGD-binding site on GPIIIa that was different from the proposed dodecapeptide-binding site between residues 296 and 314 of GPIIb provided the basis for the initial hypothesis that the binding of the RGD and dodecapeptide sequences were not mutually exclusive. However, direct competition binding studies have demonstrated that the binding of the dodecapeptide can be inhibited by RGD peptides (82). Furthermore, the dodecapeptide sequence can inhibit the binding of von Willebrand factor and fibronectin to platelets, despite the absence of the dodecapeptide sequence in these adhesive molecules (82). The RGDF sequence at residues 95–97 in the Aα-chain resides in a "coiled coil" domain and may not be in a conformation that is accessible to GPIIb/IIIa (80). Removal of the carboxyl terminus of the fibrinogen Aα-chain by partial plasmin degradation results in the loss of the RGDS sequence at residues 572–574 (fibrinogen fragment X) but not the dodecapeptide sequence. Platelets adhere to microtiter wells coated with fragment X, whereas endothelial cells cannot adhere (11). The differential binding of platelets and endothelial cells to fragment X suggests that the RGD sequence is not required for platelet adhesion mediated by GPIIb/IIIa, but the binding of endothelial cells to fibrinogen via the vitronectin receptor ($\alpha_v\beta_3$) requires the RGD sequence located between residues 572–574 (11).

The role of platelet recognition of fibrinogen RGD sequences adhesion and aggregation is unclear. Even though the dodecapeptide is required for the recognition of fibrinogen by GPIIb/IIIa, it has been postulated that the binding of fibrinogen to platelets may be multiphasic and other interactions between ligand and receptor may occur (83,84). One proposed mechanism for ligand binding is that a single binding site on GPIIb/IIIa acts as a high-affinity ligand-docking site (84). Once initial contact is achieved, other ligand-binding sites with weaker affinities may contribute in a cooperative manner to increase the overall stability of the interaction between GPIIb/IIIa and fibrinogen. Sequential utilization of ligand-binding sites may account for the observation that fibrinogen binding to GPIIb/IIIa is initially reversible, but after 60 min becomes irreversible and insensitive to dissociation by EDTA (85). In this model, the dodecapeptide sequence may act as the high-affinity docking sequence required for initial contact, and recognition of RGD sequences may increase the binding avidity.

GPIIb/IIIa-MEDIATED PLATELET SPREADING AND PROTEIN TRAFFICKING

In addition to the critical role of GPIIb/IIIa ($\alpha_{IIb}\beta_3$) in platelet aggregation, this receptor is crucial for platelet spreading and protein trafficking (8,10,85,86). Platelet spreading occurs via the interaction of GPIIb/IIIa ($\alpha_{IIb}\beta_3$) with adhesive glycoproteins in the subendothelial matrix. Resting platelets can adhere to immobilized fibrinogen on the vascular matrix via their GPIIb/IIIa ($\alpha_{IIb}\beta_3$) receptors after initial contact is established through the platelet GPIb-IX receptor with von Willebrand factor (1,14). Once initial contact is established, the platelets are activated and spread in a process that is dependent on GPIIb/IIIa ($\alpha_{IIb}\beta_3$). Platelet spreading is associated with extensive cytoskeletal reorganization and the appearance of membrane-based structures analogous to focal adhesions (87).

The GPIIb/IIIa ($\alpha_{IIb}\beta_3$) receptor also functions in protein trafficking (8) in the transport of plasma fibrinogen into the platelet α-granules where it is concentrated. A number of integrin receptors circulate to and from the plasma membrane (5,6) and GPIIb/IIIa ($\alpha_{IIb}\beta_3$) can move from the plasma membrane to the α-granules carrying molecules of plasma fibrinogen (88,89). Platelet α-granules contain factors that are involved in platelet activation and coagulation (1). Fibrinogen comprises 10% of the protein content found in α-granules (1). Since megakaryocytes do not synthesize fibrinogen, it has been proposed that plasma fibrinogen is internalized into α-granules by endocytosis (89). Studies performed with the snake venom GPIIb/IIIa antagonists termed "disintegrins" demonstrated that the endocytosis of plasma fibrinogen is mediated by the GPIIb/IIIa receptor (89–91). The involvement of GPIIb/IIIa for the internalization of plasma fibrinogen is strengthened by the observation that patients with Glanzmann thrombasthenia typically have markedly reduced platelet fibrinogen in their α-granules (92). The internalization of plasma fibrinogen appears to be mediated by an actively cycling pool of GPIIb/IIIa receptors that translocate to the α-granule membrane upon endocytosis (90,91). Since the fibrinogen γ-chain variant that contains a disrupted dodecapeptide sequence and comprises 10% of total plasma fibrinogen has not been detected in platelet α-granules, the dodecapeptide sequence appears to be required for endocytosis (93). The role of platelet fibrinogen may be to mediate platelet aggregation by increasing the local concentration of fibrinogen at the site of injury.

Evidence has been presented suggesting that GPIIb/IIIa-mediated uptake of fibrinogen does not require receptor activation (89,90). Studies performed on unstimulated platelets with the snake venom disintegrin, applaggin, demonstrated that endocytosis of plasma fibrinogen occurs in an activation-independent manner that does not require exposure of high-affinity ligand-binding sites on GPIIb/IIIa (91). Resting platelets can adhere to immobilized fibrinogen (81,94), raising the possibility that the interactions required for the binding of resting platelets to immobilized fibrinogen may be similar to the interactions for the activation-independent uptake of fibrinogen by GPIIb/IIIa. The adhesion of resting platelets to immobilized fibrinogen may be due to low affinity interactions with GPIIb/IIIa or to the exposure of fibrinogen neoepitopes due to immobilization on a surface (81,83,85). Another possibility is that a small number of GPIIb/IIIa receptors with ligand-binding sites in a high-affinity binding conformation exist on the cell surface.

ACTIVATION OF GPIIb/IIIa RECEPTORS

The activation of the GPIIb/IIIa ($\alpha_{IIb}\beta_3$) receptor occupies a central role in platelet physiology (1,95). On resting platelets, this receptor does not bind fibrinogen with high affinity and platelet aggregation does not occur. Following platelet activation by a variety of physiologic agonists including thrombin, thromboxane A_2, and epinephrine, GPIIb/IIIa appears to undergo a conformational change resulting in the exposure of ligand-binding sites. The evidence for this event is as follows: (1) a complex-dependent mAb, PAC-1, binds to GPIIb/IIIa on activated, but not resting platelets (96); (2) following platelet activation, the on-rate of the complex-dependent mAb, 7E3 (which binds to GPIIb/IIIa on both resting and activated platelets and inhibits platelet adhesion and aggregation) increases threefold, indicating that the 7E3 epitope becomes more accessible (97); and (3) a change in orientation of the extracellular domains of GPIIb/IIIa receptors has been detected by fluorescence resonance energy transfer studies (98).

The signal transduction events induced by agonist stimulation that modulate the affinity of GPIIb/IIIa are known as "inside-out" signaling (95,99). Many agonists bind to specific G protein–coupled receptors expressed on the surface of platelets and activate signaling pathways. These pathways result in GTP-binding protein and serine-threonine kinase activation, increased phospholipid metabolism, tyrosine phosphorylation, and changes in intracellular calcium concentrations and pH. The cytoplasmic domains of GPIIb and GPIIIa appear to play a role in modulating the conformation of GPIIb/IIIa after agonist stimulation (43,100,101). The domains are small and do not contain catalytic sites, but the ability of the GPIIb and GPIIIa cytoplasmic domains to mediate inside-out signaling was demonstrated by expression studies performed in CHO cells (100). Deletion of a highly conserved amino acid motif, glycine–phenylalanine-phenylalanine–lysine–arginine (GFFKR), in the cytoplasmic domain of GPIIb resulted in the expression of GPIIb/IIIa receptors that constitutively bound soluble fibrinogen and the activation dependent mAb PAC-1. Charged residues in the cytoplasmic domains of GPIIb and GPIIIa may form a salt bridge that keeps GPIIb/IIIa in a default, low-affinity binding conformation (95,102). This "broken hinge" model (102) suggests that disruption of the interactions between the GPIIb and GPIIIa cytoplasmic tails may regulate the induction of a high-affinity ligand-binding conformation of GPIIb/IIIa (103).

The binding of fibrinogen to activated GPIIb/IIIa receptors results in additional events termed "outside-in" signaling (95). Ligand-occupancy of the GPIIb/IIIa receptor is necessary for platelet aggregation. This binding interaction also results in the oligomerization of GPIIb/IIIa receptors and the localization of clustered receptors to focal adhesion plaques (104,105). The cytoplasmic tail of GPIIIa mediates binding to cytoskeletal proteins, such as talin and α-actinin (106). This results in the reorganization of actin filaments, which may strengthen adhesion. Several tyrosine kinases are found in association with the focal adhesion plaques, such as focal adhesion kinase (pp125[fak]), pp60[c-src], and pp75[syk] (107). Activation and phosphorylation of these tyrosine kinases results in the rapid phosphorylation of multiple substrates that may be involved in the events of platelet adhesion and aggregation.

GPIIIa ALLOANTIGEN IN CARDIOVASCULAR DISEASE

The GPIIb/IIIa receptor is a major target for antiplatelet antibodies responsible for immune-mediated thrombocytopenias (108). Polymorphisms within both subunits constitute well-defined diallelic alloantigen systems that give rise to neonatal alloimmune thrombocytopenia purpura (NAITP) and post-transfusion purpura (PTP). The most frequently encountered alloantigen is the human platelet antigen (HPA)-1 system (also designated P1[A]) (108). This polymorphism results from a T to C base change in GPIIIa exon 2 resulting in a Leu33Pro substitution in the amino terminal end of the polypeptide chain. The allele expressing Leu33 is designated HPA-1a and the allele expressing Pro33 is designated HPA-1b. In Caucasians, the phenotype frequency for HPA-1a is 97.9% and for HPA-1b it is 26.5% (108). The HPA-1 alloantigen system has recently been implicated as a risk factor for patients with premature cardiovascular disease in which the patient population at risk more commonly expresses the HPA-1b phenotype (109). The expression of a proline residue at this site affects the three-dimensional structure of the receptor complex, but no specific functional mechanism has been described that would explain the predisposition to vascular disease.

GLANZMANN THROMBASTHENIA

The role of the GPIIb/IIIa ($\alpha_{IIb}\beta_3$) receptor in platelet aggregation was elucidated by characterization of the naturally occurring inherited mutations in patients with the bleeding disorder Glanzmann thrombasthenia (110,111). This rare, inherited recessive bleeding disorder is characterized by a quantitative or qualitative abnormality of GPIIb (α_{IIb}) or GPIIIa (β_3). Patients with Glanzmann thrombasthenia have a lifelong bleeding diathesis characterized by mucocutaneous bleeding, defective clot retraction, absence of platelet adherence to and spreading on glass, and absence of platelet aggregation in response to physiologic agonists (110,111). These patients rarely experience spontaneous central nervous hemorrhage despite their having markedly prolonged bleeding times throughout their lives (110). The dysfunctional GPIIb/IIIa ($\alpha_{IIb}\beta_3$) receptor can be either absent or present on the platelet surface but the platelets of all patients with Glanzmann thrombasthenia are functionally abnormal in that they do not aggregate in response to physiologic agonists such as ADP, thrombin, or epinephrine.

The identification of the genes encoding GPIIb and GPIIIa enabled determination of the molecular defects causing Glanzmann thrombasthenia. Among the first mutations that were identified at the molecular level were in Iraqi-Jewish and Arab populations in Israel (112). An 11 base pair deletion within exon XII of the GPIIIa gene was found in the Iraqi-Jewish population and a 13 base pair deletion, including a splice acceptor site, in exon IV of the GPIIb gene in the Arab population were identified. Both of these mutations affect biosynthesis of the GPIIb/IIIa complex resulting in greatly reduced surface expression. The platelets from these two patient populations were utilized in another study that identified a quick way of determining if mutations were present in the gene encoding GPIIb or GPIIIa (13). This study took advantage of the fact that platelets also express $\alpha_v\beta_3$ vitronectin receptors that utilize the same β_3-chain as GPIIb/IIIa ($\alpha_{IIb}\beta_3$). Patients lacking both GPIIb/IIIa ($\alpha_{IIb}\beta_3$) and $\alpha_v\beta_3$ receptors have defects in GPIIIa (β_3), whereas patients who lack GPIIb/IIIa ($\alpha_{IIb}\beta_3$) but have $\alpha_v\beta_3$ vitronectin receptors have defects in GPIIb (α_{IIb}). In recent years, 17 GPIIb (α_{IIb}) and 15 GPIIIa (β_3) (22–25,30,72–75,112–132) genetic defects responsible for Glanzmann thrombasthenia have been identified. Missense and nonsense mutations, deletions, and insertions in exons and introns have been identified, as well as mutations in splice acceptor and splice donor sites. The correlation of the phenotype of the disease with the identification of the genotype has provided important insights into the biogenesis of the subunits and the ligand-binding properties of the receptor. This disease provides a paradigm for the inhibition of GPIIb/IIIa ($\alpha_{IIb}\beta_3$) receptors in cardiovascular disease by pharmacologic agents (133,134).

INHIBITORS OF THE GPIIb/IIIa ($\alpha_{IIb}\beta_3$) RECEPTOR

Due to the key role of platelets in thrombus formation (135), inhibition of platelet aggregation is a natural target for antithrombotic therapy. In particular, therapy targeting the GPIIb/IIIa ($\alpha_{IIb}\beta_3$) receptor is attractive since (1) the receptor is platelet specific (1,10), (2) all physiologic agonists activate the receptor by generating a high-affinity ligand conformation (1,10), (3) platelet adhesion remains intact after selective blockade of the receptor, thus allowing some contribution to hemostasis without causing vaso-occlusion (134); and (4) patients with Glanzmann thrombasthenia who lack functional receptors have moderate to severe mucocutaneous hemorrhage, but rarely experience spontaneous central nervous bleeding (110).

The clinical benefit of platelet-inhibitor therapy in patients with ischemic heart disease was proved with aspirin (134). The use of aspirin, however, is limited because only one pathway of platelet activation, thromboxane-A_2-mediated platelet aggregation, is blocked. New drugs that inhibit fibrinogen binding to GPIIb/IIIa ($\alpha_{IIb}\beta_3$) receptors are being developed (133,134). These drugs inhibit platelet aggregation irrespective of the activation pathway of the receptor complex. Anti-GPIIb/IIIa murine mAbs inhibit the in vitro biding of fibrinogen to platelets and inhibit platelet aggregation (136). One such anti-GPIIb/IIIa antibody, designated 7E3 (97), was designed as a therapeutic agent in which a chimeric Fab fragment (c7E3) was created by molecular techniques (137). This fragment contains the original murine variable region domain (antigen-binding portion of the antibody molecule) and the first constant region domain of a human antibody. The Fc portion of the murine antibody was removed for in vivo studies to decrease the likelihood of clearance of antibody-coated platelets from the circulation by macrophages bearing Fc receptors (136,137). In addition to anti-GPIIb/IIIa function, the 7E3 antibody inhibits the function of the $\alpha_v\beta_3$ vitronectin receptor (13). The c7E3 antibody is a potent inhibitor of platelet aggregation in vitro and in vivo, with almost complete inhibition of aggregation when $\geq 80\%$ of the receptors are blocked (136).

Animal studies using c7E3 demonstrated inhibition of platelet thrombus formation while platelet adhesion remained relatively intact (136,138). These studies led to the Phase III Evaluation of c7E3 for the Prevention of Ischemic Complications (EPIC) trial (139). In this double-blind trial, patients undergoing coronary angioplasty or atherectomy, and at high risk of suffering an ischemic complication, were eligible for the study. All patients received standard medical therapy including aspirin and high-dose heparin. Patients were randomized to receive a bolus injection of c7E3, a bolus injection of antibody followed by a 12-hour infusion, or placebo. The primary endpoint of the study, monitored within 30 days, was death, myocardial infarction, or urgent intervention including repeat atherectomy, bypass surgery, stent replacement, or balloon pump insertion. The results of the study showed that the group receiving a bolus administration of c7E3 followed by a 12-hour infusion had 35% fewer adverse events. Patients enrolled in this study were followed for six months with a modified endpoint including death, myocardial infarction, and all revascularization procedures (140). The decrease in ischemic events and revascular procedures of the bolus plus infusion group was sustained throughout the entire six month period. The results of this study provided strong support for the hypotheses that (1) GPIIb/IIIa receptor inhibition is more effective that aspirin in preventing platelet thrombi, and (2) platelet-dependent thrombi are major contributors to ischemic heart disease.

In the EPIC study, heparin was not weight adjusted and bleeding events were more common in the c7E3-treated group than in the control group (139). An analysis of these events indicated a relationship between bleeding risk and the dose of heparin administered per kilogram of body weight. Follow-up studies using lower doses of heparin and weight adjustment of doses demonstrated a dramatic reduction in major bleeding in 7E3-treated patients (141). Additional trials are being analyzed to assess whether the drug will benefit all patients undergoing coronary angioplasty or atherectomy and patients with unstable angina who are candidates for coronary angioplasty or atherectomy (142). A number of peptide and nonpeptide inhibitors of GPIIb/IIIa patterned after the RGD recognition sequence, some of which are orally active, are currently under study and some have been tested in large Phase III studies with promising results. In conclusion, the use of c7E3 as anti-GPIIb/IIIa therapy has been shown to be protective against ischemic complications following coronary angioplasty or atherectomy in human patients. This drug is the first antiplatelet agent of proved efficacy that was developed from the advancements in our understanding of platelet physiology. The studies demonstrate the beneficial effect of anti-GPIIb/IIIa therapy and provide the basis for the continued development of antiplatelet therapy for the treatment and prevention of thrombotic vascular disease.

REFERENCES

1. Ware AJ, Coller BS. Platelet morphology, biochemistry, and function. In: Beutler E, Lichtman MA, Coller BS, Kipps TJ, eds. Williams hematology, 5th ed. New York: McGraw-Hill, 1995:1161–1201.
2. Yangsoo J, Lincoff AM, Plow EF, Topol EJ. Cell adhesion molecules in coronary artery disease. J Am Coll of Cardiol 1994; 24:1591–1601.
3. Peerschke, EIB. Platelet glycoproteins. Functional characterization and clinical applications. Am J Clin Pathol 1992; 98:455–463.
4. Nurden AT. Polymorphisms of human platelet membrane glycoproteins: Structure and clinical significance. Thromb Haemostas 1995; 74:345–351.
5. Hynes RO. Integrins: a family of cell surface receptors. Cell 1987; 48:549–554.
6. Hynes RO. Integrins: Versatility, modulation, and signaling in cell adhesion. Cell 1992; 69:11–25.
7. Takahashi N, Takahashi Y, Putnam FW. Periodicity of leucine and tandem repetition of a 24-amino acid segment in the primary structure of leucinerich α_2-glycoprotein of human serum. Proc Natl Acad Sci USA 1985; 82:1906–1910.
8. Coller BS, Seligsohn U, West SM, Scudder LE, Norton KJ. Platelet fibrinogen and vitronectin in Glanzmann thrombasthenia: Evidence consistent with specific roles for glycoprotein IIb/IIIa and and $\alpha_v\beta_3$ integrins in platelet protein trafficking. Blood 1991; 78:2603–2610.
9. Ginsberg MH, Loftus JC, Plow EF. Cytoadhesins, integrins, and platelets. Thromb Haemostas 1988; 59:1–6.
10. Phillips DR, Charo IF, Parise LV, Fitzgerald LA. The platelet membrane glycoprotein IIb-IIIa complex. Blood 1988; 71:831–843.
11. Cheresh DA, Berliner SA, Vincente V, and Ruggeri ZM. Recognition of distinct adhesive sites on fibrinogen by related integrins on platelets and endothelial cells. Cell 1989; 58:945–953.

12. Wagner CL, Mascelli MA, Neblock DS, Weisman HF, Coller BS, Jordan RE. Analysis of GPIIb/IIIa receptor number by quantitation of 7E3 binding to human platelets. Blood 1996; 88:907–914.

13. Coller BS, Cheresh DA, Asch E, Seligsohn U. Platelet vitronectin receptor expression differentiates Iraqi-Jewish from Arab patients with Glanzmann thrombasthenia. Blood 1991; 77:75–83.

14. Roth GJ. Developing relationships: Arterial platelet adhesion, glycoprotein Ib, and leucine-rich glycoproteins. Blood 1991; 77:5–19.

15. Modderman PW, Admiraal LG, Sonnenberg A, von dem Borne AEGKr. Glycoproteins V and Ib-IX form a noncovalent complex in the platelet membrane. J Biol Chem 1992; 267:364–369.

16. Nurden AT, Caen JP. An abnormal platelet glycoprotein pattern in three cases of Glanzmann's thrombasthenia. Br J Haematol 1974; 28:253–260.

17. Jennings LK, Phillips DR. Purification of glycoproteins IIb and III from human platelet plasma membranes and characterization of a calcium-dependent glycoprotein IIb-III complex. J Biol Chem 1982; 257:10458–10466.

18. Phillips DR, Agin PP. Platelet plasma membrane glycoproteins: Evidence for the presence of nonequivalent disulfide bonds using nonreduced-reduced two-dimensional gel electrophoresis. J Biol Chem 1977; 252:2121–2126.

19. Poncz M, Eisman R, Heidenreich R, Silver SM, Vilaire G, Surrey S, Schwartz E, Bennett JS. Structure of the platelet membrane glycoprotein IIb. Homology to the α subunit of the vitronectin and fibronectin membrane receptors. J Biol Chem 1987; 264:12596–12603.

20. Dupperray A, Berthier R, Chagnon E, Ryckewaert JJ, Gonsberg MH, Plow EF. Biosynthesis and processing of platelet GPIIb/IIIa in human megakaryoctes. J Cell Biol 1987; 104:1665–1673.

21. Calvette JJ. Clues for understanding the structure and function of a prototypic human integrin: The platelet glycoprotein IIb/IIIa complex. Thromb Haemostas 1994; 72:1–15.

22. Poncz M, Rifat S, Coller BS, Newman PJ, Shattil SJ, Parrella T, Fortina P, Bennett JS. Glanzmann thrombasthenia secondary to a Gly273Asp mutation adjacent to the first calcium-binding domain of platelet glycoprotein IIb. J Clin Invest 1994; 93:172–179.

23. Wilcox DA, Wautier JL, Picard D, Newman PJ. A single amino acid substitution flanking the fourth calcium binding domain of α_{IIb} prevents the maturation of the $\alpha_{IIb}\beta_3$ integrin complex. J Biol Chem 1994; 269:4450–4457.

24. Wilcox DA, Paddock CM, Lyman S, Gill JC, Newman PJ. Glanzmann thrombasthenia resulting form a single amino acid substitution between the second and third calcium-binding domains of GPIIb: Role of the GPIIb amino terminus in integrin subunit association. J Clin Invest 1995; 95:1553–1560.

25. Basani RB, Vilaire G, Shattil SJ, Kolodziej MA, Bennett JS, Poncz M. Glanzmann thrombasthenia due to a two amino acid deletion in the fourth calcium-binding domain: Demonstration of the importance of calcium-binding domains in the conformation of $\alpha_{IIb}\beta_3$. Blood 1996; 88:167–173.

26. Shattil SJ, Brass LF, Bennett JS, Pandhi P. Biochemical and functional conse-

quences of dissociation of the platelet membrane glycoprotein IIb-IIIa complex. Blood 1985; 66:92–98.

27. Gulino D, Boudignon C, Zhang L, Concord E, Rabiet MJ, Marguerie G. Ca^{2+} binding properties of the platelet glycoprotein GPIIb ligand-interacting domain. J Biol Chem 1992; 267:1001–1007.

28. Calvette JJ, Henschen A, Gonzalez-JRodriguez J. Assignment of disulphide bonds in human platelet GPIIIa. A disulphide pattern for the β subunit of the integrin family. Biochem J 1991; 274:63–71.

29. Wippler J, Kouns WC, Schlaeger EJ, Kuhn H, Hadvary P, Steiner B. The integrin $α_{IIb}β_3$, platelet glycoprotein IIb-IIIa, can form a functionally active heterodimer complex without the cysteine-rich repeats of the $β_3$. J Biol Chem 1994; 269:8754–8761.

30. Loftus JC, O'Toole TE, Plow EF, Glass A, Frelinger AL III, Ginsberg MH. A $β_3$ integrin mutation abolishes ligand binding and alters divalent cation-dependent conformation. Science 1990; 249:915–918.

31. Lee J-O, Rieu P, Arnaout MA, Liddington R: Crystal structure of the A domain from the α subunit of integrin CR3 (CD11/CD18). Cell 1995; 80:631–638.

32. Rosa, J-P, Bray PF, Bayet O, Johnston GI, Cook RG, Jackson KW, Shuman MA, McEver RP. Cloning glycoprotein IIIa cDNA from human erythroleukemia cells and localization of the gene to chromosome 17. Blood 1988; 72:593–600.

33. Fitzgerald LA, Steiner B, Rall SC, Lo SS, Phillips DR Protein sequence of endothelial glycoprotein IIIa derived from a cDNA clone. Identity with platelet glycoprotein IIIa and similarity to "integrin." J Biol Chem 1987; 262:3936–3939.

34. Heidenreich R, Eisman R, Surrey S, Delgrasso K, Bennett JS, Schwartz E, Poncz M. Organization of the gene for platelet glycoprotein IIb. Biochemistry 1990; 29:1232–1244.

35. Zimrin AB, Gidwitz S, Lord S, Schwartz E, Bennett JS, White GC, Poncz M. 1990. The genomic organization of platelet glycoprotein IIIa. J Biol Chem 1990; 265:8590–8595.

36. Duperray A, Troesch A, Berthier R, Chagnon E, Frachet P, Uzan G, Marguerie G. Biosynthesis and assembly of platelet GPIIb-IIIa in human megakaryocytes: Evidence that assembly between pro-GPIIb and GPIIIa is a prerequisite for expression of the complex on the cell surface. Blood 1989; 74:1603–1611.

37. Rosa J-P. McEver RP. Processing and assembly of the integrin, glycoprotein IIb-IIIa, in HEL cells. J Biol Chem 1989; 264:12596–12603.

38. O'Toole TE, Loftus JC, Plow EF, Glass AA, Harper JR, Ginsberg MH. Efficient surface expression of platelet GPIIb-IIIa requires both subunits. Blood 1989; 74:14–18.

39. Kolodziej MA, Vilaire G, Rifat S, Poncz M, Bennett JS. Effect of deletion of glycoprotein IIb exon 28 on the expression of the platelet GPIIb/IIIa complex. Blood 1991; 78:2344–2353.

40. Dupperray A, Berthier R, Chagnon E, Ryckewaert JJ, Ginsberg MH, Plow EF. Biosynthesis and processing of platelet GPIIb-IIIa in human megakaryoctes. J Cell Biol 1987; 104:1665–1673.

41. Bresnahan PA, Leduc R, Thomas L, Thorner J, Gibson H, Brake L, Barr AJ, Thomas G. Human *fur* gene encodes a yeast KEX2-like endoprotease that cleaves Pro-β-NGF in vivo. J Cell Biol 1990; 11:2851–2859.

42. Kolodziej MA, Vilaire G, Gonder D, Poncz M, Bennett JS: Study of the endoproteolytic cleavage of platelet glycoprotein IIb using oligonucleotide-mediated mutagenesis. J Biol Chem 1991; 266:23499–23504.

43. O'Toole TE, Loftus JC, Du X, Glass AA, Ruggeri ZM, Shattil SJ, Plow EF, Ginsberg MH: Affinity modulation of the $\alpha_{IIb}\beta_3$ integrin (Platelet GPIIb-IIIa) is an intrinsic property of the receptor. Cell Regulation 1990; 1:883–893.

44. Peerschke EI, Zucker MS, Grant RA, Egan JJ, Johnson MM. Correlation between fibrinogen binding to human platelets and platelet aggregability. Blood 1980; 44:841–847.

45. Weiss HJ, Hawiger J, Ruggeri ZM, Turritto VT, Thiagarajan P, Hoffman T. Fibrinogen-independent platelet adhesion and thrombus formation on subendothelium mediated by glycoprotein IIb-IIIa complex at high shear rate. J Clin Invest 1989; 83:288–297.

46. Davie EW, Fujikawa K, Kisiel W. The coagulation cascade: Initiation, maintenance, and regulation. Biochemistry 1991; 30:10363–10370.

47. Doolittle RF. Structural aspects of the fibrinogen-fibrin conversion. Adv. Protein Chem 1973; 27:1–109.

48. Doolittle RF. The structure and evolution of veterbrate fibrinogen. Ann NY Acad Sci 1983; 408:13–27.

49. McKee PA, Rogers LA, Marler E, Hill RL. The subunit polypeptides of human fibrinogen. Arch. Biochem. Biophys. 1966; 116:271–279.

50. Kant JA, Fornance AJ Jr, Saxe D, Simon MI, McBride OW, Crabtree GR. Evolution and organization of the fibrinogen locus on chromosome 4: Gene duplication accompanied by transposition and inversion. Proc Natl Acad Sci USA 1985; 82:2344–2348.

51. Weisel JW, Chandrasekaran N, Vilaire G, Bennett JS. Examination of the platelet membrane glycoprotein IIb-IIIa complex and its interaction with fibrinogen and other ligands by electron microscopy. J Biol Chem 1992; 267:6637–16643.

52. Nossel HL, Hurlet-Jensen A, Liu CY, Koehn JA, Canfield RE. Fibrinopeptide release from fibrinogen. Ann NY Acad. Sci. 1983; 408:269–278.

53. Schwartz ML, Pizzo SV, Hill RL. Human factor XIII from plasma and platelets. J Biol Chem 1973; 248:1395–1407.

54. Lucas MA, Fretto LJ, McKee P. The relationship of fibrinogen structure to plasminogen activation and plasmin activity during fibrinolysis. Ann. NY Acad. Sci. 1983; 408:71–96.

55. Kloczewiak M, Timmons S, Lukas TJ, Hawiger J. Platelet receptor recognition site on human fibrinogen. Synthesis and structure-function relationship of peptides corresponding to the carboxy-terminal segment of the γ chain. Biochemistry 1984; 23:1767–1774.

56. Doolittle RF, Watt KWK, Cottrell BA, Strong DD, Riley M. The amino acid sequence of the α-chain of human fibrinogen. nature 1979; 280:464–468.

57. Kloczewiak M, Timmons S, Hawiger J. Localization of a site interacting with human platelet receptor on carboxy-terminal segment of human fibrinogen gamma chain. Biochem Biophys Res Commun. 1982; 107:181–187.

58. Kloczewiak M, Timmons S, Hawiger J. Recognition site for the platelet receptor that is present on the 15-residue carboxy-terminal fragment of the gamma

chain of human fibrinogen and is not involved in the fibrin polymerization reaction. Thromb Res 1983; 29:249–255.

59. Pierschbacher MD, Ruoslahti E. Cell attachment activity of fibronectin can be duplicated by small synthetic fragments of the molecule. Nature 1984; 39:30–33.

60. Ginsberg MH, Pierschbacher MD, Ruoslahti E, Marguerie G, Plow EF. Inhibition of fibronectin binding to platelets by proteolytic fragments and synthetic peptides which support fibroblast adhesion. J Biol Chem 1985; 260:3931–3926.

61. Haverstick DM, Cowan JF, Yamada KM, Santoro SA. Inhibition of platelet adhesion to fibronectin, fibrinogen, and von Willebrand factor substrates by a synthetic tetra-peptide derived from the cell-binding domain of fibronectin. Blood 1985; 66:946–952.

62. Plow EF, Pierschbacher MD, Ruoslahti E, Marguerie GA, Ginsberg MH. The effect of Arg-Gly-Asp containing peptides on fibrinogen and von Willebrand factor binding to platelets. Proc Natl Acad Sci 1985; 82:8057–8061.

63. Gartner TK and Bennett JS. The tetrapeptide analogue of the cell attachment site of fibronectin inhibits platelet aggregation and fibrinogen binding to activated platelets. J Biol Chem 1985; 260:11891–11894.

64. Pytela R, Pierschbacher MD, Ginsberg MH, Plow EF, Ruoslahti E. Platelet membrane glycoprotein IIb/IIIa: Member of a family of Arg-Gly-Asp-specific adhesion receptors. Science 1986; 231:1559–1562.

65. Beer J, Springer KT, Coller BS. Immobilized Arg-Gly-Asp (RGD) peptides of varying lengths as structural probes of the glycoprotein IIb/IIIa receptor. Blood 1992; 79:117–128.

66. D'Souza SE, Ginsberg MH, Matsueda GG, Plow EF. A discrete region in a platelet integrin is involved in ligand recognition. Nature 1991; 350:66–68.

67. Alemany M, Concord E, Garin J, Vinçon M, Giles, A, Marguerie G, Gulino D. Sequence 274-368 in the β_3-subunit of the integrin $\alpha_{IIb}\beta_3$ provides a ligand recognition and binding domain for the γ-chain of fibrinogen that is independent of platelet activation. Blood 1996; 87:592–601.

68. D'Souza SE, Ginsberg MH, Burke TA, Lam SC-T., Plow Ef. Localization of an Arg-Gly-Asp binding site within an integrin adhesion receptor. Science 1988; 242:91–93.

69. Ginsberg MH, Lightsey A, Kunicki TJ, Kaufmann A, Marguerie GA, Plow EF. Divalent cation regulation of the surface orientation of platelet membrane glycoprotein IIb. Correlation with fibrinogen binding function and definition of a novel variant of Glanzmann's thrombasthenia. J Clin Invest 1986; 78:1103–1111.

70. Charo IF, Nannizzi L, Phillips DR, Hsu MA, Scarborough RM. Inhibition of fibrinogen binding to GP IIb-IIIa by a GP IIIa peptide. J Biol Chem 1991; 266:1415–1421.

71. Steiner B, Trzeciak A, Pfenninger G, Kouns W. Peptides derived from a sequence within β_3 integrin bind to platelet $\alpha_{IIb}\beta_3$ (GPIIb/IIIa) and inhibit ligand binding. J Biol Chem 1993; 268:6870–6873.

72. Lanza F, Stierlé A, Fournier D, Morales M, Andre G, Nurden AT, Cazenave JP. A new variant of Glanzmann's thrombasthenia (Strasbourg I). Platelets with functionally defective glycoprotein IIb-IIIa complexes and a glycoprotein IIIa^{214}Arg→^{214}Trp. J Clin Invest 1992; 89:1995–2004.

73. Djaffer I and Rosa J-P. A second case of variant of Glanzmann's thrombasthenia due to a substitution of platelet GPIIIa (integrin β_3) Arg 214 by Trp. Hum Mol Genet 1993; 2:2179–2180.

74. Bajt ML, Ginsberg MH, Frelinger ALIII, Berndt MC, Loftus JC. A spontaneous mutation of integrin $\alpha_{IIb}\beta_3$ (platelet glycoprotein IIb-IIIa) helps define a ligand binding site. J Biol Chem 1992; 267:3789–3794.

75. Newman PJ, Weyerbusch-Bottum S, Visetin GP, Gidwitz S, White GCII. Type II Glanzmann thrombasthenia due to a destabilizing amino acid substitution in platelet membrane glycoprotein IIIa. Thromb Haemst 1993; 69:1017 (Abst).

76. Kouns WC, Steiner B, Kunicki TJ, Moog S, Jutzi J, Jennings LK, Canzenave JP, Lanza F. Activation of the fibrinogen binding site on platelets isolated from a patient with the Strasbourg I variant of Glanzmann's thrombasthenia. Blood 1994; 84:108–1115.

77. Hawiger J, Timmons S, Kloczewiak M, Strong DD, Doolittle RF. γ and α chains of human fibrinogen possess sites reactive with human platelet receptors. Proc Natl Acad Sci 1992; 79:2068–2071.

78. Wolfenstein-Todel C and Mosesson MW. Carboxy-terminal animo acid sequence of a human fibrinogen γ chain variant (γ'). Biochemistry 1981; 20:6146–6149.

79. Peerschke EIB, Francis C, Marder VJ. Fibrinogen binding to human blood platelets: Effect of γ chain carboxyterminal structure and length. Blood 1986; 67:385–390.

80. Farrell DH, Thiagarajan P, Chung DW, Davie EW. Role of fibrinogen α and γ chain sites in platelet aggregation. Proc Natl Acad Sci 1992; 89:10729–10732.

81. Kieffer N, Fitzgerald A, Wolf D, Cheresh DA, Phillips DR. Adhesive properties of the β_3 integrins: Comparison of GPIIb-IIIa and the vitronectin expressed in human melanoma cells. J Cell Biol 1991; 113:451–461.

82. Lam SC-T, Plow EF, Smith MA, Andrieux A, Ryckwaert JJ, Marguerie G, Ginsberg MH. Evidence that Arginyl-Glycyl-Aspartate peptides and fibrinogen γ-chain peptides share a common binding site on platelets. J Biol Chem 1987; 262:947–950.

83. Peerschke EIB. The platelet fibrinogen receptor. Sem. In Hematol. 1985; 4:241–259.

84. Plow EF, D'Souza SE, Ginsberg MH. Ligand binding to GPIIb-IIIa: A status report. Sem In Thromb and Hemost 1992; 18:324–332.

85. Peerschke EIB. Glycoprotein IIb and IIIa retention on fibrinogen-coated surfaces after lysis of adherent cells. Blood 1993; 82:3358–3363.

86. Harrison P: Platelet α-granular fibrinogen. Platelets 1992; 3:1–10.

87. Burridge K, Fath K, Kelley T, Nuckolls G, Turner N: Focal adhesion: Transmembrane junctions between the extracellular matrix and the cytoskeleton. Annu Rev Cell Biol 1988; 4:487–525.

88. Harrison P, Wilbourn B, Debili N, Vainchenker W, Breton-Gorius J, Lawrie AS, Masse J-M, Savidge GF, Cramer EM: Uptake of plasma fibrinogen into the alpha granules of human megakaryocytes and platelets. J Clin Invest 1989; 84:1320–1324.

89. Handagama P, Scarborough RM, Shuman MA, Bainton DF: Endocytosis of fi-

brinogen into megakaryocyte and platelet α-granules is mediated by $\alpha_{IIb}\beta_3$ (Glycoprotein IIb-IIIa). Blood 1993; 82:135–138.

90. Wencel-Drake JD. Plasma membrane GPIIb/IIIa. Evidence for a cycling receptor pool. Am J Pathol 1990; 136:61–70.

91. Wencel-Drake JD, Frelinger ALIII, Dieter MG, Lam SC-T. Arg-Gly-Asp-dependent occupancy of GPIIb/IIIa by applaggin: evidence for internalization and cycling of a platelet integrin. Blood 1993; 81:62–69.

92. Coller BS, Seligsohn U, Peretz H, Newman PF. Glanzmann thrombasthenia: New insights from an historical perspective. Sem In Hematol 1994; 31:301–311.

93. Francis CW, Nachman RL, Marder VJ. Plasma and platelet fibrinogen differ in γ chain content. Thromb Haemost 1984; 51:84–88.

94. Coller BS. Interaction of normal, thrombasthenic, and Bernard-Soulier platelets with immobilized fibrinogen: Defective platelet-fibrinogen interaction in thrombasthenia. Blood 1980; 55:169–178.

95. Shattil SJ, Ginsberg MH, Brugge JS. Adhesive signaling in platelets. Curr Opin Cell Biol 1994; 6:695–704.

96. Taub R, Gould RJ, Garsky VM, Ciccarone TM, Hoxie J, Friedman PA, Shattil SJ. A monoclonal antibody against the platelet fibrinogen receptor contains a sequence that mimics a receptor recognition domain in fibrinogen. J Biol Chem 1989; 264:259–265.

97. Coller BS. A new murine monoclonal antibody reports an activation-dependent change in the conformation and/or microenvironement of the platelet glycoprotein IIb/IIIa complex. J Clin Invest 1985; 76:101–108.

98. Shatti SJ, Hoxie JA, Cunningham M, Brass LF. Changes in the platelet membrane glycoprotein IIb-IIIa complex during platelet activation. J Biol Chem 1985; 260:11107–11114.

99. Ginsberg MH, Du X, Plow EF. Inside-out integrin-signalling. Curr Opin Cell Biol 1992; 4:766–771.

100. O'Toole TE, Mandelman D, Forsyth J, Shattil SJ, Plow EF, Ginsberg MH. Modulation of the affinity of integrin $\alpha_{IIb}\beta_3$ (GPIIb-IIIa) by the cytoplasmic domain of α_{IIb}. Science 1991; 254:845–847.

101. O'Toole TE, Katagiri Y, Faull RJ, Peter K, Tamura R, Quaranta V, Loftus JC, Shattil SJ, Ginsberg MH. Integrin cytoplasmic domains mediate inside-out signal transduction. J Cell Biol 1994; 124:1047–1059.

102. Hughes, P. E., Diaz-Gonzalez, F., Leong, L., Wu, C., McDonald, J. A., Shattil, S. J., and Ginsberg, M. H. Breaking the hinge. A defined structural constraint regulates integrin signaling. J Biol Chem 1996; 271:6571–6574.

103. Chen Y-P, O'Toole TE, shipley T, Forsyth J, LaFlamme SE, Yamade KM, Shattil SJ, Ginsberg MH. "Inside-out" signal transduction inhibited by isolated integrin cytoplasmic domains. J Biol Chem 1994; 269:18307–18310.

104. Pelletier, A. J., Kunicki, T. J., Ruggeri, Z. M., and Quaranta, V. The activation state of the integrin $\alpha_{IIb}\beta_3$ affects outside-in signals to cell spreading and focal adhesion kinase phosphorylation. J. Biol. Chem.1995, 270:18130–18140.

105. Ylänne, J., Huuskonen, J., O'Toole, T. E., Ginsberg, M. H., Virtanen, I., and Gahmberg, C. G. Mutation of the cytoplasmic domain of the integrin β_3 subunit.

Differential effects on cell spreading, recruitment to adhesion plaques, endocytosis, and phagocytosis. J Biol Chem 1995; 270:9550–9557.

106. Golden A, Brugge J, and Shattil, SJ. Role of platelet membrane glycoprotein IIb-IIIa in agonist-induced tyrosine phosphorylation of platelet proteins. J Cell Biol 1990; 111:3117–3127.

107. Richardson A, Parsons JT. Signal transduction through integrins: a central role for focal adhesion kinase? BioEssays 1995; 17:229–236.

108. Kunicki TJ and Newman PJ. The molecular immunology of human platelet proteins. Blood 1992; 80:1386–1404.

109. Weiss EJ, Bray PF, Tayback M, Schulman SP, Kickler TS, Becker LC, Weiss JL, Gerstenblith G, Goldschmidt-Clermont PJ. A polymorphism of a platelet glycoprotein receptor as an inherited risk factor for coronary thrombosis. N Eng J Med 1996; 334:1090–1094.

110. George JN, Caen JP, Nurden AT. Glanzmann's thrombasthenia: The spectrum of clinical disease. Blood 75:1383–1395, 1990.

111. Coller BS. Inherited disorders of platelet function. In: Bloom AL, Forbes CD, Thomas DP, Tuddenham EGD, eds., Haemostatis and thrombosis, 3rd Ed. Edinburgh: Churchill Livingstone, 1994:721–766.

112. Newman PJ, Seligsohn U, Lyman S, Coller BS. The molecular genetic basis of Glanzmann thrombasthenia in the Iraqi-Jewish and Arab populations in Israel. Proc Natl Acad Sci USA 88;3160–3164, 1991.

113. Burk CD, Newman PJ, Lyman S, Gill J, Coller BS, Poncz M. A deletion in the gene for glycoprotein IIb associated with Glanzmann's thrombasthenia. J Clin Invest 87:270–276, 1991.

114. Li L, Bray PF: Homologous recombination among three intragene Alu sequences causes an inversion-deletion resulting in hereditary bleeding disorder Glanzmann thrombathenia. Am J Hum Genet 53:140–149, 1993.

115. Djaffar I, Caen JP, Rosa J-P. A large alteration in the human platelet glycoprotein IIIa (integrin β_3) gene associated with Glanzmann's thrombasthenia. Human Mol Genet 2:2183–2185, 1993.

116. Peretz H, Rosenberg N, Usher, S, Graff E, Newman PJ, Coller BS, Seligsohn U. Glanzmann's thrombasthenia associated with deletion-insertion and alternative splicing in the glycoprotein IIb gene. Blood 85:414–420, 1995.

117. Wang R, Ambruso DR, Newman PJ. Truncation in the cytoplasmic domain of integrin β_3 subunit confers an inactivated state to the $\alpha_{IIb}\beta_3$ complex in a variant type of Glanzmann thrombasthenia. Blood 84:244a, 1994 Abstr.

118. Chen Y-P, Djaffar I, Pidard D, Steiner B, Cieutat A-M, Caen JP, Rosa J-P. Ser-752 → Pro mutation in the cytoplasmic domain of integrin β_3 subunit and defective activation of platelet integrin $\alpha_{IIb}\beta_3$ (glycoprotein IIb-IIIa) in a variant of Glanzmann thrombasthenia. Proc Natl Acad Sci USA 89:10169–10173, 1992.

119. Simsek S, Heyboer H, de Bruijne-Admiraal LG, Goldschmeding R, Cuijpers HThM, von dem Borne AEGKr. Glanzmann's thrombasthenia caused by homozygosity for a splice defect that leads to deletion of the first coding exon of the glycoprotein IIIa mRNA. Blood 81:2044–2049, 1993.

120. Jin Y, dietz HC, Nurden A, Bray PF. Single-strand conformation polymorphism

analysis is a rapid and effective method for the identification of mutations and polymorphisms in the gene for glycoprotein IIIa. Blood 82:2281–2288, 1993.

121. Vinciguerra C, Trzeciak MC, Philippe N, Frappaz D, ReynaudJ, Dechavanne M, Negrier C. Molecular study of Glanzmann thrombasthenia in 3 patients issued from 2 different families. Thromb Haemostat 1994; 74:822–827.

122. Skogen B, Wang R, McFarland JG, Newman PJ. A two base deletion in exon 4 of the PI allelic form of GPIIIa: Implications for the correlation of serologic versus genotypic analysis of human platelet alloantigens. Blood 1994; 84:244a.

123. Kato A, Yamamoto K, Miyazaki S, Jung SM, Moroi M, Aoki N. Molecular basis for Glanzmann's thrombasthenia (GT) in a compound heterozygote with glyco-protein IIb gene: A proposal for the classification of GT based on the biosynthetic pathway of glycoprotein IIb-IIIa complex. Blood 1992; 79:3212–3218.

124. Gu JM, Xu WF, Wang XD, Wu QY, Chi CW, Ruan CG. Identification of a nonsense mutation at amino acid 584-Arginine of platelet glycoprotein IIb in patients with type I Glanzmann thrombasthenia. Br J Haemotol 1993; 83:442–49.

125. Iwamoto S, Nishiumi E, Kajii E, Ikemoto S. An exon 28 mutation resulting in alternative splicing of the glycoprotein IIb transcript and Glanzmann's thromb-asthenia. Blood 1994; 83:1017–1023.

126. Tomiyama Y, Kashiwagi H, Kosugi S, Shiraga M, Kanayama Y, Kurata Y, Matsuzawa Y. Abnormal processing of the glycoprotein IIb transcript due to a nonsense mutation in exon 17 associated with Glanzmann's thrombasthenia. Thromb. Haemostas 1995; 73:756–762.

127. Schlege N, Gayet I, Morel-Kopp M-C, Wyler B, Hurtaud-Roux M-F, Kaplan C, McGregor J. The molecular genetic basis of Glanzmann's thrombasthenia in a Gypsy population in France: Identification of a new mutation on the α_{IIb} gene. Blood 1995; 86:977–982.

128. Chen FP, Coller BS, Weiss HJ, Xu L-Z, French DL. Glanzmann thrombasthe-nia due to a glycoprotein IIb missense mutation Leu214Pro. Thromb Haemostas 1995; 73:1191(abstr).

129. Bourre F, Peyruchaud O, Bray P, Combrié R, Nurden P, Nurden AT. A point mutation in the gene for platelet GPIIb leads to a substitution in a highly con-served amino acid located between the second and third Ca^{++}-binding domain. Blood 1995; 86:452a(abstr).

130. Kirchmaier CM, Westrup D, Becker-Hagendorff, K, Just M, Jablonka B, Seifried E. A new variant of Glanzmann's thrombasthenia (Frankfurt I). Thromb Haemostas 1995; 73:1058(abstr).

131. Peyruchaud O, Nurden AT, Bourre F. Use of PCR-SSCP to screen the exons of the GP IIb and GP IIIa genes of a variant with Glanzmann's thrombasthenia: A mutation in the nucleotide sequence for the GFFKR cytoplasmic domain of the integrin subunit α_{IIb} (GP IIb). Thromb Haemostas 1995; 73:1189(abstr).

132. Grimaldi CM, Chen F-P, Scudder LE, Coller BS, French DL. A Cys374Tyr homozygous mutation of platelet glycoprotein IIIa (β_3) in a Chinese patient with Glanzmann's thrombasthenia. Blood 1996; 88:1666–1675.

133. Coller BS. Blockade of platelet GPIIb/IIIa receptors as an antithrombotic strat-egy. Circulation 1995; 92:2373–2380.

134. Coller BS. Antiplatelet agents in the prevention and therapy of thrombosis. Ann Rev Med 1992; 43:171–180.

135. Davies MJ. Pathology of arterial thrombosis. Br Med Bull 1994; 50:789–802.

136. Coller BS, Scudder LE, Beer J, et al. Monoclonal antibodies to platelet GPIIb/IIIa as antothrombotic agents. Ann NY Acad Sci 1991; 614:193–213.

137. Tcheng JE, Ellis SG, George BS, et al. Pharmacodynamics of chimeric glycoprotein IIb/IIIa integrin antiplatelet antibody Fab 7E3 in high-risk coronary angioplasty. Circulation 1994; 90:1757–1764.

138. Coller BS. Inhibitors of the platelet glycoprotein IIb/IIIa receptor as conjunctive therapy for coronary artery thrombolysis. Coronary Art Dis 1992; 3:1016–1029.

139. The EPIC Investigators. Use of a monoclonal antibody directed against the platelet glycoprotein IIb/IIIa receptor in high-risk coronary angioplasty. N Eng J Med 1994; 330:956–961.

140. Topol EJ, Califf Rm, Anderson K, et al. Randomized trial of coronary intervention with antibody against platelet IIb/IIIa integrin for reduction of clinical restenosis: results at six months. Lancet 1994; 343:881–886.

141. Lincoff AM, Tcheng JE, Bass TA, et al. A multicenter, double-blind pilot trial of standard versus low dose weight-adjusted heparin in patients treated with platelet GPIIb/IIIa receptor antibody c7E3 during percutaneous coronary revascularization. J Am Coll Cardiol 1995; 25:80A(abstr).

142. Ferguson JJI. EPILOG and CAPTURE trials halted because of positive results. Circulation 1996; 93:637.

143. Shattil SJ, Ginsberg MH, Brugge JS. Adhesive signaling in platelets. Current biol 1994; 6:695–704.

144. Ruoslahti E. Integrin. J Clin Invest 1991; 87:1–5.

145. Farrell DH, Thiagarajan P, Chung DW, Dave EW. Role of fibrinogen α and γ chain sites in platelet aggregation. Proc Natl Acad Sci 1992; 89:10729–10732.

Appendix: Genetic Cardiovascular Disease

Disease	Cardiac Phenotype(s)	Gene Name or Locus	References[a]
Velocardiofacial	Conotruncal defects	22q11, 10p13, ?	8,18–20, A
DiGeorge	Conotruncal defects	22q11, 10p13, ?	4,5,7–10, A
Williams	Supravalvular AS, branch PS	Microdeletions including the elastin gene at 7q11	45,46
Familial SVAS	Supravalvular AS	Elastin	43,44
Marfan	Aortic root dilation, mitral valve prolapse	Fibrillin1	B
Ehlers-Danlos IV	Aortic dilation	Collagen, type III	C
Noonan	PS, Ao Coartct., PDA, hypertrophic cardio-myopathy	12q2	57
Watson	PS	NF1	63,64
Familial TAPVR	Total anomalous pulmonary venous return	4p13–q12	72
Holt-Oram	ASD, VSD, hypoplastic LH	12q2, ?	53–55
Ellis–van Creveld	ASD	4p16	D
X-linked heterotaxy	Heterotaxy	Xq24–27	75
Autosomal recessive heterotaxy	Heterotaxy	Connexin43	73
Familial hypertrophic cardiomyopathy			
CMH1	Hypertrophic cardiomyopathy	Myosin heavy chain	E
CMH2	Hypertrophic cardiomyopathy	Cardiac troponin-T	F
CMH3	Hypertrophic cardiomyopathy	α-tropomyosin	F
CMH4	Hypertrophic cardiomyopathy	Cardiac myosin binding protein-C	G
CMH5	Hypertrophic cardiomyopathy	?	H
CMH6	Hypertrophic cardiomyopathy with Wolff-Parkinson-White	7q3	I

Familial dilated cardiomyopathy

X-linked	Dilated cardiomyopathy with elevated CPK	Dystrophin	J
	Fetal infantile	Xq28	K
Autosomal dominant	Dilated cardiomyopathy with arrhythmias and AV block	1p11–q11	L
	Dilated cardiomyopathy	1q32	M
	Dilated cardiomyopathy with sinus node dysfunction and SVT	3p25–p22	N
	Dilated cardiomyopathy	9p13	O
	Dilated cardiomyopathy with mitral valve prolapse	10q21–q23	P

Familial arrhythmogenic right ventricular dysplasia

ARVD	14q23–q24	Q
"Concealed" ARVD	1q42–43	R

Familial long-QT syndrome

Type 1	LQTS	KVLQT1 (potassium channel)	S
Type 2	LQTS	HERG	T
Type 3	LQTS	SCN5A (sodium channel)	U
Type 4	LQTS with sinus bradycardia	4q25–q27	V

Progressive familial heart block

[a]Numbered references refer to references in Chapter 6, "Congenital Heart Disease: Gene Defects and Molecular Biologic Studies," by Bruce D. Gelb. Lettered references are as follows:

A. Daw SCM, Taylor C, Kraman M, Call K, Mao J, Schuffenhauer S, Meitinger T, Lipson T, Goodship J, Scambler P. A common region of 10p deleted in DiGeorge and velocardiofacial syndromes. Nature Genet 1996; 13:458–460.

B.1. Lee B, Godfry M, Vitale E, Hori H, Mattei M-G, Sarfarazi M, Tsipouras P, Ramirez F, Hollister DW. Linkage of Marfan syndrome and a phenotypically related disorder to two different fibrillin genes. Nature 1991; 352:330–334.

B.2. Maslen CL, Corson GM, Maddox BK, Glanville RW, Sakai LY. Partial sequence of a candidate gene for the Marfan syndrome. Nature 1991; 352:334–337.

B.3. Dietz HC, Cutting GR, Pyeritz RE, Maslen CL, Sakai LY, Corson GM, Puffenberger EG, Hamosh A, Nanthakumar E, Curristin S, Stetten G, Meyers DA, Francomano CA. Marfan syndrome caused by a recurrent de novo missense mutation in the fibrillin gene. Nature 1991; 353:337–339.

C.1. Superti-Furga A, Gugler E, Gitzelmann R, Steinmann B. Ehlers-Danlos syndrome type IV: a multi-exon deletion in one of the two COL3A1 alleles affecting structure, stability, and processing of type III procollagen. J Biol Chem 1988; 263:6226–6232.

C.2. Superti-Furga A, Steinmann B, Ramirez F, Byers PH. Molecular defects of type II procollagen in Ehlers-Danlos syndrome type IV. Hum Genet 1989; 82:104–108.

D. Polymeropoulos MH, Ide SE, Wright M. Goodship J, Weissenbach J, Pyeritz RE, Da Silva EO, Ortiz De Luna RI, Francomano CA. The gene for the Ellis–van Creveld syndrome is located on chromosome 4p16. Genomics 1996; 35:1–5.

E. Geisterfer-Lowrance AAT, Kass S, Tanigawa G, Vosberg H-P, McKenna W, Seidman CE, Seidman JG. A molecular basis for familial hypertrophic cardiomyopathy: A β cardiac myosin heavy chain gene missense mutation. Cell 1990; 62:999–1006.

F. Thierfelder L, Watkins H, MacRae C, Lamas R, McKenna W, Vosberg H-P, Seidman JG, Seidman CE. α-tropomyosin and cardiac troponin T mutations cause familial hypertrophic cardiomyopathy. Cell 1994; 77:701–712.

G.1. Watkins H, Conner D, Thierfelder L, Jarcho JA, MacRae C, McKenna WJ, Maron BJ, Seidman JG, Seidman CE. Mutation in the cardiac myosin binding protein-C gene on chromosome 11 cause familial hypertrophic cardiomyopathy. Nature Genet 1995; 11:434–437.

G.2. Bonne G, Carrier L, Bercovic J, Cruaud C, Richard P, Hainque B, Gautel M, Labeit S, James M, Beckmann J, Weissenbacuh J, Vosberg H-P, Fiszman M, Komajda M, Schwartz K. Cardiac myosin binding protein-C gene splice acceptor site mutation is associated with familial hypertrophic cardiomyopathy. Nature Genet 1995; 11:438–440.

H. Hengstenberg C, Charron P, Beckmann JS, Weissenbach J, Isnard R, Komajda M, Schwartz K. Evidence for the existence of a fifth gene causing familial hypertrophic cardiomyopathy (abstract). Am J Hum Genet 1993; 53:A1013.

I. McRae CA, Ghaisas N, Kass S, Donnelly S, Basson CT, Watkins HC, Anan R, Thierfelder LH, McGarry K, Rowland E, McKenna WJ, Seidman JG, Seidman CE. Familial hypertrophic cardionmyopathy with Wolff-Parkinson-White syndrome maps to a locus onchromosome 7q3. J Clin Invest 1995; 96:1216–1220.

J. Towbin JA, Hejtmancik JF, Brink P, Gelb B, Zhu XM, Chamberlain JS, McCabe ERB, Swift M. X-linked dilated cardiomyopathy: Molecular genetic evidence of linkage to the Duchenne muscular dystrophy (dystrophic gene at the Xp21 locus). Circulation 1993; 87:1854–1865.

K. Gedeon AK, Wilson MJ, Colley AC, Sillence DO, Mulley JC. X-linked fatal infantile cardionmyopathy maps to Xq28 and is possibly allelic to Barth syndrome. J Med Genet 1995; 32:383–388.

L. Kass S, MacRae C, Graber HL, Sparks EA, McNamara D, Boudoulas H, Basson CT, Baker PB III, Cody RJ, Fishman MC, Cox N, Kong A, Wooley CF, Seidman JG, Seidman CE. A gene defect that causes conduction system disease and dilated cardiomyopathy maps to chromosome 1p1–1q1. Nature Genet 1994; 7:546–551.

M. Durand J-B, Bachinski LL, Bieling LC, Czernuszewicz GZ, Abchee AB, Yu QT, Tapscott T, Hill R, Ifegwu J, Marian AJ. Localization of a gene responsible for familial dilated cardiomyopathy to chromosome 1q32. Circulation 1995; 92:3387–3389.

N. Olson TM, Keating MT. Mapping a cardiomyopathy locus to chromsome 3p22-p25. J Clin Invest 1996; 97:528–532.

O. Krajinovic M, Pinamonti B, Siagra G, Vatta M, Severini GM, Milasin J, Falaschi A, Camerini F, Giacca M, Mestroni L; The Heart Muscle Disease Study Group. Linkage of familial dilated cardiomyopathy to chromosome 9. Am J Hum Genet 1995; 57:846–852.

P. Bowles KR, Gajaski R, Porter P, Goytia V, Bachinski L, Roberts R, Pignatelli R, Towbin JA. Gene mapping of familial autosomal dominant dilated cardiomyopathy to chromosome 10q21-23. J Clin Invest 1996; 98:1355–1360.

Q. Rampazzo A, Nava A, Danieli GA, Buja G, Daliento L, Fasoli G, Scognamiglio R, Corrado D, Thiene G. The gene for arrhythmogenic right ventricular cardiomyopathy maps to chromosome 14q23-q24. Hum Molec Genet 1994; 3:959–962.

R. Rampazzo A, Nava A, Erne P. Eberhard M, Vian E, Slomp P, Tiso N, Thiene G, Danieli GA. A new locus for arrhythmogenic right ventricular cardiomyopathy (ARVD2) maps to chromosome 1q42-43. Hum Molec Genet 1995; 4:2151–2154.

S. Wang Q, Curran ME, Splawski I, Burn TC, Millholland JM, VanRaay TJ, Shen J, Timothy KW, Vincent GM, de Jager T, Schwartz PJ, Towbin JA, Moss AJ, Atkinson DL, Landes GM, Connors TD, Keating MT. Positional cloning of a novel potassium channel gene: KVLQT1 mutations cause cardiac arrhythmias. Nature Genet 1996; 12:17–23.

T. Curran ME, Splawski I, Timothy KW, Vincent GM, Green ED, Keating MT. A molecular basis for cardiac arrhythmia: HERG mutation cause long QT syndrome. Cell 1995; 80:795–803.

U. Wang Q, Shen J, Splawski I, Atkinson D, Li Z, Robinson JL, Moss AJ, Towbin JA, Keating MT. SCN5A mutations associated with an inherited cardiac arrhythmia, long QT syndrome. Cell 1995; 80:805–811.

V. Schott J-J, Charpentier F, Peltier S, Foley P, Drouin E, Bouhour J-B, Donnelly P, Vergnaud G, Bachner L, Moisan J-P, Le marec H, Pascal O. Mapping of a gene for long QT syndrome to chromosome 4q25-27. Am J Hum Genet 1995; 57:1114–1122.

W. Brink PA, Ferreira A, Moolman JC, Weymar HW, van der Merwe P-L, Corfield VA. Gene for progressive familial heart block type I maps to chromosome 19q13. Circulation 1995; 91:1633–1640.

Index

A23187, 188
Action potentials, 173, 197, 198
Activin receptor, 351
Adenoassociated viruses, 388, 389
Adenoviruses, 383, 386–388
Adenyl cyclase, 165, 167
β-adrenergic receptors, 171
Akt/PKB kinase, 301, 302
α-actin promoter, skeletal, 343, 345
α-actin, skeletal, 351
α1-receptor antagonist, 219
αvβ3 integrin, 411, 415, 490, 491,
    492, 504
  endothelial cells, 490
  vascular smooth muscle cells, 490
Amiodarone, 208
Angiogenesis, 394
Angiopeptin, 417
Angiotensin II, 292, 309, 311–313,
    339, 457
Angiotensin II receptor (AT1R), 309–
    314, 353
Antiarrhythmic drugs, 174, 187
  class I antiarrhythmic therapy, 187
  class III antiarrhythmic drugs, 205
Antibody production, 44

Anticoagulants, 461
Antiplatelet agents, 460, 504
Antisense mRNA, 416
Antisense oligonucleotides, 346, 391
Antithrombins, 461
Aorta, 432
Apolipoprotein B, 472, 475–483
  ARP-1, 475
  degradation, 480
  gene, 475
  lysosomal inhibitors, 482
  mRNA processing, 476
  mRNA translation, 476, 477
  postsecretory control, 483
  posttranslational regulation, 478–480
  promoter, 475
Apolipoproteins, 471, 472, 474
AP-1, 343, 457, 458
Apoptosis, 413, 415
Arterial balloon injury
  porcine, 449, 455, 461
  primates, 461
  rabbit, 406, 407, 449, 450, 455, 456
  rat, 406, 407, 413, 449, 450, 454, 455
Arterial injury, 489
Aspirin, 460, 504

Atherogenesis, 472
Atheromas, 452
Atherosclerosis, 447–449, 453, 458, 460, 489
AT-1 cells, 95
Atrioventricular septal defects, 116
Atrioventricular valves, 346
Autosomal recessive heterotaxy, 518

Bigylcan, 411

Calcium channels 237–246
  α1 subunits, 237
  β subunits, 245
  L type, 241, 243
  N type, 241
  P type, 241
  S4 region, 241
  T type, 241
Calcium-induced calcium release, 252
Calcium release channels, intracellular, 251–266
  channel accessory protein, 260
  foot structures, 252
  RyR1, 254, 258
  RyR2, 254
  triad junction, 252
cAMP, 243
Cardiac hypertrophy, 263
Cardiac morphogenesis, 345
Cardiac muscle (see Myocardium)
Cardiac myoblasts, 346
Cardiac myocytes, 67, 90–93, 97, 263, 328, 329, 332, 333, 343, 344, 351, 355, 357
Cardiomyopathy
  doxorubicin, 265
  familial dilated, 518
  familial hypertrophic, 518
  idiopathic dilated, 264, 282
  ischemic, 264
Carvedilol, 418
CATCH syndrome, 112–115
CCAAT box, 7
CDC25, 298

CEK (see Fibroblast growth factor receptors)
Cell-mediated gene transfer, 381
Charybdotoxin, 209
Cholesterol, 471, 472, 475
Cholesterol via cholesteryl ester transfer protein (CETP), 474
Chondroitin sulfates (CSPGs), 409–412
Chromosomes, 3, 6
Chylomicrons, 472, 473, 479
Clotting factors, 449, 451
  factor VII/VIIa, 451, 453, 454, 456
  factor IX/IXa, 451, 453
  factor X/Xa, 448, 459, 461
Coagulation, 449–451, 459, 460, 496, 497
Codons, 11
Collagens, 116, 404, 410, 431, 518
  type I, 404
  type III, 518
  type VI, 116
Congenital contractural arachnodactyly (CCA), 433, 441
Congenital heart defects, 111
Connexin 43, 122
Coronary artery disease (CAD), 471, 479
Counteradhesive matrix proteins, 410, 412
  laminin, 410, 412
  SPARC (osteonectin), 410, 412
  tenascin, 410, 412
  thrombospondin, 410, 412
Cromakalim, 219
β-cyclodetrin tetradecasulfate, 417

Decorin, 411
Delayed rectifier, 206, 208
Dermatan sulfate proteoglycans (DSPGs), 409–411
Developmental regulation, 240
Dextrocardia, 123
Diabetes and streptozotocin, 477
Diacylglycerol (DAG), 311
Diastolic tone, 263
Differential display of mRNA, 61–62

DiGeorge, 112, 518
Dihydropyridine receptor, 237
Direct injection of genetic material, 69,
    70
DNA (deoxyribonucleic acid), 1, 3
    adenine, 2
    Chargaff's rules, 2
    chromosomes, 3
    cytosine, 2
    deoxyribonucleotides, 3
    double helix, 2
    genomic, 49
    guanine, 2
    labeling, 23, 25, 26,
    nick translation, 25
    phage, 48
    plasmid isolation and microplasmid
        prep, 46
    plasmid isolation and midiprep, 47
    plasmid isolation and miniprep, 46
    plasmid isolation and superminiprep,
        47
    preparation, 13
    purines, 2
    pyrimidines, 2
    random hexamer labeling, 25
    restriction endonucleases 17
    restriction mapping, 20
    supercoiling, 21
    thymine, 2
DNA polymerase, 4, 26, 35
    Klenow fragment, 26
DNA sequencing, 22–25, 63
    Maxam and Gilbert method, 22
    Sanger and Coulson method, 23, 25
DNA synthesis, measurements in vivo,
    407
Down's syndrome (trisomy 21), 116
Drosophila, 351

EBP (tropoelastin binding protein), 432
EGF motifs, 434, 435, 438–440
Egr-1, 457
Ehlers-Danlos IV, 518
eIF-4E (eukaryotic initiation factor 4E),
    301, 313

Elastic fibers, 432
Elastin, 118, 432, 433, 518
Elastogenesis, 433
Ellis–van Creveld, 518
Embryonic stem (ES) cells, 96, 97
Emilin, 433
Encainide, 175
Endothelial cells, 333, 405
Endothelin, 342
Enhancers, 5, 129
EPIC trial, 505
Epidermal growth factor (EGF), 307, 338
Epidermal growth factor receptor
    (EGF-R), 298, 306, 307, 311
ERK (extracellular signal regulated
    kinase), 300, 301, 305–308, 312,
    313
ERK kinase (MEK), 300, 307
Escherichia coli, 13
Excitation-contraction coupling, 239,
    245, 264
Extracellular matrix (ECM), 401–419,
    431–433, 439, 440, 490, 492,
    496, 498

FAK (focal adhesion kinase), 304, 312,
    315, 503
Familial arrhythmogenic right ventric-
    ular dysplasia, 518
Familial combined hyperlipidemia,
    (FCHL), 474, 483, 484
Familial long-QT syndrome, 519
Familial supravalvular aortic stenosis
    (SVAS), 116, 518
Familial total anomalous pulmonary
    venous return (TAPVR), 121, 518
Fibrillin, 432–441, 518
    genes, 435, 436
    mutations, 439–441
    fibrillin-like protein (FLP), 434
Fibrin, 448–451, 458–461, 497
    deposition, 394, 450, 455, 460
Fibrinogen, 493, 496–499, 501, 505
    internalization, 501
Fibrinolytic system, 458, 460

Fibroblast growth factor (FGF), 306,
307, 328, 332, 333, 335, 343–346,
349, 353, 357, 408
Fibroblast growth factor receptor (FGF-
R/FGFR) 308, 330, 334–336, 346,
349, 350, 357
FGFR1 knockout mice, 346
Fibroblasts, 303, 313, 333
Fibronectin, 132, 410, 411, 490, 491,
493, 496, 498, 499
FK506, 258, 418
FK506-binding protein, 258
FKBP12, 258, 340, 418
Flecainide, 175
c-*fos*, 73, 75, 314, 342, 343, 345
Fyn, 261

GAL4, 56
GATA-4, 98, 99
Gel electrophoresis, 20
Gene, 1
structure, 8
therapy 379, 380
transduction, 385
transfer vectors, 382, 383
Genetic code, 11
Genome, 7
Glanzmann thrombasthenia, 501, 503,
504
Glycoprotein Ib (GPIb), 492, 493, 501
Glycoprotein IIb/IIIa (GPIIb/IIIa), 460,
489–506
GPIIb gene, 495, 504
GPIIIa gene, 495, 504
G proteins, 161–171, 294, 297, 299, 302
G protein receptor kinase (GRK), 309
G protein-coupled receptors, 294
Grb-2, 336, 296, 298, 299
GTPase, 163, 304
GTPase activators, 297, 340
Guanine nucleotide binding protein, 161
Guanine nucleotide exchange factors,
297–299
Guanylate cyclase, 141

Heart failure, 240, 263, 264, 327, 347

Helix–loop–helix proteins, 343
Heparan sulfate proteoglycans (HSPG),
332, 409–411, 472
Heparin, 332, 408, 409, 460, 461, 505
High-density lipoprotein (HDL), 474,
475
HDL-binding receptor (SR-B1), 474
Hirudin, 461
His-Purkinje system, 198
HMGCoA reductase inhibitors, 483
Holt-Oram, 518
Hox-1.5, 125–126
Hypertrophy, cardiac, 342, 351, 353, 355

"Immediate-early" genes, 342, 355
Immunophillin, 258
Infection with viral vectors, 385
Inositol trisphosphate (IP3), 260, 311,
312
IP3-induced intracellular calcium
release, 262
Insulin-like growth factor (IGF), 307,
328, 336–338, 346, 347, 353, 357
IGF-binding properties (IGFBP),
336, 337
IGF-I knockout mice, 346
Insulin-like growth factor receptor
(IGFR), 130, 308, 330, 337–339,
346, 347, 355, 357
IGF2R knockout mice, 347
Integrins, 132, 490, 491, 492
Intimal hyperplasia, 393, 401, 418,
448, 450, 461
Introduction of genetic material into the
vessel wall, 382
IRS-1, 296, 308, 338
Ischemia, 357
Isosorbide dinitrate, 141

JAK (Janus kinase), 294, 295, 314
JAK phosphorylation, 294
JNK/SAPK 300, 306
c-*jun*, 342, 343

K+ channels (*see* Potassium channels)
Kartagener syndrome, 123

Lidocaine, 176
Linkage analysis, 440, 441
Lipids, 472, 472
Lipoproteins, 471, 472
  lipoprotein lipase, 472, 483
  metabolism, 471, 472
Liposomes, 391, 392
Low-density lipoprotein (LDL), 459,
  471, 473, 474, 475, 483

Macrophages, 472
MAP (mitogen-activated protein), 300
MAP kinase phosphatase-1 (MKP-1),
  305, 306
MAP kinase phosphatase-2 (MKP-2),
  306
MAP kinase phosphatase-3 (MKP-3),
  306
MAPK (mitogen-activated protein kinase)
  superfamily
  JNK/SAPK 300, 306
  MAPK, 169, 170, 299, 300, 303, 305,
    306, 312, 335, 339
  MEK (ERK kinase), 170, 300, 307
  SAPK kinase (MEK-4, SEK) 300
Marfan syndrome (MFS), 432, 433,
  438–440, 518
  aortic dissection, 438, 439
  mitral valve prolapse, 438
Matrix metalloproteinases (MMPs),
  412–414
  collagenases, 412–414
  gelatinases, 412–414
  stromelysins, 412–414
MCM-1 cells, 95
MEK (ERK kinase), 170, 300, 307
Mesoderm, 96
Mexiletine, 187
mMcrofibrils, 432, 433, 436, 438, 440
  microfibrillar sheet, 432
  microfibril assembly, 436–438
  microfibril-associated glycoprotein
    (MAGP), 433
Microsomal triglyceride transfer
  protein (MTP), 479–481, 483

Migration assays
  artificial matrices, 404
  Boyden chamber, 402, 408, 415,
    417, 418
  circular outgrowth assay, 402
  collagen gels, 404, 416, 417
  in vivo, 407
  Teflon "fences", 403
  "wound and scrape", 403
Mitogenesis, 303
Molecular cloning, 33, 45, 53–62
  differential display of mRNA, 61–62
  differential screening, 57, 60
  expression cloning, 53, 55
  expression cloning in COS cells, 54
  expression cloning in oocytes, 45
  subtractive cloning, 59
  yeast two-hybrid system, 56
Molecular conjugates as gene transfer
  vectors, 390
Molecular probes, 36, 37
  cDNA probes, 36
  cRNA probes, 37
  oligonucleotide probes, 37
Monoclonal antibody 7E3, 502, 505,
  506
Monoclonal antibody PAC-1, 502
c-*myb*, 393
c-*myc*, 342, 343, 393
N-*myc*, 127
Myocardial contractility, 266
Myocarditis, 356
Myocardium, 328, 329, 335, 340, 342,
  349, 351
Myosin heavy chain, 72

Na$^+$ channels (*see* Sodium channels)
Na$^+$/K$^+$ exchanger (*see* Sodium/
  potassium exchanger)
Neointima (*see* Intimal hyperplasia)
Neonatal alloimmune thrombocytopenic
  purpura (NAITP), 502
NF-1 343, 518
NFκB, 457, 458
Nitrendipine, 237
Nitric oxide (NO), 141

Nitric oxide synthases (NOS), 142
  endothelial NOS, 145
  inducible NOS, 144
  neuronal NOS, 143
  NO synthase knockout mice, 152
Nitroglycerin, 141
Nkx2-5/Csx, 126
Nodal, 346
Nonviral gene transfer vectors, 389–391
Noonan syndrome, 120, 518
Northern blot analysis, [*see* RNA (and
  Northern hybridizations)]
Nucleosomes, 6

Okazaki fragments, 4
Osteopontin, 405, 415–417
Osteopontin antisense mRNA, 416

PAK, 299
Patch-clamp technique, 237
Pax-3, 127
Paxillin, 312
Peptide growth factors, 327
Percutaneous transluminal coronary
  angioplasty (PTCA), 392, 393,
  401, 447, 449, 460
Phospholipase C, 164, 168, 295, 307,
  311–313, 335, 336
Phosphoserine/phosphothreonine
  phosphatases (PSPases), 305
Phosphotyrosine binding (PTB)
  domain, 295, 296
PI 3-kinase, 295, 296, 301, 302, 307,
  336–338
Pinacidil, 219
Plaque, 448, 449, 453, 454, 456, 460
Plaque rupture, 448, 449, 454, 456, 460
Plasmin, 458, 459
Plasminogen, 458
Plasminogen activator inhibitor-1
  (PAI-1), 458
  adventitia, 458
  intima, 458
  macrophages, 458
  media, 458
  VSMC, 458

Plasminogen activator inhibitor-2
  (PAI-2), 459
Platelet adhesion, 490, 504
Platelet adhesion receptors, 490–506
Platelet aggregation, 490, 492, 496, 499,
  503, 505
Platelet α-granules, 501
Platelet deposition, 394, 449, 450, 460
Platelet-derived growth factor (PDGF),
  129, 292, 299, 301–303, 306–308,
  312, 315, 408, 411, 418, 448, 456,
  457
  anti-PDGF antibodies, 408, 417
Platelet-derived growth factor receptors
  (PDGF-R), 301–303, 307, 308, 312
Platelets, 448–450, 460, 489–506
Platelet spreading and protein trafficking,
  500, 501
Pleckstrin homology (PH) domain,
  295, 296, 299, 301
Polymerase chain reaction (PCR), 38
Polyribosomes, 13
Posttransfusion purpura, 502
Potassium channels 169, 197–222
  CIR, 213
  GIRK1, 213
  I_{Kr}, 205
  I_{Ks}, 205, 208
  IRK1, 212
  K_{ACh} channels, 213
  K_{ATP} channels, 215, 216, 218
  Kir3.1, 213
  Kir3.4, 213
  K_1 channels, 211
  K_{to}, 201
  Kv1.5, 208, 221
  maxi K^+, 28, 209
  minK, 208
Pressure overload, 353
Primer extension, 41
Probes (*see* Molecular probes)
Progressive familial heart block, 518
Promoters, 5
Protein kinase A (PKA), 189, 243, 306
Protein kinase C (PKC), 189, 297, 301,
  304, 306, 312, 313
  14-3-3 family, 296, 300

Protein phosphatases, 305, 306
Protein tyrosine kinases (PTK), 291–316
Protein expression in insect cells, 44
p21 (*see* Ras)
pyk2, 304

Raf, 297, 299, 300, 303, 306, 313, 335,
    339
Raf kinase, 298, 300, 306
Rapamycin, 258, 418
Rapid amplification of cDNA ends
    (RACE), 40
Ras, 297–302, 306, 313, 336, 339–343
Ras-GAP, 297, 299, 307
Receptor protein tyrosine kinases, 295,
    296, 298–301, 313, 314, 336
Repetitive sequences, 7
Replication fork, 7
Restenosis after angioplasty, 392, 393
Retinoic acid receptors, 127
Retroviruses, 382–385, 416
Reverse cholesterol transport, 474
Reverse transcriptase, 18, 35
RGD sequences, 415, 497–499, 506
RGS (regulators of G-protein signaling),
    297
Ribozymes, 391, 392
RNA (ribonucleic acid), 1, 16
    blot hybridizations, 28, 42
    5′ capping, 9
    heterogeneous nuclear RNA (hnRNA),
        9
    in vitro synthesis, 42
    isolation of total RNA, 16
    measurement by A260/A280 ratios, 16
    messenger RNA (mRNA), 5, 16
    poly A$^+$, 9, 34
    polymerases 7, 9
    ribosomal RNA (rRNA), 9
    splicing, 9
    transfer RNA (tRNA), 9
RNAse, 15
RNAse protection assays, 41, 29
Ryanodine receptor (*see* Calcium
    release channels)

SAPK kinase (MEK-4, SEK) 300
Saxitoxin, 175
"Scavenger receptor", 474
Ser/Thr kinase, 331
Serum response factor (SRF), 344
S4 domain/segment, 177, 182, 241
sf9 cells, 256
Shc, 296, 299, 307, 313, 335, 336,
    338
Shprintzen syndromes, 112
"Sicilian Gambit," 220
Silencers, 5
SkA promoter, 344
Sodium channels, 173–191
    phosphorylation, 189
Sodium nitroprusside, 141
Sodium/potassium exchanger, 275–286
    alternative splicing, 284
    calcium binding sites, 280
    calcium regulatory domain, 280
    signal peptide, 280
Sos, 297–299
Southern blot hybridization, 26
Spectroscopy, 15
Sp1, 344.457
Src, 303, 304, 311, 312, 314, 315, 335
    C Src Kinase (Csk) 303
    Src kinase, 261, 302, 303
    Src-related kinases, 302
Src homology 2 (SH2) domain, 295,
    296, 302–304, 307, 308, 311,
    312, 335, 338
Src homology 3 (SH3) domain, 295,
    296, 302, 303, 304
SRF, 343, 345
S6 kinase, 302
S6 protein, 313
Stat (signal transducers and activators of
    transcription) proteins, 294, 314
Stretch-activated ion channels, 355
Subconductance states, 259
Sulfonylureas, 216
Supravalvular aortic stenosis (SVAS),
    116, 518
SV40 T antigen, 94

TEF-1, 343–345
Terminal cisternae, 253
Tetralogy of Fallot, 114
Tetrodotoxin, 175
Thrombin, 408, 409, 448, 456, 457,
    458, 461, 497
Thrombosis/thrombus, 393, 447–452,
    456, 458, 460, 489, 505
Thyroid hormone, 72
Tissue factor, 448–460, 452–457
    in adventitia, 454
    antigen/protein, 451–453
    in arterial media, 454
    in endothelial cells, 456, 457
    in endothelium, 454
    in fibroblasts, 456
    gene regulation, 457, 458
    immunohistochemistry, 451–454
    in situ hybridization, 451, 454
    in monocyte/macrophages, 452, 454,
        456–458
    mRNA, 451, 452, 454, 456, 457
    promoter, 457, 458
    in vessel injury, 454
Tissue factor pathway inhibitor (TFPI),
    456, 459, 461
    in endothelial cells 459
Tissue inhibitors of metalloproteinases
    (TIMPs), 413
Tissue plasminogen activator (t-PA),
    394, 458, 459
Torsade de pointes, 221
Transcription, 4, 8
Transcription factors, 355
Transferrin, 390
Transforming growth factor β (TGFβ),
    328–332, 335, 340–357, 408, 409,
    411
    TGFβ-deficient mice, 356
    TGFβ overexpressing transgenic
        mice, 357
    TGF binding protein (TGFbp), 435,
        438
Transforming growth factor β receptors
    (TβR), 329–332, 349–353

Transgenic animals, 77, 125
Translation, 8
Transmembrane topography, 179, 255,
    262
Transplantation, 356
Transverse tubule, 252
Triggered rhythms/arrhythmias, 200,
    206
Triglycerides, 472, 479
Tropoelastin, 432
Tyrosine kinase, 335
Tyrosine phosphorylation 291–316, 335,
    338

Urokinase-type plasminogen activator
    (uPA), 458, 459

Vascular cell adhesion molecule
    (VCAM-1), 130, 490
    VCAM-1 knockout mice, 130
Vascular endothelial growth factor
    (VEGF), 357, 393, 394
Vascular smooth muscle cells (VSMC),
    291–316, 357, 393, 401–419, 448,
    452, 454–458, 461, 472
    adhesion, 416
    chemotaxis, 402
    migration, 402–409, 411, 417, 418
    migration, inhibition of, 417
    proliferation, 407, 409
Velocardiofacial syndrome, 112, 113,
    518
Verapamil, 188
Very-low-density lipoprotein (VLDL),
    473, 474, 476, 478, 479, 481, 483
Vitronectin, 410, 411, 490–493, 496,
    498
Vitronectin receptor (see αvβ3 integrin)
Voltage-dependent calcium channels
    (VDCC), 237
von Willebrand factor, 492, 493, 496,
    498, 499, 501

Watson syndrome, 120, 518
Western blot analysis, 44

Williams syndrome, 117, 518
Wnt gene, 345
WT-1, 127

Xenopus
  embryos, 345, 346, 349

[*Xenopus*]
  oocytes, 180, 256

X-linked heterotaxy syndrome, 123, 518

Zoxide, 219

About the Editors

ANDREW R. MARKS is the Irene and Dr. Arthur M. Fishberg Professor of Medicine (Cardiology); Director of the Cardiology Training Program; and Associate Professor of Medicine, Molecular Biology, and Physiology and Biophysics at Mount Sinai School of Medicine, New York, New York. The author or coauthor of over 55 professional papers and book chapters and the holder of two U.S. patents, he is a Fellow of the American College of Cardiology and a member of the American Heart Association, the American Society for Biochemistry and Molecular Biology, the American Society for Cell Biology, the Biophysical Society, and the American Society of Clinical Investigation, among other organizations. Dr. Marks received the B.A. degree (1976) in biochemistry and English from Amherst College, Massachusetts, and the M.D. degree (1980) from Harvard Medical School, Boston, Massachusetts.

MARK B. TAUBMAN is the Dr. Arthur M. Fishberg Professor of Medicine (Cardiology); Associate Professor of Molecular Biology; and Codirector, Section of Molecular and Cellular Cardiology; Mount Sinai School of Medicine, New York, New York. A member of the American Heart Association, the International Society on Thrombosis and Hemostasis, and the American Society of Hypertension, among other organizations, he is the author or coauthor of over 50 professional papers. Dr. Taubman received the B.A. degree (1972) in biochemistry from Columbia University, New York, New York, and the M.D. degree (1978) from the New York University School of Medicine, New York, New York.